Interventional Critical Care

Dennis A. Taylor • Scott P. Sherry
Ronald F. Sing
Editors

Interventional Critical Care

A Manual for Advanced Care Practitioners

Foreword by
W. Robert Grabenkort and Ruth Kleinpell

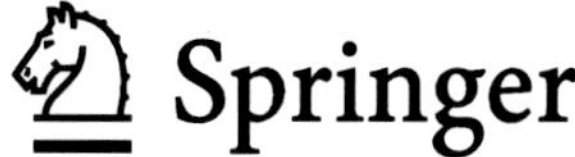

Editors
Dennis A. Taylor
Carolinas HealthCare System
Charlotte, NC, USA

Scott P. Sherry
Department of Surgery
Oregon Health and Sciences University
Portland, OR, USA

Ronald F. Sing
Carolinas HealthCare System
Charlotte, NC, USA

ISBN 978-3-319-25284-1 ISBN 978-3-319-25286-5 (eBook)
DOI 10.1007/978-3-319-25286-5

Library of Congress Control Number: 2016944159

This Springer imprint is published by Springer Nature
The registered company is Springer International Publishing AG Switzerland

Foreword

"By failing to prepare, you are preparing to fail."

Benjamin Franklin

Increasingly, hospital systems and healthcare leaders are incorporating advanced practice providers to supply a 24/7 clinician presence in the intensive care unit (ICU). Nurse practitioners (NPs) and physician assistants (PAs) are an increasingly important component of the nation's healthcare provider pool, and it has been identified that the addition of NPs and PAs to ICU teams is a strategy to meet ICU workforce needs. As NPs and PAs assimilate into this new role, guidance is needed to assume proficiency in the role through mentoring and self-study. This text, *Interventional Critical Care: A Manual for Advanced Care Practitioners*, is a needed resource for these practitioners. In providing instruction on many of the technical skills needed to practice in the acute and critical care environment, the text is a useful reference for novice as well as experienced practitioners. The scope of content covers topics related to essential aspects including credentialing, patient safety considerations, billing and coding for procedures, as well as a review of a number of invasive skills commonly performed in the management of acute and critically ill patients. The insightful chapters are designed specifically for NPs and PAs to assist in learning the procedural techniques performed by the bedside critical care provider. Each chapter is authored by an experienced practitioner describing not only the technical aspects of the procedure but also the clinical indications and pertinent practical considerations. The editors have done a thorough job in choosing a wide range of procedures, and the chapter authors are seasoned practitioners who have performed the skills and share their expertise. This text will undoubtedly be an essential reference for NPs and PAs practicing in the ICU setting. We thank the editors for having the foresight to work on preparing the text and the chapter authors for sharing their knowledge and expertise to enhance NP and PA roles in the ICU.

Atlanta, GA, USA — W. Robert Grabenkort, PA, MMSc, FCCM
Chicago, IL, USA — Ruth Kleinpell, PhD, ACNP-BC, FCCM

Preface

Over the past 10 years, the utilization of advanced practice providers (APPs) in both the intensive care unit (ICU) and operating room (OR) has increased dramatically. With this surge in specialty providers, many educational programs have had difficulty providing the necessary didactic, psychomotor and affective skills, and experiences. These are skills that are necessary for the APP working in these areas and for facility credentialing and privileging that would allow APPs to practice to the full extent of their license and ability. In many cases, the lack of clinical experiences has contributed to this gap. While APPs are very well grounded in the pathophysiology, pharmacology, and physical assessment of patient care, they may have not been exposed to the indications, contraindications, and technical aspects of performing many of these critical skills.

To fill this knowledge gap, we have envisioned and created a textbook that focuses on improving the knowledge and education of the APP in critical care procedures and skills. The editors and chapter authors of this text were recruited from facilities and programs from across the United States. They all actively practice in the ICU and OR and are considered content experts in their respective fields. All chapters are authored by an APP and/or physician. The majority of all authors are also designated as Fellows of the American College of Critical Care Medicine (FCCM). They have made significant contributions to patient care and the Society of Critical Care Medicine (SCCM).

We hope you will enjoy reading and using this text as a reference in your daily practice in the ICU setting. It has been a pleasure working with all of the chapter authors and contributors. We, the editors, would like to express our appreciation to Patricia Hevey, Sonya Hudson, and Sarah Landeen at Carolinas HealthCare System for their contributions to editing and coordinating the efforts of this work. We also express our appreciation to Michael Koy at Springer Publishing for all of his contributions and work on this project.

Charlotte, NC, USA — Dennis A. Taylor, DNP, ACNP-BC, FCCM
Portland, OR, USA — Scott P. Sherry, MS, PA-C, FCCM
Charlotte, NC, USA — Ronald F. Sing, DO, FCCM

Contents

Part X Special Procedures and Concepts

Part I

Administrative Considerations

1 The Multidisciplinary ICU Team

Dennis A. Taylor, Scott Sherry, and Ronald F. Sing

1.1 Introduction

Many highly educated and experienced personnel staff the intensive care unit. This chapter will describe the education and roles of many of these staff. There have been significant discussions in the literature regarding communication, direction, and coordination of these care teams. Each discipline brings a unique perspective to bear on patient care and contributes to the healing and recovery process.

In addition, patient monitoring and ventilation options are better addressed in the ICU setting. More sophisticated ventilators located in the ICU provide better ventilation and oxygenation options.

Many facilities have adopted "crew resource management or CRM" communication techniques from the aviation profession to facilitate the use of checklists and patient hand-off at change of shifts.

1.2 Critical Care ICU Physicians

In both the medicine and surgery fields, there are physicians who specialize in the treatment of critically ill and injured patients. These physicians often complete a specialized Fellowship in Critical Care Medicine after they complete their medical education and residency programs. There are specialty boards that address practice in this very intensive environment. Critical care medicine is concerned with the diagnosis, management, and prevention of complications in patients who are severely ill and who usually require intensive monitoring and/or organ system support. Critical care medicine fellowships provide advanced education to allow a fellow to acquire competency in the subspecialty with sufficient expertise to act as a primary intensivist or independent consultant.

The educational preparation for these surgical professionals includes 4 years of medical education, 6 years of a surgical residency program, and a 1- to 2-year postgraduate fellowship in critical care and/or surgery. The preparation for those working in a medical ICU includes

D.A. Taylor, DNP, ACNP-BC, FCCM (✉)
R.F. Sing, DO, FACS, FCCM
Carolinas HealthCare System, Charlotte, NC, USA
e-mail: dennis.taylor@carolinashealthcare.org; ronald.sing@carolinashealthcare.org

S. Sherry, MPAS, PA-C, FCCM
Department of Surgery, Oregon Health and Science University, Portland, OR, USA
e-mail: sherrys@ohsu.edu

D.A. Taylor et al. (eds.), *Interventional Critical Care*, DOI 10.1007/978-3-319-25286-5_1

4 years of medical education, 4–5 years of specialized medical education in pulmonary medicine, and then a fellowship in critical care medicine as well.

1.3 Critical Care Advanced Clinical Practitioners

Critical Care Advanced Clinical Practitioners, or ACPs, are physician assistants or nurse practitioners who are educated to care for the acutely ill or injured patient in the ICU setting. They have 2 years of postgraduate education in advanced practice nursing or physician assistant studies. They typically have a board certification in the adult to gerontology acute care population of patients. Many have completed a postgraduate fellowship program that focuses on the care of the ICU patient.

The Critical Care ACP has a minimum of a master's degree in nursing or physician assistant studies. Many also have doctoral terminal degrees and some postdoctoral education. They are typically credentialed and privileged (state and facility specific) to perform high-risk, low-volume, and high-acuity procedures such as:

Advanced airway management including emergent cricothyrotomy
Placement of central venous lines (with and without ultrasound)
Placement of arterial monitoring lines
Placement and removal of chest tubes
Thoracentesis and paracentesis
Placement of dialysis catheters
Placement of pulmonary artery monitoring catheters
Complex wound management including debridement
Functioning as a surgical first assistant
Focused abdominal sonography for trauma (FAST) exams

1.4 Clinical Pharmacists (PharmD)

Critical care clinical pharmacists are a vital contributor to patient outcomes. They often guide antibiotic stewardship, sedation, and pain control guidelines utilized in the critical care settings. They are often participants in multidisciplinary rounds and are a great resource for teaching in educational settings.

The profession of pharmacy evolved over the last century from a discipline that focused on pharmaceutical products into one that primarily focuses on the patient and the optimal delivery of pharmaceutical care. The curricula in most pharmacy colleges and universities have changed significantly to reflect this transformation. Courses in pharmacotherapeutics, pharmacokinetics, pathophysiology, human anatomy and physiology, physical assessment, and pharmacoeconomics have been added to prepare graduates for careers as clinicians. Furthermore, pharmacy graduates can pursue additional training by completing residencies or fellowships in their areas of interests, which can include critical care [1].

1.5 Registered Respiratory Therapists (RRT/RCP)

Respiratory therapists provide the hands-on care that helps people recover from a wide range of medical conditions [2]. Registered respiratory therapists are found:

- In hospitals giving breathing treatments to people with asthma and other respiratory conditions
- In intensive care units managing ventilators that keep the critically ill alive
- In emergency rooms delivering life-saving treatments
- In operating rooms working with anesthesiologists to monitor patients' breathing during surgery
- In air transport and ambulance programs rushing to rescue people in need of immediate medical attention

Respiratory therapists are considered the go-to experts in their facilities for respiratory care technology. But their high-tech knowledge isn't just limited to the equipment they use in their jobs. They also understand how to apply high-tech devices in the care and treatment of patients, how to assess patients to ensure the treatments are working properly, and how to make the care changes necessary to arrive at the best outcome for the patient.

The combination of these skills—hands-on technical know-how and a solid understanding of respiratory conditions and how they are treated—is what sets respiratory therapists apart from the crowd and makes them such a crucial part of the healthcare team [3].

Respiratory therapy programs are anywhere from 2 to 6 years in length resulting in an associate's degree to a master's degree upon completion. In addition, there are now many doctoral-level programs in respiratory therapy [6].

1.6 Physical Therapists

Physical therapists are a valued part of the healthcare team. They work with patients to help restore function, improve mobility, relieve pain, and prevent or limit permanent physical disabilities of patients. They also restore, maintain, and promote overall fitness and health. A physical therapist will examine patient's medical histories and perform tests to measure patient's strength, range of motion, balance, coordination, posture, muscle performance, respiration, and motor function. Physical therapists then develop plans describing a treatment strategy. In addition, they also help to develop fitness and wellness-oriented programs to prevent the loss of mobility before it occurs [4].

Physical therapist education programs integrate theory, evidence, and practice along a continuum of learning. Physical therapists usually need a master's degree from an accredited physical therapy school and a state license. Only master's degree and doctoral degree physical therapy schools are accredited. The Commission on Accreditation of Physical Therapy Education (CAPTE) accredits entry-level academic programs in physical therapy.

Physical therapist education programs include both classroom and laboratory instruction. Physical therapist training programs include foundational science courses, such as biology, anatomy, physiology, and cellular histology. Other physical therapist classes include exercise physiology, neuroscience, biomechanics, pharmacology, pathology, and radiology/imaging, as well as behavioral science courses, such as evidence-based practice and clinical reasoning. Some of the clinically based physical therapist courses include medical screening, examination tests and measures, diagnostic process, therapeutic interventions, outcomes assessment, and practice management.

Physical therapist schools also provide student with supervised clinical experience. This may include clinical rotations which enable supervised work experience in areas such as acute care, ICU, and orthopedic care.

1.7 Occupational Therapists

Occupational therapists and occupational therapy assistants help people across the lifespan participate in the things they want and need to do through the therapeutic use of everyday activities (occupations) [7]. Common occupational therapy interventions include helping children with disabilities to participate fully in school and social situations, helping people recovering from injury to regain skills, and providing supports for older adults experiencing physical and cognitive changes. Occupational therapy services typically include:

- An individualized evaluation, during which the client/family and occupational therapist determine the person's goals
- Customized intervention to improve the person's ability to perform daily activities and reach the goals
- Outcome evaluation to ensure that the goals are being met and/or make changes to the intervention plan

Occupational therapy services may include comprehensive evaluations of the client's home and other environments (e.g., workplace, school), recommendations for adaptive equipment and training in its use, and guidance and education for family members and caregivers [8]. Occupational therapy practitioners have a holistic perspective, in which the focus is on adapting the environment to fit the person, and the person is an integral part of the therapy team [5]. Occupational therapy programs are anywhere from 4 to 6 years. Postgraduate residencies in specialized areas are also common.

1.8 Speech and Language Pathologists

Speech pathologists, officially called speech-language pathologists and sometimes called speech therapists, work with people who have a variety of speech-related disorders. These disorders can include the inability to produce certain sounds, speech rhythm and fluency problems, and voice disorders. They also help people who want to modify accents or who have swallowing difficulties. Speech pathologists' work involves assessment, diagnosis, treatment, and prevention of speech-related disorders [9].

In most states, one must have a master's degree in speech-language pathology to practice. Some states will only license speech pathologists that have graduated from a program that is accredited by the Council on Academic Accreditation in Audiology and Speech-Language Pathology. Coursework includes anatomy, physiology, the nature of disorders, and the principles of acoustics. Students receive supervised clinical training. Doctoral program are very common in this area as well.

References

1. Papadopoulos J, Rebuck JA, Lober C, Pass SE, Seidl EC, Shah RA, Sherman DS. The critical care pharmacist: an essential intensive care practitioner. Pharmacotherapy. 2002;22(11):1484–8.
2. American Association for Respiratory Care [Internet]. Irving: AARC; c2015. Available from: https://www.aarc.org/careers/what-is-an-rt/rts-at-work/ [cited 24 Apr 2015].
3. American Association for Respiratory Care [Internet]. Irving: AARC; c2015. Available from: https://www.aarc.org/careers/what-is-an-rt/equipment-use/ [cited 24 Apr 2015].
4. Physical Therapist Education and Schools [Internet]. Available from: http://www.physicaltherapistcareers.net/physical-therapist-job-description.php [cited 24 Apr 2015].
5. The American Occupational Therapy Association, Inc. [Internet]. Bethesda: AOTA; c2015. Available from: http://www.aota.org/About-Occupational-Therapy.aspx [cited 24 Apr 2015].
6. Healthcare Careers [Internet]. Foster City: QuinStreet, Inc.; c2003–2015. Available from: http://www.health-care-careers.org/respiratory-therapy-career-training.html [cited 24 Apr 2015].
7. Physical Therapist Education and Schools [Internet]. Available from: http://www.physicaltherapistcareers.net/physical-therapist-education.php [cited 24 Apr 2015].
8. American Physical Therapy Association [Internet]. Alexandria: APTA; c2015. Available from: http://www.apta.org/AboutPTs/ [cited 24 Apr 2015].
9. About Careers [Internet]. About.com; c2015. Available from: http://careerplanning.about.com/od/occupations/p/speech_path.htm [cited 24 Apr 2015].

The Surgical Setting: ICU Versus OR

2

Gena Brawley, Casey Scully, and Ronald F. Sing

As both volume and acuity of hospital populations continue to swell, so does the need for surgical services. Many healthcare systems across the country have found it increasingly difficult to meet those growing needs. Specialization of surgical procedures, lengthy operations, and elective surgeries creates a competition for time in the operating room (OR) that further complicates the already stressed need [1]. Furthermore, advancements in surgical critical care allow for higher complexity and higher-acuity patients to survive longer periods of time and require multiple operative procedures. Often there are multiple patients in the ICU (intensive care unit) with open body cavities that require a staged return to the OR for closure. Unfortunately, there is little ongoing development of strategies and processes to meet the patient's surgical needs in a setting other than the OR. Out of this necessity, the trend toward the ICU as a surrogate operative setting has been developed.

To establish the suitability of the ICU to meet the patient's surgical needs, it is important to understand the requirements of the OR. This ensures that the quality of care is maintained despite the setting the patient is being treated in.

G. Brawley, ACNP-BC (✉) • C. Scully, PA-C
R.F. Sing, DO, FCCM
Carolinas HealthCare System, Charlotte, NC, USA
e-mail: Gena.Brawley@carolinashealthcare.org;
Casey.Scully@carolinashealthcare.org;
Ron.Sing@carolinashealthcare.org

Caregivers and providers must keep in mind the patients' clinical needs and clinical status are not different because of the location of procedures; the change requires a heightened need for communication and coordination to limit risk.

An important consideration for performing surgery in the ICU versus operating room is the setup of the room and the ability to perform that procedure in the space provided. The bed is central in the OR as it is in many ICUs with monitoring in place at the head of the bed. Supplies are often readily available in the OR and are easily accessible for operative interventions. The ICU has a stock of supplies that are often used for general nursing care. The ICU's supply of operative equipment is often limited due to space and cost. Many times supplies for bedside procedures will be delivered from the operating room to the ICU (see Figs. 2.1 and 2.2).

One important component is the prerequisite of the "Universal Protocol." This protocol dictates that a pre-procedure verification process occurs prior to the start of the procedure. This includes the site being properly marked when laterality is applicable and that a timeout be performed prior to sedation given for the procedure. The timeout must include the patient's name, procedure to be performed, and any applicable information. The timeout must be verified by the performing provider responsible for sedation. During the timeout, other activities and conversations must be suspended so that all present team members can confirm the patient and procedure.

D.A. Taylor et al. (eds.), *Interventional Critical Care*, DOI 10.1007/978-3-319-25286-5_2

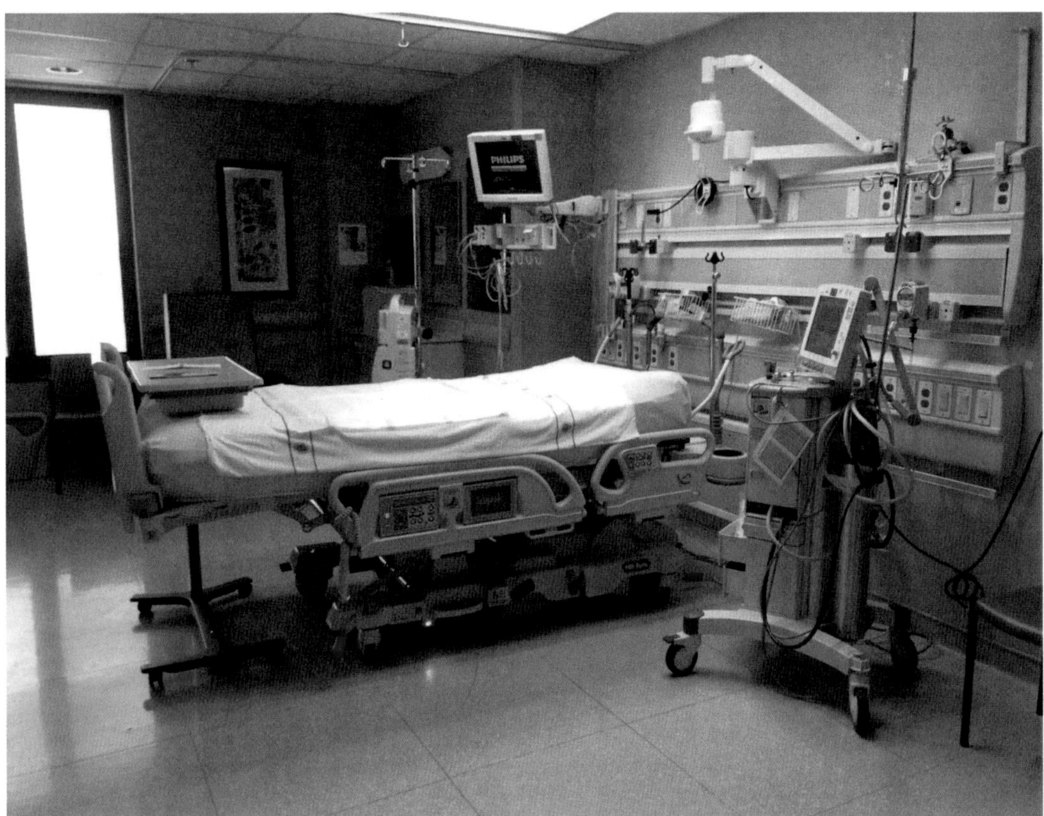

Fig. 2.1 Standard ICU set up including bed, monitor, and ventilator

The Joint Commission delegates that safety practices be in place to ensure the prevention of surgical errors. This includes the Universal Protocol that ensures a proper timeout, verification of procedures and patient, and marking of the surgical site [2]. This occurs whether the setting is the ICU or the OR and must be performed regardless of the surgical scene. The Joint Commission also ensures that standards of sterility are maintained, that appropriate dress for the OR is maintained, and that foot traffic is minimized to maintain sterility and minimize distraction. Many ORs have strict guidelines to ensure that they comply with these recommendations; however, with variation in the bedside OR setting, it can be easy to neglect the full process. Special efforts must be made to maintain the proper procedures despite the circumstances.

Another important aspect of the pre-procedure verification check is to ensure that informed consent is obtained. The goal of this consent is to establish mutual understanding and agreement between the patient or surrogate and the provider who is responsible for the procedure. Informed consent implies that the patient or their decision maker has been fully described the procedure with all material risks, benefits, and alternatives.

Preparation of the patient also needs to be considered. A thorough review of the patient's history, potential complications that could arise due any comorbidity, the current condition, and current status prior to any operation should be considered. Recent anticoagulants and home medications such as aspirin and direct thrombin inhibitors may change the coagulation state of the patient, and without direct access to cross-matched or uncrossmatched blood and blood products on hold, hemorrhage could ensue. Special attention should also be given to patients with liver and renal dysfunction while undergoing an operative procedure either for the OR or

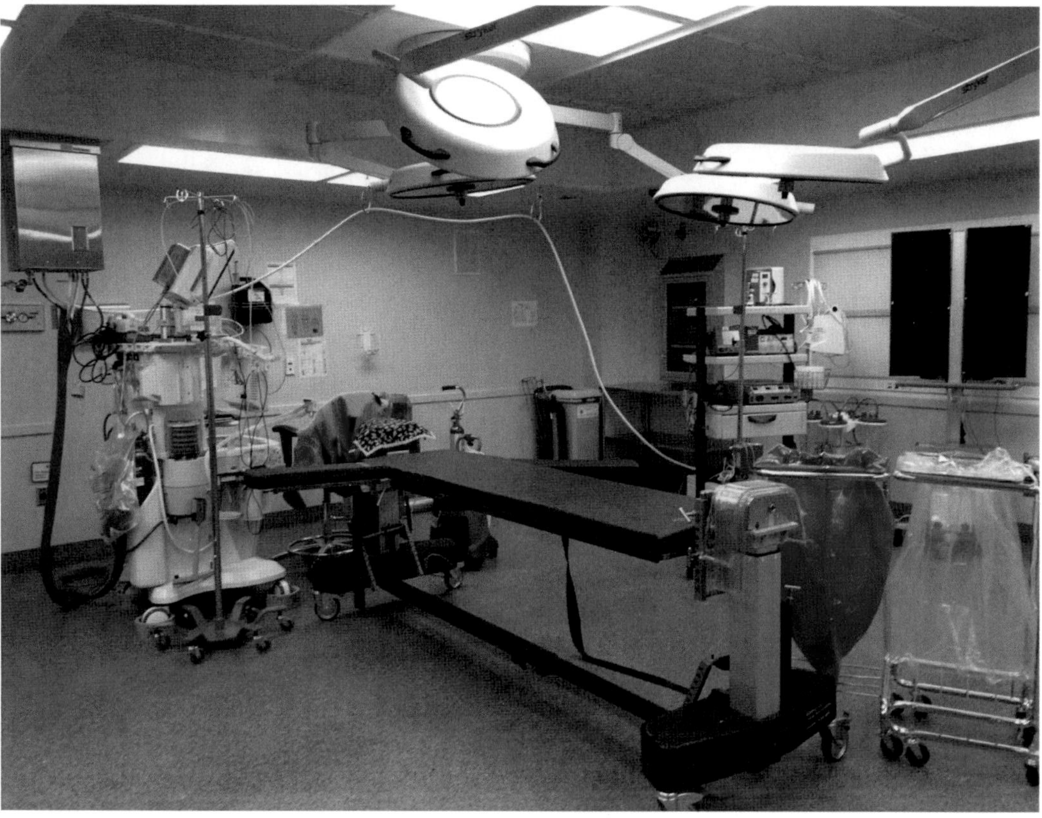

Fig. 2.2 Standard operating room setup

bedside procedure. Furthermore, preparation should be made for the sedation of the patient prior to the procedure. Enteral nutrition should be held due to the risk of aspiration; a sedation or anesthetic plan should be ordered and in place, as well as a backup plan. Patients could have hypermetabolic states and may require additional medications for desired sedative level as well as side effects from sedation. The surgeon and support staff should be prepared with fluid and potential vasopressors should a vasodilatory response occur after administration of sedation, pain medications, and/or paralytic. This is paramount to avoid potential unfavorable hypoperfusion and hemodynamic compromise (see Fig. 2.3).

Some proposed benefits of bringing operative careto the patient's bedside include timeliness, safety, and cost.

2.1 Timeliness

Many surgical services recognize the need to manage an increasing patient population. Both the increasing volume and acuity often exceed the capabilities of standard management. A strategy to streamline efficient care is to transition some of the operative care to the bedside. This decreases OR room requirements and anesthesia services, thereby decreasing wait times and giving the provider more efficiency in their day. Often cases can be scheduled at the bedside alternately with OR cases to minimize the wait between procedures. This is particularly true with bedside procedures that require minimal deviation from standard care. More complex procedural needs will often require the equipment and staff of the OR and

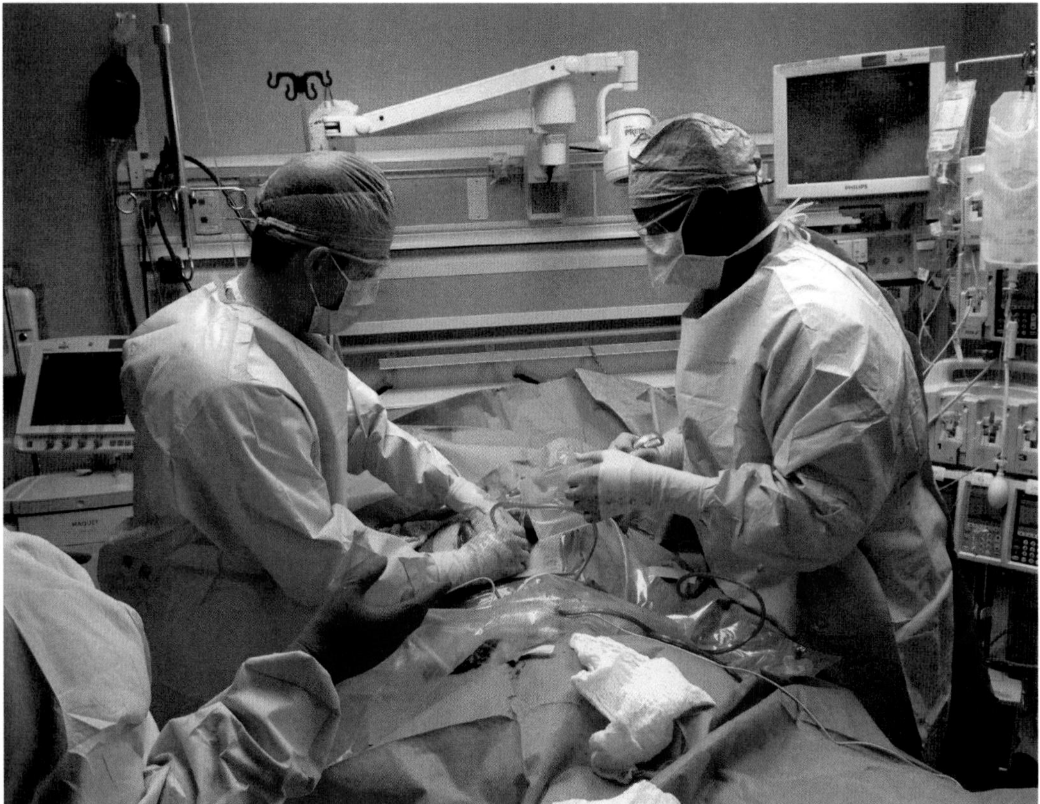

Fig. 2.3 Bedside laparotomy in the ICU

may be subject to the same delays as the case actually being scheduled in the OR.

2.2 Safety

Another noted benefit of using the ICU as the operative setting is that this limits the patient's transport requirements. This is particularly beneficial when the patient is crucially ill and either their hemodynamic instability or significant equipment requirements make their transport on and off the unit exceedingly difficult. "Road trips" can have adverse outcomes such as unintentional equipment removal and alterations in patient's hemodynamic stability. Additionally, transport on and off the unit requires staffing removal from their intended assignments and could potentially affect the care of other critically ill patients if the transports are lengthy or frequent. Szems et al. observed ICU patients that were ventilated and underwent intrahospital transport, despite the high severity of illness, the occurrence of problems related to the transport, were minor and only found to have a rate of 5 %. Most often the common complications of the transport included tubing, connections, and temporary disconnection of support line. That being said, specific attention needs to be focused on advanced ventilator support and the patient requiring high levels of positive end expiratory pressures (PEEP) that can result in a decreased recruitment with multiple disconnections required with transfers [3].

2.3 Cost

With our changing healthcare economy, the need to deliver cost-effective care to even the complicated surgical patient is a growing consideration. OR procedures entail the additional room and equipment charges as well as anesthesia fees. This result of moving some operative cases to the bedside can have a significant cumulative savings.

2.4 Potential Issues when the ICU Is an OR

2.4.1 OR Staff

One potential issue with the need to perform operative interventions at the bedside is the limitations of OR staffing ratios. Traditionally, staffing is determined by the number of OR rooms running, volume, and timing of cases. When emergent or semi-emergent cases present to the OR, the resources needed to meet this demand, including staffing, must be reevaluated and redistributed to fit the needs of the schedule. It is important that these needs not significantly disrupt the set scheduled operating room day unless truly emergent.

The OR is a very protocol-driven setting. It is arranged in a consistent manner to allow for quick location and access to anticipated and frequently needed supplies. Bringing the OR staff to the ICU bedside can drive down comfort and efficiency. This often requires the ICU bedside nurse to assist with more than hemodynamic monitoring of the patient.

2.4.2 ICU Staff

ICU nurses are not specifically trained to assist with bedside procedures or operative interventions. Their role is generally to assess the patient's hemodynamic status and tolerance of the procedure. Additionally not being in the OR setting generally means the absence of anesthesia support to assist with the hemodynamic and ventilator care of the patient during the procedure. The primary concern of the provider performing the procedure is the operative intervention at hand. Often this means their role is expanded to include the total hemodynamic management of the patient as well as surgical technique. Having respiratory therapy and bedside nursing available and able to support the patient is essential to the successful bedside operation. The more experienced the staff often the more smoothly their support during tense cases.

2.4.3 Equipment

The ideal ICU OR mimics the setup of the actual OR including its layout and access to supplies. For bedside procedures, supplies can often be gathered from stock on the ICU floors. Most critical care units keep sterile supplies, gloves, drapes, and trays for specific surgical procedures often performed or needed emergently. For more complex interventions, supplies often have to be requested and delivered from the OR. This requires transport and setup of the supplies at the ICU bedside. Sterile OR back tables can be delivered fully stocked as if they were remaining in the OR suite; however, these must be staffed to facilitate access as well as maintain correct counts for surgical safety. Some specific equipment necessities such as the radiology, Doppler, ultrasound, electrocautery, and others must be acquired and set up in the ICU. The attainment of these specialty resources often requires communication and timing. The ability to properly use these devices can be affected by personnel experience, availability, and the layout of the room. Some ICU rooms may not be able to accommodate specific procedural needs. A study completed at Yale University from August 2002 to June 2009 looked at the ICU as an operating room for patients on the Emergency General Surgery census. They compared ICU and operative databases specifically focusing on mode of ventilation, type of anesthesia used, and adverse outcomes. They found advanced ventilation was used increasingly from 2002 to 2007 and 2008 from 15 to 40 %, and most cases were performed under deep sedation [1]. Also, they noted that advanced ventilation may have influenced the choice of operative location. Unexpected issues that were noted during the ICU operations included recurrent hemorrhage, need for specific instrumentation not present during initial planning, space, and device failure (see Figs. 2.4, 2.5, and 2.6) [4].

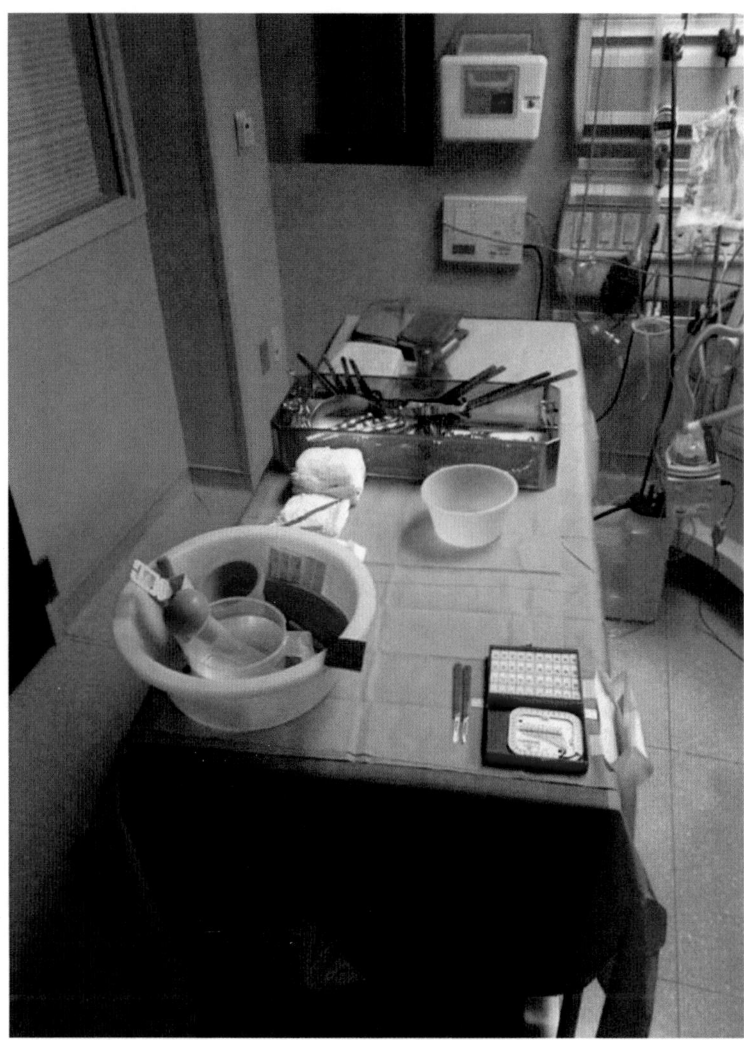

Fig. 2.4 Back table setup in the ICU

2.4.4 Backup

A very important consideration for the provider in the bedside OR setting is to anticipate backup plans that may need to be implemented should unforeseen circumstances arise. In the OR there is the possibility of extra staffing that can be shifted to accommodate the needs of an increasingly difficulty or increasingly unstable patient. Often at the bedside, experienced OR staff is limited, and additional surgical support may be delayed by location challenges. The surgeon or provider must know their available resources and when to call for backup early to ward off adverse outcomes. Specific issues that should be anticipated and require preplanning include unexpected hemorrhage, patient hemodynamic instability, need for specific instrumentation, and potential for device failure. Often finesse in managing these unforeseen circumstances comes from experience and comfort in operating outside of the standard OR suite. This builds confidence and eases one's ability of how to react.

A final backup plan would necessitate the transition of the patient to the OR suite when the procedures can no longer be safely performed at the bedside. This requires quick decision-making and staffing accommodations as well as maintenance of sterility when transitioning care settings.

Bedside procedures performed are as follows:

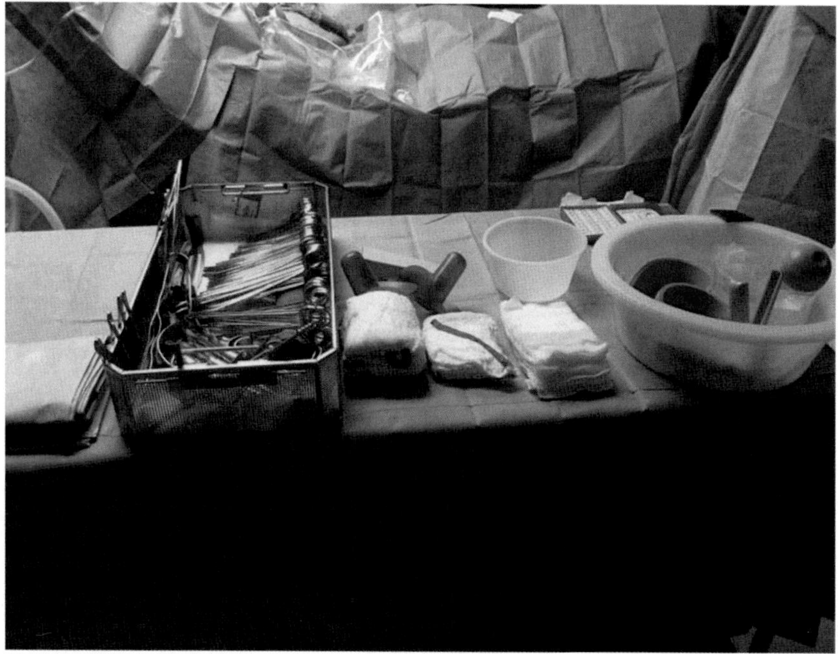

Fig. 2.5 Back table setup in the ICU aside prepped and draped patient

Emergent

- Cricothyroidotomy
- Tracheostomy
- Tube thoracostomy
- Resuscitative thoracostomy
- Decompression of abdomen in setting of abdominal compartment syndrome
- External fixation
- Fasciotomy
- Uncontrolled hemorrhage

Urgent

- Pericardial drainage
- Reopening of exploratory laparotomy in setting of open peritoneum
- Ultrasound-guided drainage of abscess
- Ultrasound-guided thoracentesis
- Ultrasound-guided paracentesis
- Lumbar puncture

Elective

- Percutaneous tracheostomy
- Percutaneous endoscopic gastrostomy tube
- IVC filter placement
- Various endoscopic procedures

2.5 Bedside Anesthesia

Critically ill patients are subjected to noxious stimuli, unpleasant experiences, and discomfort from general disease states. There are varying degrees of consciousness and memory during the critical state and stay in the ICU. Extra care and attention needs to be focused toward providing comfort in this patient population as well as perioperatively. A number of measures can be taken to provide reduction of the experience of pain, anxiety. Examples of the procedures listed above all require an amount of sedation and analgesic medication; however, there are no set guidelines that determine what is the most appropriate, and it is often left up to the surgeon and ICU team involved in the procedure. Guidelines have been developed by the American Society of Anesthesiologists on nonoperating room anesthetizing locations that offer recommendations on equipment, oxygen, suctioning, and emergency equipment such as

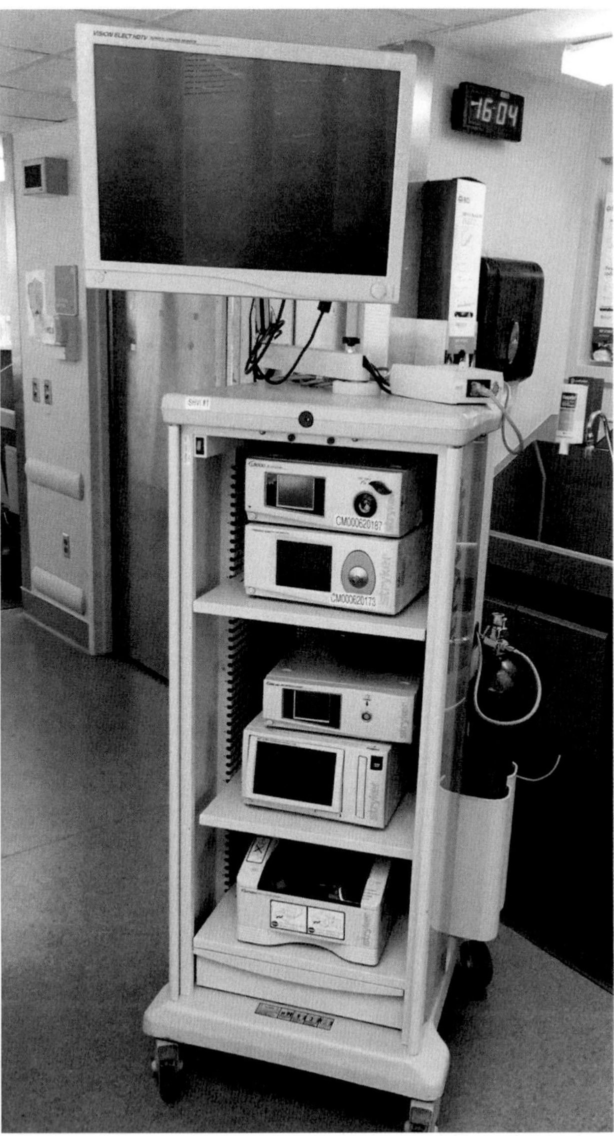

Fig. 2.6 Portable laparoscopic tower, for bedside laparoscopic use

crash cart with defibrillator [5]. This also describes potential monitoring needs and monitoring, which is present in the ICU setting. As previously mentioned, care needs to be taken in interpreting these monitors and action for the negative effects of anesthetic provided. Anesthetic options are limited in the ICU, and adequate gas systems are not available, yet many considerations need to be made and plans individualized when choosing sedation, paralytics, and analgesics [6]. Guidelines for sedation and analgesia in the ICU are present, yet limited surrounding the ICU as an operating room.

Again, it is essential to consider the patient's current state and condition when choosing anesthesia for the procedure. As mentioned above, each medication has caveats on potential harmful effects if not chosen with the patient's history, disease state, and metabolism potential of the individual [7].

2.6 The IVC Filter: A Case Study of Transition to the Bedside

The IVC filter was developed to lower the risk of fatal PE in patients with a DVT of the lower extremity who cannot be anticoagulated or who have a recurrence while on anticoagulation. When indicated the IVC filter is placed after obtaining access to the patient venous circulatory system. This is often obtained by femoral access and cannulation with filter placement into the inferior vena cava under fluoroscopy guidance. Fluoroscopy is necessary to guide appropriate placement in just above the renal veins.

Previously, this technique required the patient's transport to the operative suite or interventional radiology for fluoroscopy guidance. As skill and familiarity with the procedure developed, the trend to move the procedure to the bedside for patients who could not tolerate transport began to emerge. Currently, common practice includes IVC filter placement safely at the bedside with the use of a C arm from the radiology department and a radiology technician for equipment operation. This process facilitates the prompt placement of filters and avoids the potential complications of transporting this frequently unstable patient population.

2.7 Summary

With the growing demand for procedural services and the increasing demand of facilities to accommodate this growth, it is increasingly necessary to use various resources to care for the surgical patient. One such shift is the transition of operative care to the bedside, in essence creating an OR out of the ICU. Over the last several decades, procedures previously performed in the OR, interventional radiology, and the cardiac cath lab can now be performed without incidence at the patient's bedside. Following in these footsteps is the transition of both routine and emergent operative care to the bedside. The benefits of efficiency and cost have been demonstrated; however, the provider must be cognizant of the limitations of the ICU and have a keen knowledge of their facility resources and the ability to successfully perform surgery outside of its previously prescribed area. Recommendations for surgical procedures performed in the ICU are reserved for emergent and simple or routine cases that have adequate preparation and planning.

References

1. Piper GL, et al. When the ICU is the operating room. J Trauma Acute Care Surg. 2013;74(3):871–5.
2. Joint Commission Standards: Universal Protocol. Retrieved from http://www.jointcommission.org/standards_information/up.aspx (2015).
3. Szem JM, et al. High risk intrahospital transport of critically ill patients: safety and outcome of the necessary "road trip". Crit Care Med. 1995;23:1660–6.
4. Bare P. The intensive care unit: the next generation operating room. In: Britt LD et al., editors. Acute care surgery: principals and practice. New York, NY: Springer; 2007. p. 106–23.
5. American Society of Anesthesiologist: Statement on Nonoperating Room Anesthetizing Locations. Retrieved from http://www.asahq/~/media/site/ASAHQ/files/resources/standards-guidelines (2013).
6. Booij LHDJ. Is succinylcholine appropriate or obsolete in the intensive care unit? Crit Care Med. 2001;5(5):245–6.
7. Oliveria Martins F, et al. Bedside surgery in the ICU. In: Kuhlen R, editor. Controversies in intensive care medicine. Berlin: MVW; 2008. p. 449–60.

that the lost art of using "anatomic markings" should not be forgotten [2]. Ultrasound guidance for catheterization of the internal jugular vein compared to landmark techniques has shown advantages over landmark technique [25]. Different individuals acquire the necessary knowledge and skills at different rates. It is recommended that a minimum number of 10 ultrasound-guided vascular access procedures be supervised to demonstrate competency in the technique. Utilizing the ultrasound can decrease the incidence of unintentional injury to the carotid artery, decrease the risk of causing a pneumo- or hemothorax, and improve direct visualization of the guidewire for proper placement in the vein [26].

Process improvements can help to eliminate serious adverse events, which include traditional training methods, simulation training, and the effective use of checklists [27]. Procedural experience, training, and complications vary among trainers. Experience does not equal expertise, especially when new technology is introduced.

3.2.3 Retained Foreign Objects

When performing an invasive procedure, "unintended retained foreign objects" (URFOs) can result in a sentinel adverse event. Objects most commonly left behind include:

1. Soft goods, such as sponges and towels
2. Small miscellaneous items, including unretrieved device components or fragments (such as broken parts of instruments), stapler components, parts of laparoscopic trocars, guidewires, catheters, and pieces of drains
3. Needles and other sharps
4. Instruments, most commonly malleable retractors [28]

3.2.4 Surgical Fires

An estimated 600 surgical fires occur on a yearly basis and can result in devastating outcomes. Most importantly, SURGICAL FIRES ARE PREVENTABLE MEDICAL ERRORS!

Surgical fires can occur if all three elements of the fire triangle are present:

1. Ignition source (e.g., electrosurgical units (ESUs), lasers, and fiber-optic light sources)
2. Fuel source (e.g., surgical drapes, alcohol-based skin preparation agents, the patient)
3. Oxidizer (e.g., oxygen, nitrous oxide, room air) [29]

Identification of a high-risk fire case should be identified prior to a procedure. These same fires can easily occur in the critical care setting, procedural setting, and other settings where patient care is rendered.

3.2.5 Teamwork Models

An important aspect of care rendered in the ICU revolves around understanding safety and error prevention strategies, teamwork, and team leadership [30]. The incorporation of evidence-based teamwork tools [e.g., TeamSTEPPS, crew resource management (CRM)] can enhance communication, performance, knowledge, and overall attitude. TeamSTEPPS is an evidence-based set of teamwork tools aimed at optimizing patient outcomes by improving communication and teamwork skills. The four primary teamwork skills include (1) leadership, (2) communication, (3) situation monitoring, and (4) mutual support. Teamwork outcomes are enhanced by (1) performance, (2) knowledge, and (3) attitude. If there is a concern that a safety error can occur, it is recommended to "stop the line."

Several interventions to overcome personal barriers can be implemented. The two-challenge rule is used when an initial assertive statement is ignored. If a statement is repeated twice, the team member can be challenged and acknowledge that they heard the concern. In addition, TeamSTEPPS also uses an assertive statement called CUS. The pneumonic CUS stands for: I am **C**oncerned! I am **U**ncomfortable! This is a **S**afety Issue! If there is a conflict that is not resolved, then mutually supported escalation to a supervisor or more senior colleague should occur [31].

Crew resource management emphasizes a safe and consistent delivery of care through respectful teamwork [32]. CRM incorporates Teamwork Skills and Hardwired Safety Tool Workshops resulting in implementation of tools and the development of metrics.

Both TeamSTEPPS and CRM focus on principles that treat everyone with respect. They fully support you when you speak up in the interest of patient safety and do not allow any retaliation for expression of concerns.

3.3 The Culture of Safety

"Huddles" are friendly and casual types of discussion that exist prior to a procedure being performed. Discussions can include staffing, equipment needs, and other requirements for the procedure. Important procedural elements in the checklist should minimally include conducting a pre-procedure verification—the correct patient, the correct procedure, and the correct site—marking the procedural site, and performing the time-out. Risk assessments can be integrated into the pre-procedural checklist. The recommended steps in preparation for a procedure can include:

- Identification of the medications being utilized in a procedure. Each basin or syringe should be clearly labeled with the medication or solution that it contains.
- A discussion on how sharps (scalpels, needles, etc.) may be handled (neutral basin) is important.
- An instrument count prior and after a procedure should be incorporated.
- If an insertion kit contains a guidewire for line placement, that guidewire must be accounted for on completion.
- Proper disposal of equipment, supplies, and contaminants is also required.

During the "time-out," everyone stops what they are doing and pays attention to the reader who usually uses a preapproved script. A source document is usually present, and other methods of patient verification may include matching the patient's identification band and date of birth.

The time-out process requires the participation of every member in the procedural area. Agreement may focus on known allergies, medications, blood products, and potential concerns and also include minimally the correct patient, the correct site, and the correct procedure to be performed. Each member in the room will verify these elements by saying that they agree, one at a time. This gives the opportunity of every member to "speak up" if there is a patient safety concern.

If a second procedure is to be performed, then an additional time-out is required. If there is a concern with a safety issue or during the prepping and draping of the patient due to a contamination issue, an outside reviewer can stop the procedure. The safety issue needs to be addressed before moving on.

Upon completion of the procedure, a "debrief" should take place. The debrief should describe what went well, what didn't go well, and what can "the team" do to improve the next time. If all are in agreement, the debrief is completed and recorded. If there is disagreement, with no resolution, a concern report may be filed. A safety committee will assign a safety assessment code score upon receiving a concern report. This assessment compares the probability to the severity of the event as low, medium, or high risk. The concern report is then forwarded to an administrative team to review the issue and meet with the team involved. Many times the issue revolves around equipment, instrumentation, environment, possibly behavior, and other issues. An organization that utilizes a non-punitive approach helps to evaluate whether actions were acceptable or unacceptable.

Other multidimensional approaches can help to minimize errors and improve clinical and economical effectiveness in the ICU [9]. Team cross-check during multidisciplinary rounds can focus on specific quality initiatives. The development of hardwired tools with key indicators that impact outcomes is an important element of the process and has demonstrated improvements in further understanding necessary tasks and procedures [33].

The concept of closed loop communication helps to avoid misunderstandings.

An example includes a hand-off communication tool that provides essential patient management information and especially allows two-way communication with the ability of the receiver to ask specific questions regarding the patient, procedures, test, etc. Other ways of verification include confirming the message by a read back and the sender confirms by saying "yes." If the sender does not get a reply, the statement is repeated until the loop is closed with the appropriate "yes" response. If the response were incorrect, the sender would say negative [31].

SBAR is a communication tool used to transmit critical information.

Situation: What is going on with the patient?
Background: What is the clinical content or context?
Assessment: What do I think the problem is?
Recommendation and Request: What would I do to correct it?

Other communication measures that can be incorporated include a "callout," where critical information can be read out loud by an outside reader informing all members of the team during emergent situations [31].

The Swiss cheese model of accident causation identifies that a series of successive layers of defenses, barriers, and safeguards can result in unintended losses simply due to active failures and associated latent conditions. The image of multiple pieces of Swiss cheese helps to identify the system failures or medical mishaps that occur under the best of intentions [34].

Not being aware of what is going on in the periphery can be labeled as "tunnel vision." A procedural example deals with "fiber-optic cord capacitance." During a laparoscopic procedure, the focus is on the tip of the cautery or laser. For example, little-to-no attention is placed on the fiber-optic cord, which may cause thermal injury to a vital structure. The same can occur when observing a monitor. The focus can be on an individual hemodynamic measure instead of addressing all the findings and understanding the complete picture.

Finally, behavioral errors can lead to an error by slips (human error), taking shortcuts (risky behavior) and blatantly ignoring required safety steps (reckless behavior) [35]. A high anxiety environment should never occur. Recognizing that one is having difficulty in performing a procedure does not mean failure. Escalation protocols should be clearly identified. Many times escalating an issue is not an indication of shame or failure.

3.4 Cognitive Aids

Cognitive aids help to guide users to perform tasks and decrease the number of errors with performance. They are especially helpful in stressful situations where complex steps and possible omissions can occur. "The main difference from guidelines, protocols or standard operating procedures is that they are to be used while the task is being performed [36]."

Recommendations are:

1. Its content must be derived from "best practice" guidelines or protocols.
2. Its design should be appropriate for use in the context of the emergency situation.
3. It should be familiar, in a format that has been used in practice and training.
4. It should also assist other team members to perform their task in a coordinated manner [36].

3.5 Checklists

Healthcare professionals are now increasingly using different approaches to improve patient safety and quality outcomes. Methods to reduce patient harm and eliminate medical errors are being monitored in the form of the checklist. Atul Gawande, MD, in his book, *The Checklist Manifesto*, reviews the positive impact of checklists used in many fields, including healthcare. According to Dr. Gawande, "the volume and complexity of what we know has exceeded our individual ability to deliver its benefits correctly, safely, or reliably. Knowledge has both saved us and burdened us" [37].

In the medical setting, checklists can promote process improvement and increase patient safety. Having a formalized protocol will reduce errors caused by lack of information and inconsistent procedures. Checklists have improved processes for patient care in intensive care and trauma units. Along with improving patient safety, checklists create a greater sense of confidence that the process is completed accurately and thoroughly. Working collaboratively with the World Health Organization (WHO), Dr. Gawande examined how a surgical safety checklist was implemented and tested in eight hospitals worldwide. With this checklist, major postsurgical complications at the hospitals fell 36 % and deaths decreased by 47 % [37]. Even with this successful trial, based on several studies, the standardization of surgical processes should not be limited to the operating room as the majority of surgical errors (53–70 %) occur outside the operating room, before or after surgery. This would ensure that a more substantial improvement in safety could be achieved possibly by targeting the entire surgical pathway [38].

In another study, two surgical teams participated in a series of simulated emergencies. Each team performed 8 simulated operations in which one or more crises existed. The teams were randomly selected and managed 4 scenarios with a checklist and 4 from memory alone. Checklist use during operating room crises resulted in nearly a 75 % reduction in failure to adhere to critical steps in management. Every team performed better when the crisis checklists were available. Survey responses stated that the checklists made the team feel better, were easy to use, and could be used in a real-life emergent situation, and if there was an intraoperative emergency, they would want the checklist to be used [39].

Ariadne Labs is a Joint Center for health systems innovation at Brigham and Women's Hospital and Harvard School of Public Health. The researchers are devoted to designing scalable solutions that drive better care at the most critical moments in people's lives everywhere. A Crisis Checklists Download Registration form is available to customize the crisis checklists for specific facility usage [40].

The Stanford Emergency Manual is an excellent aid for perioperative critical events. This is a free perioperative emergency manual that contains several critical events as well as crisis management resource key points.

The researchers provide reasons for implementing an emergency manual:

1. In simulation studies, integrating emergency manuals results in better management during operating room critical events
2. Pilots and nuclear power plant operators use similar cognitive aids for emergencies and rare events, with training on why and how to use them
3. During a critical event, relevant detailed literature is rarely accessible
4. Memory worsens with stress and distractions interrupt planned actions.
5. Expertise requires significant repetitive practice, so none of us are experts in every emergency [41].

The use of checklist training can be integrated with TEAMSTEPPS or crew resource management (CRM). In the operating room, the intensive care units, procedural areas, and other venues, these safety tools can be implemented.

3.6 Conclusion

Chassin [42] notes that after nearly 14 years since the Institute of Medicine report (IOM), "To Err is Human: Building a Safer Health System," there is still a widespread overuse of services, there is a need for more effective strategies and tools to address management complexities in healthcare, and the cultures of most American hospitals and healthcare organizations need change. Leadership's adherence to safe practices needs to eliminate intimidating behavior that does not allow for accurate reporting and results in unsafe conditions.

"Challenges for the future include continued improvement in our systems of care and inclusion of patient safety training in standard educational curricula for health professionals [43]."

Online learning or blended learning models may be a necessary direction to actually go beyond the walls and provide the type of asynchronous learning supported by current evidence-based and peer-reviewed literature [44].

Since "human infallibility is impossible, the only chance to keep human errors from hurting patients is by creating collegial interactive teams" [45].

References

1. Institute of Medicine. To err is human: building a safer health system. Washington, DC: The National Academies Press; 1999.
2. Conlon T, Boyer D. The future of inexperience: a challenge and an opportunity. Crit Care Med. 2013;42(4):994–5.
3. Institute of Medicine. Crossing the quality chasm: a new health system for the 21st century. Washington, DC: The National Academies Press; 2001.
4. Berwick DM, Calkins DR, McCannon CJ, Hackbarth AD. The 100,000 lives campaign: setting a goal and a deadline for improving health care quality. JAMA. 2006;295(3):324–7.
5. National Quality Forum (NQF). Serious reportable events in health-care-2011 update: a consensus report. Washington, DC: NQF; 2011.
6. The Joint Commission (TJC). Retrieved 8 Sep 2014 from www.jointcomission.org
7. AHRQ–Agency for Healthcare Research and Quality. Quality tool—modified early warning system (MEWS). Retrieved 3 July 2014 from http://www.innovations.ahrq.gov/content.aspx?id=2631 (2014).
8. Valetin A, Capuzzo M, Guidet B, Moreno RP, Dolanski L, Bauer P, Metnitz PG. Patient safety in intensive care: results from the multinational sentinel events evaluation (SEE) study. Intensive Care Med. 2006;32(10):1591–8.
9. Moreno RP, Rhodes A, Donchin Y. Patient safety in intensive care medicine: the declaration of Vienna. Intensive Care Med. 2009;35:1667–72. Pg 1660.
10. Sexton JB, Berenholtz SM, Goeschel CA, Watson SR, Holzmueler CG, Thompson DA, Hysy RC, Marsteller JA, Schumacker K, Pronovost PJ. Assessing and improving safety climate in a large cohort of intensive care units. Crit Care Med. 2011;39(5):934–9.
11. de Vries EN, Ramrattan MA, Smorenburg SM, Gouma DJ, Boermeester MA. The incidence and nature of in-hospital adverse events: a systematic review. Qual Saf Health Care. 2008;17:216–22.
12. Schulman P, Roe E, van Eeten M, de Bruijne M. High reliability & the management of critical infrastructures. J Conting Crisis Manag. 2004;12(1):14–28.
13. Chassin MR, Loeb JM. The ongoing quality improvement journey: next stop, high reliability. Health Aff. 2011;30(14):559–68.
14. Hines S, Luna K, Lofthus J, et al. Becoming a high reliability organization: operational advice for hospital leaders. Rockvill, MD: Agency for Healthcare Research and Quality; 2008. http://www.ahrq.gov/professionals/quality-patient-safety/quality-resources/tools/hroadvice/hroadvice.pdf. Accessed 14 July 2014.
15. IHI—Institute for Healthcare Improvement Failure Modes and Effects Analysis (FMEA) Tool. Retrieved 14 June 2014 from http://www.ihi.org/resource/Pages/Tools/FailureModesandEffectsAnalysisTool.aspx (2014).
16. Bassily-Marcus A. Early detection of deteriorating patients: leveraging clinical informatics to improve outcome. Crit Care Med. 2014;42(4):976–8.
17. Gardner-Thorpe J. The value of modified early warning score (MEWS) in surgical in-patients: a prospective observational study. Ann R Coll Surg Engl. 2006;88(6):571–5.
18. Churpek M, et al. Using electronic health record data to develop and validate a prediction model for adverse outcomes in the wards. Crit Care Med. 2014;42(4):841–8.
19. Huh JW, Lim CM, Koh Y, Lee J, Jung YK, Seo HS, Hong SB. Activation of a medical emergency team using an electronic medical recording-based screening system. Crit Care Med. 2014;42(4):801–8.
20. Kleinpell R, Buchman TG. The value and future of patient-centered outcomes research. Critical Connections. 2 April 2014.
21. Papadakos PJ. Training health care professionals to deal with an explosion of electronic distraction. Neurocritical care. New York: Springer; 2012.
22. O'Grady NP, Alexander M, Burns LA, E. Patchen Dellinger, Garland J, Heard SO, Lipsett PA, Masur H, Mermel LA, Pearson ML, Raad II, Randolph A, Rupp ME, Saint S, the Healthcare Infection Control Practices Advisory Committee (HICPAC). Guidelines for the prevention of Intravascular- catheter related infections. 2011. Available at https://www.premierinc.com/safety/topics/guidelines/downloads/bsi-guidelines-2011.pdf
23. Song Y, Messerlian AK, Matevosian RM. Case report: a potentially hazardous complication during central venous catheterization: lost guidewire retained in patient. J Clin Anesth. 2012;24:221–6.
24. Roux D, Reignier J, Guillaume T, Boyer A, Hayon J, Souweine B, Papazian L, Mercat A, Bernardin F, Combes A, Chiche J-D, Diehl J-L, Cheyron D, L'Her E, Perrotin D, Schneider F, Thuong M, Wolff M, Zeni F, Dreyfuss D, Ricard J-D. Acquiring procedural skills in ICUs: a prospective multicenter study. Crit Care Med. 2014;42(4):886–95.
25. Karakitsos D, Labropoulos N, Groot ED, Patrianakos AP, Kouraklis G, Poularas J, Samonis G, Tsoutsos DA, Konstadoulakis MM, Karabinis A. Real-time ultrasound-guided catheterization of the internal jugular vein: a prospective comparison with the landmark technique in critical care patients. Crit Care. 2006;10(6):R162.

26. Troianos CA, Hartman GS, Glas KE, Skubas NJ, Eberhardt RT, Walker JD, Reeves ST. Councils on intraoperative echocardiography and vascular ultrasound of the American Society of Echocardiography. J Am Soc Echocardiogr. 2011;24(12):1291–318.
27. Weiss CH, Baker DW. The evolving application of implementation science in critical care. Crit Care Med. 2014;42(4):996–7.
28. Sentinel Event Alert, Issue 51. Retrieved 27 July 2014 from http://www.jointcommission.org/assets/1/6/SEA_51_URFOs_10_17_13_FINAL.pdf
29. FDA—Preventing Surgical Fires. Retrieved 19 July 2014 from http://www.fda.gov/Drugs/DrugSafety/SafeUseInitiative/PreventingSurgicalFires (2014).
30. Reader TW, Flin R, Mearns K, Cuthbertson BH. Developing a team performance framework for the intensive care unit. Crit Care Med. 2009;37(5):1787–93.
31. TeamSTEPPs. Retrieved 7 Sep 2014 from www.teamstepps.ahrq.gov
32. Crew Resource Management (CRM). Retrieved 7 Sep 2014 from www.saferpatients.com/services/crew-resource-management-training
33. Dingley C, Daugherty K, Derieg MK, Persing R. Improving patient safety through provider communication strategy enhancements—advances in patient safety: new directions and alternative approaches. Vol. 3: performance and tools. Rockville, MD: Agency for Healthcare Research and Quality (US); 2008.
34. Perneger TV. The Swiss-cheese model of safety incidents: are there holes in the metaphor. BMC Health Serv Res. 2005;5:71.
35. InFocus—The Quarterly Journal for Health Care Practice and Risk Management. The future of training for patient safety and quality. Retrieved 7 July 2014 from http://www.fojp.com/sites/default/files/InFocus_Summer12.pdf
36. Marshall S. The use of cognitive aids during emergencies in anesthesia: a review of the literature. Anesth Analg. 2013;117:1162–71.
37. Gawande A. The checklist manifesto. New York, NY: Metropolitan Books; 2010.
38. Griffen FD, Stephens LS, Alexander JB, et al. The American college of surgeons closed claims study: new insights for improving care. J Am Coll Surg. 2007;204:561–9.
39. Arriaga A, Bader A, Wong J, Lipsitz S, Berry W, Ziewacz J, Hepner DL, Boorman DJ, Pozner CN, Smink DS, Gawande A. Simulation-based trial of surgical-crisis checklists. N Engl J Med. 2013;368:3.
40. Crisis Checklists Project Registration Form. Retrieved 27 July 2014 from http://www.projectcheck.org/crisis-checklist-download.html
41. Stanford Anesthesia Cognitive Aid Group. Emergency manual: cognitive aids for perioperative critical events. Creative Commons BY-NC_ND. 2013.
42. Chassin M. Improving the quality of health care: what's taking so long. Health Aff. 2013;32(10):1761–5.
43. Patterson J, et al. Infection control in the intensive care unit: progress and challenges in systems and accountability. Crit Care Med. 2010;38(Suppl):S265–268.
44. Burns J. Transforming critical education and career development for the 21st century-time to move beyond the walls. Crit Care Med. 2014;42(4):1017–8.
45. Nance JJ. Why hospitals should fly—the ultimate flight plan to patient safety and quality care. Boseman, MT: Second River Healthcare Press; 2012.

4 The Administrative Process: Credentialing, Privileges, and Maintenance of Certification

Todd Pickard

4.1 Introduction

This chapter will focus on the processes for credentialing, privileging, and maintenance of certification. The advanced care practitioner will be able to understand the differences between credentialing and privileging as well as the importance of each process. The role of state laws, regulatory agencies, and accreditation agencies will be discussed to provide the context of these processes. The chapter will conclude with a discussion on the role of certification and maintenance of certification as it pertains to compliance with regulatory and accrediting agencies, competency, and patient safety.

Before discussing the various processes in this chapter, it is crucial to define them for clarity. Many times the processes of credentialing, privileging, and maintenance of certification are confused or combined into one concept. However, there are three distinct and separate processes that happen to be interrelated as they all apply to patient care and competency.

T. Pickard, MMSc, PA-C (✉)
The University of Texas MD Anderson Cancer Center, 1515 Holcombe, Unit 1418, Houston, TX 77030, USA
e-mail: tpickard@mdanderson.org

Credentialing is a formal process that has both internal and external regulatory requirements for reviewing the "credentials" of an applicant for clinical appointment within an institution or practice. This process is governed by internal policy, state law, external regulation, and accreditation requirements. During this process, the candidate's degrees, medical training, licensure, certifications, professional references, competency attestations, malpractice data, and insurance claims data are reviewed. This process focuses on primary source verification. The medical staff office or practice management will request documentation and will contact information sources directly such as universities, training program, previous employers, national databases, and licensing bodies [1].

Privileging is an internal process used by institutions and practices to define and approve clinical activity. This process is governed by internal policy and is referenced by state law, external regulators, and accreditation agencies. Unlike credentialing, the process for privileging is completely at the discretion of the institution or practice. The external groups merely require that there is a standard process in place and that clinicians are deemed to be competent, but they do not define what that process entails. A clinician's privileges define their scope of practice, detail the specific patient care activities that are allowed, and communicate to other members of the workforce what each provider is allowed to do within the institution or practice [2].

D.A. Taylor et al. (eds.), *Interventional Critical Care*, DOI 10.1007/978-3-319-25286-5_4

Maintenance of certification (MOC) is a process in which individual clinicians complete certain training, education, performance improvement, and self-assessment activities in order to keep certification from state or national certification agencies. This typically includes a formal examination of medical knowledge, patient care, ethics, and regulatory knowledge. The MOC process varies by each certifying agency and is typically specific to physicians, advanced practice registered nurses, and physician assistants. State and government licensing agencies typically require these profession-specific certifications for the granting of licensure. There are also certifications that are not specific to any profession such as radiation safety certification, CPR, fundamentals of critical care, pediatric advanced life support, and others. These types of certifications may be required by institutions and practices in addition to the professional certifications that are required to keep licensure. MOC is usually a requirement for continued credentialing and the grant of privileges by institutions and practices.

It is evident that these processes are interrelated, but it is also important to remember that each process has its own requirements, timeline, and review process. In general institutions and practices use these processes to fulfill both internal and external requirements to ensure that clinicians are competent, that patients are treated safely, and that quality care is provided. Accrediting agencies such as the Joint Commission require that certain elements of performance are completed during credentialing and privileging in order for an institution or practice to be accredited. Government agencies such as the Centers for Medicare and Medicaid Services (CMS) and insurance companies also require that certain conditions of participation are met before they will reimburse for patient care and other clinical services [3]. It is crucial that clinicians have an understanding of these processes and comply with requests for information, documentation, and professional references, as well as meet any training or education requirements as indicated by the institution or practice.

4.2 Credentialing

This is the first step to practice as an Advanced Care Practitioners (ACP). Any employer will need to review the education, training, certification, and previous work experience of an ACP [4]. Small practices and large institutions are required to complete this assessment at a minimum to ensure patient safety. Institutions such as hospitals and university medical centers will have a well-defined process in place that will likely be governed by bylaws and policies. Clinical practice may simply have checklists or internal guidelines. Whichever the case, it is crucial for the ACP to review the process and follow it within the timeframe allotted.

Primary source verification is a key concept within the credentialing process. Employers will go to the source of information that can verify the credentials of the ACP. This will include education, licensure, certification(s), and last employment position. Employers will contact the sources of this information directly without the need for the ACP to provide any additional information [5]. The ACP should not list any items in the credentialing packet that cannot be verified.

The review of Malpractice and Insurance Claims data will be completed at institutions and based on state requirements for reporting by the ACP. There are several national databases that provide this service for a fee. The ACP will not be asked to gather or provide this information from these national databases. However, they may be required to self-report any malpractice history or insurance claims. The ACP should be prepared to discuss each judgment, dismissal, or claim to provide the clinical details and outcomes. It is critical to be completely forthcoming with the details for any/each event. The ACP can face a negative credentialing decision if they mischaracterize or omit any information.

The ACP will be requested to furnish a substantial list of information in the credentialing application beyond education, licensure, certification, and work history. The process will include written attestations of fitness for duty and self-reporting. As previously mentioned, this will include malpractice and insurance claims. This will also include standard questions regarding health status, mental health history, physical disability, substance abuse, rehabilitation from addiction, and behavioral issues. The ACP will also be asked to describe any disciplinary issues from previous employers. While this information may seem intimate and personal, it is required by credentialing processes and based on state law, accrediting agencies, and payer's requirements for enrolling providers into their system.

Professional references are an important part of the credentialing process that will require careful consideration by the ACP. Identifying those physicians, physician assistants, and advanced practice registered nurses that have recently worked with the ACP in a clinical setting is only one aspect of professional references. It will be crucial for the ACP to ensure that those references are not only familiar with the clinical work of the ACP but can also positively speak to the competence and professionalism of the ACP. Poor feedback from professional references can significantly impact the credentialing process unfavorably.

Once the credentialing application is complete, the review process begins. This will include review by the medical staff office or practice management to ensure that the application is complete. Once the application is complete, it will then be submitted for formal review by a credentials committee that will include review from professional peers. The review process is governed by a number of guidelines that will be based on bylaws and policies as well as outside regulatory agencies [6]. There will also be a process to appeal any decisions if they are negative toward the ACP. It is important for the ACP to review the process and understand all of their options during the process. Negative credentialing decisions are reportable and discoverable. A negative credentialing decision can significantly impact future employment of an ACP.

4.3 Privileging

This is the process that governs what the clinical role or scope of practice will be for an ACP. Once an employer had accepted the credentials of an ACP, they must define what the role of the ACP will be within their organization. There is typically a standard request form that is completed by the ACP and their collaborating physician(s). This form may have a standard set of clinical activities, procedures, and patient care responsibilities, or it may be up to the ACP to define what they will need to be authorized to do in order to effectively provide patient care. The privileging request is typically reviewed by the same committee that reviews credentialing applications. It is important to remember that the ACP is not authorized to engage in any kind of patient care until they receive privileges [7].

The purpose of privileging is not only to define the clinical role of the ACP; it also ensures that there are minimum standards in training and experience for the ACP to hold each particular privilege. This is one of the most important methods for ensuring patient safety and quality of care. Typically healthcare institutions, practice groups, or hospitals will set parameters around the type of training and a minimum number of times an ACP has performed certain procedures before they will grant authority for the ACP to perform those procedures. There may be required training protocols and standard competency assessments as part of the privileging process. The ACP should maintain a log of their training and the number of each procedure that they have performed. This will greatly simplify the privileging process by providing a detailed account for review.

When an ACP has held privileges at previous institutions, having letters of attestation from supervising physician(s) is in the best interest of the ACP. These letters can be used in lieu of having to recomplete training and perform minimum numbers of procedures. It makes little sense for an ACP to spend time in this activity if they have previously held and competently performed privileges. Even with letters of attestation, some employers may require the ACP to demonstrate proficiency and competency in certain procedural privileges before granting the ACP that privilege. This should not discourage or concern the ACP. They should be willing and able to demonstrate their skill and expertise as needed.

For the advanced practice registered nurse (APRN), it is important to understand the role of the chief nursing officer (CNO) for any institution. Beyond what is required by the medical staff, bylaws, policy, or practice guidelines, the CNO has the responsibility and authority to govern nursing practice. This may be as simple as reviewing the previous experience, licensure, and certification or the APRN. However, it can include additional documentation, peer references, or specific training required for nurses within the institution such as mock code certification, population-based competency training, or age-specific competency training. The APRN should be aware of the role of the CNO and any additional requirements for clinical practice that might be required.

When applying for privileges, it will be fundamentally important for the ACP to understand the laws of the state that govern their professional practice. Typically, each state will have laws that govern the practice of APRNs and PAs. There is a great deal of variation in ACP practice laws from state to state. The ACP should never assume that what was allowed in one state will also be allowed in another state. The ACP must review the practice laws governing their profession in each and every state in which they practice. State law typically sets the maximum (the "ceiling") of professional practice for the ACP. Employers are allowed to lower the professional practice of ACPs to less than what the state allows. This could include a requirement for certain orders to have physician co-signature, limitations on independent practice, or limitations on certain procedures or clinical activities. While the ACP may not agree with these limitations, it is important to realize that this kind of limitation is allowable and a normal practice. Fortunately, most employers realize that limiting ACPs is detrimental to clinical effectiveness, patient access, and quality of care.

The privileging process is one that is continuous in nature. Simply because one was granted privileges in the past does not mean that they will continue on indefinitely. National accreditation standards, such as the Joint Commission (JC), require the institutions to review the performance and set minimum standard for the maintenance of privileges. Additionally, it is an accepted practice standard to re-privilege physicians, APRNs, and PAs every two years. During these cycles, the number of times an individual has performed certain procedures and the quality with which they were performed will be reviewed. It is worth mentioning that there are two review processes utilized: Focused Professional Practice Evaluation (FPPE) and Ongoing Professional Practice Evaluation (OPPE). The FPPE process is used when an individual is first granted privileges, receives new privileges, or has questions raised about their competence. During FPPE, the ACP will be assigned a proctor that will be responsible for evaluating the ACP performance. This evaluation will last a minimum of 6 months and can include chart review, interviews, observation, testing, and discussing performance with peers or staff [8]. Once FPPE is successfully completed, the ACP will move into the OPPE process. This requires the ongoing and current review of metrics and data that must be accumulated to assess the ACP performance in comparison to others that hold the same privileges. The purpose of OPPE is to identify outliers in clinical practice with regard to utilization of resources, adherence to practice standards, quality of care, and patient safety [9].

The ACP should review and understand all of the requirements for the privileging process, FPPE, OPPE, and re-privileging. These are typically outlined in bylaws, policies, or practice guidelines. The ACP should engage in conversations with their clinical supervisors and managers early in the process to ensure that they have the support and direction they need to be successful.

4.4 Maintenance of Certification

The certification process is the mechanism used by local and national professional certification bodies to document that ACPs have met certain standards and in some cases have passed standardized examinations. Some of these certifications, such as the Physician Assistant National Certifying Examination (PANCE), are requirements for obtaining licensure as an ACP [10]. The initial certifications are typically based on completing education in an ACP training program and then passing a standardized examination. However, maintenance certification generally requires a commitment to ongoing education, clinical practice, performance improvement, self-assessment, and other activities.

Generally speaking, certification is used as a surrogate for competency in the areas of medical knowledge and patient care. There are some certifications that are used to ensure technical competencies and knowledge of safety processes such as Radiation Safety Certification. The point of these certifications is to ensure that ACPs are exposed to a standard set of knowledge and skills related to their work of providing care to patients. As such, institutions, medical practices, licensing boards, accrediting agencies, and insurance companies have adopted these certifications as an indication that an ACP is prepared to provide care and should be reimbursed for that care.

Is it imperative that the ACP is aware of the certifications that are required for their practice and the roles they assume within each institution or practice. Additionally, they must adhere to the prescribed methods set forth by each certifying agency for the maintenance of their certifications. In most cases, this will require the ACP to complete a certain number of continuing education hours within a specified time frame or cycle. Some certifications require specific content such as ethics or pharmacology. Others simply provide general requirements that the continuing education meet certain standards and that a specified number of hours are completed within each certification cycle.

The ACP should be aware of the recent changes in physician maintenance of certification. The American Board of Internal Medicine (ABIM), for example, has created a 10-year cycle for physicians in internal medicine specialties that will require a number of areas of activity. These include: continuing education in medical knowledge, practice assessment (performance improvement), patient safety training, and passing a recertifying examination [11]. This is important for the ACP because some certification bodies such as the National Commission on the Certification of Physician Assistants (NCCPA) have adopted this MOC process. This means that ACPs can and should work with their collaborating physicians in completing MOC activity. This is particularly true for practice assessment in which the care of patients is assessed for adherence to certain standards of care, and then practice improvements are implemented. This type of activity is intended to educate participants in the area of performance improvement.

It is important that the ACP is supported in MOC activity by their institutions or practice. The ACP will need time and funds in order to participate and successfully complete the variety of educational and performance assessment activates required for MOC [12, 13]. It is a generally accepted practice that physicians, advanced practice registered nurses, and physician assistants are granted a certain number of educational days per year and a fixed amount of funding for their MOC. The ACP should discuss these benefits as part of the interview process and before they accept any position.

4.5 Summary

The ACP must be aware of the processes and requirements involved in credentialing, privileging, and maintenance of certification. As they expand their clinical skill and learn new procedures, these processes will govern their ability to provide care to their patients. Every institution and practice has internal and external requirements to ensure that providers are competent to provide safe and effective care. This also includes insurance companies and other payers that have their own sets of rules that govern who they reimburse for care and how they reimburse that care. The ACP must be informed and adhere to all of these if they wish to be successful in growing their practice, learning new procedures, and providing quality care to their patients.

References

1. Deutsch S, Mobley CS. The credentialing handbook. 1st ed. Gaithersburg, MD: Aspen; 1999.
2. Roberts A. The credentialing coordinators handbook. 1st ed. Marblehead, MA: HCPro; 2007.
3. Condition of participation: Medical staff, 42 C.F.R. Section 482.22 (2007).
4. The Joint Commission: Medical Staff, MS.06.01.03, Hospital Accreditation Standards (2014).
5. The Joint Commission: Medical Staff, MS.06.01.05, Hospital Accreditation Standards (2014).
6. The Joint Commission: Medical Staff, MS.06.01.07, Hospital Accreditation Standards (2014).
7. The Joint Commission: Medical Staff, MS.06.01.09, Hospital Accreditation Standards (2014).
8. The Joint Commission: Medical Staff, MS.08.01.01, Hospital Accreditation Standards (2014).
9. The Joint Commission: Medical Staff, MS.08.01.03, Hospital Accreditation Standards (2014).
10. American Academy of Physician Assistants [Internet]. Alexandria: The Association; c2010–2014. Available from: http://www.aapa.org/twocolumn.aspx?id=984 [cited 1 Oct 2014].
11. American Board of Internal Medicine [Internet]. Philadelphia: The Association; c2004–2014. Available from: http://www.abim.org/maintenance-of-certification/requirements.aspx [cited 1 Oct 2014].
12. American Academy of Nurse Practitioners [Internet]. Austin: The Association; c2009–2013. Available from: http://www.aanpcert.org/ptistore/control/index [cited 1 Oct 2014].
13. The Joint Commission: Medical Staff, MS.12.01.01, Hospital Accreditation Standards (2014).

5 Billing and Coding for Procedures

David Carpenter

5.1 Introduction

- Disclaimer
  - This presentation was current at the time it was submitted. It does not represent payment or legal advice.
  - Medicare policy changes frequently, so be sure to keep current by going to www.cms.gov.
  - Although every reasonable effort has been made to assure the accuracy of the information within these pages, the ultimate responsibility for the correct submission of claims and response to any remittance advice lies with the provider of services.
  - The American Medical Association has copyright and trademark protection of CPT ©.

Procedures are a common part of the critical care physician assistant (PA) and nurse practitioner (NP) practice. While a significant portion of PAs and NPs perform procedures, billing for them is less understood. Institutional billing and commercial carriers are accustomed to billing for physician services and may not understand how to bill for PAs and NPs. In addition, procedural billing is relatively complex, and descriptors are very similar for multiple procedures. Billing incorrectly carries substantial penalty. Failure to bill will lead to significant revenue loss for the PA or NP employer. Incorrect billing can carry substantial penalties from Medicare and Medicaid. By selecting the proper procedure to bill for and ensuring adequate documentation, the PA or NP can ensure their reimbursement is adequately represented.

5.2 Basis for NP and PA Billing

PA and NP procedural regulation is a complex mix of hospital bylaws, state law, and insurance company regulations. It is beyond the scope of this article to evaluate all state laws and hospital bylaws. It is incumbent on the provider to know the particular rules and regulations that govern their practice.

5.2.1 Medicare billing

Medicare has authorized PA and NP billing since 1986. The description for PA practice is included in the Medicare Benefit Policy Manual Chapter 15, Section 190 [1].

"The services of a PA may be covered under Part B, if all of the following requirements are met:

- They are the type that are considered physician's services if furnished by a doctor of medicine or osteopathy (MD/DO);

D. Carpenter, MPAS, PA-C (✉)
Emory Center for Critical Care, Atlanta, GA, USA
e-mail: david.carpenter@emoryhealthcare.org

D.A. Taylor et al. (eds.), *Interventional Critical Care*, DOI 10.1007/978-3-319-25286-5_5

- They are performed by a person who meets all the PA qualifications,
- They are performed under the general supervision of an MD/DO;
- The PA is legally authorized to perform the services in the state in which they are performed; and
- They are not otherwise precluded from coverage because of one of the statutory exclusions."

Notably two important statements are made in regard to procedures:

"Also, if authorized under the scope of their State license, PAs may furnish services billed under all levels of CPT evaluation and management codes, and diagnostic tests if furnished under the general supervision of a physician."

"The physician supervisor (or physician designee) need not be physically present with the PA when a service is being furnished to a patient and may be contacted by telephone, if necessary, unless State law or regulations require otherwise."

Taken together, these two statements authorize PAs to perform diagnostic and therapeutic procedures as authorized by state law. Furthermore, there is no requirement for direct physician oversight unless required by state law.

For NPs, the regulation is found in the Medicare Benefit Policy Manual Chapter 15, Section 200.

The rules are very similar to those of the PA. The principle difference is the use of collaboration to describe the relationship with physicians.

"The services of an NP may be covered under Part B if all of the following conditions are met:

- They are the type that are considered physician's services if furnished by a doctor of medicine or osteopathy (MD/DO);
- They are performed by a person who meets the definition of an NP (see subsection A);
- The NP is legally authorized to perform the services in the State in which they are performed;
- They are performed in collaboration with an MD/DO (see subsection D); and
- They are not otherwise precluded from coverage because of one of the statutory exclusions. (See subsection C.2.)"

In terms of collaboration:

"In the absence of State law governing collaboration, collaboration is to be evidenced by NPs documenting their scope of practice and indicating the relationships that they have with physicians to deal with issues outside their scope of practice.

The collaborating physician does not need to be present with the NP when the services are furnished or to make an independent evaluation of each patient who is seen by the NP."

Similar to the PA, the NP collaborating physician does not have to be present for a procedure. As with the PA, the state law governs scope of practice.

Finally, while other E/M services may be subject to share billing with the services performed in conjunction with the services, procedures must be billed by the provider who performed them. In terms of reimbursement, in comparison to physicians, Medicare reimburses PAs and NPs at 85 % of the agreed physician payment rate for all services including procedures.

5.2.2 Private Payer Billing

Private payer billing is in some ways more convoluted and in some ways simpler than Medicare. At the time of this chapter, the majority of insurance companies are not credentialing PAs and NPs. In this case, most insurance companies have instructed practices to bill for the PA or NP services under the supervising or collaborating physician's national provider identifier (NPI). This is generally reimbursed at the physician rate. A number of insurance companies have begun to credential PA and NPs with a variety of reimbursement rates. Whether this trend will continue is uncertain.

A common problem in ensuring private payer reimbursement is using the correct terminology when inquiring about PA and NP reimbursement. When asked if a particular insurance company reimburses for PAs or NPs, the answer is frequently "no." However, the correct way to ask this question is "how do we submit for reimbursement for a PA or NP"? The answer will generally be to submit the bill under a physician NPI.

PAs and NPs can bill for procedures in almost all circumstances. However, administrative staff may be unfamiliar with billing methods for PAs and NPs which may differ from those of physician. Close cooperation and monitoring of billing flow is a key to productive billing in the ICU.

5.3 Critical Care and Billing for Procedures

Critical care has separate billing from evaluation and management (E/M). When using the Current Procedural Technology [2] (CPT) codes 99291 (first 30–74 min critical care) and 99292 (each additional 30 min), certain procedural CPT codes are considered bundled into critical care. The list can be found in the Medicare Policy Manual Chapter 12, Section 30.6.12 [3] (Table 5.1).

Any other medically necessary procedure code may be billed separately. Also note that this only applies to critical care billing. If services are performed on E/M patients (CPT 99221–3 and 99231–3) or performed separately on the floor such as with a rapid response team, some procedures such as vascular access or gastric intubation may be reimbursable.

5.4 Vascular Access

Vascular access is one of the most common ICU procedures that PAs and NPs perform. Billing for vascular access is relatively complicated given the similar descriptions of the vascular access procedures.

5.4.1 Central Venous Access

The most common procedure is a central venous line (CVL). CVLs include both non-tunnel central venous catheters and peripherally inserted centrally catheter (PICC). Ports are also included in this category. As these are not usual ICU procedures, they are not included in this chapter. CVL is divided based on age. In addition, ICU PAs and NPs should be aware that removal of a tunneled CVL is reimbursable under codes 36589 and 36590 (depending on with or without a port). CVL repair is also reimbursable under code 36575. Finally, replacement of a CVL over a wire uses code 36580 (Table 5.2).

Particular care should be taken when using CPT codes to make sure the correct code is used.

Table 5.1 Procedures bundled into critical care (99291 and 99292) codes

Services and procedures	CPT	Description
Interpretation of cardiac output measurements	93561	Cardiac output measures
	93562	Subsequent CO measures
Chest X-ray, professional component	71010	CXR single view
	71015	Stereo CXR
	71020	2 view CXR
Blood draw for specimen	36415	Venipuncture
Blood gases and other information stored in computers	99090	Analysis of patient data
Gastric intubation	43752	NG or OG placement
Pulse oximetry	94760	Pulse oximetry
	94761	Pulse ox exercise testing
	94762	Pulse ox continuous overnight
Temporary transcutaneous pacing	92953	Transcutaneous pacing
Ventilator management	94002	Vent management initial day
	94003	Vent management subsequent
	94004	Vent management nursing home
	94660	CPAP initiation
	94662	Pentamidine inhalation
Vascular access procedures	36000	Introduction catheter into vein
	36410	Venipuncture, age 3 years or older requiring physician skill (not for routine venipuncture)
	36591	Collection of blood from port
	36600	Aterial puncture, withdrawl of blood for diagnosis

Table 5.2 Central venous access description and CPT codes

Description	CPT code
Non-tunneled central venous catheter under 5 years of age	36555
Non-tunneled central venous catheter 5 years of age or older	36556
Tunneled central venous catheter under 5 years of age	36557
Tunneled central venous catheter 5 years of age or older	36558
PICC without port or pump under 5 years of age	36568
PICC without port or pump 5 years of age or older	36569
Repair of central venous catheter without port or pump	36575
Replacement, complete, non-tunneled catheter without port or pump through same venous access	36580
Replacement, complete, PICC without port or pump, through same venous access	36584
Removal tunneled central venous catheter without port or pump	36589
Removal tunneled central venous catheter with port or pump	36590

For example, CPT 36556 describes a non-tunneled central venous catheter age 5 years or older. CPT 36558 describes a *tunneled* central venous catheter age 5 years or older. While the CPT number and description are very similar, they have different reimbursement and documentation requirements.

5.4.2 Arterial Line

Another common ICU procedure is arterial line. This is described as percutaneous arterial catheterization or cannulation for sampling, monitoring, or transfusion. The CPT code is 36620. If a cutdown is performed to get arterial access, then use CPT 36625.

5.4.3 US and Fluoroscopic Guidance

US and fluoroscopic guidance use separate codes for reimbursement. They are described as add-on codes and can only be used with another associated CPT code. In the case of ultrasound, there needs to be an associated CVL or arterial line code. In the case of fluoroscopy, it must be used with a CVL code. As mentioned above, the use of fluoroscopy must be within the PA or NPs scope of practice and state law. Use CPT 77001 for fluoroscopic guidance for central venous access device. Use CPT 76937 for ultrasound guided vascular guidance. Note this code has a very specific description:

"Ultrasound guidance for vascular access requiring ultrasound evaluation of potential access sites, documentation of selected vessel patency, concurrent real-time ultrasound visualization of vascular needle entry, with permanent recording and reporting."

This has generally been interpreted to include not only mention of the ultrasound in the procedure report but retention of an image. The image should have patient identification but can be either maintained electronically or in paper form (Fig. 5.1).

5.5 Airway Procedures

Airway procedures done by PAs and NPs commonly include emergency endotracheal intubation. Emergency cricothyroidotomy and emergency tracheotomy, while less common, are included in airway procedures. In addition, PAs may assist with percutaneous tracheotomies performing either the bronchoscopy portion (covered elsewhere) or the tracheotomy portion. Finally, a number of PAs and NPs perform either diagnostic or therapeutic bronchoscopy.

In terms of coding, CPT code 31500 is used for emergency intubation. Emergency cricothyroidotomy uses CPT 31605 (listed as tracheotomy, emergency procedure, cricothyroid membrane). Emergency tracheostomy uses CPT 31603 (tracheostomy emergency procedure, transtracheal). For planned procedures, CPT 31600 is used. For planned tracheostomy on patients under age 2, use CPT 31601. Finally, for tracheostomy changes prior to fistula formation, CPT code 31502 is used.

Bronchoscopy in the ICU can be either therapeutic to remove mucus plugs for example or diagnostic with bronchial lavage. In the case of

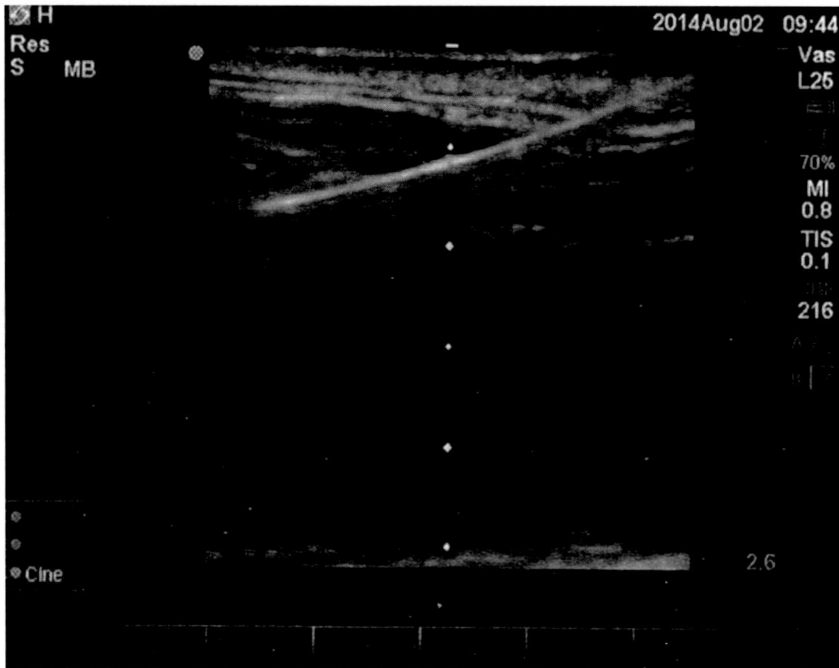

Fig. 5.1 Example of US image of CVL with wire shown

therapeutic bronchoscopy, use CPT 31622. In the case of bronchoscopy with lavage, use CPT 31624.

5.6 Chest Procedures

Chest procedures include bothopen chest tube thoracostomy as wells as thoracentesis and percutaneous placement of pleural drainage systems. This CPT range underwent major revision in 2013 and is a source of confusion. In 2013 recognizing that open chest tube thoracostomy was being incorrectly billed since both tube thoracostomy and percutaneous pleural drains were billed as a type of thoracentesis. In addition, Medicare bundled imaging guidance into the thoracentesis, and pleural drain codes recognizing the majority were being done with ultrasound.

Tube thoracostomy is reserved for open procedures which involve cutdown, blunt, or sharp dissection into the pleural space. The correct CPT code is 32551. Thoracentesis involves two separate codes. CPT 32554 is for thoracentesis needle or catheter aspiration of the pleural space without imaging guidance. CPT 32555 is for thoracentesis with imaging guidance. Similarly for percutaneous placement of pleural drains, there are two codes. CPT 32556 is for percutaneous placement of pleural drain. CPT 32557 is for percutaneous placement without imaging guidance. For bilateral procedures, please see the section on modifier codes.

5.7 Abdominal Procedures

Abdominal procedures include diagnostic or therapeutic procedures such as paracentesis or peritoneal lavage as well as enteral procedures such as percutaneous endoscopic gastrostomy (PEG) and post-pyloric NG placement. Diagnostic procedures underwent revision in 2012. Prior to this, the US code was entered separately from the paracentesis. Currently, there are two different codes depending on whether US is used. CPT 49082 covers abdominal paracentesis without imaging guidance. CPT 49083 is used with imaging guidance. These codes cover both diagnostic and therapeutic paracentesis. Providers should note that the CPT 49083 requires the provider to perform the imaging. Paracentesis that is marked by another service such as radiology uses CPT 49082. Peritoneal lavage uses CPT 49084. This included imaging guidance when performed (imaging is not required for the code).

Enteral access codes are another area of confusion. While critical care codes cover the use of nasogastric tube placement, if the tube is placed post-pyloric, then it is reimbursable. CPT 43761 covers repositioning of gastric feeding tube, through the duodenum for enteric nutrition. For placement of a PEG, the CPT is 43246 which includes upper endoscopy. If two providers perform the PEG placement, i.e., the endoscopy and percutaneous entry, then each bills code 43246 with a 62 modifier. Each provider must submit a separate procedure report.

5.8 Cardiovascular Procedures

Cardiovascular procedures commonly done in the ICU include extracorporeal membrane oxygenation (ECMO), vascular assist device management, as well as Swan-Ganz catheter placement. In 2015 ECMO codes were revamped. Codes 36822, 36960 and 33961 were deleted. In their place a set of 25 codes covering management, insertion, repositioning and decannulation were included in the CPT manual. For the purposes of this section only percutaneous ECMO is covered, for open or sternotomy cannulations see the CPT manual. ECMO initiation and management is divided by veno-venous (VV) and veno-arterial (VA). For VV initiation use CPT 33946 and 33947 for VA initiation. For management CPT 33948 (VV) and 33949 (VA) can be reported once per day. For initial cannulation CPT 33951 is reported for birth to 5 years and CPT 33952 for age 6 or older. Repositioning cannulas uses CPT 33957 for birth to 5 years and CPT 33958 for age 6 or older. Finally, decannulation uses CPT 33965 for birth to 5 years and CPT 33966 for age 6 or older. ECMO billing continues to evolve and providers should work closely with coding specialists. Critical care time unrelated to the ECMO management can be billed if it exceeds 30 minutes.

Vascular assist devices are usually inserted in the OR or cath lab and as such is outside the purview of this chapter. However, removal of these devices frequently occurs in the ICU. CPT code 33992 covers removal of a percutaneous ventricular assist device at a separate time from insertion. If this procedure is done using imaging guidance, then CPT code 33993 is used.

While Swan-Ganz catheters are used in a variety of setting, they are probably most commonly encountered in the cardiac and cardiovascular ICUs. Most Swan-Ganz catheters are placed through a vascular introducer. There is some controversy on billing for this, but the general consensus is that if the introducer is placed at the time of the Swan-Ganz, then it is part of the procedure. The CPT code for Swan-Ganz catheter is 93503 (insertion and placement of flow directed catheter) (Fig. 5.2).

5.9 Neurological Procedures

The neurological ICU is a relative newcomer to the ICU environment. However, PAs and NPs are well represented in this setting. Procedures vary depending on the institution and neurosurgical coverage, but can include lumbar puncture, lumbar drain placement, and placement of intracranial pressure (ICP) monitor such as an EVD. Lumbar punctures can include either therapeutic or diagnostic lumbar punctures. If the lumbar puncture is done for diagnostic purposes, CPT code 62270 is used. If the lumbar puncture is done for therapeutic purposes using either a needle or catheter, then CPT code 62272 is used. For a lumbar drain, the same CPT code 62272 is used as for a therapeutic lumbar puncture.

ICP monitoring can be done in the OR or the ICU. If a handheld device such as a twist drill is used, CPT code 91107 is used. If a powered device such as a power burr is used, then CPT code 61210 (burr holes for implanting ventricular catheter) is used.

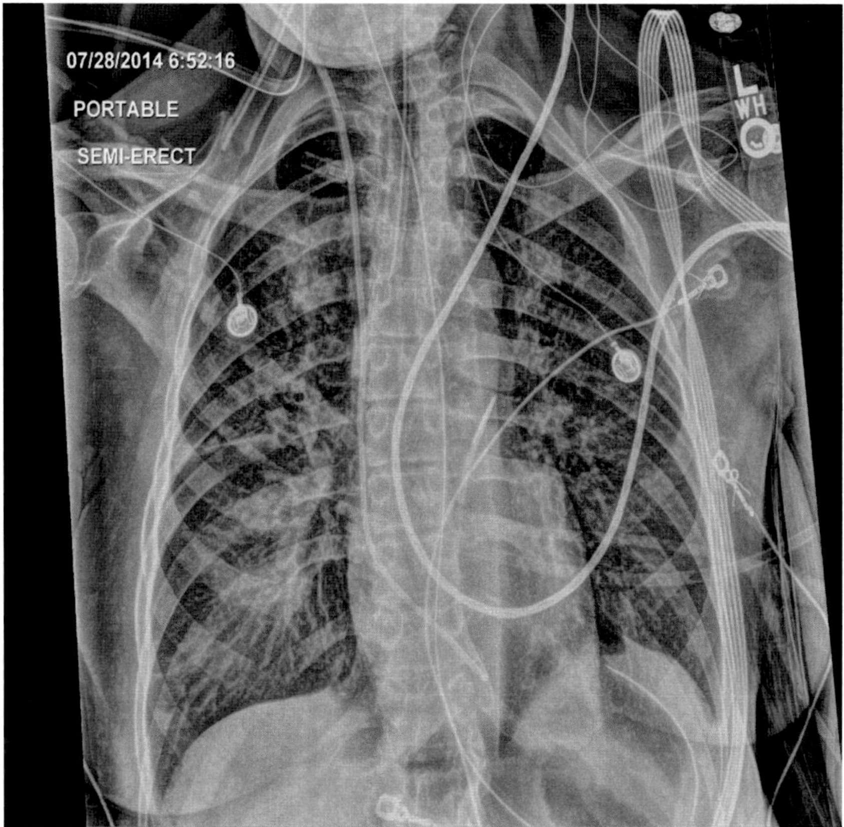

Fig. 5.2 Chest X-ray after Swan-Ganz placement

5.10 Incision and Drainage

Depending on the ICU type, incision and drainage is another common ICU procedure. There are a number of codes to use depending on the type of wound and procedures done.

Abscesses are divided into two types, simple and complex. A simple abscess uses CPT code 10060 and is a simple incision that drains on its own. A complex abscess requires a drain or packing and uses CPT code 10061.

Hematomas, seromas, or fluid collections rarely require action; however, if it is necessary to drain them, then CPT code 10140 is used.

Complex wounds which require drainage and excision of tissue with packing or drain placement use CPT code 10180.

5.11 Procedural Sedation

Conscious sedation is a common occurrence in the ICU. However, it is governed not only by state law, but by hospital bylaws. PAs and NPs doing conscious sedation in the ICU should have a firm understanding of the local legislative environment before performing conscious sedation. PAs and NPs should also ensure they follow institutional requirements for conscious sedation.

In 2006 Medicare renamed conscious sedation to conscious (moderate) sedation to clearly delineate conscious sedation from minimal (anxiolysis) sedation or deep sedation. In this spectrum, it adds clarity to use moderate sedation. When providing moderate sedation, a number of services are included and may not be reported separately:

- Assessment of the patient
- Establishment of IV access
- Administration of sedation
- Maintenance of sedation
- Monitoring
- Recovery

Moderate sedation also includes the concept of intraservice time. This starts with the administration of the sedating agent and ends with the conclusion of personal contact of the provider. This time requires continuous face-to-face contact with the patient for the entirety of the time. Note this time begins with the sedation so the assessment of the patient, although bundled into the CPT is not included in the time.

The codes depend on whether the provider giving sedation is also performing the procedure or is independently providing the sedation for the provider performing the procedure. There are also different codes depending on the age of the patient. Finally, this is a time-based code requiring a minimum time to report the code.

CPT code 99143 governs moderate sedation provided by the same provider who performs the service on a patient under the age of 5 for the first 30 min. This requires the presence of an independent trained observer to assist in monitoring the patient's level of consciousness and vital signs. This provider should have no other duties outside of monitoring the patient. CPT code 99144 is used for the same patient age 5 years or older. For each additional 15 min of moderate sedation, CPT code 99145 is used. Time is handled under CPT rules where the time is not obtained until the midpoint had been passed. For CPT code 99144, this would be 16 min, and for CPT code 99145, it would be 8 min. For example, 35 min of moderate sedation would generate a CPT code 99144 but not a 99145.

For moderate sedation done by a separate provider than the one performing the procedure, CPT code 99148, for the first 30 min, is used for patients under the age of 5. For patient 5 years or older, CPT code 99419 is used. For each additional 15 min, CPT code 99150 is used.

5.12 Surgical First Assist and Wound Care

While relatively rare, surgery is occasionally performed in the ICU. First assist in surgery is reimbursable for PAs and NPs under a number of conditions. Generally, Medicare reimburses 85 % of the first assist fee paid to surgeons (16 %) or 13.6 %. The first assist is billed under the PA or NPs NPI number with an AS modifier to indicate first assist. Medicare will then apply the appropriate discount. Other providers may or may not reimburse for first assist by PAs or NPs depending on their policies. In addition, Medicare has determined that approximately 5 % of surgeries require a first assistant. Medicare maintains a list of approximately 1900 surgical procedures for which it permits first assist. All others are excluded. Whether a particular procedure allows a first assist can be found in the Medicare Physician Fee Schedule Database.

For PAs and NPs working in an academic center, there are further rules. Medicare requires a first assist be performed by an appropriate resident unless the following conditions are met:

- No qualified resident available.
- The primary surgeon has an across-the-board policy of never utilizing residents in the care of his or her patients.
- Trauma.
- The surgeon believes that the resident is not the best individual to perform the service.

The supervising surgeon must carefully document the reason that the PA or NP was used as a first assist to avoid audits. Finally, the PA or NP must have an appropriate supervisory or collaborative agreement with the surgeon.

While wound care in the ICU is generally covered under either critical care or E/M, wound vacs are a special case. For wound vac, use CPT 97605 for wounds under or equal to 50 cm^2 and 97606 for wound greater than 50 cm^2. This charge can be applied for each application.

5.13 Coding Modifiers

As noted in the previous sections, various procedures require coding modifiers. These are two digit modifiers that are appended to the CPT code to describe specific actions. For example, bilateral chest tube placement would use CPT code 32551 with a modifier of 50 for bilateral procedures. This would be written as 32551–50. This submission would allow the provider to be reimbursed for both procedures, while submission of two 32551's would result in denial due to duplicate procedures. Common coding modifiers are:

- –25 significant, separately identifiable E/M service on the same day as a separate procedure done by the same provider
- –50 bilateral procedures
- –62 two providers

The –25 modifier is the most confusing. It is generally used when evaluation and management is done on the same day as a procedure. Generally, Medicare considers evaluation and management to be included in some procedures but allows others to be billed separately. Close coordination with the billing department on the use of this code will help avoid claims rejections.

5.14 Documentation of Procedures

Much like patient care documentation, procedural documentation helps protect the provider from risk but also communicate the course of care for the patient. Designing a documentation template helps ensure that this information is included. With the advent of electronic medical records, it is relatively easy to ensure that the documentation is complete.

At the minimum, documentation should include:

- Date and time of the procedure
- Procedure being done
- Indications for the procedure
- Sedation used
- Description of the procedure
- Any complications of the procedure

In addition for critical care patients (CPT 99291), the record should reflect that the time spent on the procedure was not included in critical care billing. For the medical record, consent should also be documented. Finally, given the penalties surrounding central line infections, consideration should be given to documenting time-out, hand washing, and sterile procedures in the procedure note.

Finally, programs should have a robust quality assurance to help identify billing problems. Routing audits should be performed of procedural documentation to ensure necessary elements are met. In addition, CPT codes should be routinely screened to ensure that the correct CPT code is used.

5.15 Conclusion

Coding and billing for procedures is a complex task. PAs and NPs generally get very little coding and billing training, and institutions used to billing for physicians may not understand the nuances of PA and NP billing or may put up obstructions when they attempt to bill. For PAs and NPs, proper CPT selection for their procedures and clear documentation is the key to reimbursement. Education for billers and coders on PA and NP capabilities will help eliminate misunderstandings. Finally, education of administration and physicians of PA and NP skills will ensure that PAs and NPs are used maximally.

Disclaimer This chapter was current as of the time it was written. It does not represent legal advice

Although reasonable effort has been made to ensure the accuracy of this chapter, the responsibility of claims submission lies with the provider.

References

1. CMS. Medicare benefit policy manual chapter 15—covered medical and other health services. 2014.
2. AMA. Current procedural terminology—standard edition. 2016.
3. CMS. Medicare claims processing manual chapter 12—physicians/nonphysician practitioners. 2014.

Part II

Airway Procedures

Airway Management in the ICU

6

Dennis A. Taylor, Alan Heffner, and Ronald F. Sing

6.1 Assessment of the Airway

Assessment of respiratory distress and subsequent need to control the airway in the ICU setting is a very common occurrence. The distinction between ventilation and oxygenation must be assessed and are both managed differently. The focus of this chapter will be on the assessment and management of the airway.

The failure to identify and recognize a difficult airway is the single most common cause of a failed airway. A failed airway may be defined as:

- Failure to maintain saturations (>90 % SpO2).
- Three failed intubation attempts.

There are four dimensions of predicting difficult airway management [1]—they include:

- Predicting difficult BVM ventilation (*MOANS*).
  - *M*=Mask seal (any difficulty with obtaining a mask seal).
  - *O*=Obesity (redundant posterior pharyngeal tissue).
  - *A*=Age>55 (loss of muscular tone).
  - *N*=No teeth.
  - *S*=Snores/stiff lungs (COPD, pneumothorax, etc.).
- Predicting difficult intubation (*LEMONS*).
  - *L*=Look externally (evaluate for trauma, landmarks).
  - *E*=Evaluate 3–3–2.
    - Three of patients' fingers between incisors (access).
    - Three fingers between tip of chin and chin–neck junction (compression space for tongue).
    - Two fingers between chin–neck junction and top of laryngeal cartilage (location of airway).
  - *M*=Mallampati score (1–4) (see Fig. 6.1).
  - *O*=Obstruction
  - *N*=Neck mobility (limited—i.e., C-collar in place).
  - *S*=Saturations (keep above 90 %).
- Predicting difficult extraglottic devices (*RODS*).
  - *R*=Restricted mouth opening (<3 cm).
  - *O*=Obstruction at larynx.
  - *D*=Disrupted/distorted anatomy.
  - *S*=Snores/stiff lungs.
- Predicting difficult surgical airway (*SMART*).
  - *S*=Surgeries (previous).
  - *M*=Mass.
  - *A*=Access difficulties (obesity).
  - *R*=Radiation (previous or current).
  - *T*=Tumor.

D.A. Taylor, DNP, ACNP-BC, FCCM (✉)
A. Heffner, MD, FCCM • R.F. Sing, DO, FACS, FCCM
Carolinas HealthCare System, Charlotte, NC 28232, USA
e-mail: dennis.taylor@carolinashealthcare.org; alan.heffner@carolinashhealthcare.org; ronald.sing@carolinashealthcare.org

D.A. Taylor et al. (eds.), *Interventional Critical Care*, DOI 10.1007/978-3-319-25286-5_6

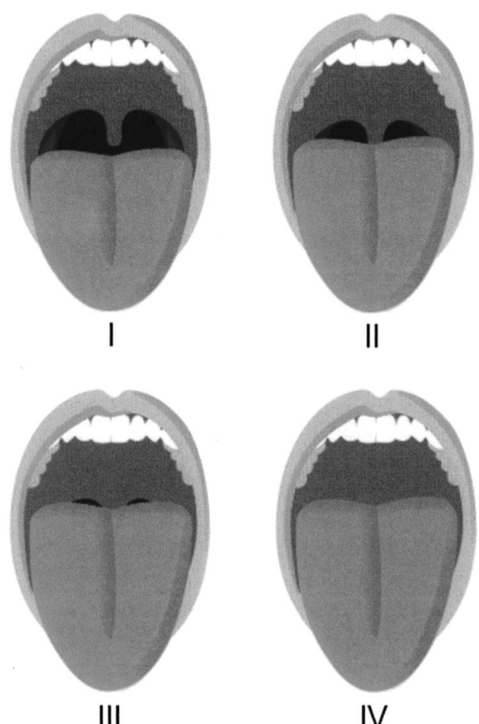

Fig. 6.1 Mallampati score. North Seattle University [Internet]. Seattle. Cited April 24, 2015. Retrieved from public domain images at: http://facweb.northseattle.edu/cduren/North%20Seattle%20AT%20Program%202011-2012%20CJ%20Duren-Instructor/ATEC%20002%20Anesthesia%20Related%20Anatomy%20and%20Physiology/Week%203/Additional%20Week%203%20Lesson%20Resources/Mallampati%20Score-Mallampati%20Classification%20Picture.png

Since 1956, clinicians have been searching for the perfect way to predict airway management difficulty. Studies have looked at various airway geometry indicators, anatomical predictors, and imaging studies. There is no one "fool proof" method.

6.2 Pharmacology Decision Points

There are multiple pharmacologic decision points when the decision has been made to perform endotracheal intubation. These include pretreatment medications, sedation medications, paralytic agents, and finally longer-acting sedatives and possible longer-acting paralytic agents.

6.3 Pretreatment Medications

The decision to use these medications is generally made by the person directing the intubation process. If being supervised for this procedure, check with the clinician responsible for the procedure and verify if they choose to use one of these medications.

The mnemonic *LOAD* may be used when considering pretreatment medications:

Lidocaine is often used when brain injury is a possibility. Dose, 1.5 mg/kg IVP (at least 3 min before the intubation procedure).

Opioid may be considered if time permits. Morphine, 5–10 mg IVP on an adult-sized patient, or fentanyl, 0.5–1 mcg/kg IV (given slowly over 1–2 min), may be omitted if patient is hypotensive (SBP<90) or dependent upon sympathetic drive for hemodynamics.

Atropine may be needed if the patient develops non-hypoxemic bradycardia; dose, 0.5–1.0 mg IV; may be repeated if needed.

Defasciculating dose of a noncompeting neuromuscular paralytic.

6.4 Sedation/Induction Medications

Common induction medications used for rapid sequence intubation (RSI) include:

Etomidate—0.3 mg/kg IV, best hemodynamic profile, short acting.

Versed—0.1 mg/kg IV.

Ativan—5–10 mg IV on an adult-sized patient, longer acting.

Ketamine—1.5 mg/kg IV, used in patients with asthma.

Propofol—1.5 mg/kg IV, monitor for hypotension.

6.5 Paralytics

Paralytics come in two varieties:

Depolarizing (succinylcholine).

Non-depolarizing (rocuronium and vecuronium are examples).

6.6 Depolarizing Muscle Paralytics

Succinylcholine is actually two-acetylcholine molecules linked together. It has a rapid onset (30–60 s) and relatively short half-life (3–5 min). It is metabolized by the enzyme acetylcholinesterase. There are some populations that have an acetylcholinesterase deficiency. In those cases, the effects of succinylcholine may last longer. The primary advantage of using succinylcholine is that if you are unable to get the patient intubated, with its short half-life, the medication will be metabolized, and the patient should resume spontaneous respirations within 3–5 min.

The dose of succinylcholine is 1.5 mg/kg. The dose is never reduced. It has no effect on hemodynamics.

There are some contraindications to using succinylcholine. They include:

- History of malignant hyperthermia.
- Burns >5 days—until healed.
- Crush injury to large muscle mass >5 days.
- Spinal cord injury/stroke with hemi- or paraplegia >5 days to 6 months.
- Neuromuscular disease.
- History of hyperkalemia/dialysis patients.

6.7 Non-Depolarizing Paralytics

There are many choices. Two will be covered here. Rocuronium is the paralytic of choice when succinylcholine is contraindicated. It has an onset of 60 s and a half-life of 30–45 min. It is given at a dose of 1.0 mg/kg IV push after the administration of an appropriate induction agent has been administered.

The second non-depolarizing agent that may be given is vecuronium. It has an onset of 3 min and a half-life of 60–75 min. The intubation dose of vecuronium is 0.15 mg/kg IV push after the administration of an appropriate induction agent has been administered.

6.8 The RSI Procedure

The RSI procedure has been described as the seven "Ps" [2]. They are:

- *P*reparation.
  - Monitors (ECG, SpO2, EtCO2, BP), IV access, equipment, suction.
- *P*reoxygenation.
  - 3 min of 100 % FiO2 (or 8 vital capacity breaths).
- *P*retreatment.
  - Lidocaine (if suspected head injury or asthma)—3 min before intubation to be effective.
  - Opioid (fentanyl for CV disease or head injury).
  - Atropine (ready for non-hypoxemic bradycardia).
  - Defasciculating dose of paralytic.
- *P*aralysis—induction agent and muscular paralytic given rapid IV push.
  - Remember—if no opioid was given, the induction agent and muscular paralytic have no effect on pain sensation.
- *P*rotection and positioning.
  - Sniffing position and cricoid pressure.
- *P*lacement of airway.
  - Confirm endotracheal tube placement with EtCO2, SpO2, breath sounds bilaterally, no sounds over epigastrium; secure the endotracheal tube.
- *P*ost-intubation management.
  - Additional longer-acting sedation and muscular paralysis if needed; consider pain medication, hemodynamic and oxygenation monitoring, and appropriate ventilator settings.

6.9 Indications for Intubation

Poor anticipated clinical course.

Glasgow Coma Scale of 8 or less.

Failure to maintain adequate oxygenation and/or ventilation.

6.10 Contraindications for Intubation

Patient able to maintain airway patency, ventilation, and oxygenation.

6.11 Complications

Hypotension.
Failed recognition of an esophageal intubation.
Damage to airway structures during attempt.
Damage to teeth.

6.12 Intubation Equipment

Oxygen, suction, oropharyngeal or nasopharyngeal airways (Figs. 6.2 and 6.3).
Monitoring equipment (ECG, SpO2, B/P, respiratory rate, ETCO2).
Bag valve mask and/or non-rebreather oxygen mask.
Endotracheal tubes.
For most adult patients, consider sizes 7.0, 7.5, and 8.0.
Endotracheal tube stylet.
Laryngoscope handle (contact versus fiber optic) Fig. 6.4.
Laryngoscope blade.
Macintosh (curved) sized 0–4 (adults usually 3 or 4) Fig. 6.5.
Miller (straight) sized 0–4 (adults usually 3 or 4) Fig. 6.6.
10 ml syringe (for ET tube cuff).
Commercial ET tube holder or ET tape.
Color metric capnometer or qualitative end-tidal CO2 monitor.
Gum elastic bougie.

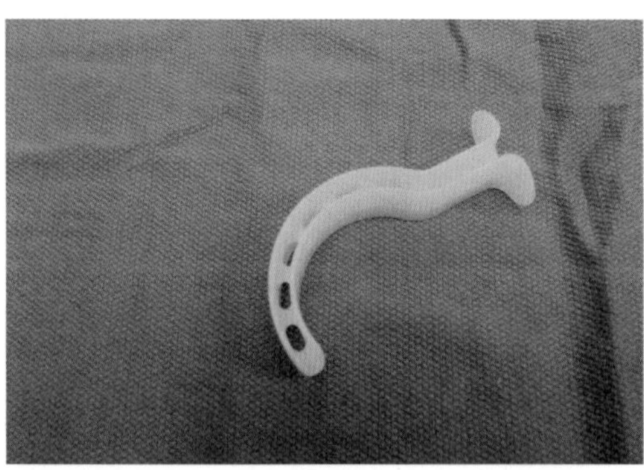

Fig. 6.2 Oropharyngeal airway

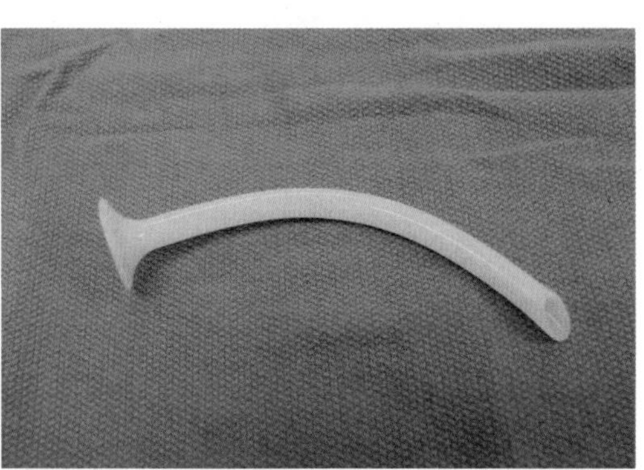

Fig. 6.3 Nasopharyngeal airway

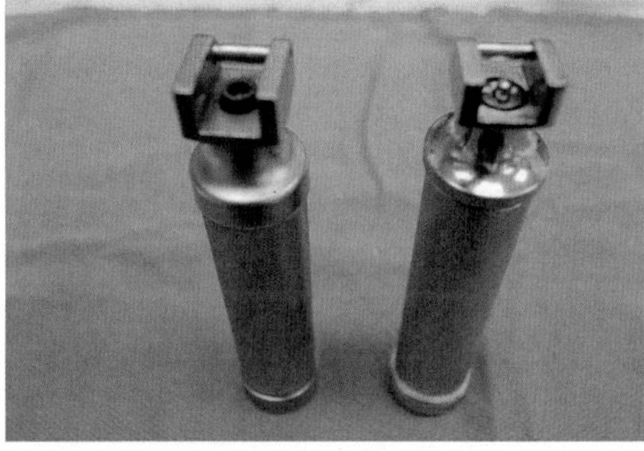

Fig. 6.4 Fiber optic on the *left* and contact on the *right* (note green band) (no green band)

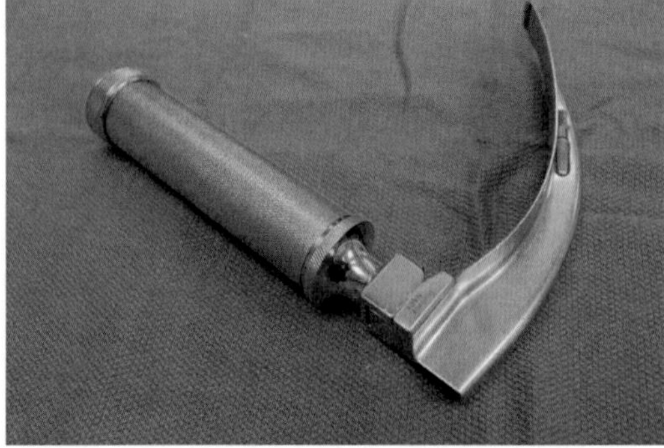

Fig. 6.5 Macintosh blade

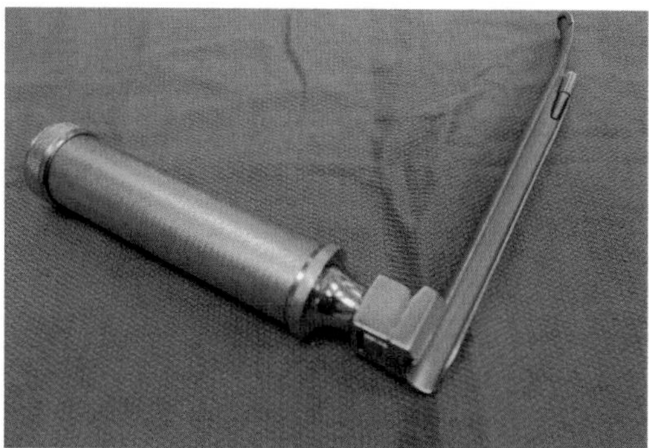

Fig. 6.6 Miller blade

6.13 Procedure

1. Assure patient is connected to appropriate monitors and adequate IV access is achieved. Assemble equipment and suction.
2. If the patient is breathing at an adequate rate and volume, assure appropriate preoxygenation by utilizing a non-rebreather mask for at least 3 min (Fig. 6.7). If the patient is not breathing at an adequate rate or volume (minute ventilation), assist ventilations with a BVM device after placing an oropharyngeal or nasopharyngeal airway and applying cricoid pressure to reduce the incidence of gastric insufflation (Fig. 6.8). Preoxygenate with 100 % oxygen for a minimum of 3 min or 8 vital capacity breaths (Figs. 6.9 and 6.10).
3. If the intubator chooses to use a pre-intubation medication such as lidocaine, opioid, atropine, or a defasciculating dose of a neuromuscular blocker, now is the time to administer these medications.
4. The selection and dosage of the sedative and neuromuscular blocker should be made at this point. Remember, for hemodynamic instability (SBP<90 mmHg), the sedative should be half-dosed. The neuromuscular blocker is never given at a reduced dose. Rapid sequence induction or intubation is given its name because the sedative is given rapid IV push followed immediately by the neuromuscular blocker IV push. Check for muscle flaccidity.
5. Insert the blade of choice and sweep the tongue from right to left.

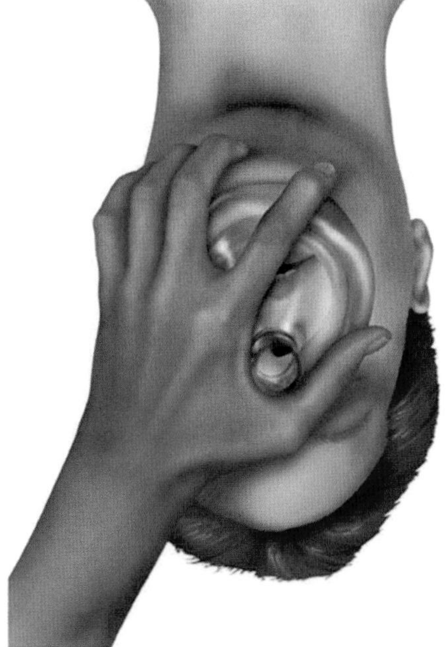

Fig. 6.7 Assure good mask seal

   (a) If the Macintosh (curved) blade is used, the tip of the blade is placed at the base of the tongue (Fig. 6.11), and the mandible is displaced anteriorly until the epiglottis is raised to easily visualize the vocal cords.
   b. If the Miller (straight) blade is used, the tip of the blade is placed under the epiglottis (Fig. 6.12) and is used to elevate the epiglottis to visualize the cords.
6. The endotracheal tube, with stylet in place and not extending beyond the tip of the ETT, is placed in the trachea under direct visualization. The ETT is placed at a depth of approximately three times the size of the ETT. For example, if placing an 8.0 ETT, it should be inserted to a depth of 24 cm at the teeth or lips. The stylet is removed, the cuff inflated, and confirmation assured by one of the following methods: ETCO2 capnography, colorimetric capnography, auscultation of bilateral breath sounds and no sounds over the epigastrium with bag-assisted ventilations, or condensation in the ETT. Wave form qualitative capnography is considered the "gold standard" for proof of correct placement.

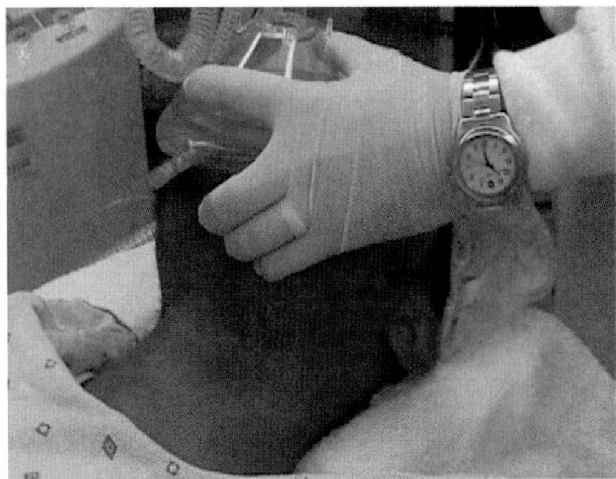

Fig. 6.8 Thumb and Index finger form the letter C; other three fingers form the letter E

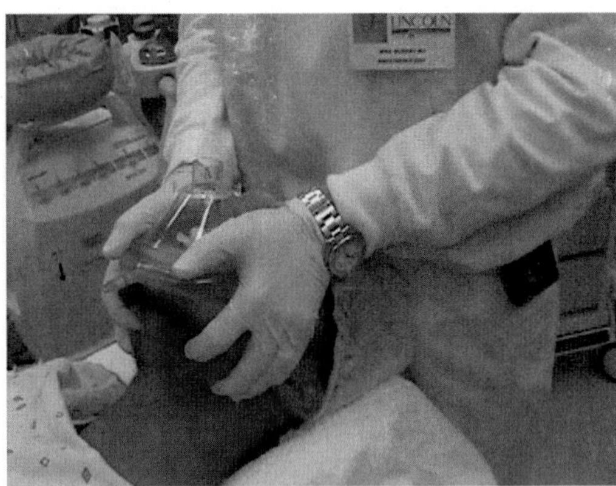

Fig. 6.10 Jaw-thrust and mask seal

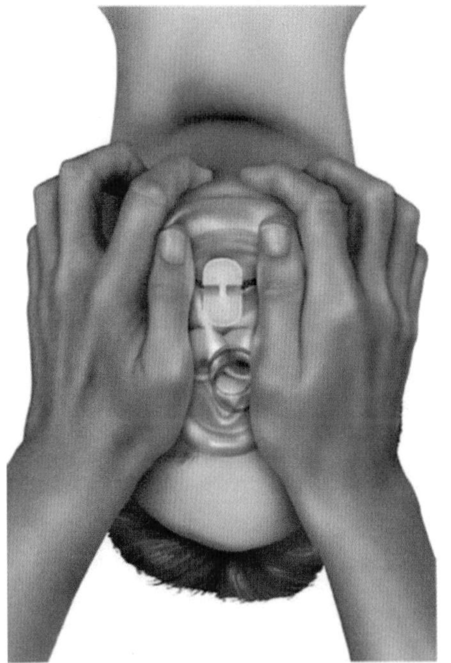

Fig. 6.9 Assure good seal - two hand technique

7. Once correct placement is confirmed, the ETT should be secured with a commercial ETT tube holder or ETT tape. A post-intubation chest X-ray should be ordered to confirm correct depth of the ETT.

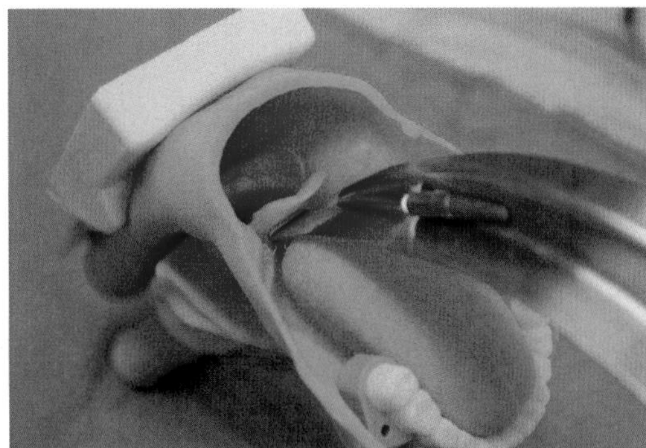

Fig. 6.11 Macintosh blade at base of tongue

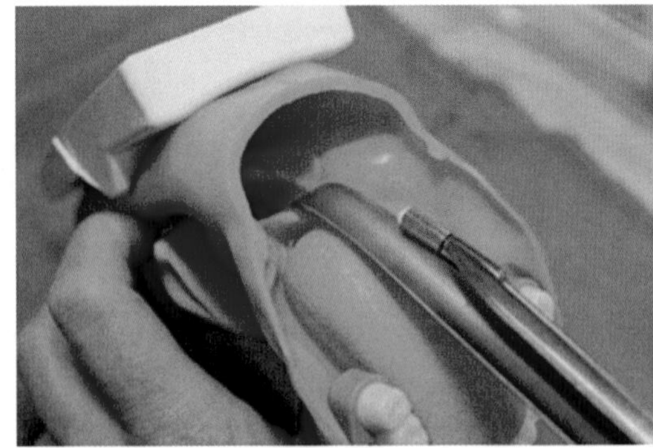

Fig. 6.12 Miller blade lifting the epiglottis

6.14 Summary

Only after a comprehensive airway assessment has been completed and the provider has determined the risks and benefits of RSI should the procedure be performed. It is just as important to recognize which patient to proceed with the RSI procedure as to whom not to. Airway management is very similar to the game of Chess—the provider must be thinking three and four steps ahead. If this fails, what is plan B and plan C? In many cases, it is wise for the provider to already have prepared the equipment that will be needed in the event of failing to secure the airway for those patients that have been deemed difficult. This is often referred to as a "double setup."

Failure to recognize an esophageal intubation in a timely fashion can be fatal. When in doubt regarding airway placement, nothing beats direct laryngoscopy to assure correct tube placement. In the following chapter, we will discuss rescue airway devices and their use.

References

1. Walls R, Murphy M. The difficult and failed airway. In: Walls R, Murphy R, editors. Manual of emergency airway management. Philadelphia: Wolters Kluwer Lippincott Williams & Wilkins; 2012. p. 9–21.
2. Walls R. Rapid sequence intubation. In: Walls R, Murphy R, editors. Manual of emergency airway management. Philadelphia: Wolters Kluwer Lippincott Williams & Wilkins; 2012. p. 221–32.

Rescue Airway Techniques in the ICU

7

Dennis A. Taylor, Alan Heffner, and Ronald F. Sing

7.1 Introduction

First-time intubation success rates in the hospital setting average 80 % [1]. There may be many causes for the failed airway. Some of these include poor body habitus, restricted mouth opening, anteriorly located airway anatomic structures, obesity, pregnancy, and genetic anatomic anomalies. Other causes may be failure to predict a difficult airway and/or failure to plan and have setup for a first-attempt failure.

7.2 Indications

Failure to secure an endotracheal tube in the trachea on the third attempt or failure to maintain oxygen saturations above 90 % constitutes a failed airway and may necessitate the utilization of a rescue airway device.

D.A. Taylor, DNP, ACNP-BC, FCCM (✉)
A. Heffner, MD, FCCM • R.F. Sing, DO, FACS, FCCM
Carolinas HealthCare System, Charlotte, NC, USA
e-mail: dennis.taylor@carolinashealthcare.org;
alan.heffner@carolinashhealthcare.org;
ronald.sing@carolinashealthcare.org

7.3 Contraindications

There are no contraindications to utilizing any of the rescue airway devices with the exception of the emergent cricothyrotomy. A cricothyrotomy should only be used in can't ventilate, can't oxygenate situations where a rescue device has also failed.

7.4 Equipment

1. Endotracheal tube introducer a.k.a. gum elastic bougie

   The ETI is a long (60 cm) narrow (5 mm) device with a fixed 40° bend at the distal end (coude tip) Figs. 7.1 and 7.2. The ETI is held with the tip pointed upward—upon visualization of the epiglottis, the tip is directed under the epiglottis and advanced. As the ETI is advanced, it will enter the trachea, and the coude tip will rub against the anterior portion of the trachea. This will produce a vibration as the tip rubs against the anterior tracheal rings. Tracheal placement can also be confirmed by a hard stop at approximately 40 cm of insertion. Placement in the esophagus will not result in a hard stop. The endotracheal tube is then placed over the ETI while the intubator keeps the laryngoscope in place.

D.A. Taylor et al. (eds.), *Interventional Critical Care*, DOI 10.1007/978-3-319-25286-5_7

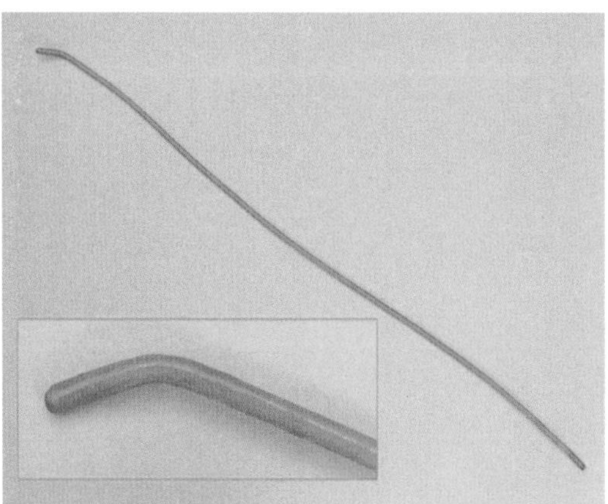

Fig. 7.1 Gum elastic bougie. Coude tip in the insert picture

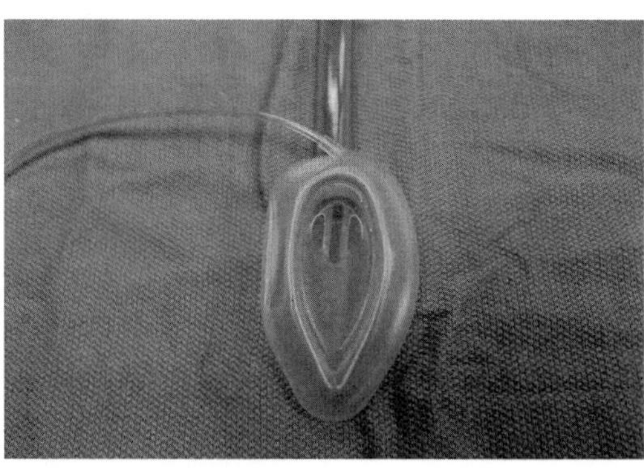

Fig. 7.3 LMA bottom view

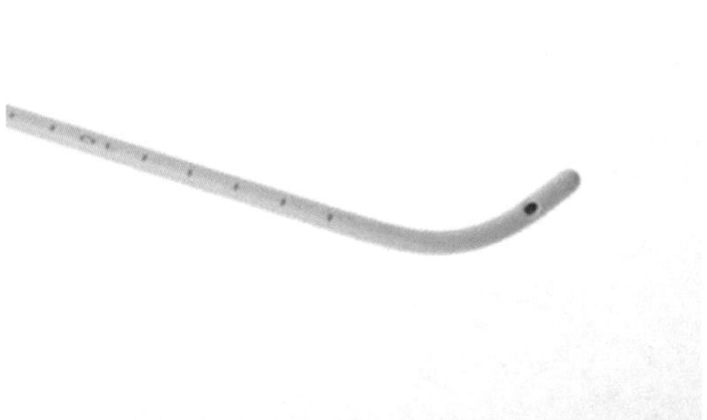

Fig. 7.2 Example of coude tip. [2]

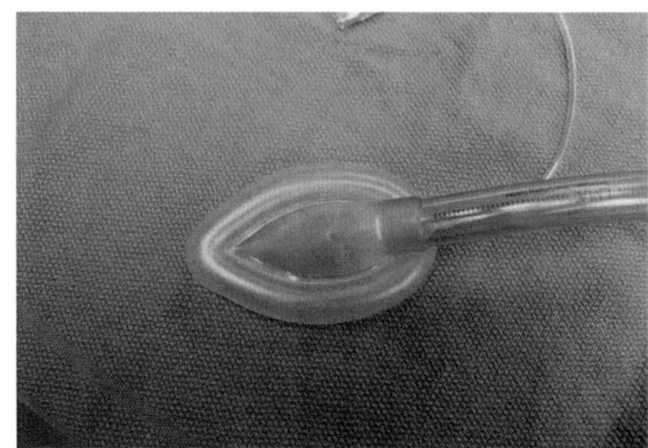

Fig. 7.4 LMA top view

2. Extraglottic devices (EGDs)
   a. Laryngeal mask airway (LMA) Figs. 7.3, 7.4

      LMAs come in a variety of Fig. 7.19 sizes that typically depend upon the patient's weight. For adults, the typical scale is a size 3 for 30–50 kg, size 4 for 50–70 kg, and size 5 for>70 kg. The LMA is inserted as follows:

   1. Completely deflate the cuff. Lubricate the cuff with a water-soluble lubricant.
   2. Open the airway by using the head-tilt maneuver. A jaw-lift maneuver is often used and is beneficial.
   3. Insert the LMA into the mouth with the laryngeal surface directed caudally and the tip of your index finger resting against the cuff-tube junction. Press the device onto the hard palate, and advance it over the back of the tongue as far as the length of index finger will allow (Fig. 7.5). Then use your other hand to push the device into its final seated position, allowing the natural curve of the device to follow the natural curve of the oropharynx (Fig. 7.6).
   4. Inflate the collar with air (20–40 ml depending upon the size of the LMA or until there is no leak with bag ventilation).

   b. King LT (laryngotracheal) airway

      The King LT airway is a latex-free single-lumen silicone laryngeal tube with oropharyngeal and esophageal low-pressure cuffs, with a ventilation port located between the two cuffs. The King LT is sized by height (see package for guidance) (Figs. 7.7 and 7.8). They come in two varieties, blind distal tip (King LT, LT-D)

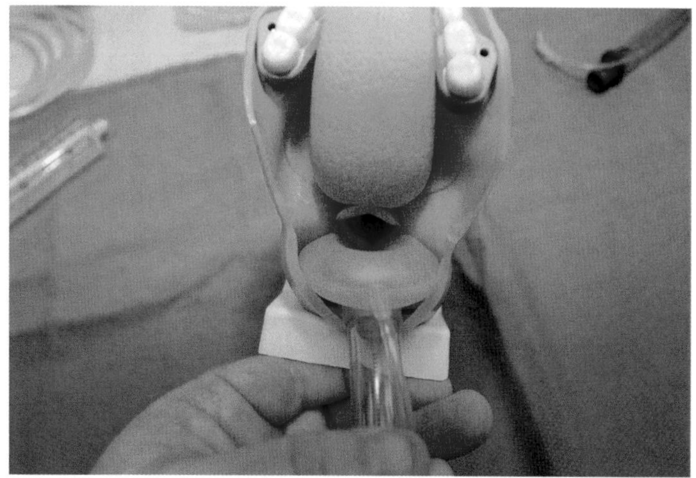

Fig. 7.5 LMA seal over epiglottis

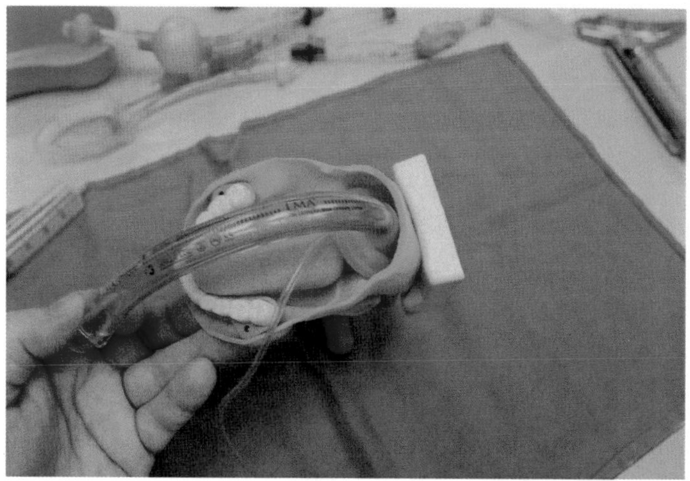

Fig. 7.6 LMA seated in place with cuff inflated

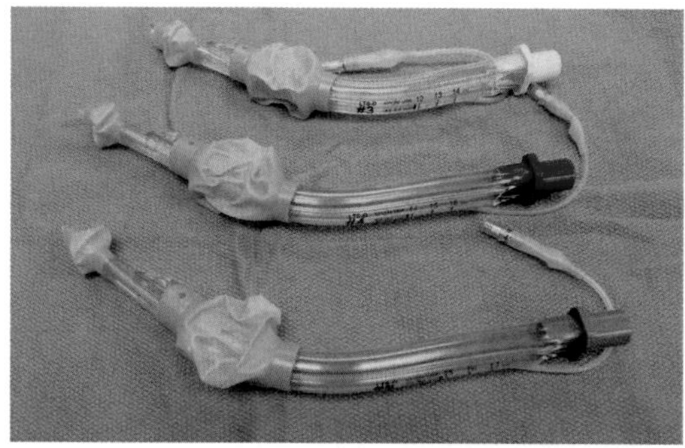

Fig. 7.7 King LT in different height based sizes

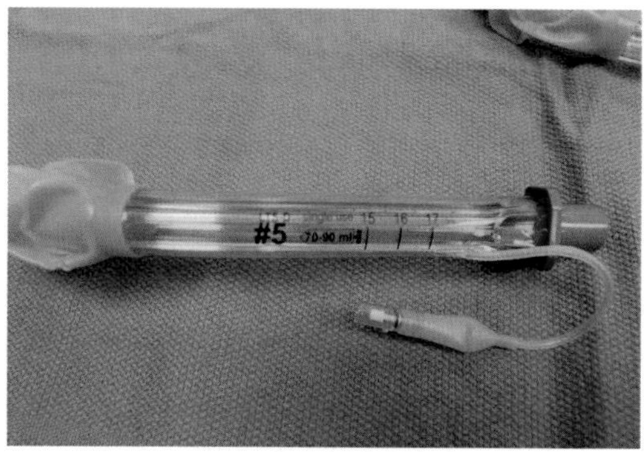

Fig. 7.8 King LT #5 - one port fills both balloons

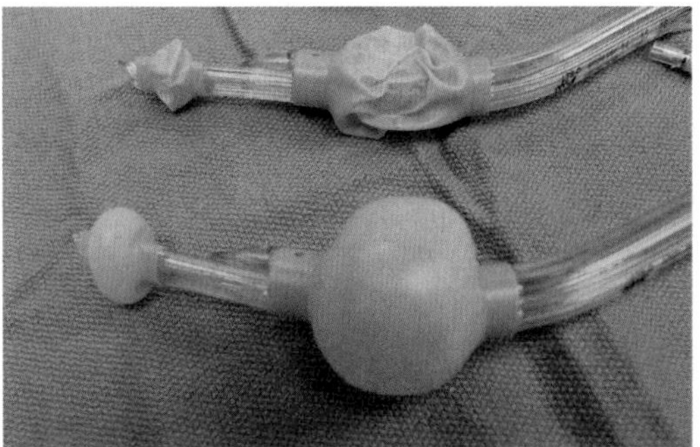

Fig. 7.9 King LT - top, deflated; bottom, inflated

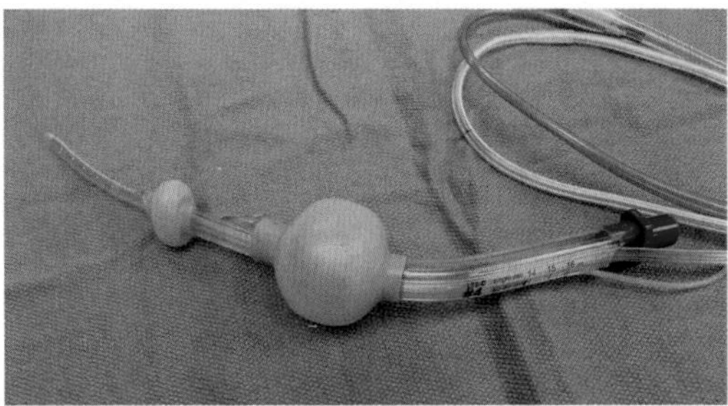

Fig. 7.10 NG tube through distal port

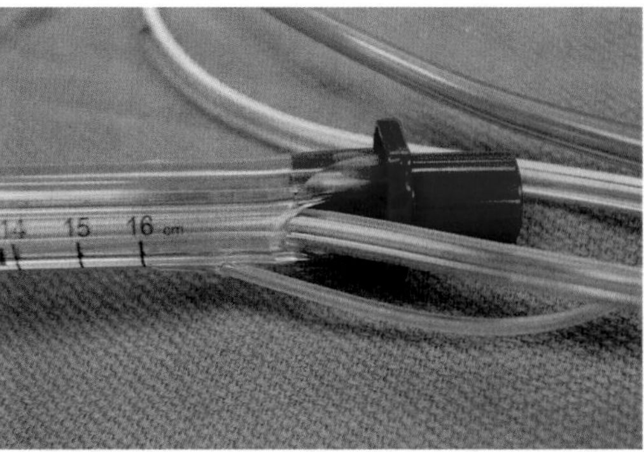

Fig. 7.11 NG tube entry port

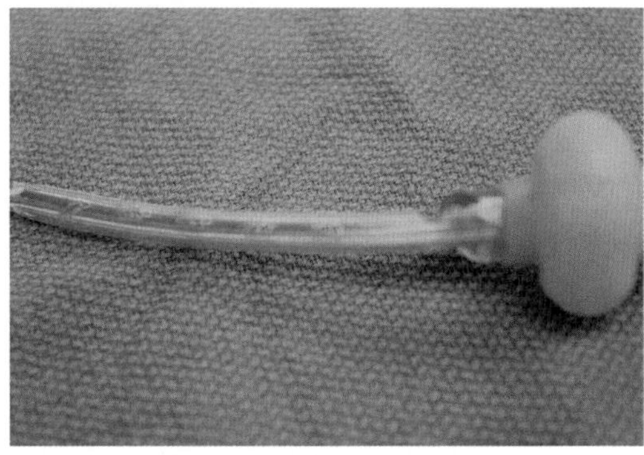

Fig. 7.12 NG tube exits distal tip of King LT

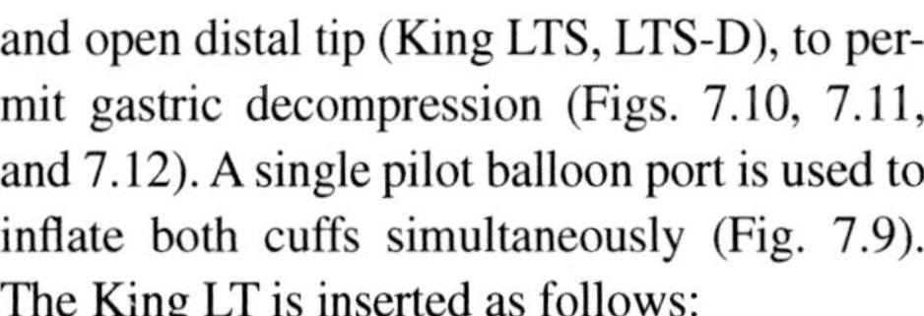

and open distal tip (King LTS, LTS-D), to permit gastric decompression (Figs. 7.10, 7.11, and 7.12). A single pilot balloon port is used to inflate both cuffs simultaneously (Fig. 7.9). The King LT is inserted as follows:

1. The King LT is designed to go only into the esophagus. The airway is opened with a head-tilt maneuver (Fig. 7.13).
2. It is advanced until definitive resistance is felt or the colored flange touches the incisors.
3. The cuffs are inflated simultaneously with a single pilot bulb. The amount of air is dependent upon the size of the King LT airway (see device for exact amount) (Fig. 7.14 and 7.15).
4. Use a bag device to ventilate the patient. If an air leak is encountered, reassess the amount of air in the cuffs.

3. Video laryngoscopy
   a. GlideScope video laryngoscope (Fig. 7.16)
   b. GlideScope cobalt/cobalt AVL
   c. GlideScope ranger
   d. Storz C-MAC (Fig. 7.17)

Procedure:

1. Prepare the equipment.
   - Plug into power source.
   - Use handle/blade cover as needed.
   - Use specific stylette for equipment.
   - Load stylette into endotracheal tube (Fig. 7.18).
   - Test ETT cuff.
   - Have suction available.
   - Appropriately preoxygenate and premedicate.
2. Look into the mouth.
3. Place the blade in the midline of the tongue (do not sweep the tongue as you would in the traditional intubation process).
4. Watch the video screen and visualize anatomic landmarks.
5. Place the ETT tube through the cords.
6. Confirm placement and secure the ETT.

4. Surgical airway options

Open cricothyrotomy

Needle cricothyrotomy

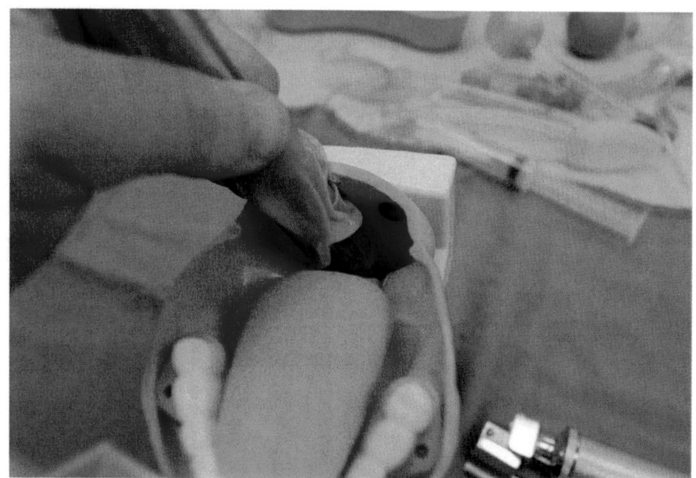

Fig. 7.13 Blind insertion of King LT

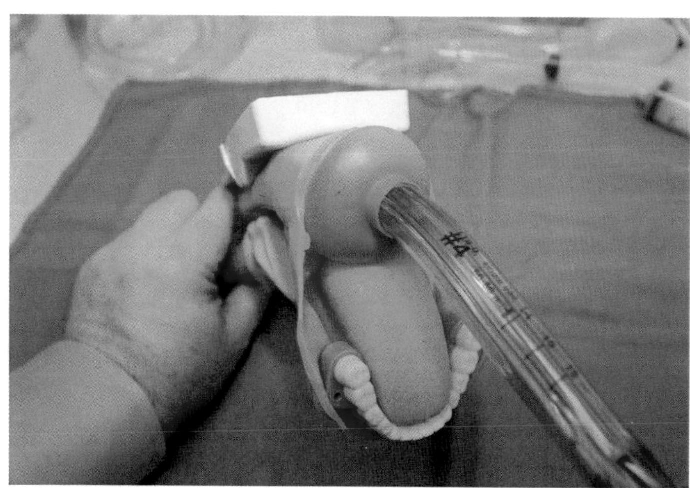

Fig. 7.14 King LT cuffs inflated

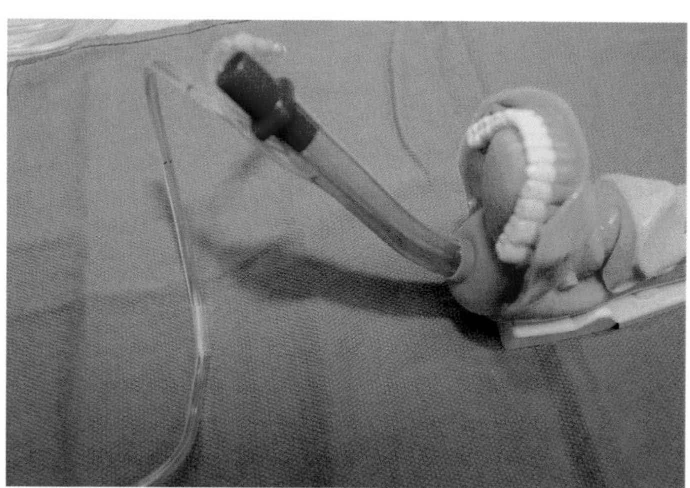

Fig. 7.15 King LT with NG tube in place

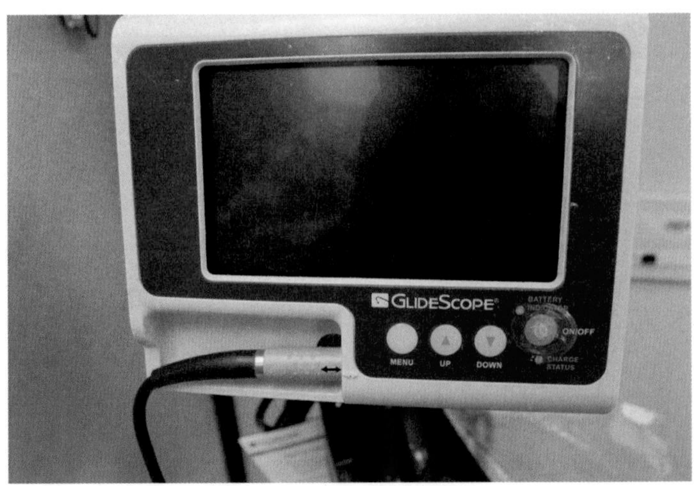

Fig. 7.16 Glidescope video laryngoscope

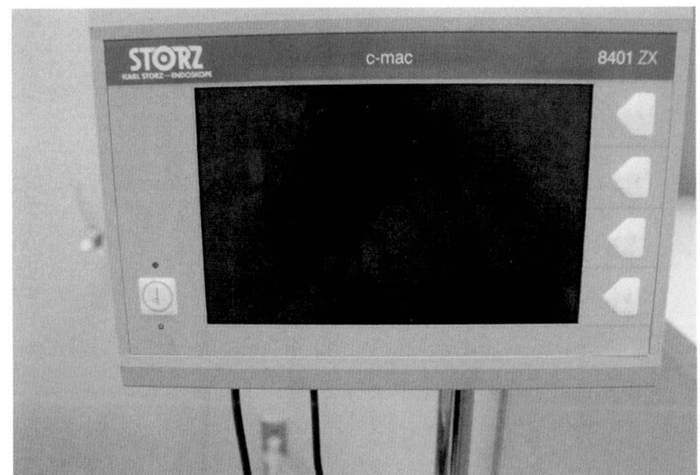

Fig. 7.17 Storz C-MAC video laryngoscope

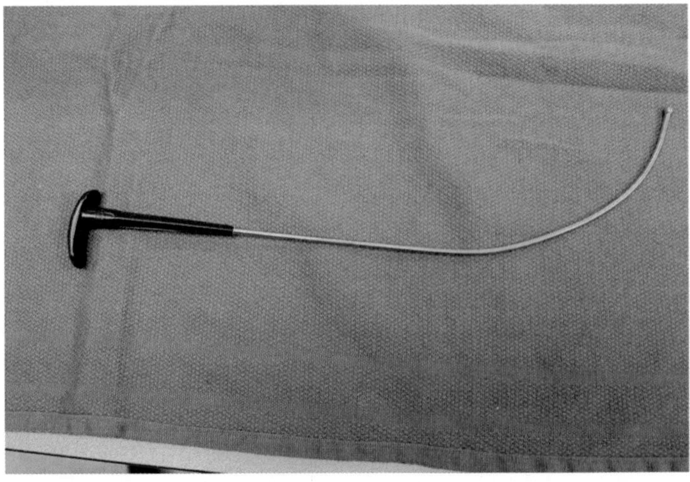

Fig. 7.18 Stylette for Glidescope

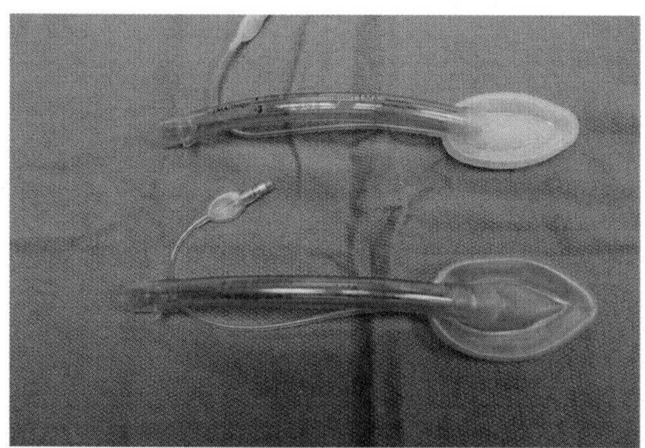

Fig. 7.19 Different sizes of LMA

7.5 Summary

It has been said that the difficult airway is something you predict and the failed airway is something you experience. There are many new devices being introduced annually that may be used to secure the failed airway. Remember, if you are able to ventilate and oxygenate, you have time to consider your rescue airway options. In the unfortunate event of the failure to oxygenate and ventilate, a quick decision to perform a surgical airway may be a lifesaving decision for the patient.

References

1. Kim C, Kang HG, Lim TH, Choi BY, Shin YJ, Choi HJ. What factors affect the success rate of the first attempt at endotracheal intubation in emergency departments? Emerg Med J. 2013;30(11):888–92.
2. Retrieved from http://trade.indiamart.com/details.mp?offer=7814041091

8 Emergency Airway: Cricothyroidotomy

Christopher A. Mallari, Erin E. Ross, and Ernst E. Vieux Jr.

8.1 Introduction

The primary purpose of a cricothyroidotomy is to establish an emergent rescue airway when standard and traditional techniques have failed. Traditional techniques include bag valve mask (BVM), laryngeal mask airway (LMA), laryngoscope, and video assist device. The inability to oxygenate, ventilate, and intubate the patient utilizing standard equipment and techniques is the indication to perform the next step, which is cricothyroidotomy. The ability to perform the procedure is a lifesaving intervention. The procedure is preferred over emergent tracheostomy due to the speed of which it can be performed, ease of landmark identification, and superficial and avascular nature of the cricothyroid membrane [1–3]. The specific technique used will vary depending on the provider comfort level, experience level, and equipment available. It most commonly performed in the intensive care unit, emergency department, trauma bay, operating room, and the prehospital setting. All providers who are responsible for managing an airway should be familiar with these techniques. Failure to perform this lifesaving intervention will likely lead to severe hypoxemia, respiratory arrest, cardiac arrest, severe anoxic brain injury, and death.

Cricothyroidotomy should not be confused with tracheostomy as they are two different procedures and have different indications. There are non-emergent indications for cricothyroidotomy, but this chapter will focus on the emergent indications for lifesaving airway establishment. Tracheostomy has also been described for emergent airway establishment, but is reserved for severe laryngeal fracture [1, 4].

8.2 Background/History

Cricothyrotomy was described in the medical literature in the mid-1800s. In the early 1900s, Dr. Jackson popularized the technique he referred to as "high tracheostomy"; however, this was thought to contribute to long-term complications such as subglottic stenosis [3]. In the 1970s, Brantigan and Grow revisited Dr. Jackson's research and found very low incidence of subglottic stenosis. This procedure is recognized as the standard technique for an emergency rescue airway [3].

C.A. Mallari, MS, PA-C (✉)
System Intensive Care Services, Lee Memorial Health System, 13681 Doctors Way, Fort Myers, FL 33912, USA
e-mail: chris@chrismallari.com

E.E. Ross, MMSc, PA-C • E.E. Vieux Jr., MD, FACS
Department of Trauma Surgery and Critical Care, Lee Memorial Health System, 2780 Cleveland Ave, Fort Myers, FL 33901, USA
e-mail: erinpac@comcast.net

D.A. Taylor et al. (eds.), *Interventional Critical Care*, DOI 10.1007/978-3-319-25286-5_8

8.3 Anatomic Review

Understanding the anatomy of the neck is crucial to successfully performing the procedure and to decrease potential complications. Superiorly, the thyroid cartilage forms the laryngeal prominence on the anterior neck also known as the "Adams apple." (Fig. 8.1) Inferiorly, the cricoid cartilage forms a firm, complete ring in the anterior neck and it is easily palpable. The cricothyroid membrane is located inferior to the thyroid cartilage and superior to cricoid cartilage. (Fig. 8.2) It is subcutaneous in location and composed of dense fibrous tissue. There are no major vessels, muscle layers, or nerves surrounding this membrane. In an average adult, the membrane can be found in the anterior midline and one third the distance from the angle of the mandible to the sternal notch.

It is important to understand that anatomical variations may exist. Distortion of normal anatomy may occur with obesity or disease processes, such as tumors, abscess, trauma, edema, or hematoma [5]. In children, the cricothyroid membrane is more superior and in infants the thyroid cartilage will not be as evident [5].

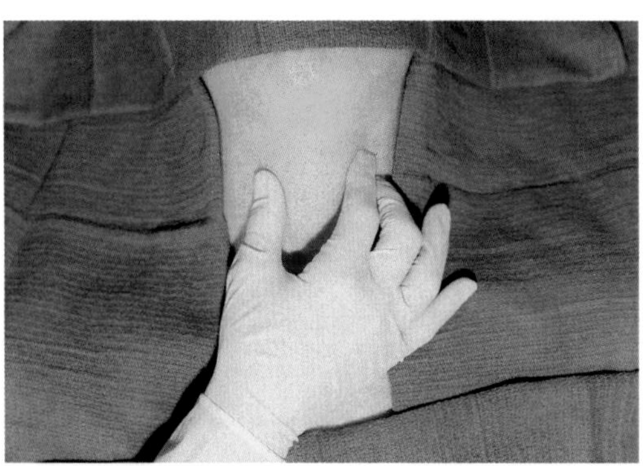

Fig. 8.1 Thyroid Cartilage (Superiorly)

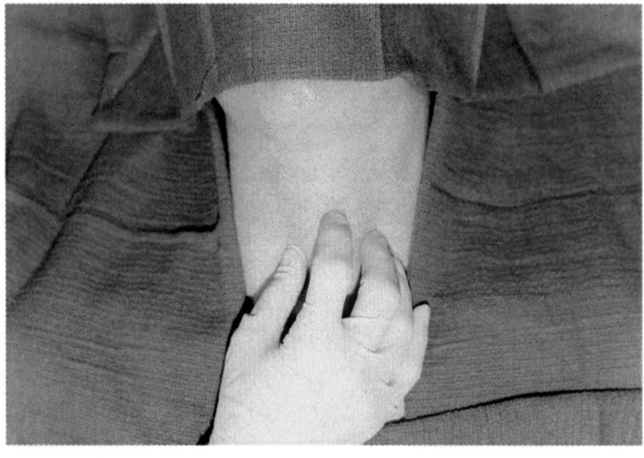

Fig. 8.2 Cricoid Cartilage (Inferiorly)

8.4 Indications

1. Failure/unsuccessful oral or nasal endotracheal intubation
2. Severe facial trauma
3. Laryngospasm
4. Airway obstruction from foreign body
5. Massive emesis/hematemesis/hemorrhage
6. Severe anaphylaxis/angioedema
7. Cannot intubate, cannot ventilate (CICV)

8.5 Contraindications

1. Transtracheal transection
2. Tracheal obstruction
3. Laryngeal fracture
4. Airway establishment – ETT, LMA, King tube

8.6 Relative Contraindications

1. Inability to identify landmarks due to anatomic distortion
2. Age less than 12

8.7 Procedural Types

8.7.1 Needle Cricothyroidotomy

Needle cricothyroidotomy is the procedure where a large bore needle with catheter (12–14 gauge) is placed percutaneously through the skin, subcutaneous tissue, and cricothyroid membrane into the trachea [1, 5]. The patient can then be ventilated through the catheter by either transtracheal or transtracheal jet ventilation. Transtracheal ventilation is oxygenation using a bag valve device with a 100% oxygen source for oxygen delivery or via oxygen tubing for passive ventilation. Respiratory rate is maintained with an average of 10–12 L/min for adults. Transtracheal jet ventilation is using an oxygen source that produces at least 50 psi of pressure to give high-frequency, low-volume bursts of oxygen delivery [5, 6]. This usually produces adequate oxygenation but leads to carbon dioxide retention and respiratory acidosis [2]. This can be decreased by allowing adequate exhalation time. Needle cricothyroidotomy is only a temporizing measure until a definitive airway can be established [1].

Advantages: Can be rapidly inserted with minimal and easily accessible equipment
Disadvantages: Not a definitive airway, will need additional intervention [1]
Special considerations: Preferred method in children less than 12 years of age [4]

8.8 Procedure

8.8.1 Instruments Required

1. Chlorhexidine or any type of sterile prep
2. 3–10 cc syringe half filled with saline or sterile water
3. Over the needle IV catheter, 12–14 gauge
4. Bag valve device with 100% oxygen source

8.8.2 Patient Preparation

In an emergent airway situation, rapid yet thoroughly clean the anterior neck with chlorhexidine. If time permits, drape out the neck from the chin to the sternal notch so anatomic structures and landmarks are easily identifiable.

8.8.3 Identification of Landmarks

Palpate the thyroid and cricoid cartilage. The cricothyroid membrane is located between these two landmarks.

8.8.4 Procedure

1. After patient preparation and landmark identification, have an assistant rapidly passing equipment. (Fig. 8.3)
2. Attach fluid-filled syringe to the needle.
3. Preferably using your nondominant hand, locate the cricothyroid membrane with your index finger. Stabilize the larynx between your middle finger and thumb with one hand to prevent it from moving.
4. With the other hand, insert needle attached to a syringe at the location marked previously by your index finger. (Fig. 8.4) Do this in a caudal direction bevel up at approximately 45 degree angle. While aspirating, slowly go through the subcutaneous, through the cricothyroid membrane, and into the trachea. (Fig. 8.5)

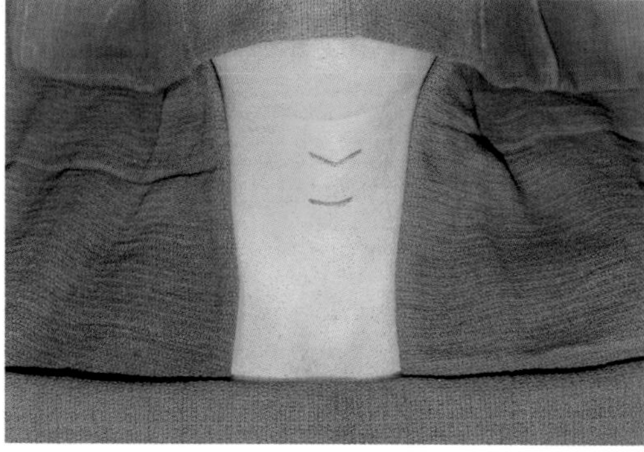

Fig. 8.3 Superior marking defines thyroid cartilage and inferior marking is the cricoid cartilage

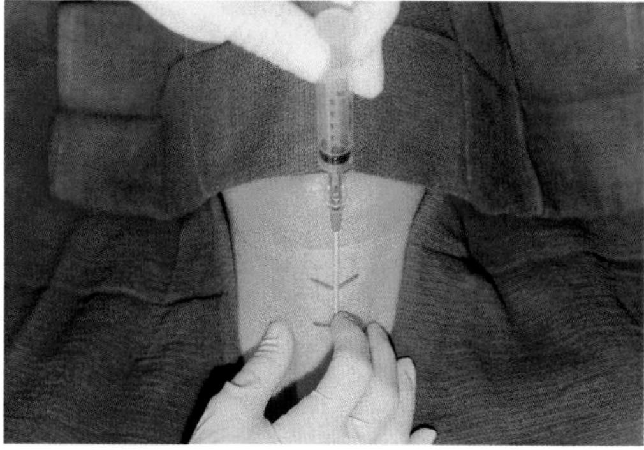

Fig. 8.4 Slowly aspirate as you advance the needle through the cricothyroid membrane

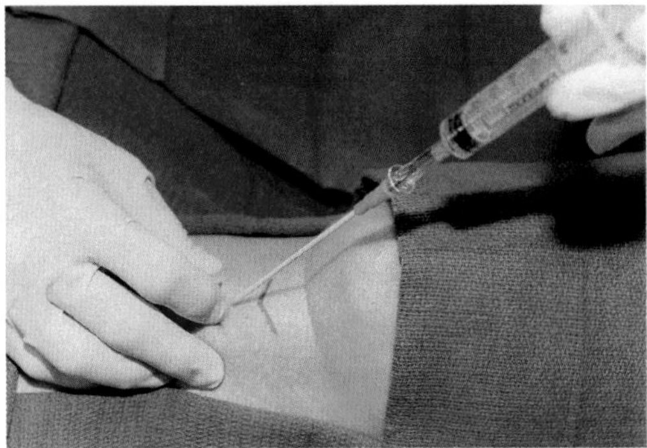

Fig. 8.5 Slowly aspirate as you advance the needle through the cricothyroid membrane

5. Once air is aspirated, stop advancing the needle. Fully advance the catheter into the trachea and remove the needle and syringe.
6. Attach a connector or adapter from a #7 endotracheal tube (ETT) directly to the catheter.
7. Attach this connector to a bag valve assist device with 100% oxygen source.
8. Ventilate the patient using respiratory rate of 5–8 per minute, and allow for long passive exhalation of carbon dioxide. This will help prevent respiratory acidosis and barotrauma.
9. If a jet insufflator is available, deliver small bursts with low volume and high-frequency oxygenation. Allow for adequate exhalation to prevent barotrauma.
10. Secure the catheter in place to prevent kinking or displacement.
11. This is only a temporizing measure and the patient will need a definitive airway.

8.8.5 Potential Complications

Perforated esophagus
Subcutaneous emphysema
Subcutaneous placement of needle/catheter
Inability to pass catheter
Kinking of catheter
Pneumomediastinum/barotrauma/pneumothorax
Bleeding
Infection

8.8.6 Procedural Pearls

Be sure to slowly advance the needle, and as soon as air is continuously aspirated, stop advancement. This avoids puncturing the back wall of trachea and potential injury to the esophagus. In addition, the advancement of the catheter can be tricky. Kinking of the catheter is a common complication that will prevent one from ventilating the patient [5]. Once the catheter is in place, hold it at all times and secure it quickly to prevent dislodgment.

8.9 Surgical Cricothyroidotomy

Surgical cricothyroidotomy is a surgical incision through the cricothyroid membrane to gain direct access into the trachea. Placement of a tracheostomy tube or endotracheal tube through the cricothyroid membrane is done so under direct visualization. Surgical cricothyroidotomy is preferred over emergent tracheostomy secondary to decreased vascularity of the cricothyroid membrane, subcutaneous location, and easily identifiable landmarks for placement [1–3].

Advantages: It is definitive airway control unlike needle cricothyroidotomy.
Disadvantages: Requires comfort and skill utilizing a scalpel.
Special considerations: Contraindicated in children less than 12 years of age due to their soft membranous cartilage and ring integrity [6].

8.10 Traditional Procedure

8.10.1 Instruments Required

1. Chlorhexidine or any sterile prep
2. Scalpel
3. Kelly clamp, +/− Trousseau dilator
4. Trach hook (if available)
5. ETT or tracheostomy tube, #5–#7
6. 5–10 cc air-filled syringe
7. 2–0 suture

8.10.2 Patient Preparation

In an emergent airway situation, rapid yet thoroughly clean the anterior neck with chlorhexidine. If time permits, drape out the anterior neck from the chin to the sternal notch so the anatomic structures and landmarks are easily identifiable.

8.10.3 Identification of Landmarks

Palpate the anterior thyroid cartilage superiorly and the firm, complete ring of the cricoid cartilage inferiorly. The membrane in between is the cricothyroid membrane.

8.10.4 Actual Procedure

1. If you are right handed, stand on the patient's right side and immobilize the larynx with thumb and middle finger of your left hand.
2. Find the cricothyroid membrane with your left index finger while continuing to immobilize. (Fig. 8.2)
3. With the scalpel, make a vertical incision 3 centimeters in length over the membrane staying in the midline of the anterior neck. (Fig. 8.6) Next, make a 1 centimeter transverse incision through the cricothyroid membrane. (Fig. 8.7)
4. If a trach hook is available, place it under the thyroid cartilage and ask an assistant to pull upward and cephalad.
5. Insert a Kelly clamp, mosquito, or Trousseau dilator into the trachea and gently widen the opening. (Fig. 8.8)
6. Insert the tracheostomy tube or endotracheal tube in a caudal fashion. (Fig. 8.9)
7. Inflate the pilot balloon. If using a tracheostomy tube, insert the inner cannula.
8. Attach tube to a bag valve device with an oxygen source and ventilate the patient with 100% oxygen.
9. Once patient is being adequately ventilated, secure the ETT or tracheostomy tube to prevent dislodgment.

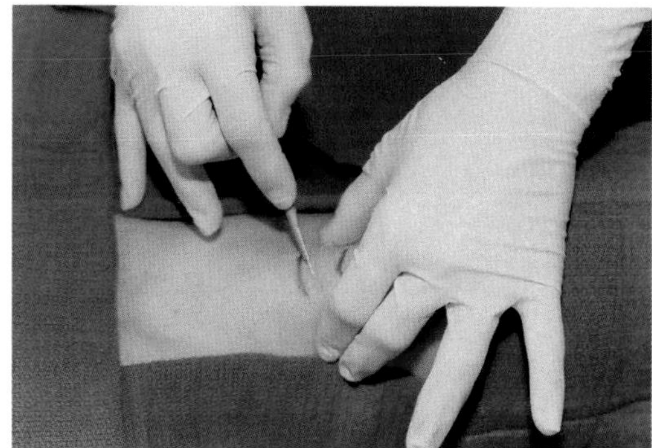

Fig. 8.7 Photo depicts simulated cricoid membrane incision

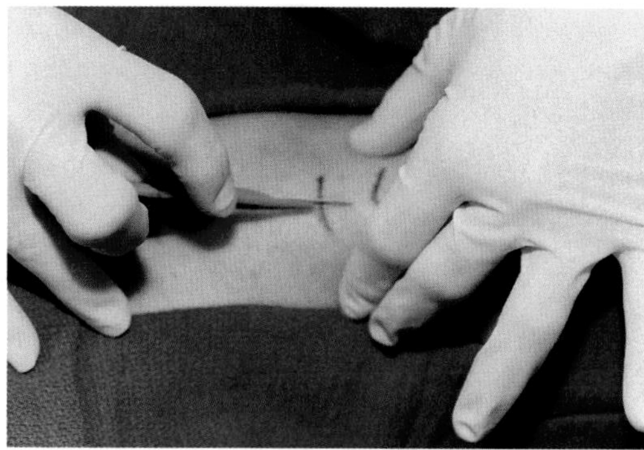

Fig. 8.6 Verticle incision through the skin

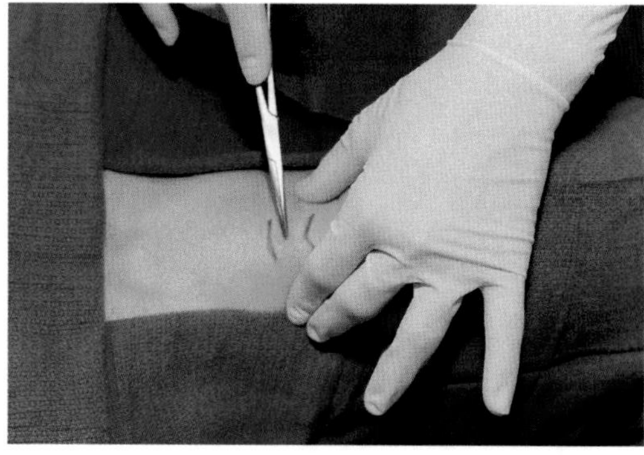

Fig. 8.8 Photo depicts simulated dilation with Kelly clamp

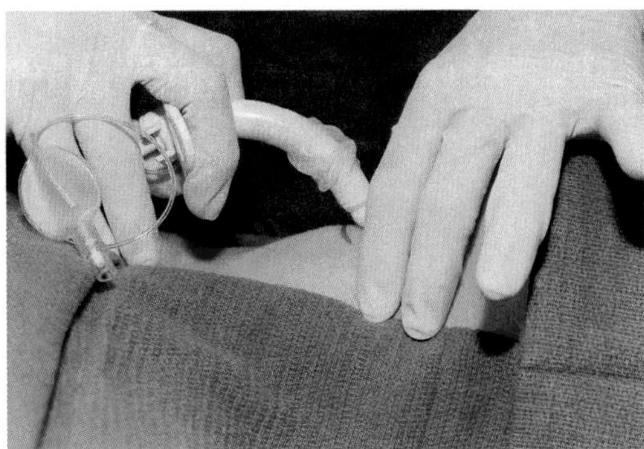

Fig. 8.9 Photo depicts direction of tracheostomy or endotracheal tube insertion

8.10.5 Potential Complications

Bleeding
Subcutaneous emphysema
Placement of endotracheal tube/tracheostomy in subcutaneous tissue
Pneumomediastinum/barotrauma/pneumothorax
Infection

8.10.6 Procedural Pearls

One must be cautious when inserting the tracheostomy tube or ETT into the airway to avoid injury to the balloon. The debate regarding conversion of a surgical cricothyroidotomy to a tracheostomy is ongoing. Literature exists to support both the ability to safely keep the surgical cricothyroidotomy in place and to convert to tracheostomy and avoid long-term complications such as tracheal stenosis.

8.11 Rapid Four-Step Surgical Cricothyroidotomy

Indications, contraindications, potential complications, patient preparation, and landmarks are unchanged from traditional surgical cricothyroidotomy.

8.11.1 Procedure [7]

1. Prep the patient and locate landmarks as previously described.
2. Immobilize the larynx with the thumb and middle finger of your nondominant hand. Identify the cricothyroid membrane with your index finger.
3. With your dominant hand, make a transverse stab incision with a #11 scalpel through the skin and cricothyroid membrane.
4. Insert a trach hook inferiorly in this procedure, under the cricoid cartilage (opposite the traditional procedure), and gently pull in a caudal direction.
5. Insert tracheostomy tube or ETT into the opening and in a caudal direction.

8.12 Percutaneous and Dilator Cricothyroidotomy Kits

Percutaneous dilator kits are commercially available from a variety of vendors. Two main types include a one-step dilator system and the other utilizes a Seldinger technique.

Advantages: Commercial kits have all the necessary equipment to complete the procedure.
Disadvantages: Kit may not be readily available or easy to find by staff.

8.13 Procedure

8.13.1 Patient Preparation

In an emergent airway situation, rapid and thoroughly clean the anterior neck with chlorhexidine. Drape out the neck so anatomic structures and landmarks are easily identifiable.

8.13.2 Identification of Landmarks

Palpate the thyroid and cricoid cartilage. The cricothyroid membrane is between these two landmarks.

8.13.3 Actual Procedure

This procedure will vary depending on commercial kit utilized by the institution. Commercial kits have quick picture instructions and more detailed instructions.

8.13.4 Potential Complications

Perforated esophagus
Subcutaneous emphysema
Subcutaneous placement of needle
Inability to pass wire into trachea
Placement of endotracheal tube/tracheostomy tube in subcutaneous tissue
Pneumomediastinum/barotrauma/pneumothorax
Bleeding
Infection

8.13.5 Procedural Pearl

During an airway emergency is not the time to familiarize yourself with the location of the kit or the assembly and technique used in your commercial kit [6]. It is important to review the location and the instructions several times throughout the year.

8.14 Summary

When traditional airway management techniques are failing, cricothyroidotomy will be the lifesaving intervention to establish an airway. This procedure is a rescue airway to either buy time (needle cricothyroidotomy) or to establish a definitive airway (surgical cricothyroidotomy). The specific type of procedure will depend on the primary operator's comfort level and experience. Although this procedure is performed infrequently, it is a vital tool for lifesaving intervention in a true airway emergency. All providers managing an airway should understand and be ready to perform this rescue intervention.

References

1. Advanced Trauma Life Support - Student Course Manual. 9th ed. Chicago; American College of Surgeons; 2012.
2. Scaletta TA, Schaider JJ. Emergent management of trauma. 2nd ed. New York, NY: McGraw-Hill; 2001.
3. Rhem CG, Wanek SM, Gagnon EB, et al. Cricothyroidotomy for elective airway management in critically ill trauma patients with technically challenging neck anatomy. Critical Care. 2002;6(6):531–5.
4. Tintinalli JE, Kelen GD, Stapczynski JS. Emergency medicine: a comprehensive study guide. 5th ed. New York, NY: McGraw-Hill; 2000.
5. Mittal MK, Stack AM, Wiley JF. Needle cricothyroidotomy with percutaneous transtracheal ventilation. 2014. www.UpToDate.com
6. Peitzman AB, Rhodes M, Schwab CW, et al. The trauma manual: trauma and acute care surgery. 3rd ed. Philadelphia: Lippincott Williams & Wilkins; 2008.
7. Brofeldt BT, Panacek EA, Richards JR. An easy cricothyrotomy approach: the rapid four-step technique. Acad Emerg Med. 1996;3(11):1060–3.

Percutaneous Dilatational Tracheostomy

9

Peter S. Sandor and David S. Shapiro

Abbreviation List

ACF	Anterior cervical spine fixation
AORN	Association of periOperative Registered Nurses
BMI	Body mass index
BVM	Bag-valve-mask
Cm	Centimeter
CPP	Cerebral perfusion pressure
DDAVP	Desmopressin acetate
ET	Endotracheal tube
FFP	Fresh frozen plasma
FiO_2	Fraction of inspired oxygen
ICP	Intracranial pressure
INR	International normalized ratio
kg	Kilogram
m^2	Meter squared
mcg	Microgram
mg	Milligram
min	Minute
ml	Milliliter
mm	Millimeter
mm Hg	Millimeter of mercury
MV	Mechanical ventilation
PDT	Percutaneous dilatational tracheostomy
PEEP	Positive end expiratory pressure
PTT	Partial thromboplastin time
RCP	Respiratory care practitioner
RN	Registered nurse

P.S. Sandor, RRT, MHS, PA-C (✉)
Department of Surgery, Saint Francis Hospital and Medical Center, 114 Woodland Street, Hartford, CT 06105, USA
e-mail: Psandor@Stfranciscare.org

D.S. Shapiro, MD, FACS, FCCM
Saint Francis Hospital and Medical Center, 114 Woodland Street, Hartford, CT 06105, USA
e-mail: DShapiro@Stfranciscare.org

9.1 Introduction (Fundamentals)

The endotracheal tube is the preferred method for airway maintenance in the short duration. Poor patient comfort and airway complications limit its long-term utility, leading to an increase in the need for tracheostomy for both airway protection and chronic respiratory failure [1]. As a result, Cook Critical Care (Bloomington, IN) collaborated in the development of a single-use bedside percutaneous dilatational tracheostomy (PDT) kit [2]. Since that time, several devices have been developed from a variety of manufacturers, with slight variations in both technique and methodology [3].

PDT is now a commonly performed critical care procedure. It has fewer complications than traditional open tracheostomy and has gained wide acceptance as the preferred method for semi-elective and elective tracheostomy [4]. When compared to open tracheostomy, PDT has the benefit of bedside placement with less perioperative complications [5]. Bedside placement

D.A. Taylor et al. (eds.), *Interventional Critical Care*, DOI 10.1007/978-3-319-25286-5_9

requires fewer resources and completely eliminates the need for transport of critically ill patient, which, in this population, carries a "mishap" rate of 33 % [6]. Avoiding the operating room also eliminates financial and time expenditures (including room times and personnel) which can also reduce cost [7, 8].

Advanced care providers of critical care services should be capable of performing PDT with attending oversight. Though uncomplicated in experienced hands, airway-related complications can be disastrous. Proper patient selection, meticulous attention to technique, proper practitioner training, and education are crucial to maximize success. PDT requires at least two trained proceduralists working together, and both must possess appropriate experience before independent involvement in either the cervical operator or the bronchoscopist role. In experienced hands, PDT is a better alternative to open tracheostomy with fewer procedural complications and equivalent long-term outcomes.

9.2 Indications

PDT is indicated in patients who require long-term airway management and/or protection or in patients who are unable to wean from mechanical ventilation via endotracheal tube. Many approaches are documented on the timing of tracheostomy, but consensus exists that patients should undergo tracheostomy if mechanically ventilated for, or anticipated to require mechanical ventilation for, longer than 10–14 days [9–12]. Particular patient populations, including those with severe stroke or traumatic brain injuries, have been shown to benefit from earlier tracheostomy [13, 14].

9.3 Contraindications

PDT is a very well-tolerated procedure, but there are some patients who may not be ideal candidates. Concerns about tracheostomy site, body habitus, concurrent injury, or overall medical condition may contribute. Relative contraindications include:

- Infection or skin/soft tissue pathology at tracheostomy site.
- Hemodynamic instability—initiation of analgesics, anxiolytics, and paralytic medication may result in irreversible hypotension.
- BMI > 35 kg/m^2—larger patients may have pre-cervical soft tissue that is too thick for the standard tracheostomy tube to traverse, resulting in incomplete or poor cannulation of the trachea and high risk for inadvertent decannulation; extra long tracheostomy tubes may be required.
- Cervical spine instability and/or fracture—to minimize the risk of complications such as pneumonia, early tracheostomy should be attempted once patients are medically stable [15]. Ordinarily, hyperextension facilitates landmark identification and palpation of the first few tracheal rings; in the absence of hyperextension, percutaneous method should be aborted unless landmarks are clearly identifiable. Removal of the rigid cervical collars should only be performed after chemical paralysis and in-line spine stabilization. In patient requiring anterior cervical instrumentation/fixation (ACF), tracheostomy can safely be performed as soon as 2 days after surgery. In a retrospective review of 1184 ACFs, 1.7 % of patients required postoperative tracheostomy which resulted in no documented postoperative wound infections [15]. Similarly, Northrup revealed that ACF can also be performed safely *after* tracheostomy with similar safety [16].
- Previous tracheostomy—PDT may still safely be performed utilizing the same tract. However, tissue bleeding can be more difficult to control, so dissection should be avoided.
- Elevated intracranial pressure—early tracheostomy in traumatic brain injury has been demonstrated to be beneficial, but maintaining intracranial pressure (ICP) <20 mmHg and cerebral perfusion pressure (CPP) >65 mmHg is important to avoid secondary brain injury. Patients should initially be evaluated by lowering the head of bed to flat and reassessing ICP and CPP with the patient in the supine

position; if elevation of ICP occurs and compromises cerebral perfusion, the procedure should be postponed.
- Severe hypoxemia—patients who require PEEP >10 cmH_2O or FiO_2>0.60 to prevent hypoxia should have PDT postponed. Changes in mean airway pressures and alveolar recruitment could occur during percutaneous tracheostomy or bronchoscopy, resulting in worsening hypoxia.
- Coagulopathy—patients with coagulopathy (INR >1.5) should be treated with fresh frozen plasma, factor concentrates, or other therapies either before or during the procedure. Thrombocytopenia of <50,000/mm^3 should be treated with platelets or desmopressin acetate (DDAVP) as clinically indicated.
- Unfractionated heparin infusion—the infusion should stop 3–6 h prior to starting the procedure to allow for normalization of the partial thromboplastin time (PTT). It is also prudent to reassess PTT prior to the procedure. Following PDT, it is safe to restart the heparin infusion within the first 3–6 h post procedure.

In addition, the manufacturers [2] include contraindications to the percutaneous method, including:

- Emergent airway settings
- Thyromegaly
- Non-palpable cricoid cartilage/absent landmarks
- Pediatric patients
- Non-intubated patients
- Positive end expiratory pressure (PEEP) >20 cmH_2O
- Uncorrected coagulopathy

9.4 Resources Required

Though PDT does not require the logistics and resources used in an open tracheostomy, two capable proceduralists are necessary. One proceduralist is responsible for the bronchoscopy and orotracheal airway management, while the second proceduralist is responsible for the tracheostomy procedure. In addition, a respiratory care practitioner (RCP) is required for maintaining the existing airway as well as changing endotracheal tube position as needed during the procedure. Some RCPs prefer to ventilate by bag-valve-mask device; however, mechanical ventilation can be used as long as the RCP remains at the bedside. An experienced ICU nurse (RN) is also required to administer medications, maintain accurate documentation, and assure the patient's monitoring and ICU level of care are unperturbed.

9.4.1 Monitoring

As in any critical care setting, patients must be maintained on continuous telemetry with a bedside monitor. Vital sign assessments and monitoring should be performed frequently during the bedside procedure, which is essential to avoid morbidity or mortality. Oxygen saturation, heart rate, and blood pressure should be monitored continuously. End-tidal carbon dioxide monitoring is helpful to confirm adequate ventilation. Monitoring equipment integrity must be considered before beginning the procedure.

Pulse oximetry should be utilized continuously. Poorly attached probes, dysfunctional devices, and diaphoretic patients could result in inaccurate data and should be remedied prior to any airway manipulation. Additionally, any variation in oxygen saturation should be met with immediate attention. A bronchoscope in the endotracheal tube can increase airway pressures which can result in low tidal volumes, hypoventilation, and hypoxia. Preemptive hyperoxygenation is important to minimize desaturation. Any decrease in oxygen saturation should be met with immediate cessation of bronchoscopy, removal of bronchoscope, and reassessment of the patient. If oxygen saturation does not return to baseline, consideration should be made to abort the procedure and reassess the patient.

Heart rate is an important indicator of pain and/or anxiety in a paralyzed patient. Analgesics and sedatives should be dosed reasonably and judiciously with any indication of pain. Bradycardia is an ominous sign if associated with hypoxemia or pulse oximetry that has been interpreted as "not accurate." If bradycardia occurs, abort the procedure and reevaluate the airway immediately. Bradycardia can also be a response to vagal stimulation, especially in patients with spinal cord injury and/or brain injury. Patients with neurological injuries may benefit from chronotropes or vasopressors.

Blood pressure must also be continuously monitored. Hypertension is most commonly associated with pain or agitation and should be treated with analgesia or sedation. Hypotension is a common response to sedation and paralysis and usually responds to a fluid bolus. Significant hypotension should be met with a head-to-toe patient examination, evaluating for other diagnoses, including complicating pneumothorax or hemorrhage. Frequently, patients may become hypotensive immediately following the procedure as stimulation is minimized. This often resolves after sedation is lightened.

9.4.2 Equipment

- Cook Critical Care (Bloomington, IN) Ciaglia Blue Rhino® percutaneous tracheostomy tray.
- Shiley™ percutaneous tracheostomy tube with disposable inner cannula.[1]
- Sterile gowns and full barrier precaution devices, including gloves, cap, and mask for each participant.
- Chlorhexidine solution applicator device.
- 15 mm angled dual-access swivel adaptor.
- Bag-valve-mask (BVM) apparatus.
- 5 mm or smaller bronchoscope with cart, screen imaging is required given the need for both providers to visualize the trachea.
- Bedside table.
- Towel, pad, or other "rolls" to assist with hyperextension (unless contraindicated).
- Sterile water, approximately 100 ml.

In addition to the list above, an intubation tray and a surgical/open tracheostomy tray should be available.

9.5 Performing the Procedure

The Cook Critical Care (Bloomington, IN) Ciaglia Blue Rhino® Advanced Percutaneous Tracheostomy Set and technique will be explained here. Other devices, including the Portex® Griggs Forceps Kit, Cook Critical Care® Blue Dolphin Kit, Surgitech/Fresenius (Runcorn, Cheshire, UK) Rapitrach, and Rusch-Thermo Fisher® (Waltham, MA) PercuTwist (2002), each have similar yet distinct techniques.

Before any procedure is undertaken at the bedside, a formal "time-out procedure" should be performed. A "time-out procedure" consists of correctly stating the patient's identity (with name band and medical record number), confirms the exact procedure, and verifies procedural consent with providers. This not only identifies the patient but also demonstrates a unified goal for the team of providers.

Step 1: After proper patient selection, patient or proxy authorization, and site marking, a briefing is held to assure proper equipment, personnel, documentation, and other needs are met (according to institutional standard). Subsequently, the institutional Association of periOperative Registered Nurses (AORN) recommended "time-out" is performed. Once the time-out is complete, the patient may undergo supplemental sedation. Propofol (initially 0.05–0.5 mg/kg IV initial bolus with maintenance of 25–50 mcg/kg/min) or intermittent midazolam bolus (1–2 mg intravenous given every 3–5 min) should be used initially to achieve adequate sedation. Once sedation is at an appropriate level, analgesia should be provided with opiate analgesia, such as fentanyl (0.5–2 mcg/kg dosed every 3–5 min). Once a stable sedation level is achieved and patient's vital signs remain stable, a single dose of cisatracurium besylate (0.15–0.2 mg/kg IV) is recommended for chemical paralysis. Fentanyl is recommended for its short duration of action with minimal hemodynamic effects. Propofol is preferred for its short half-life, but patients may become hypotensive due to its vasodilatory

1 *The Shiley™ brand is specially designed for compatibility with the Blue Rhino insertion kit, including a tapered distal tip and inverted cuff shoulder for easier insertion* [2].

effects, especially in those with severe inflammatory response or distributive shock. After initiation of the procedure, further doses of analgesia or sedation should be provided every 3–5 min based upon perceived pain and agitation.

Step 2: The patient and bed position are both important. The patient's headboard should be removed if present, and the bed must be moved to provide space to accommodate both the bronchoscopic provider and respiratory care practitioner. The right-handed cervical operator should be positioned at the patient's right and on the left for the left handed. After the stable anesthetic plane is established, the head of bed is lowered so the patient is in a supine position, and a rolled pad or towel is placed beneath the patient's scapulae with sufficient elevation to permit hyperextension (Fig. 9.1). The occiput should remain on the mattress, foam ring, or small pillow. Absorptive pads should be used to avoid spillage of blood, preparatory solution, or irrigation on the bed linens. Hyperextension allows for slight cephalad projection of the trachea, permitting palpation of the tracheal rings. Reexamination of the neck should be performed by inspection and palpation. A systematic approach is best: palpate the thyroid cartilage and move inferiorly in a stepwise fashion locating the cricothyroid membrane, the cricoid cartilage, and the first and second tracheal rings. The ideal location for the needle puncture will be either in the first or second tracheal ring interspaces.

Step 3: The bed height is adjusted to accommodate both the bronchoscopist and operator. The bronchoscopist should ready the bronchoscope, including checking for suction and image quality. The operator should ready the PDT tray and equipment by first checking for package integrity and expiration date. The PDT tray is opened and, under sterile conditions, placed on a bedside table or Mayo stand. About 25–50 ml of sterile water is poured into the largest cavity in the Blue Rhino tray (Fig. 9.2). The *EZ-Pass®* hydrophilic coating is activated by sterile water or saline [2]. The operator should cleanse his/her hands and don a sterile gown, cap, mask, and gloves. The properly sized Shiley percutaneous tracheostomy tube is then opened and placed on the sterile tray. The tracheostomy balloon may be tested by institutional or practice standard. The bedside table or Mayo stand may be positioned over the patient for convenient access.

Step 4: The removable inner cannula will usually be found in the tracheostomy when the package is opened—this should be removed and placed in a convenient location, as the patient

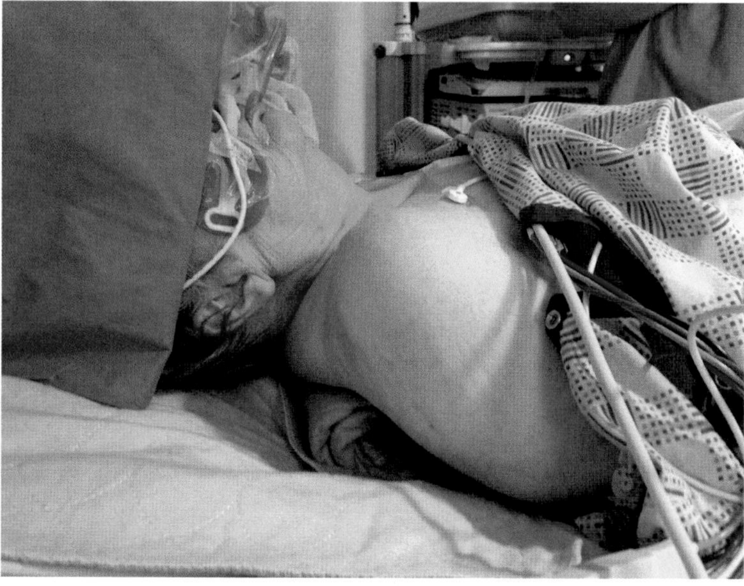

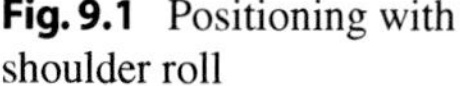

Fig. 9.1 Positioning with shoulder roll

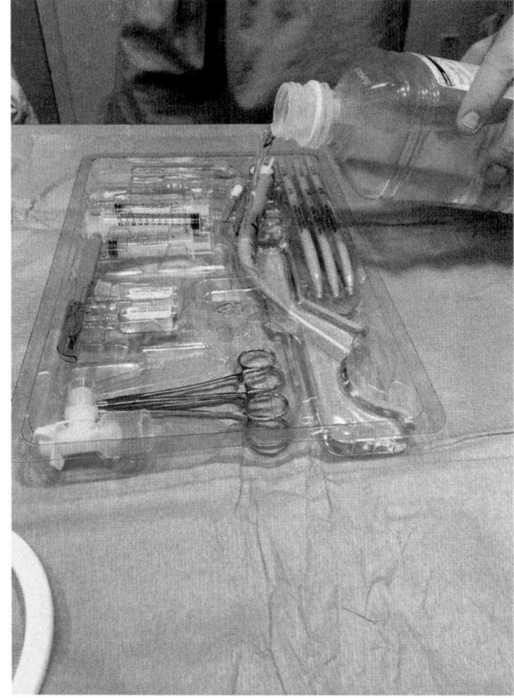

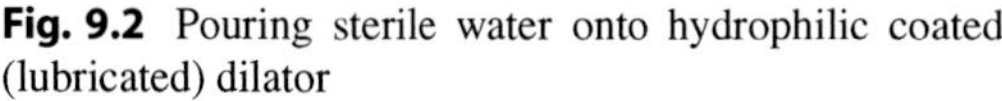

Fig. 9.2 Pouring sterile water onto hydrophilic coated (lubricated) dilator

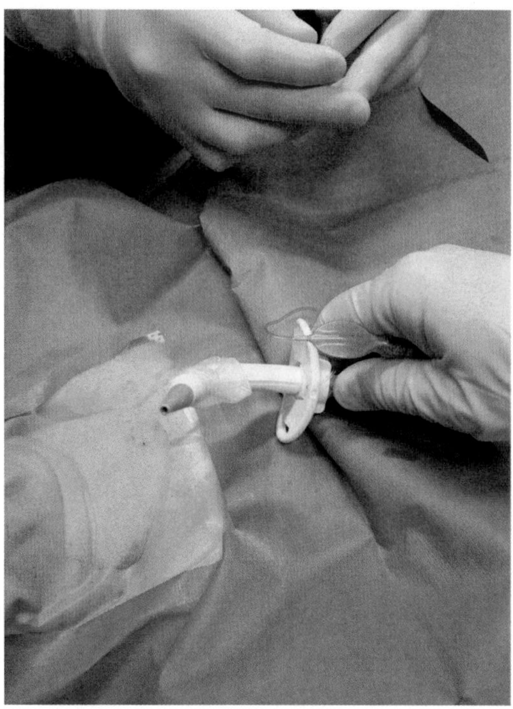

Fig. 9.3 Trach with loading dilator

cannot be ventilated without the inner cannula as a conduit. The tracheostomy tube should then be lubricated and the appropriately sized blue loading dilator inserted to the appropriate distance; approximately 2 cm of dilators tapered end should protrude through the distal portion of the tracheostomy (Fig. 9.3). Three *loading* dilators are included with the Cook PDT kit: 24 French (F), 26 F, and 28 F (Fig. 9.4). They correspond to size 4, size 6, and size 8 Shiley tracheostomy tubes, respectively. The white guiding catheter should be inserted into the narrow end of the Blue Rhino® *taper* dilator until the safety ridge is reached and all should be moistened with water (Fig. 9.5).

The patient's neck is then prepped with chlorhexidine solution and permitted to dry. Then the sterile drape, included in the Ciaglia kit, is applied making certain the center of the hole of the drape is located over the thyroid cartilage and sternal notch (Fig. 9.6).

Step 5: A syringe is prepared with *10 ml of the 1.5 % lidocaine with epinephrine* which is located in the disposable tray. Secure the 25

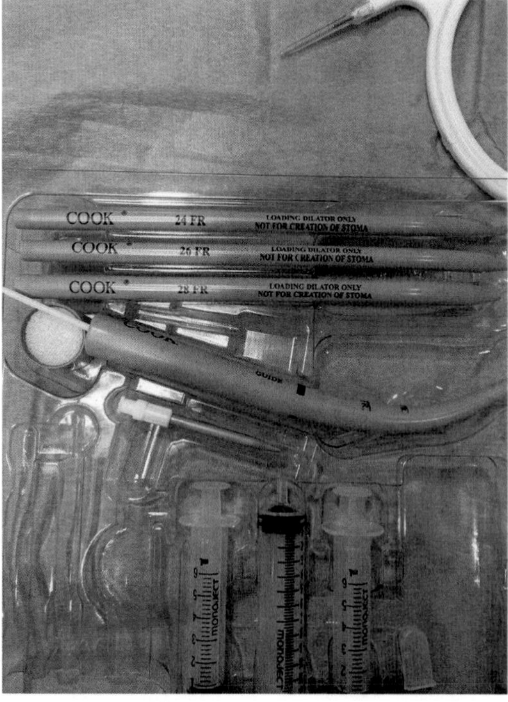

Fig. 9.4 Loading dilators

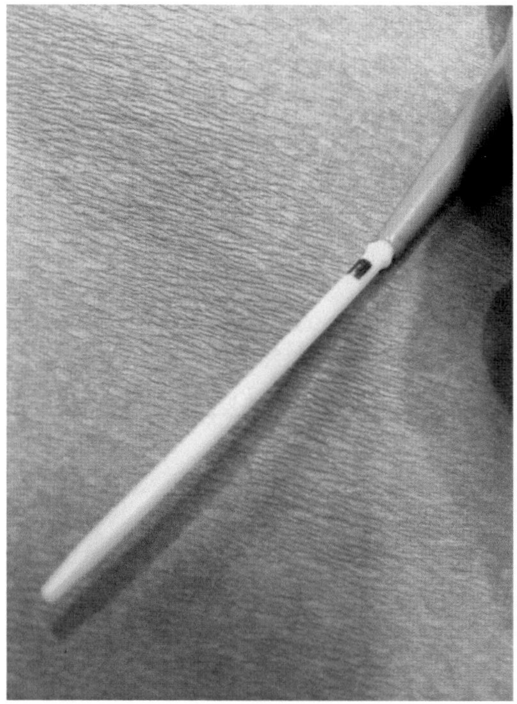

Fig. 9.5 Guiding catheter within tapered dilator

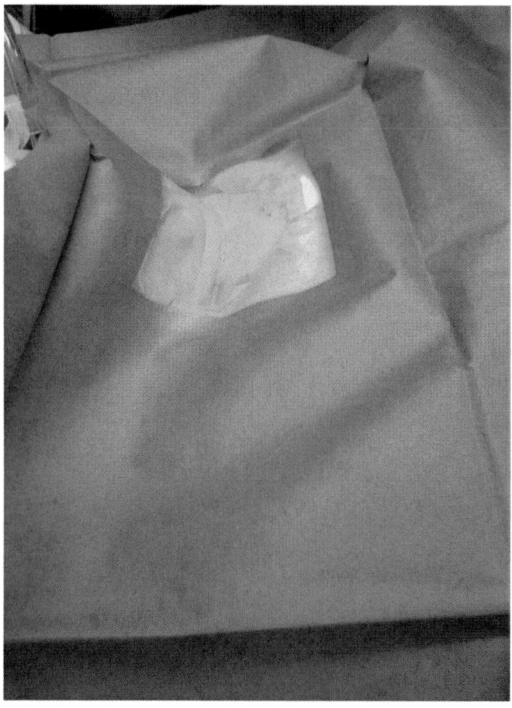

Fig. 9.6 Neck prepped and draped

gauge needle in place on this syringe. All sharps should be secured in the red and white foam sharp device cup.

Step 6: With the patient adequately sedated and paralyzed, the respiratory care practitioner should remove the patient from mechanical ventilation (MV) and manually ventilated with 100 % inspired oxygen. A 15 mm dual-access angled swivel adaptor should be attached to the endotracheal tube to allow for bronchoscopy and ventilation simultaneously.

Step 7: The bronchoscopist will apply a small amount of water-soluble lubricant to the scope shaft. The RCP will secure the endotracheal tube (ET) during the bronchoscopy. Prior to initiation of the procedure, the bronchoscope is advanced through the ET to the level of the carina. This will confirm that the bronchoscope could be advanced through the ET conduit. Significant secretions or concretions should be noted. Care should be taken not to injure the tracheal mucosa. Formal bronchoscopy is delayed until after tracheostomy is completed. During the procedure, the bronchoscope should be left within the endotracheal tube lumen and should only be utilized during the actual procedure to avoid hypoventilation and hypoxia.

Step 8: With the airway now secure, landmarks are identified, including the sternal notch, cricoid cartilage, etc. With the nondominant hand's thumb and middle finger, the trachea is secured in the midline, allowing use of the index finger to palpate the tracheal rings. First, inject 5–10 ml of the local anesthetic. Skin bleeding is usually minimized with an epinephrine-containing solution. Then, a vertical incision is made, approximately 1.5–2 cm in length, through the skin only, avoiding the deeper structures of the neck. This incision is centered about 2–3 cm superior to the sternal notch. A vertical incision is chosen to provide flexibility in the final location of the tracheotomy. This vertical incision allows for extension in either direction if needed. It can also avoid skin bleeding as most skin vascular structures are vertically located.

Step 9: Once the incision is completed, the thumb and middle finger of the operator's nondominant (superior) hand are placed on either side of the incision and used to center the trachea in the midpoint of the incision and visualize soft tissues (Fig. 9.7). To better palpate the tracheal rings, some prefer to develop a small plane through the soft tissues of the neck using a small hemostat. In order to avoid unnecessary bleeding, dissection should be midline, minimal, controlled, and blunt (Fig. 9.8).

Step 10: The bronchoscopist and respiratory care practitioner work together to withdraw the ET to a level just below the vocal cords. The bronchoscope is first inserted to the level of the carina. Prior to withdrawing the endotracheal tube, transillumination (in a darkened room, withdrawing the bronchoscope from carina to the proximal ET, observe for transillumination in the incision—this measured distance should be noted) can help predict the proper distance to withdraw the ET tube (Fig. 9.9). As a rule of thumb, 18 cm is a reasonable distance to begin in most adult patients. As the respiratory care practitioner prepares to withdraw the ET, the bronchoscopist should readvance the scope so the tip is just above the carina. Caution must be utilized to avoid premature extubation. Without deflating

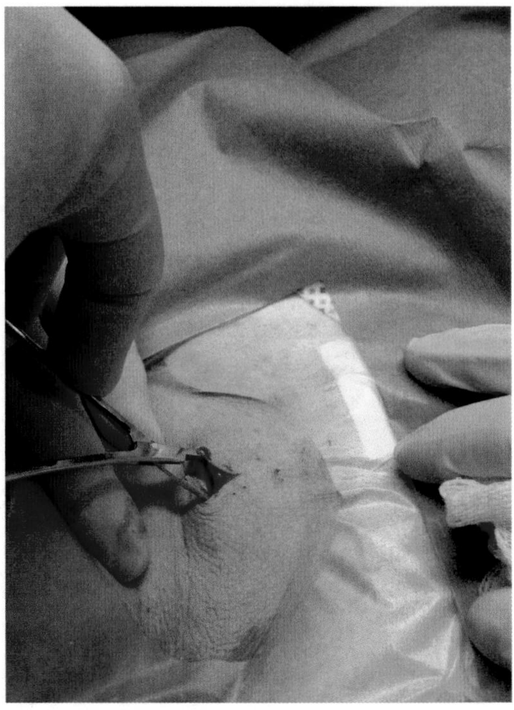

Fig. 9.8 Hemostat dilating soft tissue following skin incision

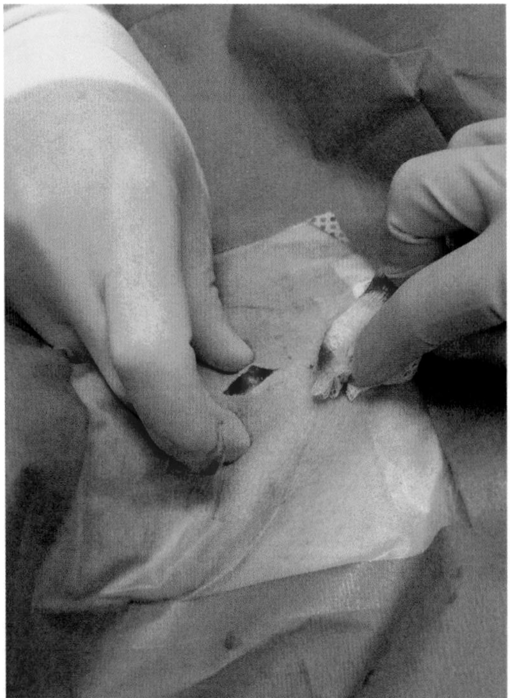

Fig. 9.7 Initial incision

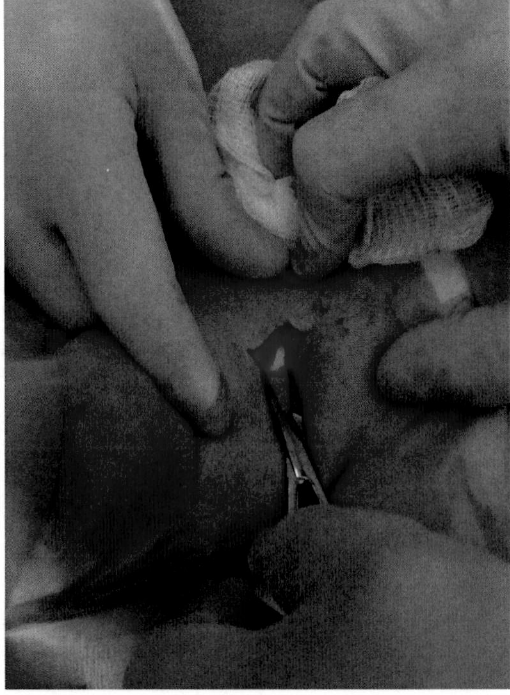

Fig. 9.9 Tracheal transillumination with bronchoscope

the ET tube cuff (to minimize aspiration of oral secretions), the RCP withdraws the ET the measured transilluminated distance. Remember, the bronchoscope should be maintained at the level of the carina during the ET withdrawal process. This allows the bronchoscope to be used as a "bougie" for re-intubation in the event of premature extubation. The RCP should resecure the tube at the new position. Once resecured, the bronchoscope should be retracted into the ET. Maintaining the bronchoscope inside the ET will prevent an inadvertent needle injury to the costly bronchoscope.

Step 11: Now that the incision has been created and the ET in proper position, tracheal puncture with the 15 gauge introducer needle is now performed. The 15 gauge introducer needle may be used without a syringe or may be attached to the hub of a 10 ml syringe containing 2–3 ml of water or saline (this allows for a better grasp of the needle, and bubbles in the syringe may help confirm tracheal placement). With the thumb and middle finger of the nondominant hand securing the trachea and retracting the skin edges, the index finger of the same hand should be used to identify the landmark of the first or second tracheal ring space. The dominant hand should grasp the needle in the middle of the shaft and placed into the midline of the tracheal incision, aiming inferiorly with the bevel facing up. The tip should be advanced into the trachea with the bronchoscope visualizing tracheal entry (Fig. 9.10). The needle should be advanced into the midpoint of the trachea. Handling the needle in the mid-shaft can prevent deep needle penetration, minimizing posterior tracheal wall injury. The needle should enter the trachea at the 12 o'clock position; however, anywhere from 10 o'clock to 2 o'clock is acceptable. Once the needle is confirmed in the trachea, immediately insert the flexible stainless steel J-wire through the needle, visualizing its entry into the tracheal lumen, and subsequently remove the needle (Fig. 9.11).

Step 12: The blue 14 French introducer dilator (Fig. 9.12) should next be advanced over the wire and passed through the puncture site three times. The wire and introducer dilator are visualized bronchoscopically. The blue 14 French dilator is then removed while leaving the guidewire in place. It is imperative to always maintain control of the guidewire.

Step 13: The large tapered dilator containing the inner 8 French white guiding catheter is then threaded onto the guidewire. When handling the tapered dilator, it should be grasped firmly behind the "skin level" line since the hydrophilic coating makes the distal end of the dilator slippery. It is then advanced over the guidewire and followed bronchoscopically. The white guiding catheter's safety ridge should be abutting the tip of the

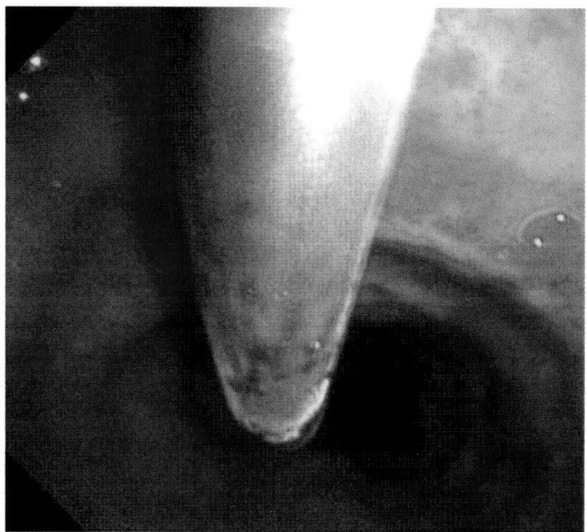

Fig. 9.10 Access needle visualized in trachea

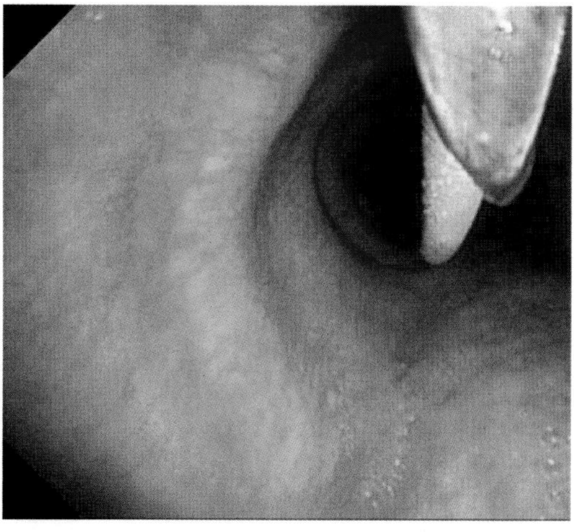

Fig. 9.11 Bronch visualizing wire (*green*) advancing into trachea

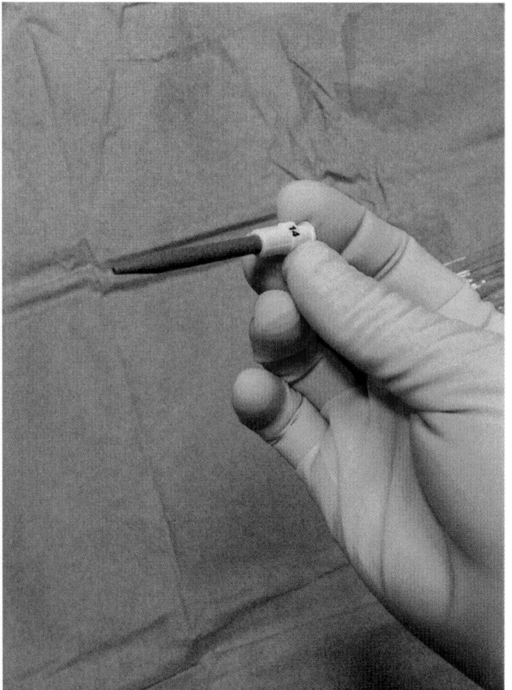

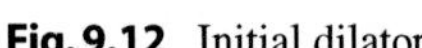

Fig. 9.12 Initial dilator

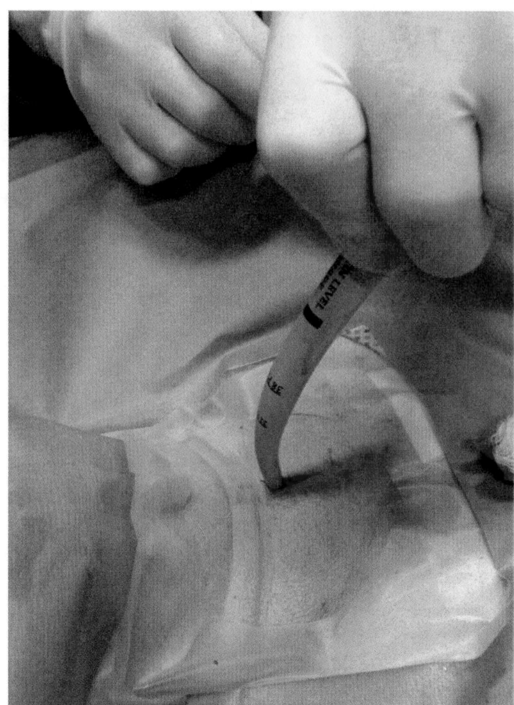

Fig. 9.13 Taper dilator being inserted

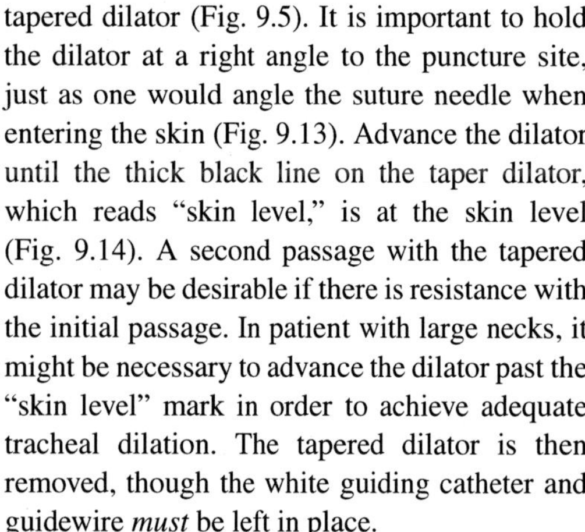

tapered dilator (Fig. 9.5). It is important to hold the dilator at a right angle to the puncture site, just as one would angle the suture needle when entering the skin (Fig. 9.13). Advance the dilator until the thick black line on the taper dilator, which reads "skin level," is at the skin level (Fig. 9.14). A second passage with the tapered dilator may be desirable if there is resistance with the initial passage. In patient with large necks, it might be necessary to advance the dilator past the "skin level" mark in order to achieve adequate tracheal dilation. The tapered dilator is then removed, though the white guiding catheter and guidewire *must* be left in place.

Step 14: Once the tapered dilator is removed, advance the tracheostomy tube with blue loading dilator as one unit over the white guiding catheter and guidewire. Again, care should be taken to abutt the saftey ridge of the white guiding catheter to the tip of the loading dilator. With gentle pressure, the tracheostomy/dilator unit should enter the trachea at a right angle, allowing the curve of the tracheostomy to advance naturally. Avoid forcing the device

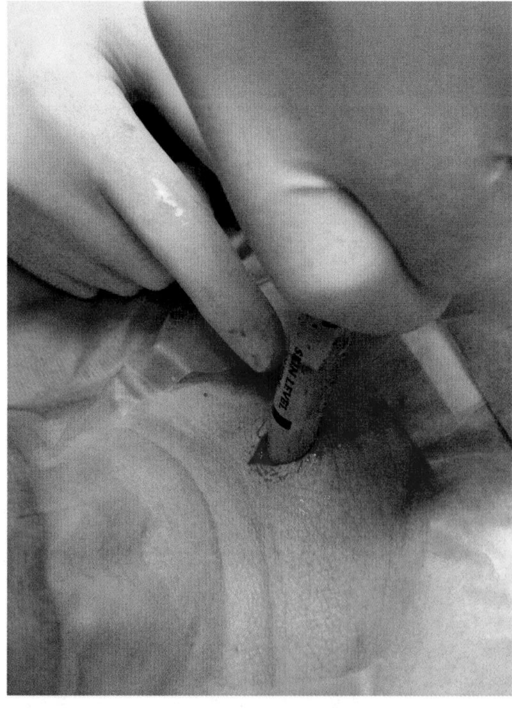

Fig. 9.14 Taper dilator being advanced to skin mark

through the incision, as too much pressure will bend the wire and white guiding catheter, permitting false passage into an extratracheal path or damaging the posterior tracheal wall. There will be some resistance when the deflated cuff of the tracheostomy tube is advanced through the anterior tracheal wall. This will be followed by an immediate loss of resistance. This should always be completed under bronchoscopic guidance confirming the cuff inside the trachea (Fig. 9.15).

Step 15: Once the tracheostomy/dilator unit is in the trachea, the operator should hold the tracheostomy in place while removing the dilator, white guiding catheter, and guidewire. The tracheostomy inner cannula should be immediately inserted and the cuff inflated (Fig. 9.16). The bronchoscope and 15 mm angled swivel adaptor should be removed from the ET and attached to the tracheostomy. Next, the bronchoscope is advanced through the tracheostomy to confirm endotracheal placement above the carina. The operator should secure and maintain control of the tracheostomy at all times.

Step 16: The tracheostomy should be secured appropriately with the institution's preferred securing device. The twill tracheostomy ties should be avoided, as they can result in inappropriately high pressure onto the skin of the neck. Similarly, suturing of the tracheostomy is not recommended as sutures can result in both pressure-related skin changes and ulceration. Additionally, sutures are not proven to prevent tracheostomy dislodgement [17]. If sutures are preferred or dictated by institutional standard, removal is advocated on post-procedure day 3 to avoid pressure-related skin changes.

Once the tracheostomy is secured, the patient should be reconnected to mechanical ventilation. Chest radiography may be the standard at some institutions, though it is not required unless complications or concern arise. Proper placement is confirmed by end-tidal carbon dioxide monitoring, vital signs, physical exam, bronchoscopy, and/or chest radiography. Vital signs should be continually monitored with the post-procedure guideline of the institution.

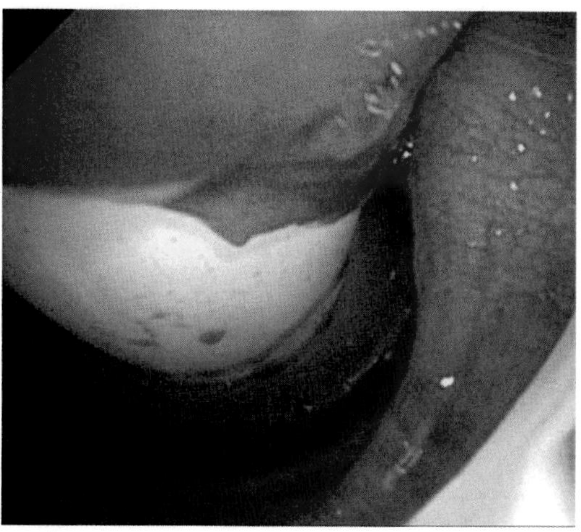

Fig. 9.15 Bronch confirming trach tube balloon within trachea

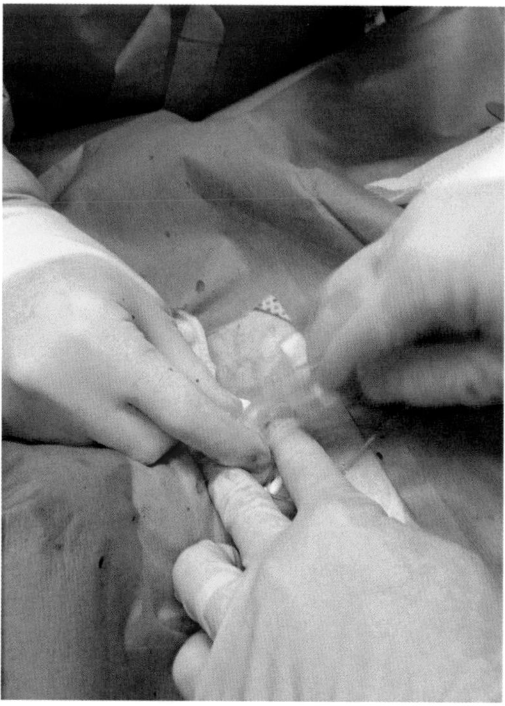

Fig. 9.16 Inner cannulae being inserted

9.6 Procedural Complications

Though percutaneous tracheostomy is a bedside procedure, it is not without associated serious risk. Proper patient selection, training, and experience will avoid most complications. Some complications will occur, including death (0.16–0.4 %), major bleeding (0.1 %), pneumothorax (0.2 %), posterior tracheal perforation (1.6 %), and loss of airway [18, 19]. The experienced use of bronchoscopy minimizes the incidence of airway loss and posterior tracheal wall injury, and though some providers prefer PDT without bronchoscopy, it is highly recommended [20]. Conversion to an open technique should always be available, either at the bedside or the operating room, as it remains the gold standard for tracheostomy.

Minor perioperative complications are quite manageable. The most commonly encountered complication is skin bleeding. If blunt dissection is minimized and bleeding is noted from the skin edge, the insertions of the PT will usually result in tamponade [21]. Visible bleeding is occasionally noted from small anterior skin vessels and may be controlled with 4–0 or 3–0 absorbable suture on a tapered needle.

Hypoxia is uncommon and minimal despite the use of bronchoscopy. If hypoxia occurs, immediate removal of the bronchoscope will usually improve oxygenation. Resume the procedure only when hypoxemia resolves.

9.7 Delayed Complications

Intermediate and late complications are difficult to accurately quantify and are infrequent. Tracheostomy tube occlusion, dislodgement, or cuff malfunction has a combined incidence of 0.3–0.8 % [17, 18]. In the event of tracheostomy dislodgement, secure an airway with either immediate replacement of the tracheostomy or by oral endotracheal intubation. Replacement of a dislodged tube in the first 72–96 h post-op may be met with difficulty in the absence of a defined tract. Oral endotracheal intubation should not be delayed if the tracheostomy cannot be easily and immediately replaced. Smaller-sized tracheostomy or endotracheal tubes may be placed into the tracheostomy site if re-intubation is not immediately available; this should only be performed by experienced providers. Extratracheal placement of a tube cannot only worsen airway obstruction, and it can result in a severe vascular, aerodigestive, or other tissue injuries.

While overall tracheal stenosis rates are noted to be 1.7 % [17], clinically evident tracheal stenosis after PDT has an incidence of 0.16–0.35 %, which is comparable to open surgical tracheostomy [18, 22]. Tracheo-innominate artery fistula is a dreaded, rare complication, with an incidence of <0.35 % [18].

References

1. Gaynor EB, Greenberg SB. Untoward sequelae of prolonged intubation. Laryngoscope. 1985;95(12):1461–7.
2. Care CC. Ciaglia Blue Rhino G2 advanced percutaneous tracheostomy introducer set with EZ pass hydrophilic coating instructions for use. 2013 [cited 2014 Sep 5]. Available from: https://www.cookmedical.com/data/IFU_PDF/C_T_PTISG_REV1.PDF
3. Cools-Lartigue J, et al. Evolution of percutaneous dilatational tracheostomy—a review of current techniques and their pitfalls. World J Surg. 2013;37(7):1633–46.
4. Kornblith LZ, et al. One thousand bedside percutaneous tracheostomies in the surgical intensive care unit: time to change the gold standard. J Am Coll Surg. 2011;212(2):163–70.
5. Delaney A, Bagshaw SM, Nalos M. Percutaneous dilatational tracheostomy versus surgical tracheostomy in critically ill patients: a systematic review and meta-analysis. Crit Care. 2006;10(2):R55.
6. Smith I, Fleming S, Cernaianu A. Mishaps during transport from the intensive care unit. Crit Care Med. 1990;18(3):278–81.
7. Cobean R, et al. Percutaneous dilatational tracheostomy. A safe, cost-effective bedside procedure. Arch Surg. 1996;131(3):265–71.
8. Grover A, et al. Open versus percutaneous dilatational tracheostomy: efficacy and cost analysis. Am Surg. 2001;67(4):297–301. discussion 301–2.
9. Rumbak MJ, et al. A prospective, randomized, study comparing early percutaneous dilational tracheotomy to prolonged translaryngeal intubation (delayed tracheotomy) in critically ill medical patients. Crit Care Med. 2004;32(8):1689–94.
10. Arabi Y, et al. Early tracheostomy in intensive care trauma patients improves resource utilization: a cohort study and literature review. Crit Care. 2004;8(5):R347–52.
11. Wang F, et al. The timing of tracheotomy in critically ill patients undergoing mechanical ventilation:

a systematic review and meta-analysis of randomized controlled trials. Chest. 2011;140(6):1456–65.
12. Zagli G, et al. Early tracheostomy in intensive care unit: a retrospective study of 506 cases of video-guided Ciaglia Blue Rhino tracheostomies. J Trauma. 2010;68(2):367–72.
13. Villwock JA, Villwock MR, Deshaies EM. Tracheostomy timing affects stroke recovery. J Stroke Cerebrovasc Dis. 2014;23(5):1069–72.
14. Alali AS, et al. Tracheostomy timing in traumatic brain injury: a propensity-matched cohort study. J Trauma Acute Care Surg. 2014;76(1):70–6. discussion 76–8.
15. Babu R, et al. Timing of tracheostomy after anterior cervical spine fixation. J Trauma Acute Care Surg. 2013;74(4):961–6.
16. Northrup BE, et al. Occurrence of infection in anterior cervical fusion for spinal cord injury after tracheostomy. Spine (Phila Pa 1976). 1995;20(22):2449–53.
17. Halum SL, et al. A multi-institutional analysis of tracheotomy complications. Laryngoscope. 2012;122(1):38–45.
18. Dennis BM, et al. Safety of bedside percutaneous tracheostomy in the critically ill: evaluation of more than 3,000 procedures. J Am Coll Surg. 2013;216(4):858–65. discussion 865–7.
19. Simon M, et al. Death after percutaneous dilatational tracheostomy: a systematic review and analysis of risk factors. Crit Care. 2013;17(5):R258.
20. Kost KM. Endoscopic percutaneous dilatational tracheotomy: a prospective evaluation of 500 consecutive cases. Laryngoscope. 2005;115(10 Pt 2):1–30.
21. Silvester W, et al. Percutaneous versus surgical tracheostomy: a randomized controlled study with long-term follow-up. Crit Care Med. 2006;34(8):2145–52.
22. Dempsey GA, Grant CA, Jones TM. Percutaneous tracheostomy: a 6 years prospective evaluation of the single tapered dilator technique. Br J Anaesth. 2010;105(6):782–8.

Diagnostic and Therapeutic Bronchoscopy

10

Alexandra Pendrak, Corinna Sicoutris, and Steven Allen

10.1 Introduction

Gustav Killian, a German laryngologist, is considered to be the father of bronchoscopy. In Killian's early years of practice, he learned his technique with a laryngoscope on a servant in his own home. Prior to this, an instrument had not been inserted into the trachea due to its perceived vulnerability, and instrumenting beyond the bifurcation of the branching bronchi was not considered. He later perfected his practices on a janitor of a hospital in exchange for a small amount of money. This is where Killian discovered that it was possible to slide a tube into the trachea and advance it to the bronchi without causing bleeding. Killian reported these findings to the Society of Medical Doctors in Freiburg and was then presented with his first patient. On March 30, 1897, Killian first removed a foreign body from the right mainstem bronchus via the translaryngeal route [1]. Killian performed the first bronchoscopy using a Mikulicz-Rosenheim esophagoscope, which was only 25 cm long, and used it to remove a pork bone from the patient's right mainstem bronchus; notably, the bone could not be drawn through the lumen of the scope due to its narrow diameter of 8 mm so the bone was removed with forceps along with the tube [1]. In 1898 Killian was able to report three successful foreign body extractions at the Congress of the Southwest German Laryngologists at Eastertime in Heidelberg, which made Heidelberg the center for study of bronchoscopy. Since its early practice, bronchoscopy has evolved into a relatively safe and widely performed procedure that is performed in various inpatient and outpatient settings.

10.2 Types of Bronchoscopy

Bronchoscopy is an endoscopic procedure where an instrument is introduced into the airways and used to visualize the airways for diagnostic purposes and/or perform interventions for therapeutic purposes. The three main types of bronchoscopy relevant to the ICU provider are rigid bronchoscopy, flexible bronchoscopy, and virtual bronchoscopy.

Rigid bronchoscopy uses a rigid scope composed of an inflexible tube that encloses the telescope, light source, and channels through

A. Pendrak, MSN, ACNP-BC (✉)
Acute Care Nurse Practitioner, Department of Surgical Critical Care, 3522 Sunset Way, Huntingdon Valley, PA 19006, USA
e-mail: Alexandra.pendrak@uphs.upenn.edu

C. Sicoutris, MSN, ACNP-BC
Nurse Practitioner Department of Surgical Critical Care, Philadelphia, PA, USA

S. Allen, MD
Department of Traumatology, Surgical Critical Care, and Emergency Surgery, Philadelphia, PA, USA

D.A. Taylor et al. (eds.), *Interventional Critical Care*, DOI 10.1007/978-3-319-25286-5_10

which to work and has been used to visualize the proximal airways [2]. A rigid bronchoscope has large working channels that allow for large amounts of tissue removal such as removal of tumors. Rigid bronchoscopy has been described as the treatment of choice for hemoptysis [200 mL in 24 h], extraction of foreign bodies, biopsy of vascular tumors, dilation of tracheobronchial strictures, and placement of airway stents [3]. Rigid bronchoscopy is typically performed under general anesthesia in the operating room by a thoracic surgeon or interventional pulmonologist. Therefore, the procedures related to rigid bronchoscopy will be discussed only briefly in this chapter since they are not likely to be performed by the ICU provider.

Virtual bronchoscopy uses computer-generated pictures that are generated from computer tomography images. Virtual bronchoscopy is noninvasive and provides information about structures outside the airways such as lymph nodes. However, this form of bronchoscopy does not closely visualize mucosal abnormalities and it is not readily available for use. Like rigid bronchoscopy, this modality is not used within the ICU setting so discussion will be limited in this chapter.

Flexible bronchoscopy is the most common type of bronchoscopy and was first introduced for clinical use in 1968 as described by Sackner in 1975 [3]. Since its introduction, flexible bronchoscopy has innovated the management of a wide variety of respiratory conditions. Flexible bronchoscopy is generally performed with conscious sedation and is used to visualize the trachea, proximal airways, and segmental airways. A flexible bronchoscope contains cables that allow the tip of the scope to be flexed and extended, as well as a light source of working channel [4]. Flexible bronchoscopy is associated with fewer complications [5], is more comfortable [6], and exposes a greater proportion of the tracheobronchial tree to direct visualization than rigid bronchoscopy [7]. Because flexible bronchoscopy is the most likely form of bronchoscopy to be used in the ICU setting, it will be the primary focus of this chapter.

10.3 Indications for Bronchoscopy

10.3.1 Diagnostic Indications for Flexible Bronchoscopy

Some of the most common indications for diagnostic flexible bronchoscopy in the ICU are suspected airway obstruction, persistent atelectasis, and persistent infiltrate, as shown in Table 10.1. In patients with physical exam findings consistent with airway obstruction such as focal wheezing, abnormal pulmonary function tests, or abnormal radiologic findings, flexible bronchoscopy can be used to confirm an airway obstruction and identify the cause. In patients with persistent atelectasis, flexible bronchoscopy can be used to identify obstructing objects such as mucous plugs or foreign bodies. In patients that are unable to produce a sputum specimen for microbiological analysis, flexible bronchoscopy may be used to obtain a sample using bronchoalveolar lavage [8].

Additional indications for flexible diagnostic bronchoscopy in the ICU include hemoptysis, acute inhalation injury, or blunt chest trauma. Hemoptysis is a diagnostic indication for flexible bronchoscopy because it can identify or localize the source of bleeding. Acute inhalation injury is also a diagnostic indication for flexible bronchoscopy because it allows the provider to assess for carbonaceous debris, mucosal pallor, mucous ulceration, and mucosal erythema [9]. Blunt chest trauma is a diagnostic indication for flexible bronchoscopy because it assesses for possible lacerations of the airway, especially in the setting

Table 10.1 Bronchoscopy cart

Indications for diagnostic bronchoscopy in the ICU	Indications for therapeutic bronchoscopy in the ICU
Suspected airway obstruction	Atelectasis
Persistent atelectasis	Mucous accumulation
Persistent infiltrate	Foreign body
Hemoptysis	Endotracheal tube management
Acute inhalation injury	
Blunt chest trauma	

of pneumomediastinum and pneumothorax after trauma; furthermore, this allows the provider to visualize injuries to the membranous portion of the distal trachea or proximal mainstem bronchi and determine the severity of the injury [10].

10.3.2 Therapeutic Indications for Flexible Bronchoscopy

The most common therapeutic indications for flexible bronchoscopy in the ICU are atelectasis, mucous accumulation, foreign bodies, and endotracheal tube management. Mucous accumulation indicates therapeutic bronchoscopy for suctioning mucous through the working channel of the bronchoscope when it is severe enough to interfere with oxygenation/ventilation and results in severe atelectasis. Flexible bronchoscopy is indicated for removal of foreign bodies from the tracheobronchial tree using retrieval devices that can be passed through the working channel of the bronchoscope [11]. Another therapeutic indication for flexible bronchoscopy in the ICU is for endotracheal tube management as the bronchoscope can assist in insertion and confirm proper positioning of the tube [12].

10.4 Relative Contraindications

Bronchoscopy has the potential to cause tachycardia, bronchospasm, or hypoxemia. Therefore, bronchoscopy is *relatively* contraindicated in patients with active myocardial ischemia, decompensated heart failure, life-threatening cardiac arrhythmias, asthma, or COPD exacerbation. There is also a risk of bleeding associated with bronchoscopy but this is most likely with brushing, biopsy, or needle aspiration, which are less likely to be performed by providers in the ICU. Additional relative contraindications to be considered are patients with unstable cervical spine injuries and limited motion of the temporomandibular joint. Manipulation of the cervical spine for optimal visualization during bronchoscopy in patients with cervical spine injuries can result in spinal cord injury with any degree of extension [13]. Limited motion of the temporomandibular joint may result in difficulty with optimal positioning and visualization. Elevated intracranial pressure is a relative contraindication for bronchoscopy due to its potential to lead to intracranial hypertension and cause secondary brain injury due to localized cerebral ischemia and in some cases herniation [14].

10.5 Preparation for Procedure

In preparation for bronchoscopy, the provider must first consider the airway for the patient in regard to the optimal mode of entry of the bronchoscope. The provider must then consider the equipment necessary to successfully perform the procedure. We will focus our discussion on flexible bronchoscopy since this is the most widely used in the ICU setting. The necessary equipment for flexible bronchoscopy is commonly stored on a "bronchoscopy cart," as seen in Fig. 10.1, for quick and easy retrieval of all bronchoscopy tools in a timely manner. Other preparations must be

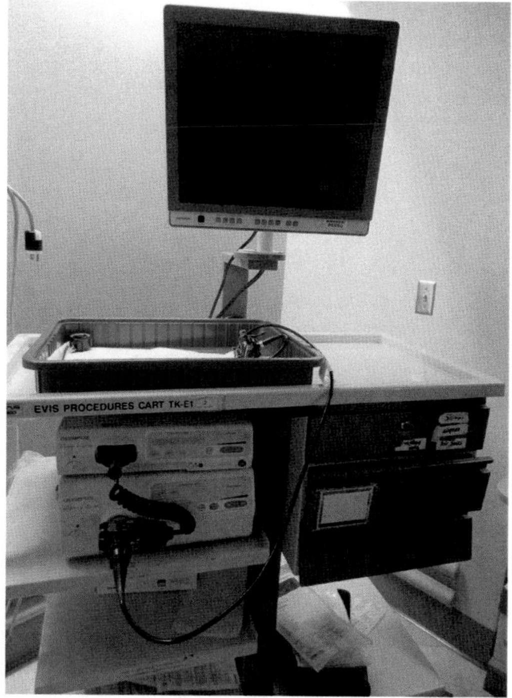

Fig. 10.1 Bronchoscopy cart

made, such as necessary monitoring with appropriate personnel and decisions for appropriate sedation and analgesia.

10.5.1 Airway

When performing either therapeutic or diagnostic bronchoscopy, the first consideration the provider must make is regarding the airway of the patient. When performing bronchoscopy on the non-intubated patient, a trans-oral approach may be taken with a bite block or a trans-nasal approach may be taken as an alternative. For intubated patients, the size of the endotracheal tube is an important consideration as the endotracheal tube should be at least 2 mm larger than the outer diameter of the bronchoscope in order to ensure adequate minute volume and to minimize barotrauma [15].

10.5.2 Personnel

The next consideration when performing bronchoscopy is the necessary personnel for successful completion of the procedure. In addition to the bronchoscopist, a nurse must be present for administration of pre-procedural medication to assist with pain control and relaxation that may consist of conscious sedation. A nurse must also be present for monitoring and recording of vital signs before, during, and after the procedure. It is also helpful for a technician, most often a respiratory therapist, to be present during a bronchoscopy for equipment setup, assistance during the procedure with collection of specimens, and cleaning the bronchoscope after the procedure. The resources and personnel available during bronchoscopy will be dependent on the standards set by individual institutions.

10.5.3 Equipment

A flexible bronchoscope is the most widely used instrument for bronchoscopy in the ICU setting. The flexible bronchoscope contains three parts: a control handle as seen in Fig. 10.2 and a flexible shaft and distal tip both seen in Fig. 10.3. The control handle is the part of the bronchoscope that is held by the bronchoscopist and contains a level to flex and extent the distal tip of the scope. The control handle also contains a suction opening and an opening through which instruments can be inserted. The distal tip of the bronchoscope is the portion that enters the patient's airway. It contains a camera and lighting component, as well as an

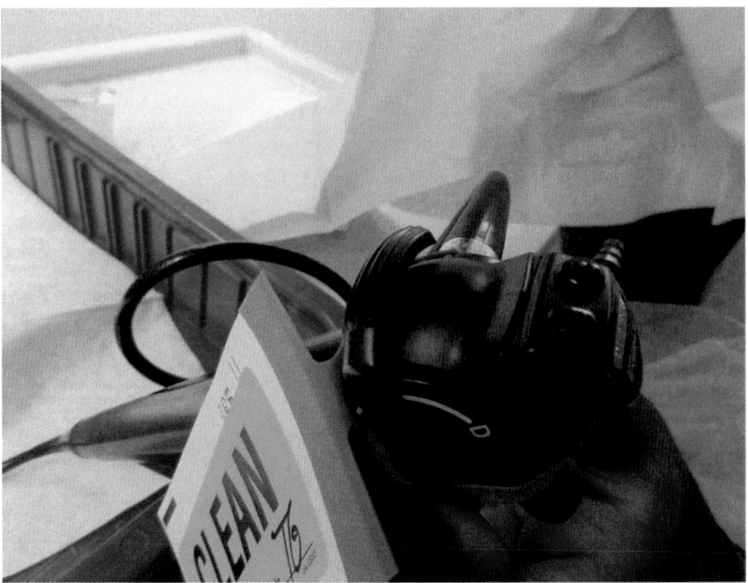

Fig. 10.2 Control handle

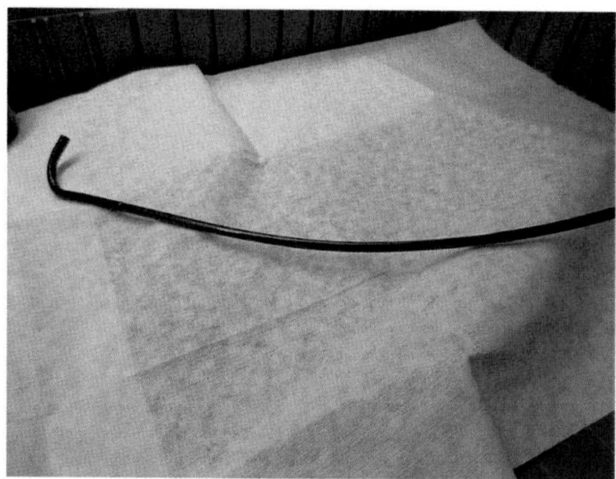

Fig. 10.3 Flexible shaft and distal tip

opening for instruments. Many flexible bronchoscopes contain a light source and image processor for fiber-optic transmission to a video processor for presentation of images. An alternative to the video-equipped flexible bronchoscope is a small portable flexible bronchoscope in which the light source is located on the scope, and an eyepiece on the handle is used to visualize the airway directly without a video monitor.

10.5.4 Premedication and Sedation

Topical lidocaine and nebulized lidocaine are two forms of topical anesthesia to consider for patient comfort when performing bronchoscopy. In the proper setting, sedation may also be considered for the comfort of the patient. A short-acting benzodiazepine such as midazolam and/or an opioid such as fentanyl are widely used agents for sedation. Lastly, the use of low-dose propofol has been established as a safe and effective form of sedation in bronchoscopy [16]. Credentials and privileges for the provider must be considered regarding the administration of mild, moderate, and conscious sedation prior to administration of sedation.

10.5.5 Other Supplies

It is helpful to consider other supplies that may be necessary when preparing for bronchoscopy so these items are readily available. A bite block is helpful when performing a bronchoscopy via the oral route in both intubated and non-intubated patients as patients' teeth may damage the bronchoscope in such a way that it may not be used until it's repaired and may prove to be very costly. Normal saline should be readily available for flushing, washing, or bronchoalveolar lavage (BAL). A specimen trap is also necessary, especially if performing BAL. Airway adjuncts such as bag valve mask, oral airways, nasal airways, and equipment for endotracheal intubation are essential, especially for non-intubated patients. Oral suction may also be a useful adjunct for managing a patient's airway. Resuscitative medications should always be available in case of hemodynamic instability.

10.5.6 Mechanical Ventilation and Oxygenation

During bronchoscopy, patients should be placed on 100 % fraction of inspired oxygen (FiO_2). Maintenance of positive end expiratory pressure (PEEP) should be considered to avoid alveolar derecruitment when performing bronchoscopy on intubated patients or patients with a tracheostomy tube. An adapter to connect the endotracheal tube or the tracheostomy appliance to a ventilator may be available to allow the flexible bronchoscope to be passed through the artificial airway and maintain PEEP.

10.6 Performing the Procedure

10.6.1 Entering the Tracheobronchial Tree

The bronchoscopist must first insert the flexible scope nasally or orally through a bite block for the non-intubated patient, or through an endotracheal tube or tracheostomy tube for the mechanically ventilated patient. In the non-intubated patient, after visualization of the vocal cords and assessment for movement, 1–2 mL of 1 % or 2 % lidocaine should be sprayed onto the vocal cords to suppress the cough reflex. If the patient is able to participate, the bronchoscopist should ask the patient to take a deep breath so that the distal tip of the bronchoscope can be passed into the trachea between the vocal cords while the patient inspires. Additional lidocaine can be sprayed inside the trachea in order to avoid coughing, anxiety, and tachypnea.

10.6.2 Airway Inspection

After passing the vocal cords, the bronchoscopist should examine the trachea, mainstem bronchi, and segmental bronchi. While initially examining the proximal airway, orientation must be established within the airway noting the cartilaginous trachea (anterior) and the membranous trachea (posterior) in order to determine left and right mainstem bronchi. The bronchoscopist must next examine and evaluate the mucosa for size, stability, and patency of the airway lumen. Assessment for mucous plugs, thick secretions, or foreign bodies within the airway is necessary in order to guide decision making for which further procedures would be most therapeutic for the patient.

10.6.3 Bronchoalveolar Lavage

BAL is the most common therapeutic procedure when performing bronchoscopy in the ICU. The bronchoscopist must first attach a specimen trap to the suction port on the bronchoscope and advance the bronchoscope until it gently wedges in a second- or third-generation segmental airway that leads to the lesion or area of interest for the bronchoscopy. Next, 20–50 mL of sterile saline is instilled into the working channel, followed by immediate application of suction to aspirate the saline. Only about half of the instilled saline will be recovered, and this sample can be sent for Gram stain and microbial culture for speciation in the case of suspected infection.

10.6.4 Bronchial Washing

Bronchial washing is a similar procedure to BAL but is less precise and does not focus on one specific airway segment. Furthermore, bronchial washing does not require the bronchoscope to be wedged and requires instillation of smaller volume of sterile saline (10–20 mL) to be instilled into the working channel. As in BAL, the saline is quickly aspirated into a specimen trap and can be sent for Gram stain and speciation. However, bronchial washing usually is contaminated by oral flora and not accurate for determining differential cell count.

10.6.5 Other Diagnostic Procedures

Bronchial brushing, endobronchial biopsy, transbronchial biopsy, and needle aspiration are diagnostic procedures that are usually performed by a thoracic surgeon or interventional pulmonologist. These procedures require certain privileges and are not likely to be performed routinely in the ICU and are beyond the scope of this chapter.

10.6.6 Post-procedure Monitoring for Complications

The patient's alertness and vital signs must be monitored until the effects of sedation have resolved, which may vary greatly depending on the methods for analgesia and sedation. The patient must be closely monitored for fatal complications such as respiratory arrest from hemorrhage and cardiac arrest from acute myocardial infarction. Some serious complications that must be considered are hypotension, bronchospasm, laryngospasm, pneumothorax, epistaxis due to nasal approach, fever, pneumonia, and vasovagal reactions. Bronchoscopy carries an overall complication rate between 0.08 and 1.08 % with pneumothorax rate of 0.16 %, hemorrhage rate of 0.12 %, and respiratory failure rate of 0.2 % [17]. Bronchoscopy mortality is extremely rare at a rate of 0.013 %, with this mortality being associated with heart disease or severe airway obstruction [18]. One must obtain a chest X-ray (usually portable) after the bronchoscopy to evaluate for the presence of a pneumothorax and hemothorax and to ensure proper endotracheal tube or tracheostomy appliance position for the patient with an artificial airway.

10.7 Conclusion

Bronchoscopy is a well-established and relatively safe procedure used frequently in the intensive care unit by both physicians and advanced practitioners. Bronchoscopy may be performed in intubated and non-intubated patients for diagnostic and/or therapeutic purposes. One must ensure safety, proper credentialing, and available personnel and monitoring when considering the appropriate analgesia and sedation for the procedure. While considered safe, one must ensure safety before, during, and after bronchoscopy to minimize morbidity and mortality and optimize the results of the procedure.

References

1. Zollner F. Gustav Killian, father of bronchoscopy. Arch Otolaryngol. 1965;82(6):656–9.
2. Bolliger CT, Mathur PN, Beamis JF, Becker HD, Cavaliere S, Colt H, et al. ERS/ATS statement on interventional pulmonology. European Respiratory Society/American Thoracic Society. Eur Respir J. 2002;19(2):356–73.
3. Sackner MA. Bronchofiberscopy. Am Rev Respir Dis. 1975;111(1):62–88.
4. Feinsilver SH, Fein A. Textbook of bronchoscopy. Baltimore, MD: Williams & Wilkins; 1995.
5. Pereira Jr W, Kovnat DM, Snider GL. A prospective cooperative study of complications following flexible fiberoptic bronchoscopy. Chest. 1978;73(6):813–6.
6. Rath GS, Schaff JT, Snider GL. Flexible fiberoptic bronchoscopy. Techniques and review of 100 bronchoscopies. Chest. 1973;63(5):689–93.
7. Kovnat DM, Rath GS, Anderson WM, Snider G. Maximal extent of visualization of bronchial tree by flexible fiberoptic bronchoscopy. Am Rev Respir Dis. 1974;110(1):88–90.
8. van der Eerden MM, Vlaspolder F, de Graaff CS, Groot T, Jansen HM, Boersma WG. Value of intensive diagnostic microbiological investigation in low- and high-risk patients with community-acquired pneumonia. Eur J Clin Microbiol Infect Dis. 2005;24(4):241–9.
9. American Burn Association. Inhalation injury: diagnosis. J Am Coll Surg. 2003;196(2):307–12.
10. Chu CP, Chen PP. Tracheobronchial injury secondary to blunt chest trauma: diagnosis and management. Anaesth Intensive Care. 2002;30(2):145–52.
11. Limper AH, Prakash UB. Tracheobronchial foreign bodies in adults. Ann Intern Med. 1990;112(8):604–9.
12. Dellinger RP. Fiberoptic bronchoscopy in adult airway management. Crit Care Med. 1990;18(8):882–7.
13. Hagberg C, Georgi R, Krier C. Complications of managing the airway. Best Pract Res Clin Anaesthesiol. 2005;19(4):641–59.
14. Kerwin AJ, Croce MA, Timmons SD, Maxwell RA, Malhotra AK, Fabian TC. Effects of fiberoptic bronchoscopy on intracranial pressure in patients with brain injury: a prospective clinical study. J Trauma. 2000;48(5):878–82. discussion 882–3.
15. Tai DY. Bronchoscopy in the intensive care unit (ICU). Ann Acad Med Singapore. 1998;27(4):552–9.
16. Grendelmeier P, Tamm M, Pflimlin E, Stolz D. Propofol sedation for flexible bronchoscopy: a randomised, non-inferiority trial. Eur Respir J. 2014;43(2):591–601.
17. Pue CA, Pacht ER. Complications of fiberoptic bronchoscopy at a university hospital. Chest. 1995;107(2):430–2.
18. Jin F, Mu D, Chu D, Fu E, Xie Y, Liu T. Severe complications of bronchoscopy. Respiration. 2008;76(4):429–33.

Part III

Vascular Access Procedures

11 Arterial Access/Monitoring (Line Placement)

Sue M. Nyberg, Daniel J. Bequillard, and Donald G. Vasquez

11.1 Introduction

Cannulation of an artery for the purpose of monitoring a patient's hemodynamic status is a common procedure in the critical care environment [1–4]. Descriptions of arterial cannulation appeared in the literature in the late 1940s through the early 1960s when Barr first described the use of an indwelling Teflon catheter in the radial artery to continuously measure blood pressure [5–7]. Continuous measurement of blood pressure through an arterial line is considered to be the most accurate measurement of systemic blood pressure and is the most common form of invasive monitoring [1, 4]. In addition to monitoring of blood pressure, the arterial line may also be used for phlebotomy when frequent laboratory studies are needed, reducing the need for repeated peripheral blood draws. Advanced practice clinicians working in the ICU commonly perform arterial cannulation [8] and therefore should have knowledge of indications and contraindications, relevant anatomy, technique, and potential complications from the procedure [1, 9].

S.M. Nyberg, MHS, PA-C (✉) • D.J. Bequillard, MPAS, PA-C • D.G. Vasquez, DO, MPH
Department of Physician Assistant, Wichita State University, Wichita, KS, USA
e-mail: Sue.Nyberg@wichita.edu

11.2 Indications

Insertion of an indwelling line into an artery is indicated in the following situations:

- Need for continuous monitoring of blood pressure in a patient with hypotension/hemodynamic instability.
- Patient receiving vasoactive medications.
- Inability to accurately monitor blood pressure by noninvasive technique (e.g., morbidly obese patient or patient with severe burns or trauma to the extremities).
- Patient requiring frequent arterial blood gases or venous blood samples (e.g., patient in respiratory failure, on mechanical ventilation or with a severe acid/base disturbance).
- To measure mean arterial pressure (MAP) when targeting a specific level is indicated (e.g., to maintain cerebral perfusion pressure following head injury) [9–12].

11.2.1 Site Selection

There are several arterial sites that may be used in the adult patient, including the radial, femoral, axillary, brachial, and dorsalis pedis [3]. The radial artery is most commonly used because of its proximity to the skin surface, ease of access, and low rate of complications [10, 13–15]. Measurement of mean arterial blood pressure in

D.A. Taylor et al. (eds.), *Interventional Critical Care*, DOI 10.1007/978-3-319-25286-5_11

radial or femoral arteries is clinically interchangeable. However, in severely hypotensive patients or during cardiopulmonary resuscitation, the femoral artery is usually the most readily palpable and accessible for successful cannulation [10]. There are no clinically significant differences in measurement of blood pressure between the radial and femoral artery, and it is not mandatory to cannulate the femoral artery, even in critically ill patients receiving high doses of vasoactive drugs [2].

Long-standing practice protocols have recommended that a patient undergoing radial or dorsalis pedis artery cannulation should have collateral flow to extremity assessed by physical examination (e.g., Allen's test), Doppler ultrasound, or pulse oximetry (modified Allen's test) [13] prior to procedure to identify potential increased risk for ischemic complication in the extremity [16]. However, several research studies conclude that the Allen's test was not useful in predicting the rare ischemic event following radial artery cannulation [4, 17, 18].

11.2.2 Anatomic Considerations

- Radial artery
  - The radial artery can be palpated just medial to the radial styloid and approximately 1–2 cm proximal to the flexor crease of the wrist. The puncture site should be approx. 1 cm proximal to the styloid process so as to keep from puncturing the transverse carpal ligament [12].
  - Collateral circulation to the hand is provided by the ulnar artery and palmar arch [3].
- Femoral
  - The femoral artery originates from the external iliac artery at the inguinal ligament. It passes under the ligament at approximately the midpoint between the anterior superior iliac spine and the pubis. It lies between the femoral nerve (laterally) and the femoral vein and lymphatics (medially) [3, 12].
  - The larger vessel diameter allows for greater longevity of the catheter compared to the radial artery [3].
  - To minimize risk for bleeding into the pelvis, the femoral artery should be accessed approximately 2.5 cm below the inguinal ligament [12].
- Dorsalis pedis
  - Although the dorsalis pedis is also relatively superficial, it may be absent (typically bilaterally) in up to 12 % of the population [10].
- Brachial
- The brachial artery can be palpated at the medial border of the antecubital fossa and is typically accessed above the antecubital crease. This artery is rarely used because of the lack of extensive collateral circulation [3]. Reported complications include ischemic occlusion and median nerve injury [3, 19].

11.3 Contraindications

Absolute contraindications (extremity cannulation): [1, 10, 12]

- Absent pulse
- Ischemic extremity
- Raynaud's syndrome
- Thromboangiitis obliterans (Buerger's disease)
- Preexisting inadequate collateral blood flow distally to the extremity
- Full-thickness burns over the cannulation site

Relative contraindications: [1, 10, 12, 20]

- Anticoagulant therapy
- Severe atherosclerosis
- Bleeding disorder
- Severe dermatitis or infection at the cannulation site
- Partial-thickness burn at the cannulation site
- Previous surgery in the area
- Synthetic vascular graft

11.4 Preparation

Insertion of an arterial line is commonly performed at the patient's bedside. After obtaining appropriate informed consent, all supplies should be gathered. The APC should ensure that appropriate informed consent is obtained from the patient/family. Prior to the procedure, a "time-out" assures correct patient identification and site selection. Full universal precautions with mask, hat, sterile gown, and gloves should be implemented by the operator, as this procedure involves potential exposure to blood (Fig. 11.1).

Equipment
- Sterile towels or drape
- 1 % lidocaine without epinephrine
- Sterile 5 cc syringe with 23 gauge needle
- Gauze pads
- Arm board
- Tape
- Chlorhexidine or povidone-iodine skin preparation solution
- Integrated arterial line kits (femoral or radial)
- Number 11 blade scalpel
- Nonabsorbable suture (3–0 or 4–0)
- Needle holder, scissors
- Occlusive dressing
- Chlorhexidine gluconate dressing (e.g., Biopatch©)

Nursing supplies
- Three-way stopcock
- Pressure transducer kit
- Pressure tubing

11.5 Procedure

There are three ways to obtain arterial cannulation: Seldinger technique [21], modified Seldinger technique using integrated kits (Fig. 11.2), and direct puncture cannulation, e.g., with an intravenous catheter [16]. For the purposes of this chapter, only the modified Seldinger technique will be described.

There is evidence that ultrasound guidance, if available, improves rate of successful cannula-

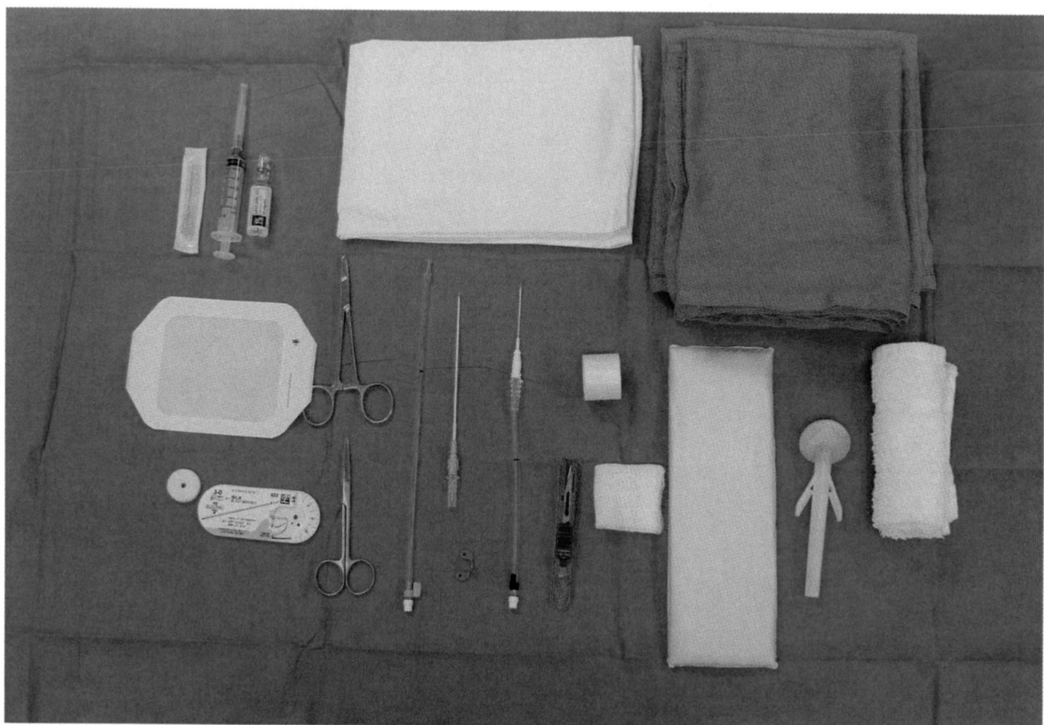

Fig. 11.1 Equipment for arterial access

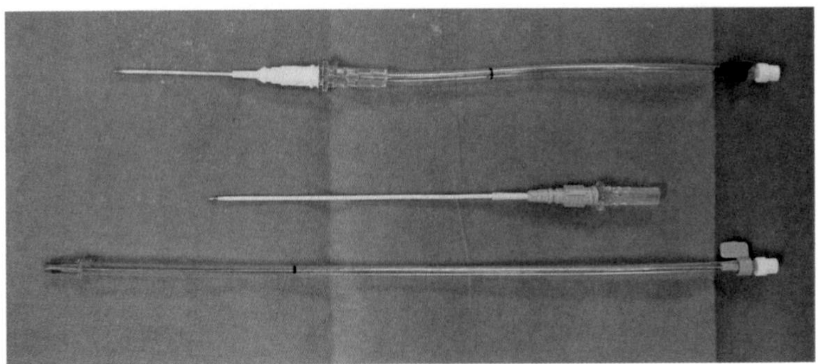

Fig. 11.2 Integrated arterial access kit

tion at first attempt [22], especially if the patient is in shock, receiving vasoconstrictive medications, or morbidly obese.

11.5.1 Radial Artery

For the radial site, the patient is usually supine or semi-recumbent. The wrist is positioned in slight dorsiflexion, with the palm up. The hand can be taped to a flat surface, such as an armboard or a bedside table. A small towel may help in the extension of the wrist (Fig. 11.3). Preparation of the arm should cover the entire ventral aspect of the forearm, as the cannulation can occur wherever the pulse is best felt along the course of the radial artery, but usually occurs just proximal to the radial styloid process at the wrist. The area is draped widely with towels, as the devices can be unwieldy due to their length, and contact with non-sterile surfaces is to be avoided.

Local infiltration with lidocaine is carried out by injecting a small weal at the anticipated puncture site. A small nick with the number 11 scalpel may facilitate passing of the needle. The operator should assume a position that allows the nondominant hand to palpate the pulse proximally and the dominant hand holding the integrated arterial catheterization device pointing proximally, at about a 30–45° angle to the surface of the forearm (Fig. 11.4).

The pulse is palpated gently by the nondominant hand so as to prevent occlusion of the target site. The needle is advance until pulsatile blood return is seen to readily enter the device. The nondominant hand then steadies the device, as it is important to maintain the needle tip inside the artery lumen. The wire is advanced into the artery lumen. Little to no resistance should be felt throughout the course of the wire advancing. Once the wire is in place, the catheter is advanced over the wire, and the needle and wire are removed together. Pulsatile flow should be seen from the catheter at this point, which is attached to the pressurized system for flushing and monitoring. Suturing of the catheter hub to the skin can now occur and ideally should be done with the local anesthetic previously injected. Following placement of a chlorhexidine gluconate dressing (e.g., Biopatch©) and locally occlusive dressing (Fig. 11.5), additional gauze dressing may be applied around the wrist and forearm to reduce likelihood of accidental dislodgement. Assess for continuing adequate distal circulation and document that the hand remains pink and warm (Fig. 11.6).

11.5.2 Femoral Artery

The approach to the femoral artery by necessity involves a supine patient with the selected leg in slight adduction and external rotation. The area prepared should be well above the inguinal fold, down to mid-thigh, and from the medial to the lateral aspects of the thigh and is similarly draped with towels.

Ultrasound guidance is particular useful in locating the femoral vessels. The acronym "NAVL" reminds the operator of the order of

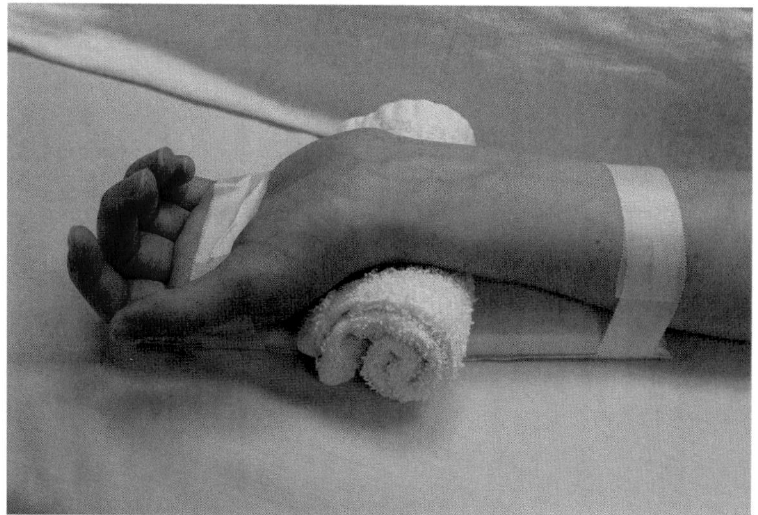

Fig. 11.3 Use of a towel roll for wrist extension

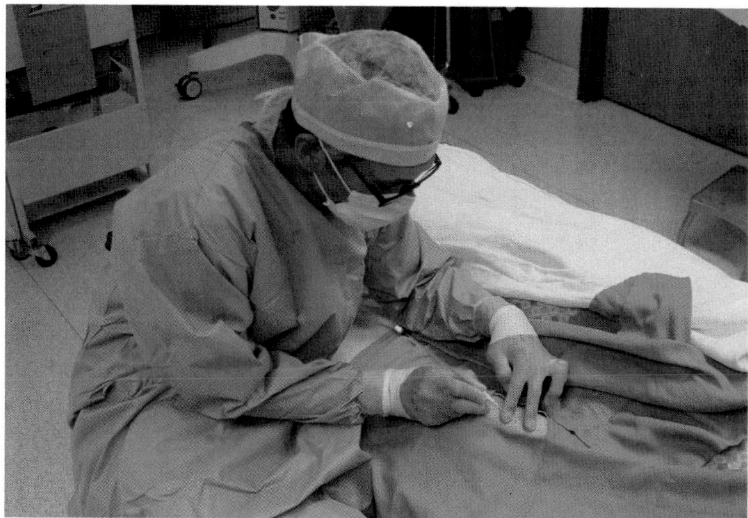

Fig. 11.4 Operator positioning for arterial access

arrangement of the femoral neurovascular bundle from lateral to medial (nerve, artery, vein, lymphatics). The nondominant hand palpates the pulse at or just below the inguinal crease, and the dominant hand guides the integrated device over the pulse, to a point approximately one to two fingerbreadths below the inguinal fold, advancing the needle at about a 45–60° angle (Fig. 11.7). A skin nick with the number 11 blade facilitates passage of the 18-ga needle-catheter-integrated device. Once blood return is obtained, insertion of the catheter proceeds similar to the radial approach, as do the securing and dressing of the catheter (Fig. 11.8). An additional suture may be placed at the other side of the hub of the pressure tubing to prevent "kinking" of the line with patient movement.

11.6 Complications

The decision to place an arterial line for patient monitoring should always be made considering the risk/benefit ratio for each patient. In the criti-

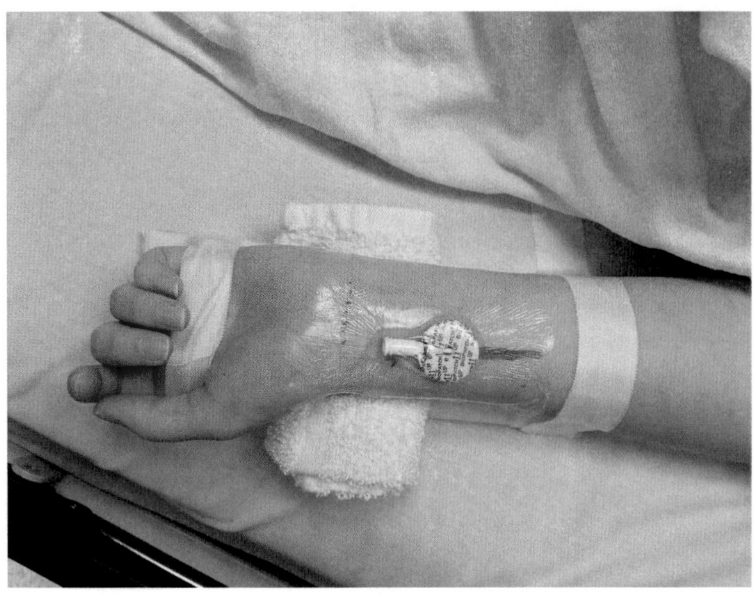

Fig. 11.5 Dressings for arterial cannulation

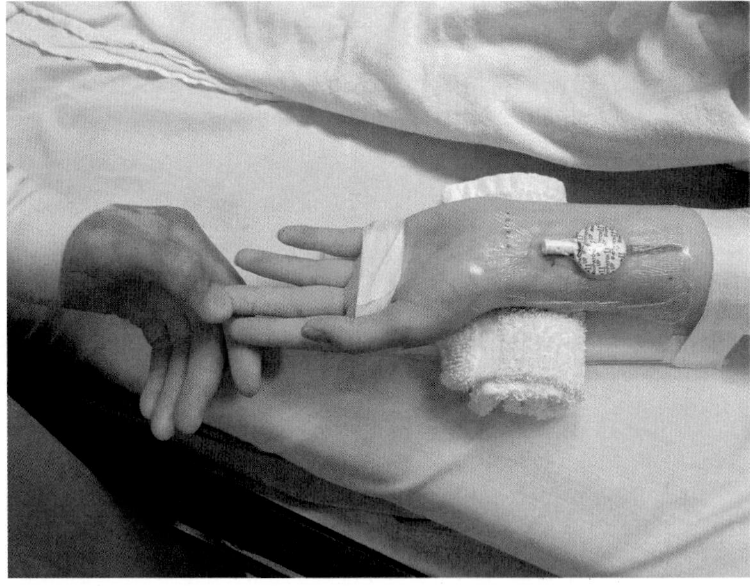

Fig. 11.6 Assessment of peripheral circulation following arterial line placement

cally ill patient, the need for accurate and timely information about respiratory and hemodynamic status may outweigh the risks based on relative contraindications. As with all invasive procedures, accurate monitoring of patient status and response is vital. A higher rate of ischemic complications has been documented in patients with preexisting vascular disease such as Raynaud's syndrome or Buerger's disease, thus the reason for listing these conditions as absolute contraindications [1, 16].

According to Scheer et al., the incidence rate for major complication (sepsis, pseudoaneurysm, or permanent ischemia) from cannulation of the radial, femoral, or axillary artery is low, occurring in less than 1 % of cases [14]. Although this clinical

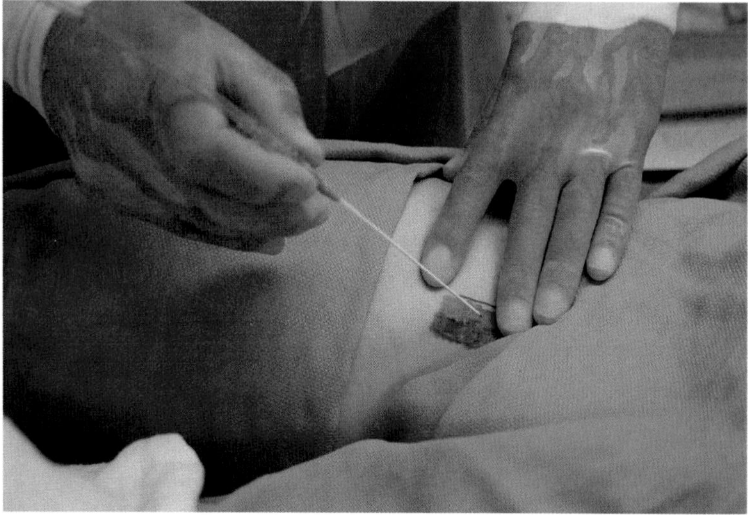

Fig. 11.7 Placement technique for femoral arterial access with arterial landmark (*red*) and venous landmark (*blue*) noted

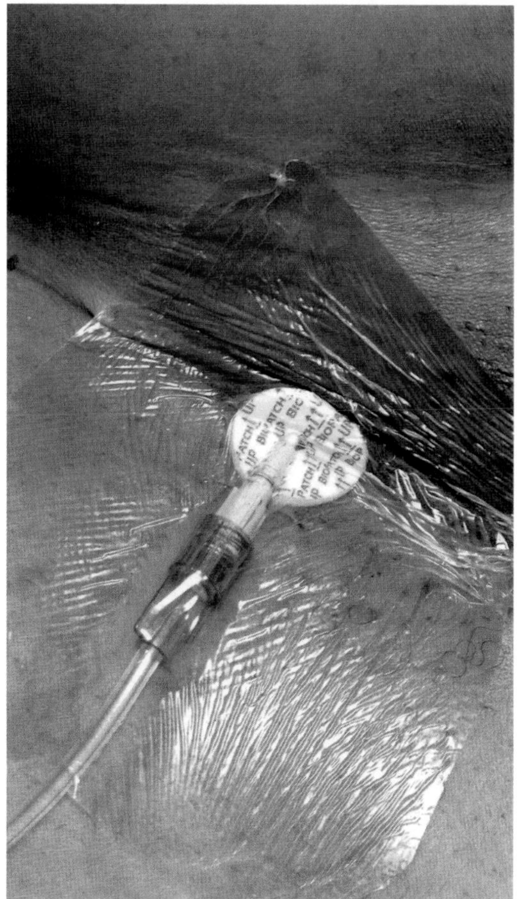

Fig. 11.8 Securing and dressing of the femoral arterial line

review indicates that arterial cannulation is generally a safe procedure, the APC should be aware of the potential complications that can occur.

Common Complications

- *Temporary arterial occlusion*
- *Hematoma*

The most common complications following radial artery cannulation include *temporary* occlusion of the artery (19.7 %) and hematoma (14.4 %). For the femoral artery, the most common complication is hematoma (6 %) followed by bleeding and temporary occlusion (both less than 2 %). Local site infections and sepsis have been reported but the incidence is generally low, and higher incidence is reported with prolonged use (generally beyond 4 days) [14]. A large study of patients in intensive care found no significant difference in infection rates between femoral and radial artery catheters [18].

Rare (<2 %) Complications: [1, 10, 12, 14]

- *Aneurysm or pseudoaneurysm (pulsatile mass)*
- *Arterial thrombosis (risk increases with longer duration of use and smaller diameter of artery)*
- *Cerebral air embolization (due to manual flushing)*

- *Significant blood loss (port valve is left open or tubing is disconnected)*
- *Nerve injury*
- *Permanent ischemic damage*
- *Artery dissection*

In summary, a large body of research suggests that arterial cannulation is a safe procedure with a very low incidence of complication.

11.7 Conclusions

Insertion of an arterial line for accurate monitoring of systemic blood pressure and to allow for frequent blood sampling is a common procedure in the intensive care unit with few complications when the patient is appropriately selected. Cannulation of the radial and femoral arteries is the most common; cannulation of the brachial or axillary artery is rare and would typically only be performed by anesthesia providers in the operating suite.

Acknowledgment The authors would like to acknowledge Wesley Medical Center, Wichita, Kansas, for their assistance in providing supplies and assistance with photographs.

References

1. Tiru BBJ, McGee WT. Radial artery cannulation: a review article. J Anesth Clin Res. 2012;3(5):1000209.
2. Mignini MA, Piacentini E, Dubin A. Peripheral arterial blood pressure monitoring adequately tracks central arterial blood pressure in critically ill patients: an observational study. Crit Care. 2006;10(2):R43.
3. Cousins TR, O'Donnell JM. Arterial cannulation: a critical review. AANA J. 2004;72(4):267–71.
4. Bowdle TA. Complications of invasive monitoring. Anesthesiol Clin North America. 2002;20(3):571–88.
5. Peterson LH, Dripps RD, Risman GC. A method for recording the arterial pressure pulse and blood pressure in man. Am Heart J. 1949;37(5):771–82.
6. Peirce II EC. Percutaneous femoral artery catheterization in man with special reference to aortography. Surg Gynecol Obstet. 1951;93(1):56–74.
7. Barr PO. Percutaneous puncture of the radial artery with a multi-purpose Teflon catheter for indwelling use. Acta Physiol Scand. 1961;51:343–7.
8. Nyberg SM, Keuter KR, Berg GM, Helton AM, Johnston AD. Acceptance of physician assistants and nurse practitioners in trauma centers. JAAPA. 2010;23(1):35–7. 41.
9. Tegtmeyer K, Brady G, Lai S, Hodo R, Braner D. Videos in clinical medicine. Placement of an arterial line. N Engl J Med. 2006;354(15), e13.
10. Fowler GC. LDA. Arterial puncture and percutaneous arterial line placement. 3rd ed. Philadelphia, PA: Elsevier Mosby; 2011.
11. Hignett R, Stephens R. Radial arterial lines. Br J Hosp Med (Lond). 2006;67(5):M86–8.
12. Freeman CJ EA. Arterial line placement. Medscape; 2014 [updated 3 June, 14 July 2014]. Available from: http://emedicine.medscape.com/article/1999586-overview.
13. Brzezinski M, Luisetti T, London MJ. Radial artery cannulation: a comprehensive review of recent anatomic and physiologic investigations. Anesth Analg. 2009;109(6):1763–81.
14. Scheer B, Perel A, Pfeiffer UJ. Clinical review: complications and risk factors of peripheral arterial catheters used for haemodynamic monitoring in anaesthesia and intensive care medicine. Crit Care. 2002;6(3):199–204.
15. Chaparro MK. Radial artery catheterism for invasive monitoring: preventing complications, a challenge in anesthesia. Colombian J Anesthesiol. 2012;40(4):262–5.
16. Arterial catheterization techniques for invasive monitoring [Internet]. Retrieved from: "http://www.uptodate.com/contents/arterial-catheterization-techniques-for-invasive-monitoring?source=machineLearning&search=arterial+catheterization+techniques&selectedTitle=1%7E150§ionRank=1&anchor=H3" \l "H3.
17. Slogoff S, Keats AS, Arlund C. On the safety of radial artery cannulation. Anesthesiology. 1983;59(1):42–7.
18. Frezza EE, Mezghebe H. Indications and complications of arterial catheter use in surgical or medical intensive care units: analysis of 4932 patients. Am Surg. 1998;64(2):127–31.
19. C. OC. Essential clinical procedures. 3rd ed. Philadelphia, PA. London: Elsevier/Saunders; 2013.
20. Mitchell JD, Welsby IJ. Techniques of arterial access. Surgery. 2004;22(1):3–4.
21. Seldinger SI. Catheter replacement of the needle in percutaneous arteriography. A new technique. Acta Radiol Suppl. 2008;434:47–52.
22. Shiloh AL, Savel RH, Paulin LM, Eisen LA. Ultrasound-guided catheterization of the radial artery: a systematic review and meta-analysis of randomized controlled trials. Chest. 2011;139(3):524–9.

12 Central Venous Catheterization With and Without Ultrasound Guidance

Ryan O'Gowan

12.1 Overview

Central venous catheter (CVC) placement is the most commonly performed procedure in the ICU with over 5 million CVC lines being placed each year in the USA alone. CVC lines first began utilization in early 1966 [1]. Their use and implementation are ubiquitous in the ICU, and routine placement has become a part of many care bundles, including early goal-directed therapy (EGDT) for sepsis. Moreover, CVC lines have become an integral part in the management of the critically ill, with CVP monitoring being a significant factor for placement [2]. They are required for a number of vasopressors, inotropic agents, antibiotics, and medications which may pose a risk of extravasation. The first reported use of ultrasound (US) technology to aid in the cannulation was in 1984. Although initially there was a lack of adoption of this vital technology, a recent survey among resident physicians has found a utilization rate of 90 % in the internal jugular site with US guidance becoming the *sine qua non* for CVC placement [3, 4]. Prior to the widespread adoption of US technology, clinicians had a significant failure rate using traditional anatomic landmarks with some authors citing a failure rate of 19.4 % [5]. Lastly, even in highly experienced operators, reliance on traditional landmark techniques may result in a sixfold increase in complication rate when more than three attempts are made at vascular access in a given site (Subclavian, Internal Jugular) [6].

R. O'Gowan, MBA, PA-C, FCCM (✉)
Surgical Critical Care, St. Vincent Hospital, Worcester, MA, USA
e-mail: ryanogowan@gmail.com

12.2 Review of Ultrasound Technology

Traditional ultrasound techniques include the use of a linear array probe and B-mode (brightness mode) ultrasound. This is in contrast to other types of probes (phased array) and modes (M or motion mode) used for indications other than CVC placement. The ultrasound machine utilizes a piezoelectric effect to utilize energy along the ultrasound crystal array to create an image of the anatomic structure of interest. Typically frequencies for procedural use operate in the range of 2–15 MHz. Variables that may be controlled include the depth and gain to create a clearer image for CVC placement. Additionally, the views utilized may consist of short axis views, long axis views, or a combination (biplanar) approach [7]. There has been some debate over the superiority of the short axis approach as opposed to the long axis approach for vessel cannulation. However, a prospective randomized study showed that success rates in the short axis group, while higher, were not statistically significant [8].

D.A. Taylor et al. (eds.), *Interventional Critical Care*, DOI 10.1007/978-3-319-25286-5_12

Although there is less of a difference in short axis vs. long axis techniques, success rates for US vs. traditional landmark techniques are drastically different with one author citing success rates of 93.9 % with US in comparison to 78.5 % using landmarks alone. Further techniques to provide for a more optimal US image of the needle include placing the bevel side down so as to be in the plane of the US transducer and the use of commercially available echogenic needle tips. Lastly, commercial needle guides may be available for utilization to facilitate optimal needle placement with an incidence angle of 30–45°.

12.3 Indications

Owing to its ubiquitous use in the critical care environment, there are a multitude of indications for the placement of a CVC catheter [9]. Hemodynamic monitoring is one of the most frequent reasons. Interestingly, some complications in SC CVC placement may actually be lower than PICC catheters. One study found that rates of thrombophlebitis were lower in SC CVC catheters when the reason for placement was TPN administration [10]. Common indications for CVC placement are outlined as follows in Table 12.1:

12.4 Contraindications

Common contraindications for CVC placement are outlined as follows in Table 12.2:

Table 12.1

Intravenous fluid administration
Hemodynamic monitoring
Total parenteral nutrition
Drug or blood product administration
Hypertonic electrolyte administration
Insertion of temporary pacing wires
Swan-Ganz catheterization
Hemodialysis access
Aspiration of air emboli

Table 12.2

Coagulopathy or TPA administration
Obstructing clot in central vein
Preexisting indwelling port or chemotherapy catheter
Pacemaker or AICD

12.5 Anatomic Locations for Catheterization and Procedure Without US Guidance

Typical anatomic locations for CVC placement include the internal jugular vein, subclavian vein, and femoral vein. Although other sites may be utilized for the placement of peripherally inserted central catheters (PICCs), their discussion is outside of the purview of this chapter and is discussed elsewhere.

Internal Jugular Site The internal jugular vein may be found beneath the digastric belly of the sternocleidomastoid muscle. The classic landmarks which delineate the borders of the carotid triangle include the sternocleidomastoid, trapezius, and the clavicle inferiorly. Traditionally, in a nonultrasound approach of the right internal jugular vein, the clinician may palpate the carotid pulse medially with their nondominant hand and insert a smaller finder needle laterally and aim at a 45° needle, inserting it in the direction of the ipsilateral nipple. It is important to initially start higher on the neck for a number of reasons. First, the internal jugular vein courses from a lateral position to the carotid to more of an anterior relationship to the vein as the internal jugular approaches the base of the neck. This relationship predisposes to possible inadvertent cannulation of the carotid artery or hematoma if posterior wall puncture (PWP) occurs. The avoidance of PWP is of tantamount importance in the placement of large bore hemodialysis CVC catheters in this site, owing to the larger dilators that are employed [11–13]. Secondly, the risk of pneumothorax increases as the insertion site moves further toward the base of the neck as the longer cannulation needle may actually penetrate the apex of the lung, which may be extended to the space above the clavicle. Relative advantages of the internal jugular vein for CVC placement include ease of access and readily visible landmarks. Relative disadvantages for CVC placement in this location include pooling of oropharyngeal secretions in intubated patients, difficulty in placing an occlusive dressing, and potential for airway compromise in the event of carotid hematoma. Failure and complication rates for traditional placement techniques in experienced vs. inexperienced operators have been listed as 11.7 % and 17.6 %, respectively [14]. In an observational study conducted in the ED setting, US in the IJ site was still safer in inexperienced operators as opposed to the SC site with a failure rate of 10 %. In that same study, complication rates of hematomas and arterial punctures were listed as 7 % and 2 %, respectively [15, 16]. Moreover, the use of ultrasound has been associated with a higher success rate (93.9 % vs. 78.5 %) and a reduced time for placement when compared with the traditional landmark technique [17–19].

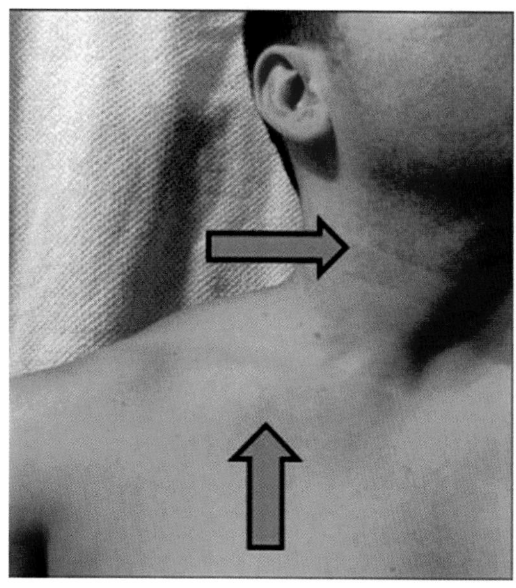

Fig. 12.1 Anatomic landmarks for IJ/SCV. Note position of clavicle/IJ points. Courtesy of the author with thanks to Saurab Joshi, MD for vessel cannulation and procedural expertise

Subclavian Site The subclavian vein may be found beneath the clavicle at the transition point between the proximal and middle third at the clavicle at the midclavicular line. Of note, the clinician may palpate this site and feel a firmness which signifies the ligament of Halsted. The optimal site of cannulation of the subclavian vein is laterally and inferiorly to this location on the clavicle (Fig. 12.1). After appropriate cleansing, anesthetic placement, and draping, the clinician may enter the skin with the needle at a thirty degree angle. With the nonneedle hand, once the needle is in the skin, the clinician then provides gentle downward pressure over the needle with their thumb and slowly advances toward the sternal notch and the contralateral shoulder. Gentle aspiration is performed until a venous flash occurs. In the event that the clinician directs the needle more caudally, they may encounter a bright red arterial flash. Additionally, great care should be taken as the risk of pneumothorax is significantly higher in this anatomic site. Loss of negative pressure on the syringe may signify entry into the pleural space and subsequent pneumothorax. For patients who are intubated, clinical signs of tension pneumothorax include an increase in peak inspiratory pressures, loss of tidal volumes, or an increase in respiratory rate. Physical examination may reveal jugular venous distention or loss of breath sounds. As with the internal jugular site, failure and complication rates for traditional placement techniques in experienced vs. inexperienced operators with the subclavian site have been listed as 7.5 % and 15 %, respectively [20]. A more detailed study of the subclavian site showed a pneumothorax rate of 2.5 % and an overall complication rate of 5.5 % [21]. Complications listed included tip misplacement, arterial puncture, inability to locate the vessel, and hemothorax. Interestingly, US guidance using either SA or LA approaches in the SC site has failed to show any meaningful reduction in complication rates [22, 23].

Femoral Site The femoral vein may be located medial to the femoral artery and below the inguinal ligament. Traditionally the clinician thoroughly cleanses the groin, drapes the patient, and anesthetizes the soft tissue. Palpating the femoral pulse, the clinician inserts the needle and syringe medially, in contradistinction to the internal jugular vein which is lateral to the pulse. Of note, it is important to cannulate the vessel below the inguinal crease, as placement above the crease may cause the needle to be inserted inadvertently into the peritoneum. Moreover, placement in an extreme medial position may cause for entry into the extralymphatic or lymphatic space. The femoral site is traditionally a site of last resort, owing to the high likelihood of contamination, vis-à-vis the groin. Instances in which the femoral site is advantageous include patients who may be coagulopathic. Although there have been few studies that specifically review the femoral vein as a primary cannulation site of choice, one study exploring US-guided cannulation in this site did show a significantly reduced number of venipuncture attempts (2.3 vs. 5.0; $P=0.0057$) and rate of complications (0 % vs. 20 %; $P=0.025$) [7]. Recall that subclavian sites may be dangerous in this case as inadvertent puncture of the subclavian artery may lead to massive hemothorax, owing to the non-compressibility of the subclavian artery. Lastly, in the event that femoral cannulation is required, it is the personal experience of the author that these femoral central venous catheters remain in place for no more than 24 h, until a definitive CVC is placed in an alternate location. Traditionally, femoral vein CVC placement is a location of last resort.

12.6 Implementation of US Guidance for CVC Placement

Ultrasound has found an expansion in utilization owing to its relatively inexpensive cost, lack of ionizing radiation, and excellent safety profile. Moreover, in its procedural implementation, there is no need for contrast. Due to this widespread adoption, many medical schools have begun implementing formal didactics and training throughout the 4-year allopathic educational model [24]. Web-based models have found widespread success in the adoption of US CVC guidance techniques for physicians in training and have improved the base of knowledge for procedural competence [25, 26]. Techniques that may be employed include either static or dynamic techniques. Static techniques are employed by operators that may not be facile in the use of probe or when a sterile probe cover is not available. By definition, static techniques rely on the operator using the probe to gain orientation to the structure of interest, marking the skin over the vein and placing the probe aside. Static techniques are less optimal as the operator may still hit the artery or penetrate the posterior wall of the vein. In contrast, dynamic techniques are superior with regard to avoiding complications [27]. However, they may be more challenging for junior operators to master. In the dynamic technique, the operator maintains the probe in the field at all times so that the needle may be visualized in the area of interest throughout the duration of vessel cannulation. This provides for a safer procedure, as inadvertent puncture of the nearby artery or the posterior wall is avoided. The author utilizes a technique where in right-sided IJ placement via US, the thenar aspect of the left hand is lightly steadied on the patient's jaw. This enables the operator to maintain the probe in an optimal perpendicular plane. A good view will reveal the IJV to be circular, whereas an off-axis view will provide an oblong appearing IJV. At this point, the operator should test for compressibility of the IJ. See Fig. 12.2 to the left.

Utilizing the dynamic technique with a short axis view, the operator then slowly advances the needle at a 30–45° angle with the bevel down, looking for a "V" indentation on the anterior aspect of the IJV. The needle is advanced until a dark red venous flash is obtained. It should be cautioned to not advance if the flash is lost, as this may signify penetration of the posterior wall of the vessel. See Fig. 12.3 for an image of the needle being introduced into the vein.

This may occur even in dynamic US placement as the angle of approach may take the needle out of the plane of the US transducer at the distal end of the vessel. Besides US, additional means of confirming the needle in the vein include utilizing a sterile length of IV tubing to

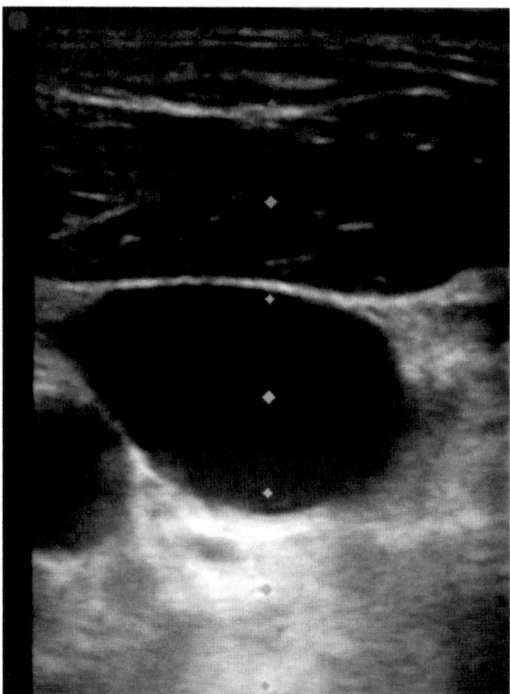

Fig. 12.2 Compressibility testing of the IJ vein. Courtesy of the author with thanks to Saurab Joshi, MD for vessel cannulation and procedural expertise

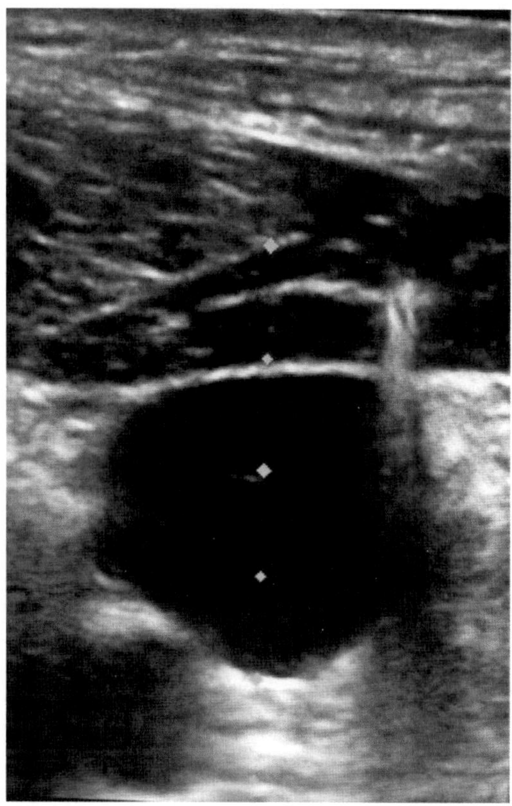

Fig. 12.3 Needle entering the internal jugular on SA view using dynamic technique. Courtesy of the author with thanks to Saurab Joshi, MD for vessel cannulation and procedural expertise

transduce central venous pressure. In the case of arterial puncture, blood flow will not cease and will climb the entire length of tubing. In venous puncture, the blood flow may rise to a certain point and then cease. Significant respiratory variation of venous flow in the transducer tubing may signify hypovolemia or pneumothorax. It should be noted that IJV CVC placement still carries a significant risk of pneumothorax, particularly if the placement occurs on the lower third of the neck. A significant review of the literature revealed a paucity of information on the use of US in the SC site. Traditionally, operators may switch to a long axis (LA) view. See Fig. 12.4.

However one prospective, randomized crossover trial failed to show an attendant increase in the success rate in US-guided SC CVC placement [28]. This is likely due to a number of reasons, among them being the fact that anatomically the SC vein courses beneath the clavicle.

12.7 Complications

A number of factors may impact complication rates in the placement of CVC lines. In research conducted at Johns Hopkins, it was noted that although operator experience of less than 25 CVC lines did not impact success rates, complication rates were higher in inexperienced operators [29]. In a comprehensive review, a number of risk factors have been elucidated, with some of the more prominent being inexperience, number of needle passes (sixfold increase in complication risk with>three needle passes), BMI>30 or<20, large catheter size (i.e., hemodialysis access catheter), or prior operation and/or radiation exposure in the area of interest [6, 30]. Rare complications may include guidewire fraying, retention, or perforation of the vena cava.

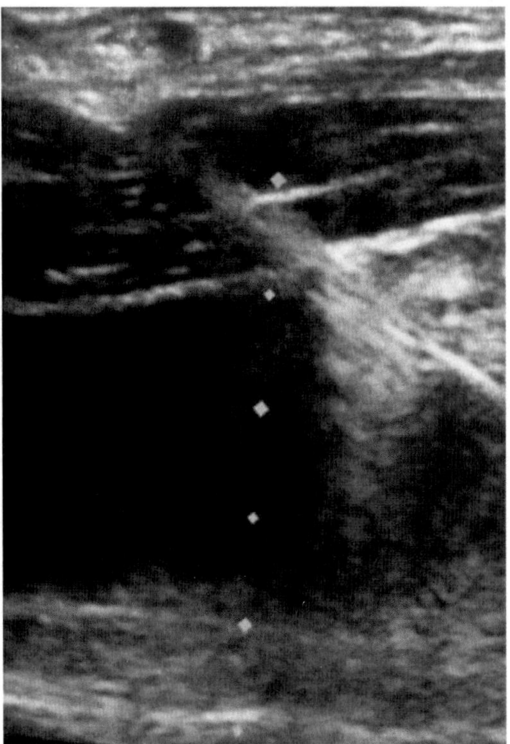

Fig. 12.4 Needle entering the vein on LA view

These complications, although rare, may require either median sternotomy or IR-guided retrieval of the retained wire [31]. Common complications for CVC placement are outlined as follows in Table 12.3:

Table 12.3

Pneumothorax
Hemothorax
Chylothorax
Hematoma
Puncture of carotid, femoral, or subclavian artery
Vessel injury, including damage to SVC or Aorta
Thoracic duct injury
CLABSI
Air embolism
Catheter fracture
Guidewire fracture
Retained catheter fragment
Retained guidewire

12.8 Process of CVC Insertion

The process of CVC insertion is best performed in a controlled environment. Clinicians are encouraged to use a pre-procedure checklist which facilitates safety and quality assurance. This provider's direct experience has been to perform the procedure with a minimum of assistance from other providers, who may be encumbered with other patient care activities.

The process is as follows for ultrasound-assisted placement of a CVC in the right internal jugular vein:

1. Obtain informed consent and discuss the risks and benefits of the procedure, as well as any potential complications. Ensure that the consent has the correct date and time. Also, if a phone consent is obtained, clearly print the name and telephone number of the consenting party. Document the type of relationship and have a witness verify and attest that you have thoroughly addressed the informed consent process.
2. Verify two forms of identification, typically patient name and date of birth. If the patient is intubated, verify with a second provider at the bedside. Also verify any allergies. Conduct a formal time-out process with the bedside nurse in attendance.
3. Gather necessary equipment including a mask and cap for each person remaining in the room during the procedure. Also gather the CVC kit, a gown, two pairs of sterile gloves, a sterile dressing kit, and sterile flushes.
4. Additionally, the ultrasound machine should be powered on, plugged in, have the correct vascular access probe connected, and should have correct settings entered for depth and gain. A sterile probe cover should be obtained. At this point, it is prudent to inform the patient of the fact that you may be resting your hand on their jaw and that a drape will cover their face during the procedure. The author simulates this motion with the patient so that they understand their optimal body positioning throughout the procedure. A baseline ultrasound view is obtained of the internal jugular vein.

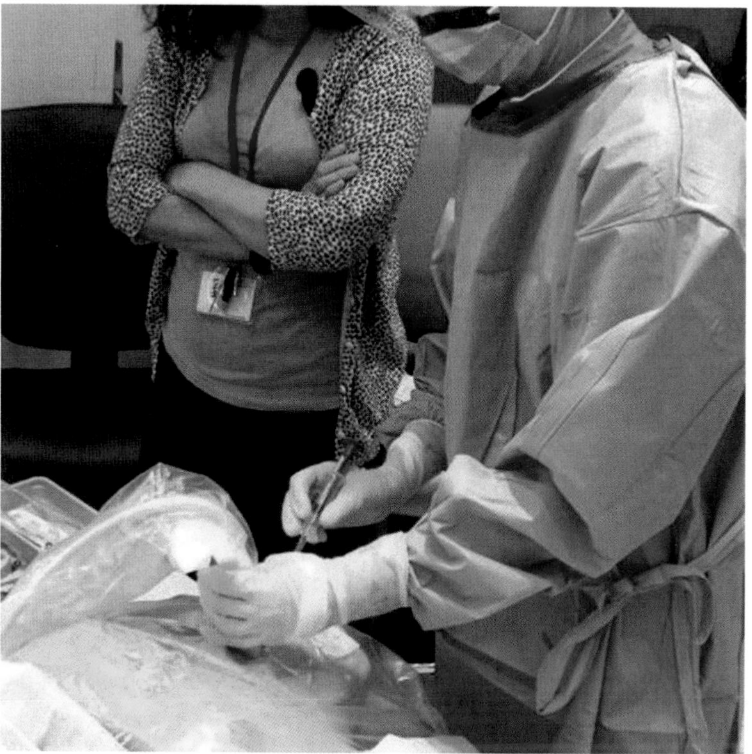

Fig. 12.5 IJ CVC placement utilizing dynamic technique

5. The bed is then placed in Trendelenburg position. If the patient has respiratory distress, this step can be deferred until after the draping process to minimize time in this position.
6. Using a skin marker, the operator marks their initials on the side of the body on which the CVC line will be placed.
7. The operator should thoroughly wash their hands for 60 s.
8. At this point the operator opens the sterile equipment and dons the gown, along with two pairs of sterile gloves. The author proposes the cover glove system as it allows for more independent preparations. The outer gloves are typically one half size larger and may be shed after draping has taken place and after the ultrasound probe has been placed in the sterile probe cover.
9. Using chlorhexidine or betadine, cleanse the area in widening concentric circles and allow the cleansed area to dry. After drying, cleanse a second time, this time with a scrubbing motion. Ensure that not only the neck, but the landmarks which encompass the subclavian site are cleansed and draped so that the SC site may be used as a secondary insertion point should IJ insertion fail.
10. Drape the patient with a sterile sheet. Most commercially available kits contain a sterile drape with a clear area for patient visibility and a circular fenestration. Place this fenestration over the IJ site, ensuring that you do not drag any contaminated patient care bed linens into the sterile field which also encompasses the upper chest.
11. If assistance is available, have your assistant hold the ultrasound probe above the opening for the sterile probe cover, and using gravity, have them gently lower the probe into the probe cover. If no assistant is available, the operator may perform this piece independently and shed the outer cover glove after carefully placing the sterile probe cover/probe assembly on the field.

12. Draw up 5 cc of 1 % lidocaine and infiltrate the soft tissues of the neck after gently aspirating the syringe.
13. At this point, organize the equipment on a sterile tray table in the order that it is used in the procedure. This ensures consistency of placement and assures an expeditious CVC placement. For junior operators, this assists them in acting as a type of prompt for the next step in the line placement process.
14. Using the provided sterile flushes included in the CVC kit, flush out all air from any attached claves, central line ports, or tubing.
15. Gently place the left hand with the probe perpendicular to the vessel in a short axis view. Steady the thenar aspect of the hand on the patient's jaw. Ensure the view with the probe matches with the anatomic positioning of the vessels, with the carotid on the medial side and the internal jugular vein on the lateral side. Gently compress the vessel and center the vein in the middle of the screen.
16. With the bevel side down, position the right hand to bring the syringe into an acute angle. Maintain the needle into the plane of the ultrasound window. While steadily advancing the needle, look for a "V" indentation on the anterior wall of the vessel while continuing to gently aspirate. Continue to keep the needle in view of the ultrasound window. If the needle bevel disappears, stop advancing with the right hand and slowly slide the left probe hand toward the base of the neck until the needle comes back into view. Once the needle is in the center of the vessel, continue to gently aspirate and drop the angle of the right hand to a shallower angle (approximately 30–45°).
17. Gently detach the syringe. If a sterile length of IV tubing is available in the kit, transduce and check blood flow.
18. Remove the tubing and introduce the guidewire. Monitor both length of guidewire and check for any dysrhythmias. Ensure that the guidewire is not put down at any time. Throughout the procedure, the operator may have to switch hands, but at no time should they put the wire down. Using ultrasound, verify the position of the guidewire in the vessel.
19. With the needle still in place over the guidewire, gently nick the skin with the number 11 blade, with the blade side up. It is important to nick the skin with the needle covering the guidewire so that the wire is not inadvertently frayed by the blade.
20. Remove the needle and advance the vessel dilator via Seldinger technique. Verify the dilator via ultrasound.
21. Remove the dilator and advance the catheter over the guidewire. Remove the guidewire and recover it into the guidewire sheath. This is in the event that the vessel needs to be recannulated for any reason. Additionally, the guidewire may potentially contaminate the field if left out.
22. Suture the catheter in position and flush all three ports with sterile saline.
23. Place a sterile dressing and mark the date and time on the dressing. Verify the needle and sharp counts with the bedside nurse.
24. Place an order for a postprocedure chest X-ray to verify the CVC line position.
25. Provide the patient/bedside nurse with education on CLABSI prevention. The CDC FAQ sheet may be found online at: http://www.cdc.gov/hai/pdfs/bsi/BSI_tagged.pdf [35].
26. Document the procedure note and document any medications given, number of attempts, complications, and results of postprocedure chest X-ray. Write an order allowing the nurse to use the CVC line and maintain a relevant operator procedure log which documents site, side, number of attempts, and complications.

12.9 Conclusions

CVC placement is a procedure which is conducted ubiquitously in a variety of critical care settings. US guidance greatly increases the likelihood of operator success. That being said, complication rates in junior operators with less than 25 line placements may still be common. Operators with <25 prior insertions cause more complications (25.2 % vs. 13.6 %, $P=0.04$), require the assistance of a senior operator more frequently, and have more completely failed attempts [32]. Best practices and good judgment should be utilized in the placement of CVC catheters, and junior operators doing 25–50 line placements have higher success rates (90 % vs. 75 %) when supervised by a more experienced operator, with a lower interim complication rate using US. Senior operators responsible for the training of individuals should utilize a number of strategies including web-based didactics, simulation, physical supervision, and frequent review of procedural logs [24–26, 32]. Although success with US guidance may be site dependent and higher in the IJ position, the long axis view utilizing a dynamic technique has a reduced likelihood of PWP [23]. With experienced operators, in the event that no US machine is available, the subclavian position may still be a safe alternative [22]. Although many studies have addressed the difference in complication rates among learners of various experience levels, some data with regard to physician assistants vs. physicians show that well-trained physician assistants have comparable complication rates when conducting invasive procedures [33, 34].

References

1. Hermosura BVL. Measurement of pressure during intravenous therapy. JAMA. 1966;195:181.
2. Gourlay D. Central venous cannulation. Br J Nurs. 1996;5(1):8–15.
3. Legler D, Nugent M. Doppler localization of the internal jugular vein facilitates central venous catheterization. Anesthesiology. 1984;60:481–2.
4. Nomura J, Sierzenski P. Cross sectional survey of ultrasound use for central venous catheter insertion among resident physicians. Del Med J. 2007; 80(7):255–9.
5. Denys B, Uretsky B. Ultrasound-assisted cannulation of the internal jugular vein. A prospective comparison to the external landmark-guided technique. Circulation. 1993;87(5):1557–62.
6. Schummer W, Schummer C, Rose N, et al. Mechanical complications and malpositions of central venous cannulations by experienced operators: a prospective study of 1794 catheterizations in critically ill patients. Intensive Care Med. 2007;33:1055–9.
7. Gibbs F, Murphy M. Ultrasound guidance for central venous catheter placement. Hosp Physician. 2006;42(3):23–31.
8. Mahler S, Wang H. Short vs. long-axis approach to ultrasound guided peripheral intravenous access: a prospective randomized study. Am J Emerg Med. 2011;29:1194–7.
9. Karakitsos D, Labropoulos N. Real -time ultrasound-guided catheterisation of the internal jugular vein: a prospective comparison with the landmark technique in critical care patients. Crit Care. 2006;10(6):1–8.
10. Cowl C, Weinstock J. Complications and cost associated with parenteral nutrition delivered to hospitalized patients through either subclavian or peripherally-inserted central catheters. Clin Nutr. 2000;19(4): 237–43.
11. Yeum C, Kim SW. Percutaneous catheterization of the internal jugular vein for hemodialysis. Korean J Intern Med. 2001;16(4):243–6.
12. Geddes C, Walbaum J. Insertion of internal jugular temporary hemodialysis cannulae by direct ultrasound guidance-a prospective comparison of experienced and inexperienced operators. Clin Nephrol. 1998;50(5):320–5.
13. Pervez A, Abreo K. Central vein cannulation for hemodialysis. Semin Dial. 2007;20(6):621–5.
14. Leung J, Duffy M. Real-time ultrasonagraphically-guided internal jugular vein catheterization in the emergency department increases success rates and reduces complications: a randomized, prospective study. Ann Emerg Med. 2006;84(5):540–7.
15. Theodoro D, Bausano B. A descriptive comparison of ultrasound-guided central venous cannulation of the internal jugular vein to landmark-based subclavian vein cannulation. Acad Emerg Med. 2010;17(4): 416–22.
16. Lampert M, Cortelazzi P. An outcome study on complications using routine ultrasound assistance for internal jugular vein cannulation. Acta Anaesthesiol Scand. 2007;51:1327–30.
17. Leung J, Duffy M. Real-time ultrasonagraphically-guided internal jugular vein catheterization in the emergency department increases success rates and reduces complications: a randomized, prospective study. Ann Emerg Med. 2006;48(5):540–7.
18. Shrestha BR, Gautam B. Ultrasound versus the landmark technique: a prospective randomized comparative study of the internal jugular vein cannulation in an intensive care unit. JNMA J Nepal Med Assoc. 2011;51(182):56–61.
19. Slama M, Novara A. Improvement of internal jugular vein cannulation using an ultrasound-guided technique. Intensive Care Med. 1997;23:916–9.
20. Sznajder J, Zveibil F. Central vein catherization. Failure and complication rates by three percutaneous approaches. Arch Intern Med. 1986;146:259–61.
21. Crozier J, McKee R. Is the landmark technique safe for the insertion of subclavian venous lines? Surgeon. 2005;3(4):277–9.

22. Mansfield P, Hohn D. Complications and failures of subclavian-vein cannulation. N Engl J Med. 1994; 331(26):1735–8.
23. Vogel J, Haukoos J. Is long-axis view superior to short axis view in ultrasound-guided central venous catheterization? Crit Care Med. 2015;43(4):832–9.
24. Baltarowich O, DiSalvo D. National ultrasound curriculum for medical students. Ultrasound Q. 2014; 30(1):13–9.
25. Grover S, Currier P. Improving residents' knowledge of arterial and central line placement with a web-based curriculum. J Grad Med Educ. 2010;2(4):548–54.
26. Mosier J, Malo J. Critical care ultrasound training: a survey of US fellowship directors. J Crit Care. 2014;29:645–9.
27. Scott L, Wax J. Use of ultrasound to guide vascular access procedures-AIUM practice guideline. American Institute of Ultrasound in Medicine. 2012:1–23
28. Bold R, Winchester D. Prospective, randomized trial of doppler-assisted subclavian vein cannulation. Arch Surg. 1998;133:1089–93.
29. Bo-Linn G, Anderson D. Percutaneous central venous catheterization performed by medical house officers: a prospective study. Cathet Cardiovasc Diagn. 1982;8:23–9.
30. Kusminsky R. Complications of central venous catheterization. J Am Coll Surg. 2007;204(4):681–96.
31. Phy M, Neilson R. Guidewire complication with central line placement. Hosp Physician. 2004; June:41–43.
32. Lennon M, Zaw N. Procedural complications of central venous catheter insertion. Minerva Anestesiol. 2012;78(11):1234–40.
33. Cox T, Parish T. A study of pneumothorax rates for physician assistants inserting central venous catheters at a large urban hospital. Internet J Allied Health Sci Pract. 2005;3(3):1–4.
34. Benham J, Culp C. Complication rate of venous access procedures performed by a radiology practitioner assistant compared with interventional radiology physicians and supervised trainees. J Vasc Interv Radiol. 2007;18:1001–04.
35. FAQs about Central Line Associated Bloodstream Infections [Internet]; 2010 [updated 2012 May 10; cited 2015 Mar 30]. Available from: http://www.cdc.gov/HAI/bsi/bsi.html. Accessed 25 Nov 2010.

13 Pulmonary Artery Catheter Insertion

Britney S. Broyhill and Toan Huynh

13.1 Introduction

Pulmonary artery catheters (PACs) were introduced in the 1970s as a means to monitor hemodynamics of critically ill patients [9]. This balloon-tipped catheter is advanced by blood flow through the right atrium and right ventricle and terminates in the pulmonary artery; this technology offers clinicians real-time pressure measurements from inside the right heart.

The use of PACs has been controversial since their inception and continues to be debated among intensivists today. Several randomized controlled trials have concluded that there is no outcome benefit in the use of PACs in high-risk surgical patients, congestive heart failure, acute lung injury, and sepsis [1, 2]. In the acute myocardial infarction cohort, evidence has shown an increased risk of mortality with the use of PACs [3].

However, in specific patient populations, the application of PACs may prove beneficial. The ATTEND trial suggested that patients with acute heart failure benefited from PAC use, especially if hypotensive or requiring inotropic support [4]. Furthermore, the use of PACs represents the standard of care in patients with severe pulmonary hypertension and those undergoing preoperative evaluation for liver transplantation [5, 6].

Regardless of the controversy, practitioners must be fully aware of the indications and the prudent application in selected patient populations. Indeed, practitioners should consider the utility of less invasive monitoring technologies as alternatives where applicable. Additionally, they should be experts in interpretation of the data provided by PACs and be comfortable translating it to guide therapy.

13.2 Indications

There is currently no evidence to suggest that the routine use of PACs results in improved patient outcomes [6]. Nevertheless, the effective use of PACs can provide a powerful tool to guide interventions in critically ill patients. In their recent review of the use of PACs, Gidwani et al. [6] recommended the following list of indications for PA catheterization in the critical care setting:

- Patients undergoing liver transplantation work-up
- Patients with cardiogenic shock receiving supportive therapy
- Patients with discordant right and left ventricular failure

B.S. Broyhill, DNP, ACNP-BC (✉)
• T. Huynh, MD, FACS, FCCM
Carolinas HealthCare System, Carolinas Medical Center, Charlotte, NC, USA
e-mail: Britney.broyhill@carolinashealthcare.org; toan.huynh@carolinashealthcare.org

D.A. Taylor et al. (eds.), *Interventional Critical Care*, DOI 10.1007/978-3-319-25286-5_13

- Patients with severe chronic heart failure requiring inotropic, vasopressor, and vasodilator therapy
- Patients with potentially reversible systolic heart failure
- Patients being evaluated for pulmonary hypertension
- Patients who are being treated for precapillary and mixed types of pulmonary hypertension to assess their response to therapy

The PAC can be used for both diagnostic and therapeutic purposes. The clinician should evaluate the goal of placement and the inherent risks to assess whether insertion benefits that particular patient. With the advent of alternative technologies in hemodynamic monitoring and evidence disputing the efficacy of PACs, there has been decreased utilization across the United States [7].

13.3 Contraindications

The advanced clinical practitioner should weigh the risks and benefits prior to insertion of the PAC. There are no absolute contraindications for this procedure but there are several relative ones.

The first relative contraindication is preexisting left bundle branch block (LBBB). An electrocardiogram should be obtained prior to the insertion of the PAC to rule out the presence of LBBB. The risk of insertion for a patient with a LBBB is that injury or interruption to the right bundle could result in complete heart block and asystole. In the event a PAC is absolutely necessary in a patient with a LBBB, the practitioner should anticipate this complication and be prepared for direct cardiac pacing.

The following is a summary of other relative contraindications for insertion:

- Right-sided heart mass (thrombus or tumor)
- Presence of pacer or defibrillator electrodes
- Severe coagulopathy or current systemic anticoagulation therapy
- Tricuspid valve prosthetic or stenosis
- Severe hypothermia

13.4 Informed Consent

Prior to beginning the PAC insertion, the practitioner must obtain informed consent from the patient or their designated surrogate decision maker. In order to properly obtain consent, the risks and benefits of the procedure must be described to the person signing the consent release.

Benefits to be discussed include accurate hemodynamic data derived from PAC in order to guide therapy. The presentation should explain that insertion will allow real-time information to the healthcare team to help direct medication and fluid delivery to the patient.

Providers should discuss the indications as well as contraindications and recommendation to proceed with the use of PAC. Risks associated with the procedure itself as well as the use of the catheter after insertion should also be disclosed.

The most common complication during insertion is cardiac arrhythmias including ectopies and tachycardias. They are usually short lived, but occur in 12.5–70 % of insertions; however, only about 3 % require antiarrhythmic therapy [2]. In addition, there is approximately a 0.5–1 % risk of pneumothorax and hemothorax during insertion.

Infection is always a risk of insertion of a foreign object into the human body. Infections can occur in the subcutaneous tissue at the insertion site, in the bloodstream, or in the heart tissue itself. Risks of bacteremia associated with PACs range from 1.3 to 2.3 % and endocarditis 2.2–7.1 % [2]. Patients with prosthetic valves are at higher risk for endocarditis [2].

Pulmonary artery rupture is perhaps the most severe complication associated with PA catheterization, although it is extremely rare with an incidence of 0.03–0.20 % [2]. Risk factors for perforation include pulmonary hypertension, hypercoagulopathy, age of greater than 60, improper catheter positioning, and improper balloon inflation [2].

As you prepare to complete the consenting process, it is important to acknowledge that there is always overall risk of death when undergoing invasive procedures to the person providing consent. In one study of critically ill patients, 4 % died from complications related to the PAC with an estimated 20–30 % with other major complications related to the catheter [8]. Clinicians should remind themselves that there is never a benign procedure.

13.5 Preparation

Prior to beginning the procedure, it is important to gather all the necessary equipment as well as to inform the bedside registered nurse who can assist during the procedure with the equipment setup (Fig. 13.1). Most intensive care units are equipped with PAC kits that contain all the necessary supplies needed for insertion; however, the provider may choose to obtain extra pressure tubing, saline flushes, sterile skin prep, and gauze sponges. The nurse will zero the monitor and add the patient-specific demographics prior to insertion so that the information is calculated correctly for the patient.

13.6 Procedure

In order to reduce the risk of bacteremia, this procedure is performed using sterile technique. All persons in the room should be required to wear masks and a surgical cap during the insertion. The provider should wear sterile gloves, gown, mask, and a surgical cap. The patient's insertion site should be prepped with chlorhexidine and draped with full-length drapes.

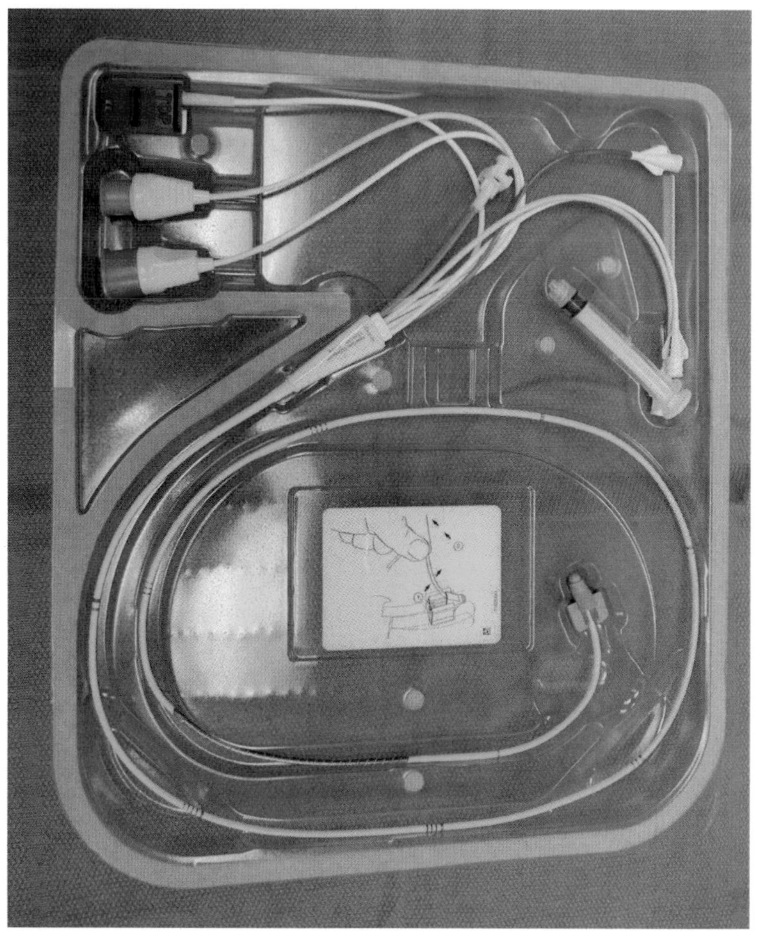

Fig. 13.1 Example of pulmonary artery insertion kit

If a transducer is not in place for the patient, then one must be placed using the Seldinger technique. The most direct insertion site for placement of the PA catheter is either the left subclavian or the right internal jugular vein; however, any insertion site including a femoral approach is appropriate. This transducer is larger in diameter than a central venous line, but is inserted similarly. During insertion, it is imperative that the provider insure that the transducer is placed in the venous vasculature. Dilation of the arterial system can be catastrophic. Using a jugular or femoral approach will allow for ultrasound confirmation prior to PAC insertion.

Once the patient is prepped and draped and the introducer is in place, the PAC itself must be tested prior to insertion. All the ports should be flushed with sterile saline and the balloon should be tested for inflation. The provider should insure that the tip is enclosed into the balloon upon inflation, and it should not extend past the balloon to prevent damage to the tissue upon insertion. The catheter should also have the protector sterile sheath covering it so that manipulations can occur via a sterile field.

As the catheter is connected to the pressure transducer and the monitor, the provider should wave the tip of the catheter to make sure it is properly connected by confirming a wave formation on the monitor. Finally, the ACP should orient the catheter so that its natural curvature is in alignment with the vasculature system depending on the insertion site.

Once the tip has been inspected and monitor connection confirmed, the catheter is inserted into the introducer until the catheter tip is about 15–20 cm from the right internal jugular or left subclavian. The catheter has measurement markings along its side to help the provider determine the length inserted into the patient. One should confirm placement in the right atrium via the waveform on the monitor (Fig. 13.2). During insertion, the provider should always reference the monitor to verify the location within the heart chambers.

Upon confirmation that the tip is in the right atrium, the balloon should be inflated. The registered nurse assisting with the procedure should state when they inflate or deflate the balloon. Once inflated, the syringe should be locked to the catheter. The provider then advances the catheter into the right ventricle which should occur around 30 cm. This position is then confirmed by the right ventricle waveform on the monitor (Fig. 13.2).

The provider continues to advance the catheter through the pulmonary valve which will be identified by a pulmonary artery waveform (Fig. 13.2), a dicrotic notch, and an increase in diastolic pressure. This typically will occur at 40 cm. As the balloon continues to float further into the pulmonary artery, it will become wedged and the tracing will flatten usually at approximately 50 cm.

The balloon should then be deflated and reinflated gently. If there is resistance felt as it is reinflated or the waveform shows signs of overwedging, balloon insertion should be stopped immediately. If the balloon is unable to be fully inflated, this could be a sign that the catheter has passed too far distally and should be deflated and pulled back about a centimeter.

Once the provider feels that the catheter is in proper position and has obtained an appropriate wedge pressure and tracing, the balloon should be deflated and the catheter secured at the length it was obtained via the locking mechanism on the device. This measurement should be recorded in the medical record for reference. A chest x-ray should be ordered to confirm proper placement and rule out complications.

13.7 Complications

During insertion, it is possible that the balloon will not float easily between the chambers of the heart. When advancing the catheter and a length of 45 to 50 cm is reached without identifying the wedge tracing, it is likely that the catheter has become curled into the right ventricle. At this point, the provider would need to deflate the balloon and pull back until the right atrial waveform can be visualized.

The provider should never withdraw the catheter without confirming that the balloon is deflated. The catheter should also never be advanced without the balloon being inflated. Doing either of these maneuvers can lead to

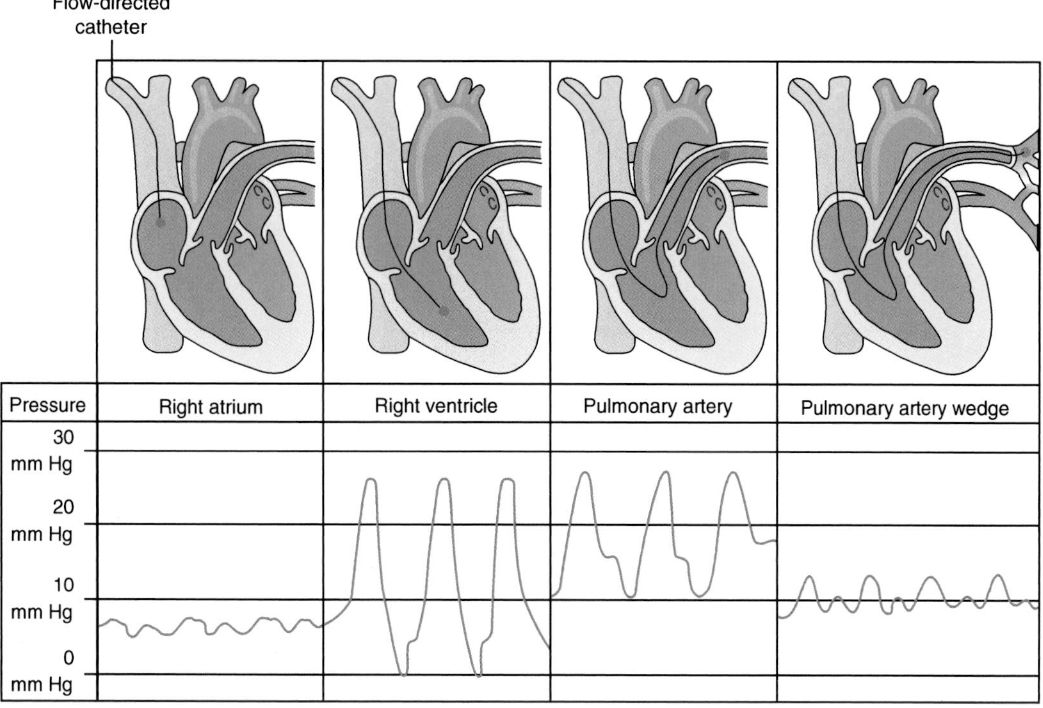

From Urden LD, Stacy KM, Lough ME: *Thelan's critical care nursing: diagnosis and management,* ed 4, St Louis, 2002, Mosby.

Fig. 13.2 Illustration of ECG tracings in relation to pulmonary artery catheter location during insertion [permission acknowledgment needed]

perforation or damage to the heart valves which is many times a fatal complication.

Finally, the clinician should be cautious when obtaining the wedge pressure to insure that the catheter has not migrated distally. As the catheter warms with the patient's body temperature, it can expand and move. Monitoring of placement by the measurement on the catheter is crucial as well as monitoring of placement via chest x-rays.

13.8 Pearls

There are several hemodynamic data directly measured by the PAC: central venous pressure (CVP), pulmonary capillary wedge pressure (PCWP), mean pulmonary artery pressure (PAP), and mixed venous oxygenation (SVO_2). Other measurements are derived from this data including cardiac output (CO), cardiac index (CI), stroke volume index (SVI), systemic vascular resistance (SVR), and pulmonary vascular resistance (PVR).

The clinician is able to utilize this information to help direct therapy for the patient. Trends of these calculations can be helpful in goal-directed therapy and in diagnostic evaluation (Table 13.1).

13.9 Conclusion

While the utilization of the pulmonary artery catheter in the intensive care unit is on the decline, there are specific populations of patients in which it is beneficial in guiding care. The advanced clinical practitioner working as an intensivist must maintain the skills of insertion and interpretation of the PAC when the need arises.

Table 13.1 Hemodynamic profiles

Hemodynamic State	CVP	PAOP	CO	CI	SVR
Normal	2–6 mmHg	8–12 mmHg	4–8 L/min	2.5–4.0 L/min/m^2	900–1300 dynes/s/cm^{-5}
Cardiogenic Shock	↑	↑	↓	↓	↑
Hypovolemic Shock	↓	↓	↓	↓	↑
Sepsis	↕	↔	↑	↑	↓
Pulmonary arterial hypertension	↑	↔	↔	↔	↑

References

1. The National Heart, Lung and Blood Institute Acute Respiratory Distress Syndrome (ARDS) Clinical Trials Network. Pulmonary-artery versus central venous catheter to guide treatment of acute lung injury. N Engl J Med. 2006;354:2213–24.
2. Evans DC, Doraiswamy VA, Prosciak MP, Silviera M, Seamon MJ, et al. Complications associated with pulmonary artery catheters: a comprehensive clinical review. Scand J Surg. 2009;98:199–208.
3. Dalen JE, Bone RC. Is it time to pull the pulmonary artery catheter? J Am Med Assoc. 1996;276(11): 916–8.
4. Sotomi Y, Sato N, Kajimoto K, Sakata Y, Mizuno M, Minami Y, Fujii K, Takano T. Impact of pulmonary artery catheter on outcome in patients with acute heart failure syndromes with hypotension or receiving inotropes: from the ATTEND Registry. Int J Cardiol. 2014;172(1):165–72.
5. Costa MG, Chiarandini P, Scudeller L, Vetrugno L, Pompei L, et al. Uncalibrated continuous cardiac output measurement in liver transplant patients: LiDCOrapidTM System versus pulmonary artery catheter. J Cardiothorac Vasc Anesth. 2014;28(3):540–6.
6. Gidwani UK, Mohanty B, Chatterjee K. The pulmonary artery catheter a critical reappraisal. Cardiol Clin. 2013;31(4):545–65.
7. Wiener RS, Welch HG. Trends in the use of the pulmonary artery catheter in the United States, 1993–2004. J Am Med Assoc. 2007;298(4):423–9.
8. Marik PE. Obituary: pulmonary artery catheter 1970 to 2013. Ann Intensive Care. 2013;3(38):1–6.
9. Swan HJ, Ganz W, Forrester J, Marcus H, Diamond G, Chonette D. Catheterization of the heart in man with use of a flow-directed balloon-tipped catheter. N Engl J Med. 1970;283:447–51.

14 Peripherally Inserted Central Catheter Placement

Christopher D. Newman

14.1 Introduction

Peripherally inserted central catheters (PICCs) have become an increasingly popular alternative to traditional percutaneous central venous lines. They require little or no sedation, can be placed at the bedside using minimal equipment, can be maintained at home, and, in the right patient population, offer lower rates of infection and other complications than traditional percutaneous central lines. This chapter describes the terminology, equipment, and techniques for the placement of PICCs. Additionally, risks, benefits, complications, and troubleshooting are discussed.

14.1.1 Definitions

Peripherally Inserted Central Catheter (PICC) A long, flexible catheter inserted percutaneously into a peripheral vein and then threaded into the central circulation such that the tip is located within the superior vena cava, inferior vena cava, or right atrium (see Fig. 14.1).

C.D. Newman, MBA, PA-C, FCCM (✉)
University of Colorado School of Medicine, Childrens Hospital Colorado, Aurora, CO, USA
e-mail: Christopher.newman@ucdenver.edu; christopher.newman@childrenscolorado.org

Obturator Wire A wire placed within the lumen of the PICC during insertion to provide additional stiffness and make advancing of the PICC through the vessels easier.

Guidewire A wire placed within the vessel that the PICC can be advanced over into the central circulation.

Introducer A sheath that is inserted into a peripheral vein, either over a needle or a dilator, through which a PICC can be inserted into the vein.

14.1.1.1 Indications

Long-Term IV Access The most common indication for a PICC is the need for IV access for >7 days, but <3 months. If access is needed for <7 days, a peripheral intravenous catheter (PIV) or percutaneous central venous line (CVL) may be preferable. If access is needed for longer than 3 months, a tunneled CVL or implantable port may be considered. PICCs can remain functional for more than a year if properly cared for, but the long-term risks and convenience issues should be a consideration in choosing access for very long-term needs.

Use of Vesicant Medications The need to administer medications not well tolerated in a

D.A. Taylor et al. (eds.), *Interventional Critical Care*, DOI 10.1007/978-3-319-25286-5_14

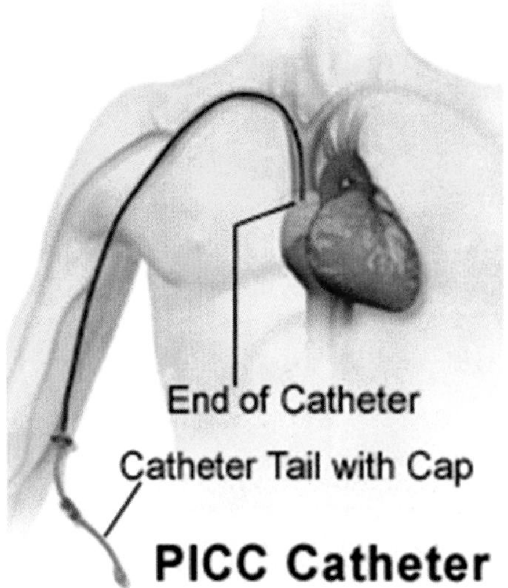

Fig. 14.1 Anatomic positioning of the PICC

peripheral vessel, such as vasoactive agents, some antibiotics, and chemotherapies, even if for <7 days, may be an indication for a PICC.

Difficult IV Access This is more controversial, but patients who have had repeated PIV failures or unsuccessful attempts, those who need repeated bloodwork, or those who, based on history, have had difficulties maintaining IV access during past hospital admissions may all benefit from PICC placement, as the deeper peripheral vessels used for PICC insertion are often less vulnerable to the conditions that can make PIV access difficult, such as dehydration, obesity, poor nutrition, etc.

Plasmapheresis In many centers, plasmapheresis can now be successfully performed using two PICCs that have a stiffened lumen suitable for high pressure injection.

14.1.1.2 Contraindications

Venous Thrombosis The presence of a venous thrombosis in any of the vessels through which the PICC will pass, such as the basilica vein, subclavian vein, or superior vena cava, is a contraindication to PICC placement. Even if the catheter can be passed beyond the thrombus, the presence of the PICC will increase the risk of both propagation of the thrombus and embolus.

End-Stage Renal Disease PICCs are generally avoided in patients that are likely to need ongoing hemodialysis because any thrombus resulting from the PICC is likely to impede the formation of fistulas used for chronic dialysis.

Anticipated Need for Fluid Resuscitation or Rapid Medication Infusion Because the lumen of a PICC is long and often narrow, the resistance to flow is higher than in a PIV or most percutaneously inserted CVLs. This makes them an inappropriate choice for rapid fluid resuscitation, massive transfusion protocols, or any other circumstance in which rapid infusion of medications (particularly high-volume medications) is indicated or likely to be needed. If no other access is available, existing PICCs can be used for these purposes, but the rate of infusion will be limited to roughly 1 l/h or slower in smaller lumen PICCs.

14.2 Preparation

PICC insertion is a sterile procedure. Appropriate handwashing, gowning, and other PPE should be donned as per institutional policy, and a "time out" should be used in the manner dictated by your institution. The patient should be supine with the head of the bed or gurney elevated approximately 30° for an upper limb insertion or flat for a lower limb insertion. If using an upper limb insertion location, the arm should be extended away from the patient and externally rotated to expose the surface of the intended insertion area. It may be necessary to use a soft restraint to assist the patient in maintaining this position. Identify and mark the point on the skin where you intend to insert your needle or PIV. Measure from this point to the axilla and then to the sternal notch. If measuring from the left, add 2 cm to this measurement. Record this measurement, as it will be the rough guide for trimming the PICC. If you intend to use a sterile tourniquet, the entire limb should now be cleaned with your sterile scrub. A sterile drape should be placed under the arm, and the tourniquet can now be loosely placed proximal to the intended insertion site. If an assistant will be utilized to tie and release the tourniquet, it should be loosely placed proximal to the intended insertion site, and then the insertion site should be cleaned with your sterile scrub. The insertion site should then be draped. Often, a clear plastic sterile fenestrated drape with adhesive on the side contacting the patient is placed over the insertion site. This may then be supplemented with sterile towels or whole body drapes, depending on your preference and institutional policy. Assemble your remaining equipment on a sterile field and place your ultrasound probe in a sterile sleeve (if using).

14.3 Procedure

14.3.1 Placement of the PICC

Choosing a PICC PICCs are available in a variety or diameters, lengths, and lumen options. They range from single lumen 1.9FR 30 cm catheters appropriate for neonates and very small babies to 6FR quad lumen 90 cm catheters for use in large adults, requiring multiple incompatible medications. There are specially designated PICCs that are certified as able to withstand the pressure created by power injectors used in radiologic procedures or plasmapheresis. PICCs with diameters of 3FR or less are often unreliable for blood return and may not be suitable if blood sampling is an indication for the PICC. In general, the smallest catheter with the fewest lumens that will meet indicated needs of the patient should be used. Increasing catheter size is associated with increased risk of thrombosis, and increased number of lumens is associated with increased infection risk. However, smaller catheters are more prone to damage, may be harder to advance through large vessels, and may not return blood reliably. In all cases, the risks and benefits of each size should be considered.

Location PICCs are most commonly inserted into either the cephalic, median basilic, or brachial veins of the arm. However, the saphenous vein (in young children who are preambulatory), popliteal vein, external jugular vein, forearm veins, and axillary vein have all been used when other options are not available. The median basilic or brachial veins are generally preferred to the cephalic vein as the tight turn and narrowing that occurs as the cephalic vein joins the axillary vein is a frequent site for phlebitis and thrombus formation. However, the cephalic vein is easier to locate (typically in the antecubital fossa) and palpate, so may be the preferred site if ultrasound guidance is not available.

Equipment PICCs are available in kits that can be as minimal as the catheter itself and an obturator wire or as comprehensive as a complete insertion kit containing all necessary drapes, devices, and materials for insertion. The equipment needed is similar to that required for percutaneous placement of a CVL. At a minimum, insertion of a PICC will require:

- A PICC.
- A device to trim the PICC to the desired length.
- If using the direct insertion technique, an obturator wire and a cannulating needle with a tear-away sheath.
- If using the modified Seldinger technique, a needle or PIV for accessing the peripheral vessel, a guidewire, and a vein dilator (with or without a tear-away introducer sheath).
- A sterile ultrasound sleeve and gel (if using ultrasound).
- A tourniquet (sterile if it will be on the field, can be nonsterile if an assistant will be tying the tourniquet outside the sterile field).
- Sterile drapes (whole body if required by your institution).
- Sterile prep (such a chlorhexidine) for cleaning insertion site.
- Tape measure (sterile) to measure from insertion site to intended tip location to aid in trimming PICC to desired length.
- Sterile flushes (saline or heparin containing, based on institutional policy).
- Caps for each lumen of the PICC (ensure caps are compatible with IV tubing system used at your institution).

- Suture material, scissors, or scalpel for cutting material and needle driver if the PICC is to be sutured in place.
- A securement device, such as a StatLock device, if the PICC will not be sutured in place.

Optional Equipment Ultrasound device for identifying peripheral vessel, guiding insertion, and (with experience) identification of PICC tip location. Several commercially available devices exist to aid in tracking the path and tip location of the PICC, often using a magnetic portion of the obturator wire and a sensor that is placed on the chest of the patient. In the operating room or radiology suite, fluoroscopy may be available for visualizing the advancement of either the guidewire or the PICC into the desired location.

Sedation Many adults and older children will tolerate this procedure with only local anesthesia. However, for many young children (and their parents) or older patients with cognitive impairment, this procedure may be both technically difficult (due to movement and crying, which can increase intrathoracic pressure and lead to more internal jugular malposition) and traumatizing to the patient. Therefore, it may be appropriate to offer anxiolysis or moderate sedation to patients undergoing PICC placement, based on the available expertise, personnel, and policies of your institution.

Insertion Once preparations are complete and all equipment is available, you can begin the insertion. There are two basic techniques for inserting a PICC—the direct introducer technique and the microintroducer (or modified Seldinger) technique. Each will be discussed separately.

Direct Introducer Technique This technique uses a needle with a tear-away sheath over it. The previously placed tourniquet is tied to enlarge the target blood vessel. The needle is inserted directly into an appropriate vessel until blood return is observed. The sheath is then advanced over the needle to its full depth. The needle is then removed, leaving a "tunnel" between the sheath opening and the vessel. Once inserted, this sheath can be capped briefly and the tourniquet should be removed. The distance between the intended insertion point (marked previously) and the actual insertion site should then be measured using your sterile measuring tape. This distance should be added or subtracted from your original measurement from intended insertion point to intended tip location. The PICC can now be trimmed to this length. Once trimmed, the PICC should be flushed with saline- or a heparin-containing solution (based on institutional policy) and an obturator wire inserted into the PICC. The obturator should terminate 1–2 cm short of the tip of the PICC to reduce the chance of vessel perforation and allow the softer PICC tip to direct the PICC towards central vessels during advancement. Once the obturator is inserted, the cap can be removed from the tear-away sheath. The PICC tip is then inserted through the sheath into the peripheral vein and slowly advanced until the PICC hub reaches the sheath. To help ensure the PICC tracks towards the central circulation, you may ask the patient to turn his or her head towards the site of insertion (or have an assistant position the patient if the patient is sedated). If ultrasound or other tracking devices are available, they can be used to determine the location of the PICC tip. Once the PICC has been inserted, the two handles of the introducer are pulled apart, and the "tear-away" sheath is torn into two pieces and removed. The PICC can then be secured to the patient using either an adhesive securement device or suturing, the wire removed, the PICC flushed, and a sterile dressing applied.

Microintroducer (Modified Seldinger) Technique This technique is similar to that employed for percutaneous CVL insertion. Once the tourniquet is applied, a needle or PIV catheter is inserted into the target vein. A guidewire is then inserted through either the needle or the PIV catheter to a depth of 10–15 cm. Unless using fluoroscopy for guidance, the guidewire should not be advanced centrally. The needle or catheter is then removed, leaving the wire. The tourniquet is then removed. A "nick" is then made with a scalpel at the point where the wire enters the skin to facilitate the introduction of a vein dilator. For the next step, several options exist:

- If fluoroscopy is available, a vein dilator can be used without an introducer sheath to dilate the tunnel between the skin and the target vein to the appropriate size for the PICC to be inserted (usually 0.5FR greater than the PICC diameter). The vein dilator is advanced over the wire in a "corkscrew" manner until it reaches the vein. The dilator is then removed.
- Some PICCs are stiff enough to advance into the central circulation without an obturator wire. In this circumstance, a vein dilator without introducer sheath can be used, identically to the way it is described above.
- In most cases, the PICC will require an obturator wire to provide sufficient stiffness to allow the tip to be advanced centrally. In these cases, special vein dilators are available that have a tear-away introducer sheath over them. The dilator is inserted under the skin and into the vein over the wire as above. However, once the vein is dilated, the dilator is detached from the tear-away introducer and removed, along with the guidewire. This leaves the introducer as a "tunnel" between the skin and the vein. This introducer should then be capped to stop blood flow.

The distance between the actual insertion point and the intended insertion point should be measured, and this distance is either added or subtracted from the original measurement from intended insertion point to desired tip location. The PICC should then be trimmed to this length, and if the introducer sheath method was used, an obturator wire is inserted. The tip of the wire should be 1–2 cm short of the PICC tip to allow for a flexible portion of the tip to help guide the catheter through vessel junctions and also to reduce the risk of perforating a vessel with the obturator wire. Once the PICC is trimmed and the obturator wire is inserted, the cap can be removed from the introducer sheath.

The PICC is then advanced through the sheath, into the vein, and is slowly introduced until the hub of the catheter touches the distal end of the introducer sheath. The two tabs of the introducer sheath can then be grasped and pulled apart. This will tear the introducer in two, allowing for it to be removed. The obturator wire can now be removed from the PICC.

If an introducer sheath was not used, the PICC is trimmed as outlined above, flushed, and then inserted over the guidewire until the hub reaches the skin. The guidewire is then removed.

The PICC is then anchored to the skin using either sutures or an adhesive securement device. Each lumen is aspirated to confirm blood return and then flushed with either saline-or a heparin-containing solution (based on individual institutional policy). The PICC insertion site is then dressed with a sterile dressing.

Use of Ultrasound Ultrasound guided PICC insertion is becoming the standard of practice, particularly in large institutions where ultrasound machines are readily available. Ultrasound offers several advantages. First, the use of ultrasound allows the inserter to access veins that are not visible or palpatable, such as the brachial vein. These veins are often larger, less damaged by PIV attempts, and less vulnerable to phlebitis. Second, the use of ultrasound reduces the number of attempts needed to access a vein, increases overall success rate, and reduces incidence of thrombophlebitis [1]. Finally, the use of ultrasound by an experienced clinician allows for the visualization of the central vessels, which facilitates identification of malpositioned PICCs. This allows for repositioning attempts under sterile conditions, reduces the number of radiographs needed to confirm placement, and reduces sedation time for patients who require sedation (see Fig. 14.2).

Confirmation Regardless of insertion technique, the gold standard for the confirmation of PICC tip location is plain film chest radiograph.

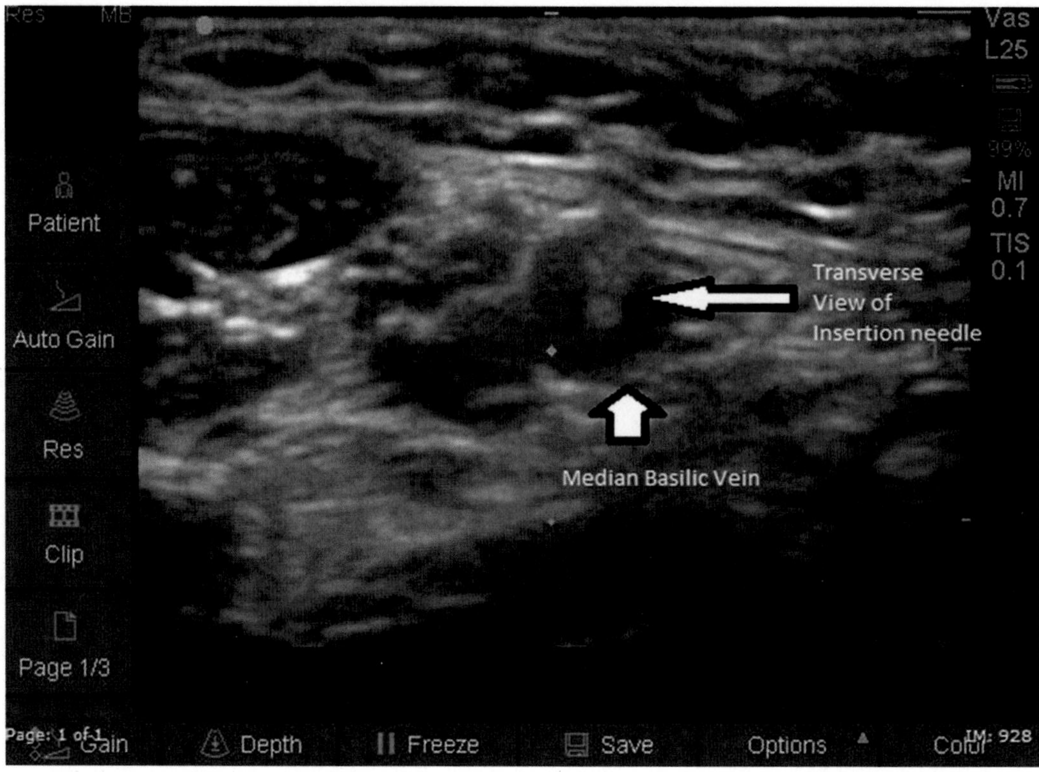

Fig. 14.2 Example of an ultrasound image used to guide the placement of the catheter for PICC insertion

The generally accepted ideal tip location is in the lower 1/3 of the superior vena cava (svc), ideally at the atriocaval junction. However, some radiologists feel that a PICC tip located in the right atrium is more "stable" and less prone to migration into the internal jugular vein than one placed in the SVC (Fig. 14.3). Conversely, many people believe (although no large-scale studies are available to demonstrate the extent of such a risk) that placement in the right atrium increases the risk of erosion into a vessel wall. One clear reason to place the PICC tip above the right atrium is the presence of ectopy. If the patient is noted to have increased premature ventricular contractions during or after PICC insertion, the PICC tip should be retracted to the SVC.

Many experienced PICC inserters will use ultrasound visualization of the internal jugular vein, subclavian vein, and SVC to visualize the PICC after insertion and prior to securing the PICC. However, this is not considered sufficient confirmation of tip location and a radiograph is still required. If the PICC is inserted under fluoroscopic guidance, a saved fluoroscopic image of the final tip location is generally considered sufficient confirmation of tip location.

14.4 Troubleshooting

Insertion If you are able to visualize or palpate an appropriate vessel but cannot cannulate it, consider the following: once an unsuccessful attempt to cannulate a vessel has been made, further attempts should be made proximal to the original site, so as to avoid cannulating a hematoma or advancing a wire through the previous insertion site. While many kits come with 20 g or larger needles or insertion catheters, many of the guidewires used will fit comfortably through a 22 g (or in some cases 24 g) PIV catheter. If you are unsuccessful using the supplied needle or PIV catheter, you can try cannulating the vessel

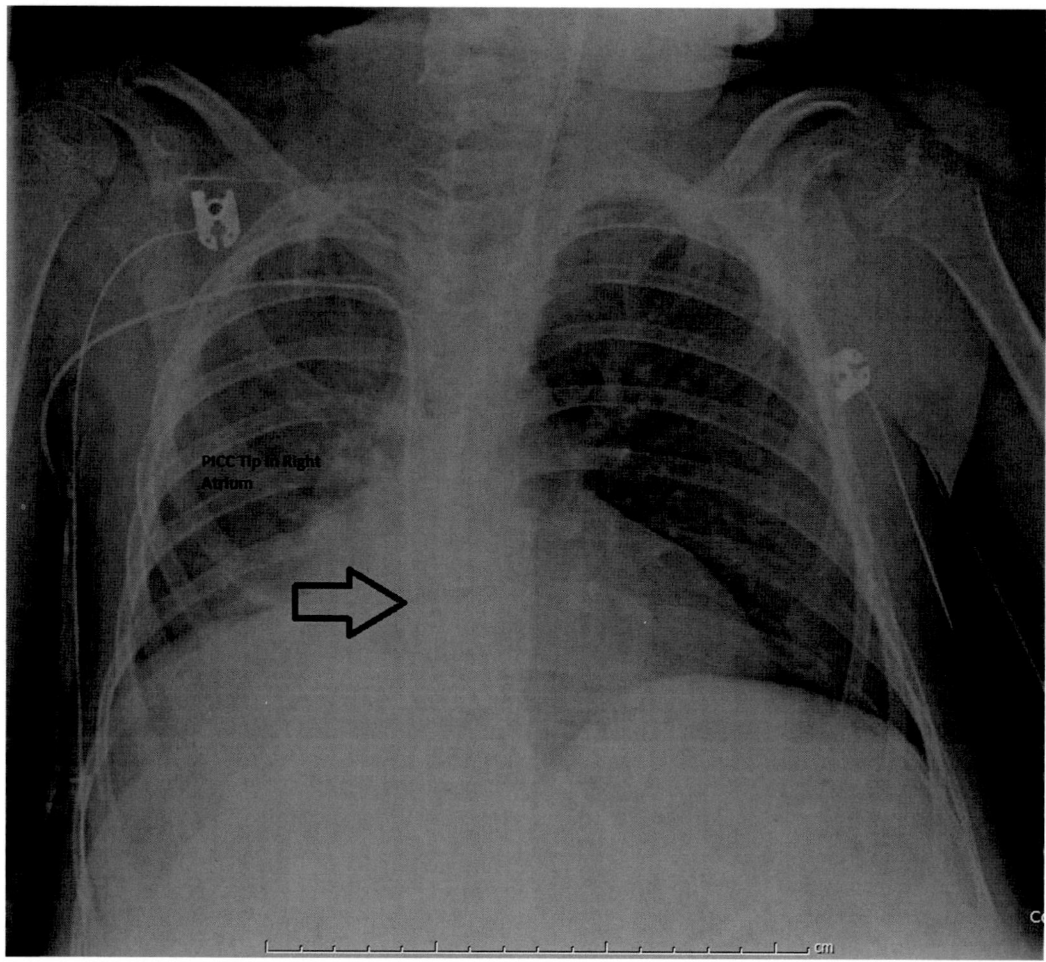

Fig. 14.3 Positioning of the PICC tip in the *right* atrium

with a smaller needle or catheter. Just be sure to confirm that your guidewire will pass through the needle or catheter you select first. If you are using ultrasound guidance and a transverse view of the vessel without success, consider using a longitudinal view of the vessel. While more technically difficult to hold during insertion, this view does allow visualization of valves, any displacement of the vessel wall by the needle, and any stenosis of the vessel at the point of attempted insertion.

Advancement If you have cannulated the vessel and inserted the PICC into the vessel but are unable to advance the PICC centrally, consider the following: advance the PICC slowly and steadily. Rapid advancement generates substantial heat through friction within the vessel, which can prompt vasospasm. If you encounter vasospasm, stop your advancement and wait a few minutes before attempting further advancement. If you encounter difficulties at the expected location of the axilla or subclavian veins, try extending the arm up and away from the patient. This sometimes helps align the vessels at the junction of the axillary and subclavian veins, allowing for passage. If this is unsuccessful, have an assistant try gently pressing on the clavicle or placing his/her hands between the shoulder blades and lifting. Some patients have a significant deflection of their subclavian vein under the clavicle which can prevent the advancement of the PICC.

If repeated attempts to advance the PICC are unsuccessful, particularly in a patient who has had previous PICCs or CVLs, a thrombus or stenosis may exist. In that case, you can either try a different limb for insertion or refer to interventional radiology, where a dye study can confirm the patency of the vessels.

Malposition The two most common malpositions of the PICC tip are in the internal jugular (IJ) vein (either ipsilateral or contralateral) and the contralateral subclavian vein. You can reduce the chance of IJ malposition during insertion by having the patient turn his/her head towards the insertion site during advancement and by having him or her take a deep breath during the last few centimeters of advancement. If the PICC tip is identified in the IJ prior to termination of the procedure (such as with ultrasound), the PICC can be retracted until out of the IJ and then reinserted. If the PICC tip migrates into the IJ or the malposition is identified after termination of the procedure, the following can be attempted to reposition the PICC. Obtain a 10 cc syringe with saline and attach it to the hub of the largest lumen of the PICC. Extend the patient's arm to 90° from the body and then raise the arm above the patient's head. This should retract the PICC tip a few centimeters. Then, flush the PICC in a rapid and pulsatile manner. This creates a "jet" of saline at the tip which can propel the PICC down into the SVC (visualize a firehose when the firefighter lets go of it and it whips around). Before you have finished flushing, drop the arm to the patient's side. This should readvance the PICC by several centimeters and ideally help guide it back into the SVC. If the PICC tip is located in the contralateral subclavian vein and the procedure has not been terminated, retract the tip to the ipsilateral subclavian vein, raise the head of the bed (if possible), and readvance. If the malposition is identified after the procedure has terminated (or the tip migration is identified on subsequent radiograph), the only practical solution is to retract the PICC until the tip rests just over the junction of the subclavian vein, IJ, and SVC. While not an ideal location, this is less likely to promote thrombosis than leaving the tip in a contralateral subclavian location.

14.4.1 Removal of the PICC

PICCs can be removed by trained nurses, either in the hospital or long-term care facility, during a clinic visit or at home for patients receiving home nursing care. To remove the PICC, the dressing is removed, the securement device (if used) or sutures are removed, and the PICC is slowly retracted until the entire PICC is removed. Prior to removal, you should confirm the length of the PICC from the insertion note (as PICCs can be trimmed to many lengths), and after removal you should confirm the PICC tip is at least as long as the recorded insertion length. The PICC may be longer than at the time of insertion, particularly if it has been indwelling for an extended period of time, as the material is designed to increase in flexibility when exposed to body heat, and adherence to vessel walls can then "stretch" the PICC. However, if the PICC measures shorter than the recorded length at insertion, the possibility that a portion of the PICC has been retained exists. This should prompt immediate referral to an interventional radiologist for further imaging and possible retrieval of retained PICC.

Once the PICC is removed, the insertion site can be dressed with an adhesive bandage. Some providers cover the insertion site with an antibiotic- or betadine-impregnated ointment prior to application of the adhesive bandage.

14.4.1.1 Complications

Infection Although PICC infections are rare (0.75/1000 catheter days, [2]), they do occur. PICCs are generally considered to have a lower overall infection rate versus percutaneously inserted CVLs. However, at least one study has demonstrated that, in high-risk hospitalized patients, the infection risk is roughly equivalent (2.1/1000 catheter days) to that of percutaneously placed CVLs [3]. This suggests that some of the association between PICCs and lower infection rates may have more to do with the types of patients who initially received PICCs rather than an innate lowering of risk due to the device or insertion site. Infection may require the removal of the device and short- or long-term courses of appropriate antibiotic therapy.

Thrombosis Although initially thought to be associated with lower risk of thrombosis than percutaneously placed CVLs, recent systematic reviews have indicated that PICCs may have a higher association with large vessel thrombus formation [4]. However, there is not an associated increased risk of pulmonary embolus. The long-term clinical significance of these thrombi is unclear. In this and other studies, most of the large vessel thrombi identified were in critically ill patients, suggesting that some of the earlier studies that suggested lower thrombus risk may have reflected the patients who initially received PICCs rather than the risk associated with the device itself or insertion site. As the use of PICCs in the acute and critical care settings increase, reevaluation of the associated complications will be necessary. Symptomatic large vessel thrombus formation may require the removal of the PICC and potentially anticoagulant therapy.

Occlusion Fibrin sheaths form on most long-term indwelling PICCs. This can result in non-thrombotic occlusion of the PICC, particularly with aspiration (due to a ball-valve effect of the sheath on the tip of the catheter). If clinically appropriate, this occlusion can be treated with the instillation of direct thrombolytic agents such as alteplase.

Phlebitis With increased use of ultrasound, insertion into deeper peripheral veins, and the increased use of the microintroducer technique, phlebitis has become a much less common complication of PICC insertion. A peripheral phlebitis not associated with thrombus will usually resolve with application of warm compresses to the affected area and use of nonsteroidal antiinflammatory medications (if clinically appropriate).

Malposition Because PICCs are generally softer and more flexible than CVLs, they are more prone to migration into unintended tip positions. The most common site of malposition is the ipsilateral internal jugular vein, although migration into the contralateral subclavian vein or migration back into the ipsilateral subclavian, axillary, or even basilica vein has been reported. Troubleshooting approaches to this malposition is addressed above, but persistent malposition may require removal or replacement of PICC.

Rupture Particularly when used in high-intensity environments, such as ICUs, PICCs can rupture. The most common site of rupture is at the catheter hub, but rupture can occur at any point. In general, this occurs when the PICC becomes occluded and pressure is exerted in an effort to instill a medication. The chance of rupture can be reduced by using only 10 cc or larger syringes for instilling medications into PICCs, as the pressure generated by larger syringes is generally insufficient to rupture the PICC wall. Ruptures of the distal catheter or hub external to the patient can sometimes be repaired using premade kits supplied by the PICC manufacturer. Internal ruptures or those close to the hub generally require the removal and replacement of the PICC.

14.5 Consideration of PICC Versus Percutaneously Placed CVL

In general, PICCs have lower reported infection rates versus percutaneously placed CVLs (0.75 versus 2.51/1000 catheter days, [2]). However, most studies comparing PICCs to CVLs have used data from PICCs that were indwelling for >7 days. There is no evidence that PICCs are safer for short-term use (<7 days) and in a critically ill patient who may require rapid or high-volume resuscitation, the percutaneously placed CVL may offer advantages that offset the theoretical reduction of infection rates in the short term.

14.6 Pearls/Pitfalls

- Advance the guidewire and catheter slowly (1–2 cm/s) as rapid advancement generates significant heat at the point where the vessel wall is in contact. This heat can cause endothelial damage and increase the risk of thrombus formation.
- If placing the PICC in an awake patient (or if an assistant is available), have him/her turn his/her head towards the side of insertion while advancing the catheter. This will slightly restrict the opening to the ipsilateral internal jugular vein and reduce the chance of malposition.
- If placing a PICC in a spontaneously breathing patient, try to perform the final 10–15 cm of catheter advancement during inhalation. Intrathoracic pressure will be at its most negative during inspiration, increasing venous return to the superior vena cava and helping direct the PICC towards the atriocaval junction. Conversely, in mechanically ventilated patients, advance during exhalation or during inhalation of an unassisted breath. Intrathoracic pressure in the mechanically ventilated patient is always positive but is the least positive during exhalation. Advancing during mechanical inhalation has a higher risk of directing the PICC tip upwards towards the internal jugular vein.

References

1. Stokowski G. The use of ultrasound to improve practice and reduce complication rates in peripherally inserted central catheter insertions: final report of investigation. J Infus Nurs. 2009;32(3):145–55.
2. Carrico R, editor. APIC text of infection control and epidemiology. 2nd ed. Washington, DC: Association for Professionals in Infection Control and Epidemiology; 2005.
3. Safdar N, Maki DG. Risk of catheter-related bloodstream infection with peripherally inserted central venous catheters used in hospitalized patients. Chest. 2005;128:489–95 [1].
4. Chopra V, et al. Risk of venous thromboembolism associated with peripherally inserted central catheters: a systematic review and meta-analysis. Lancet. 2013;382(9889):311–25. doi:10.1016/S0140-6736(13)60592-9. Epub 2013 May 20.

Intraosseous Access Techniques in the ICU

15

Dennis A. Taylor and Alan Hefner

15.1 Indications

Generally, the intraosseous route will be used for the critically ill or injured patient that quick intravenous access cannot be obtained. This is defined as three attempts or 90 seconds. Access sites for adults include the femur, tibia, and humerus.

15.2 Contraindications

- Establishment of a peripheral IV or central venous line.
- Fracture of the targeted bone.
- Previous, significant orthopedic procedures at insertion site (e.g., prosthetic limb or joint).
- IO in the targeted bone within the past 48 h.
- Infection at area of insertion.
- Excessive tissue or absence of adequate anatomical landmarks.

15.3 Equipment/Procedure

There are many commercially available devices that enable the placement of an intraosseous needle. This chapter will review and discuss the EZ-IO by VidaCare system (Figs. 15.1 and 15.2) [1].

- EZ-IO® Power Driver.
- EZ-IO® Needle Set and EZ-Connect® Extension Set.
- EZ-Stabilizer® Dressing.
- Non-sterile gloves.
- Cleansing agent of choice.
- Luer lock syringe with sterile normal saline flush (5–10 ml for adults, 2–5 ml for infant/child).
- Sharps container.
- 2 % preservative and epinephrine-free lidocaine (intravenous lidocaine).
- Intravenous fluid.
- Infusion pressure pump or pressure bag, tubing, 3-way stop cock.
- Supplies for lab samples.

D.A. Taylor, DNP, ACNP-BC, FCCM (✉)
A. Hefner, MD, FCCM
Carolinas HealthCare System, Charlotte, NC 28232, USA
e-mail: dennis.taylor@carolinashealthcare.org; alan.hefner@carolinashealthcare.org

D.A. Taylor et al. (eds.), *Interventional Critical Care*, DOI 10.1007/978-3-319-25286-5_15

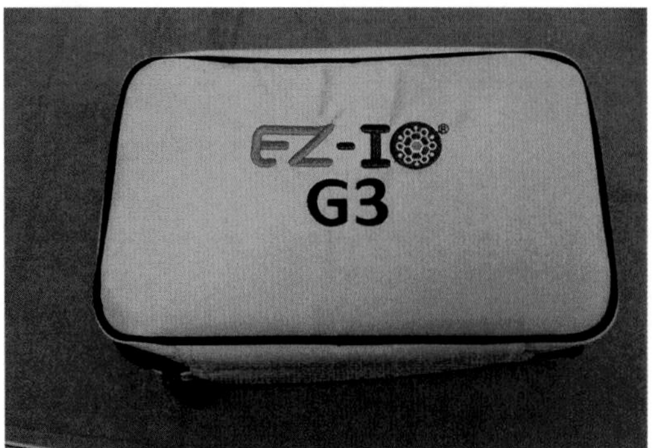

Fig. 15.1 EZ-IO Kit

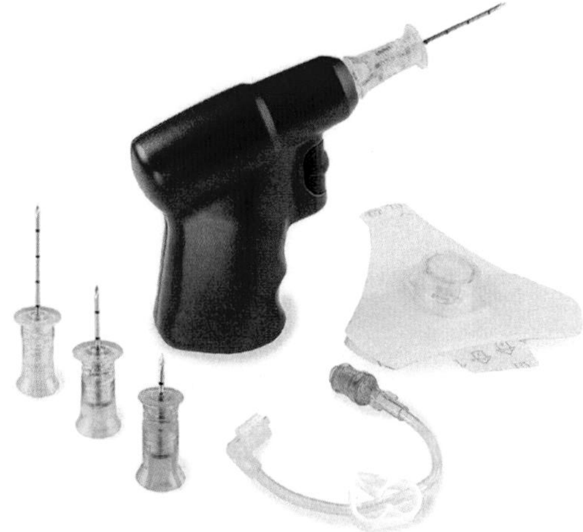

Fig. 15.2 EZ-IO Drill

15.3.1 Adult Insertion Site Identification

Proximal Humerus (Adult)

1. Place the patient's hand over the abdomen (elbow adducted and humerus internally rotated) (Fig. 15.3).
2. Place your palm on the patient's shoulder anteriorly; the "ball" under your palm is the general target area (Fig. 15.4).

   You should be able to feel this ball, even on obese patients, by pushing deeply.
3. Place the ulnar aspect of your hand vertically over the axilla and the ulnar aspect of your other hand along the midline of the upper arm laterally (Fig. 15.5).
4. Place your thumbs together over the arm; this identifies the vertical line of insertion on the proximal humerus (Figs. 15.6 and 15.7).

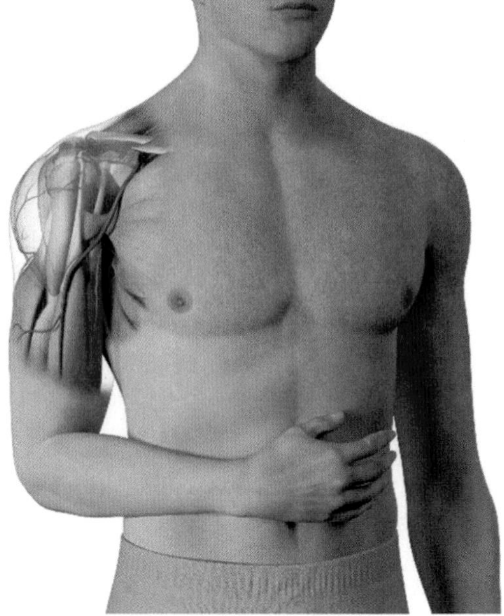

Fig. 15.3 Positioning arm

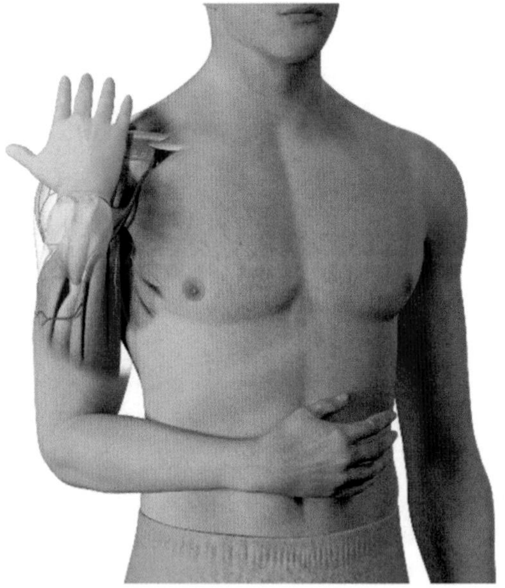

Fig. 15.4 Feeling humeral head

5. Palpate deeply up the humerus to the surgical neck.

   This may feel like a golf ball on a tee—the spot where the "ball" meets the "tee" is the surgical neck (Fig. 15.8).

   The insertion site is 1–2 cm above the surgical neck, on the most prominent aspect of the greater tubercle (Fig. 15.9).

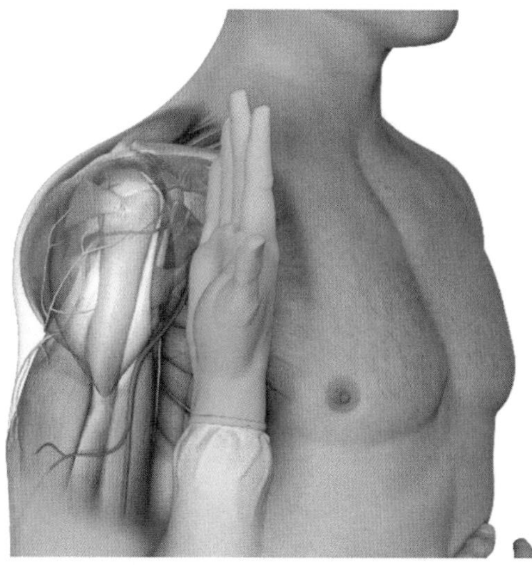

Fig. 15.5 Placement of *right* hand

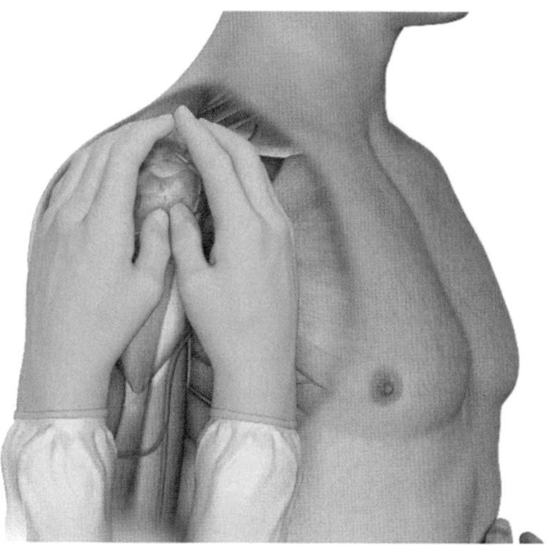

Fig. 15.7 *Vertical line* of insertion

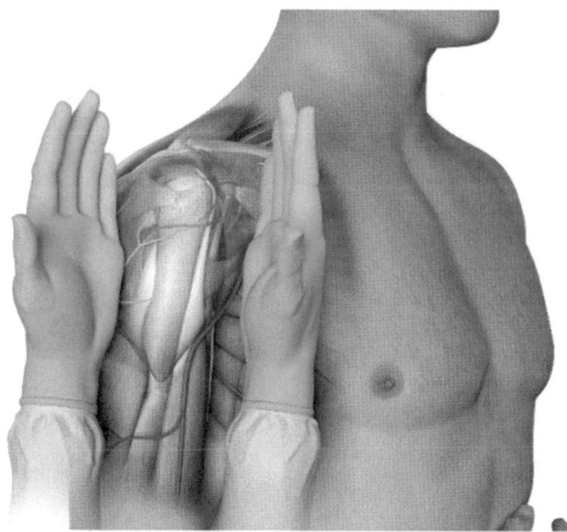

Fig. 15.6 Placement of *left* hand

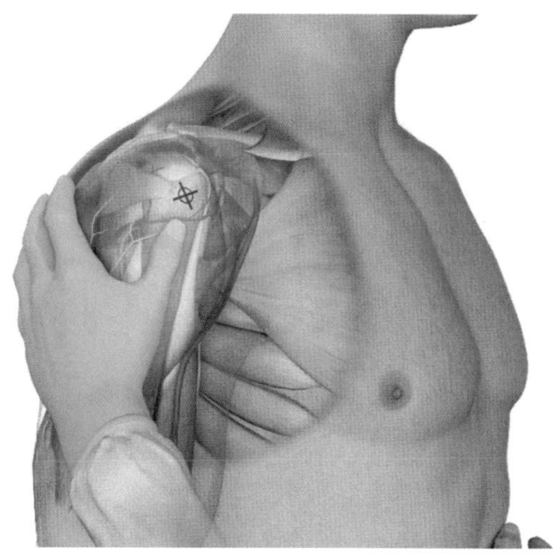

Fig. 15.8 Location of surgical neck

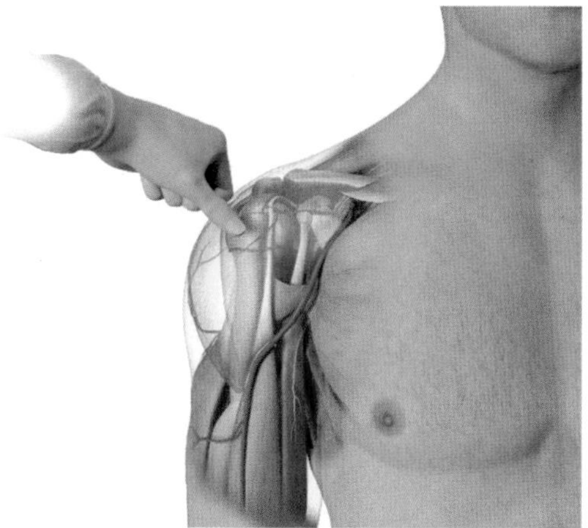

Fig. 15.9 Greater tubercle

Proximal Tibia (Adult)

1. Extend the leg.
2. Insertion site is approximately 2 cm medial to the tibial tuberosity, or approximately 3 cm below the patella and approximately 2 cm medial, along the flat aspect of the tibia (Fig. 15.10).
3. Aim the needle set at a 90° angle to the bone.
4. Push the needle set tip through the skin until the tip rests against the bone.

The 5 mm mark must be visible above the skin for the confirmation of adequate needle set length.

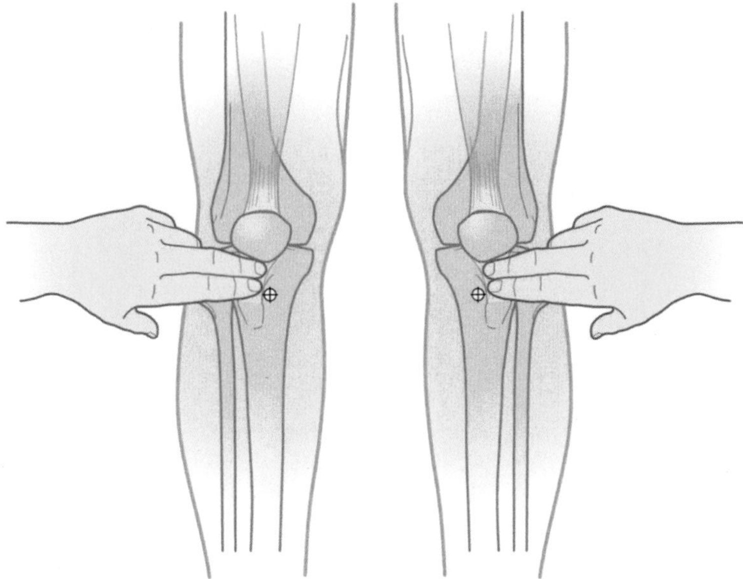

Fig. 15.10 Location of insertion—tibial tuberosity

5. Gently drill, advancing the needle set approximately 1–2 cm after entry into the medullary space or until the needle set hub is close to the skin.

Distal Tibia (Adult)

1. Insertion site is located approximately 3 cm proximal to the most prominent aspect of the medial malleolus (Fig. 15.11).
2. Palpate the anterior and posterior borders of the tibia to assure insertion site is on the flat center aspect of the bone.

15.4 Needle Set Selection

Select EZ-IO® Needle Set based on patient weight, anatomy, and clinical judgment. The EZ-IO® catheter is marked with a black line 5 mm proximal to the hub. Prior to drilling, with the EZ-IO® Needle Set inserted through the soft tissue and the needle tip touching bone, adequate needle length is determined by the ability to see the 5 mm black line above the skin.

- EZ-IO® 45 mm Needle Set (yellow hub) should be considered for proximal humerus insertion in patients 40 kg and greater and patients with excessive tissue over any insertion site.
- EZ-IO® 25 mm Needle Set (blue hub) should be considered for patients 3 kg and greater.
- EZ-IO® 15 mm Needle Set (pink hub) should be considered for patients approximately 3–39 kg.

15.5 Insertion Completion

1. Hold the hub in place and pull the driver straight off; continue to hold the hub while twisting the stylet off the hub with counterclockwise rotations; catheter should feel firmly seated in the bone (first confirmation of placement);

   Dispose of all sharps and biohazard materials using standard biohazard practices and disposal containers.

   If using the NeedleVISE® 1 port sharps block, place on stable surface and use a one-handed technique.
2. Place the EZ-Stabilizer® Dressing over the hub (Fig. 15.12).
3. Attach a primed extension set to the catheter hub; firmly secure by twisting clockwise.

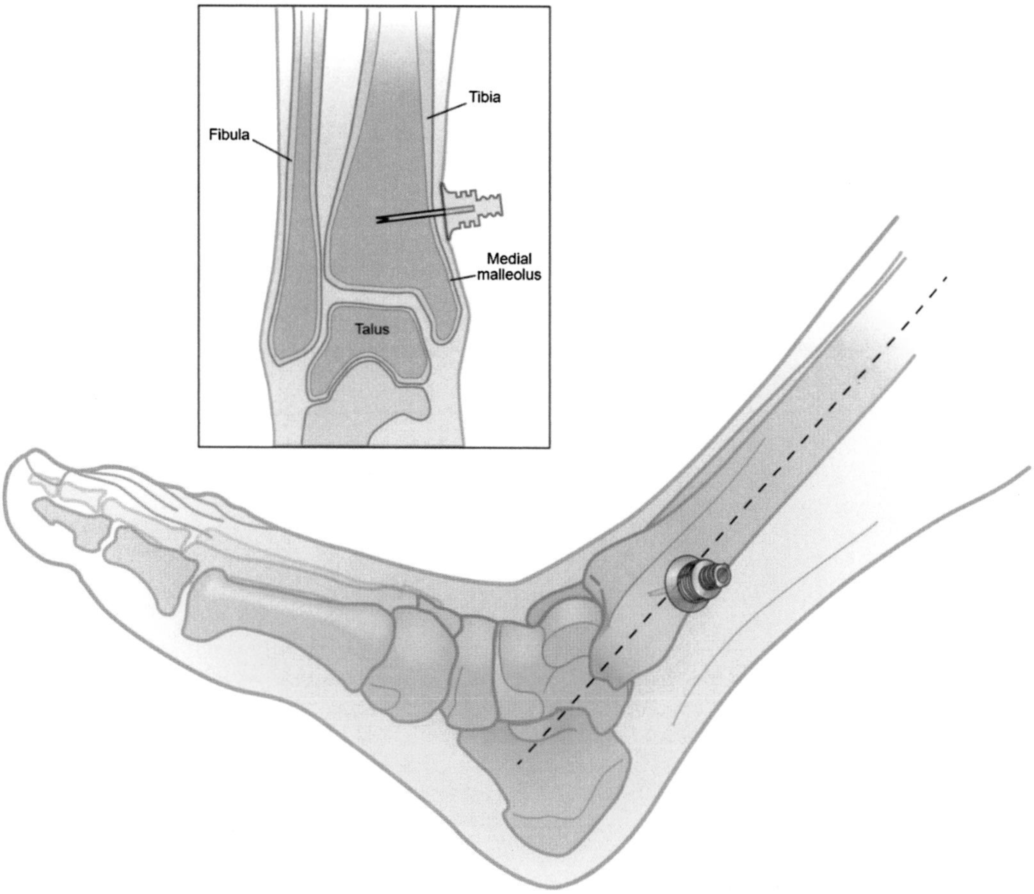

Fig. 15.11 Lateral malleolus

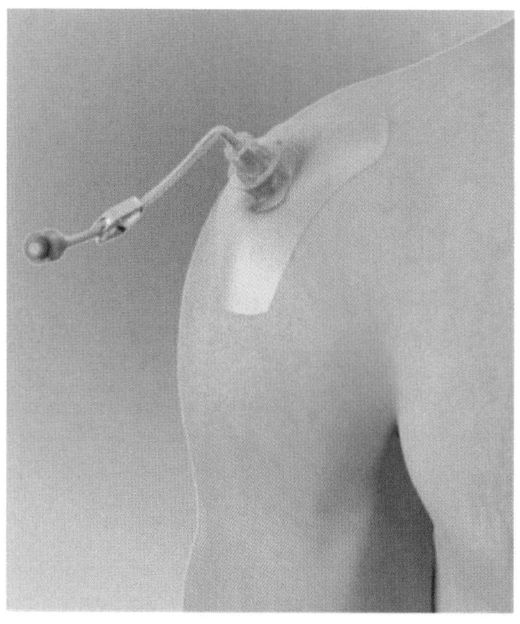

Fig. 15.12 IO with dressing in place

4. Pull the tabs off the dressing to expose the adhesive; apply to the skin.
5. Aspirate for blood/bone marrow (second confirmation of placement)[1]
6. Proceed with technique below, based on situation:
   (a) Adult (responsive to pain): recommended anesthetic.
   Observe recommended cautions/contraindications to using 2 % preservative and epinephrine-free lidocaine (intravenous lidocaine) and confirm lidocaine dose per institutional protocol
      1. Prime extension set with lidocaine.
   Note that the priming volume of the EZ-Connect® Extension Set is approximately 1.0 ml.

[1] *Inability to withdraw/aspirate blood from the catheter hub does not mean the insertion was unsuccessful.*

2. Slowly infuse lidocaine 40 mg IO over 120 s.
3. Allow lidocaine to dwell in IO space 60 s.
4. Flush with 5–10 ml of normal saline.
5. Slowly administer an additional 20 mg of lidocaine IO over 60 s.

Repeat PRN; consider systemic pain control for patients not responding to IO lidocaine.

(b) Adult: unresponsive to pain.

1. Prime extension set with normal saline.
2. Flush the IO catheter with 5–10 ml of normal saline.

If patient develops signs indicating responsiveness to pain, refer to adult recommended anesthetic technique.

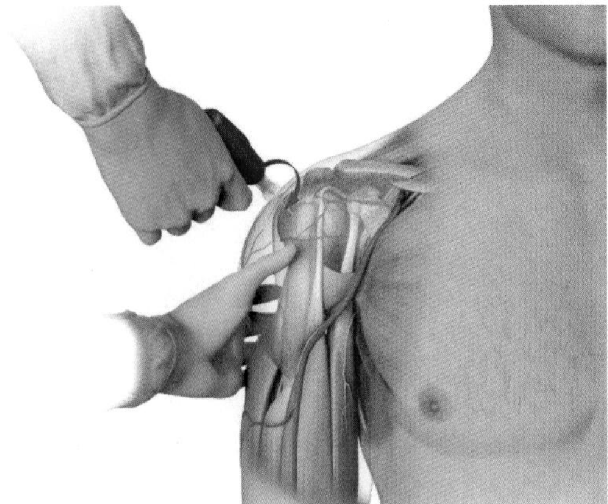

Fig. 15.13 The hub of the needle set should be perpendicular to the skin

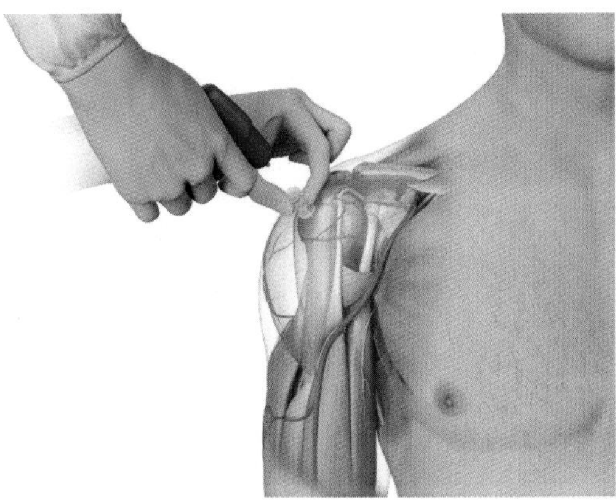

Fig. 15.14 Hold the hub in place and pull the driver straight off

15.6 Inserxtion: Adult Humerus

- Prepare the site by using antiseptic solution of your choice.
- Use a clean, "no touch" technique.
- Remove the needle cap.
- Point the needle set tip at a 45° angle to the anterior plane and posteromedial.
- Push the needle tip through the skin until the tip rests against the bone.
- The 5 mm mark must be visible above the skin for the confirmation of adequate needle length.
- Gently drill into the humerus 2 cm or until the hub reaches the skin in an adult (Figs. 15.13 and 15.14).
- Continue to hold the hub while twisting the stylet off the hub with counterclockwise rotations.
  - The needle should feel firmly seated in the bone (first confirmation of placement).
- Place the stylet in a sharps container.
- Place the EZ-Stabilizer™ dressing over the hub.
- Attach a primed EZ-Connect® Extension set to the hub; firmly secure by twisting clockwise.
- Pull the tabs off the EZ-Stabilizer dressing to expose the adhesive; apply to the skin.
- Aspirate for blood/bone marrow (second confirmation of placement).
- Secure the arm in place across the abdomen.

15.7 Removal Technique

1. Remove extension set and dressing.
2. Stabilize catheter hub and attach a Luer lock syringe to the hub.
3. Maintaining axial alignment, twist clockwise and pull straight out.
   Do *not* rock the syringe.
4. Dispose of catheter with syringe attached into sharps container.

5. Apply pressure to site as needed to control bleeding and apply dressing as indicated.

15.8 Complications

Complications may be similar to those of a peripheral IV such as infection, air embolism, infiltration, circulatory overload, allergic reactions, and thrombophlebitis. In addition, complications may also include fracture, growth plate damage, and insertion of the needle through both sides of the bone resulting in infiltration. Finally, the risk of developing a pulmonary embolism is greater due to the bone, fat, or marrow particles that may make their way into central circulation and ultimately the lungs.

15.9 Summary

Rapid venous access is often needed in the critical care area. Placement of an IO is a safe, rapid, and effective means to establish a route of medication and blood administration.

Reference

1. http://www.teleflex.com/en/usa/ezioeducation/index.html

Temporary Transvenous Pacemakers

16

Fred P. Mollenkopf, David K Rhine, and Hari Kumar Dandapantula

16.1 Introduction

The goal of this chapter is to give an overview of bedside insertion of temporary transvenous pacemaker catheters through established central venous access. Central venous access has been addressed in a previous chapter. The optimal sites of venous or sheath access (in order of preference) are right internal jugular vein, left subclavian vein, or femoral vein. The right internal jugular vein offers the most direct route to the ventricle and is associated with the highest success rate and fewest of complications [1]. Additionally, avoiding the left subclavian area leaves a clean site if the patient needs permanent pacemaker placement in the future. Using the right internal jugular (IJ) or left subclavian vein utilizes the natural curve of the pacemaker lead. These approaches have been the most successful particularly with placement of temporary floating or balloon-tipped leads. Pacemaker implantation from the femoral route can be used but is best reserved for semi-rigid leads advanced under fluoroscopic or echographic control. "J"-shaped catheters are available for femoral access that helps transition from the IVC through the tricuspid valve. Often manipulation of the lead in the right atrium or inferior vena cava is necessary to access the right ventricular (RV) apex. Femoral leads are the least stable due to possible dislodgement and are prone to infection and early deep venous thrombosis. We will describe herein temporary pacing lead insertion using the flow-directed as well as the ECG-guided bedside technique.

16.2 Indications

Temporary pacing is indicated when bradycardia causes severe hemodynamic impairment, syncope, or signs of organ malperfusion. These are primarily patients with symptomatic second or third degree AV block or significant hypotension from profound sinus bradycardia. In experienced hands, temporary pacing can be also used to suppress atrial arrhythmias, (e.g., atrial flutter) and to treat recurrent monomorphic ventricular tachycardia in patients with prolonged QT intervals. Frequently, pacing catheters are utilized following acute myocardial infarction (particularly inferior wall), either temporarily or as bridge to permanent pacemaker implantation.

F.P. Mollenkopf, PA-C (✉)
Thoracic and Cardiovascular Institute of Sparrow Hospital, 405 W. Greenlawn Ave Suite 200, Lansing, MI 48910, USA
e-mail: Fredmeds@gmail.com; fredmed@sprynet.com

D.K. Rhine, MD
Thoracic and Cardiovascular Institute of Sparrow Hospital, 405 W. Greenlawn Ave Suite 200, Lansing, MI 48910, USA
e-mail: DKRhine@hotmail.com

H.K. Dandapantula, MD
Cleveland Clinic Heart and Vascular Institute, 9500 Euclid Avenue, Cleveland, OH 44195, USA
e-mail: harikumar7@yahoo.com

D.A. Taylor et al. (eds.), *Interventional Critical Care*, DOI 10.1007/978-3-319-25286-5_16

Class I recommendations for temporary pacemaker placement include the following: [2]

- Asystole
- Symptomatic bradycardia
- Bilateral bundle branch block (or alternating BBB)
- New or indeterminate age bifascicular block
- Mobitz-type II second-degree AV block
- Complete heart block

Temporary pacing should be used for very short periods. Complications increase significantly after 24 h of use, and we feel strongly that cardiology and/or electrophysiology consultation should be sought early. When pacing is required more than 2–3 days in a pacer-dependent patient, the safest option is the insertion of an active fixation (screw-in) endocardial lead which can be externalized and connected to generator. This is the usual approach for patients undergoing device explant for endocarditis or lead infection during systemic antimicrobial therapy. The lead can be easily removed for permanent device implant following appropriate length of treatment and negative cultures [3].

It is important to emphasize that insertion of a temporary pacemaker carries a high risk of potential complications as outlined later in this chapter. The operator should be experienced in obtaining central venous access from multiple sites, have knowledge of intracardiac anatomy, and be able to recognize the difference between captured and non-captured pacing stimuli [4].

Less invasive strategies such as pharmacologic agents for acutely reversible causes as well as transcutaneous cardiac pacing should be instituted, while equipment for temporary venous pacemaker insertion is readied.

Short-term transcutaneous pacing with appropriate sedation can be lifesaving if ventricular capture is successful. It is commonly employed first in an emergency. Most defibrillators have the ability to deliver emergency external pacing via multifunction pads that can be used to perform cardioversion, defibrillation, and pacing. It is stressed to familiarize oneself with the defibrillators in the units you cover. The most frequent error in attempting to initiate either external pacing or synchronized cardioversion is failure to attach the patient ECG cable to the defibrillator unit prior to initiation. The device cannot "read" the rhythm for the pads AND pace or defibrillate simultaneously. Pacing pads are placed either in the anterior-lateral or anterior-posterior positions in a patient that has the ECG cable attached to the device as you would for a synchronized cardioversion. When pacing initiated, the default setting begins at a rate of 70 with a current (mA) of 30. Current is then increased until evidence on monitor of ventricular capture and palpable pulse is present. In bradyasystolic arrest, mA should be initiated at maximum output (~200 mA) and then decreased slowly while ascertaining ventricular capture and systemic pulse to about 10 (mA) above threshold (see threshold below). Typical transcutaneous threshold should be ≤ 80 mA. Failure to capture can be secondary to metabolic derangement (commonly acidosis), poor electrode contact, obesity, myocardial ischemia, and pneumothorax.

Transcutaneous pacing should only be instituted in the symptomatic patient. Initiating pacing in a patient with a stable escape rhythm may render that patient pacer dependent with asystole occurring upon loss of capture or termination of pacing. The limitations of external pacing are reliability and the need for continuous sedation and control of pain from skin contact (burning) and skeletal muscle contraction. Usual requirements would include a benzodiazepine/narcotic combination or use of dexmedetomidine for procedural sedation.

It should be noted that there are limited scenarios where pacing is indicated for asystolic cardiac arrest, particularly in the prehospital or emergency setting. Randomized trials have failed to show survival benefit in those situations [5]. Temporary external pacing has most success in temporary or reversible situations or until a more experienced personnel arrive to assist with transvenous wire insertion. Attempts at wire placement may often prevent or delay delivery of effective chest compressions.

16.3 Contraindications

The only absolute contraindication is failure to get consent from conscious patient. There are a number of relative contraindications to transvenous pacemaker insertion. Temporary and reversible causes of conduction disorders such as myocarditis, drug intoxication, and electrolyte disorders should be managed conservatively. Patients with profound coagulopathy or those receiving thrombolytics should be considered at increased risk for complications. These patients should be managed transcutaneously or with pharmacologic adjuncts if at all possible. In general, pacemaker insertion for asystolic and traumatic arrest does not seem to be beneficial. In patients with significant hypothermia, bradyarrhythmias are frequently present. Hypothermia can produce dramatic electrocardiographic abnormalities such as QRS widening, PR and QT interval prolongation, as well as atrial and ventricular arrhythmias. There are limited data on the need or benefit for treatment of bradycardia associated with hypothermia, and there are concerns for terminal dysrhythmias in those patients. Lastly, atrial fibrillation, multifocal atrial tachycardia, and significant AV conduction system disease are relative contraindications to transvenous *atrial* pacing, which are not usually considered in emergency situations.

16.4 Pacing Background

A basic understanding of pacemaker nomenclature includes the abbreviations for various pacing modes. The international NBG five-letter code describes pacing capabilities of any device in terms of pacing, sensing, and the response to sensing as seen in Fig. (16.1).

The first three positions relate to all types of pacing, with the latter two referring to permanent pacing only. The reader is referred to the revised NASPE/BPEG Generic Code for Antibradycardia, Adaptive-Rate, and Multisite Pacing for a more comprehensive study [6]. For the purpose of single-chamber pacing, we are only concerned with four potential combinations of code. The most common mode during initial insertion is VOO or asynchronous ventricular pacing with continuous pacing output regardless of any cardiac activity. In VVI or demand ventricular pacing, ventricular depolarization is sensed by the pacer, and the pacing

Fig. 16.1 Revised NASPE/BPEG generic code for antibradycardia, adaptive-rate, and multisite pacing. *Source*: Adapted from PACE 2002; 25: 260–264

Revised NASPE/BPEG Code for Antibradycardia Pacing*

Position I Chamber Paced	**Position II** Chamber Sensed	**Position III** Response to Sensing	**Position IV** Rate Modulation
0 = None	0 = None	0 = None	O = None
0 = None	0 = None	T = Triggered	R =Rate Modulation
V =Ventricle	V =Ventricle	I = Inhibited	-
D =Dual (A + V)	D =Dual (A + V)	D =Dual (A + V)	-

output is inhibited or withheld by the generator. Typically this mode might be used in bradycardia, or intermittent heart block or pauses, where the patient has some intrinsic rhythm. Similarly, in single-chamber pacing leads placed in the atrium only, AOO or AAI modes can be programmed.

16.5 Equipment

- Full-body sterile drape, standard sterile personal protective equipment
- Cardiac monitor (continuous), ECG machine, and code cart available
- Vascular sheath (large enough to pass catheter), typically 6Fr. diameter
- Normal saline for sheath flush
- External pacemaker (pulse generator) with pacing cable and wire connectors
- New battery in generator for every patient
- Pacemaker lead appropriate for insertion site

16.6 Pacemaker Catheters

A variety of prepackaged catheter sets are available. Most critical care and emergency units have at least one type of balloon-tipped catheter for temporary pacing. Careful review of the packaging will indicate whether the specific lead is more suitable for SVC or femoral insertion. Typically the package includes a single-lumen introducer sheath, pacing catheter, pacing wire adapters, and protective plastic sleeve. The typical catheter tray is shown below, containing the pacing catheter, syringe, and adapters that connect to pacing cable (Fig. 16.2). Note the lead adapters in the center of the tray. These are used to adapt the lead to a pacemaker cable as seen in Fig. 16.3. Use of the cable provides for less tension on the lead during placement and allows an assistant to control the pacemaker lead system away from the sterile field. The two adapters are packaged in a separate envelope in the tray. During the opening of the peel-away package, they can be lost in the drapes

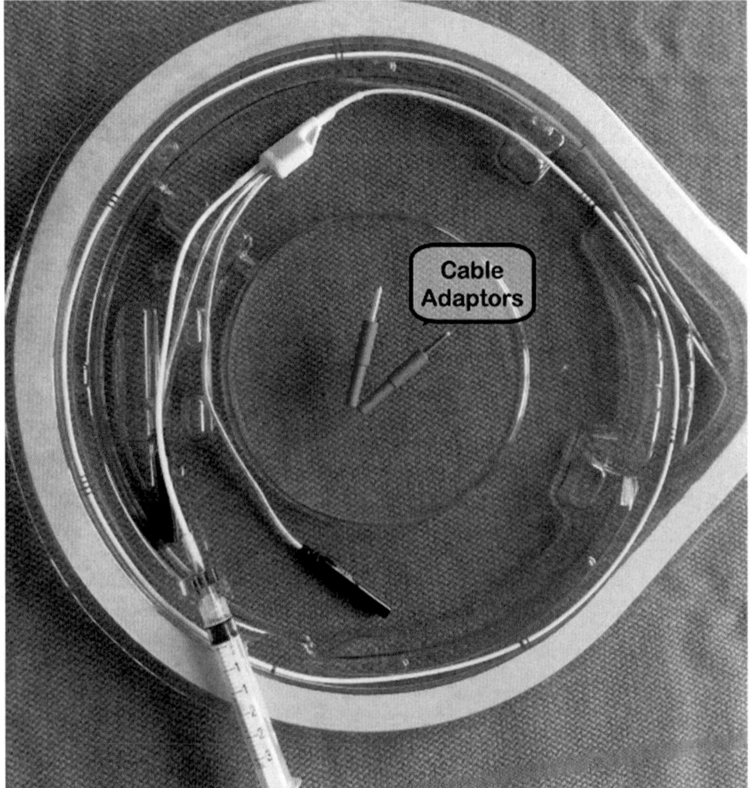

Fig. 16.2 Pacemaker tray with catheter, syringe, and adapters in *center*

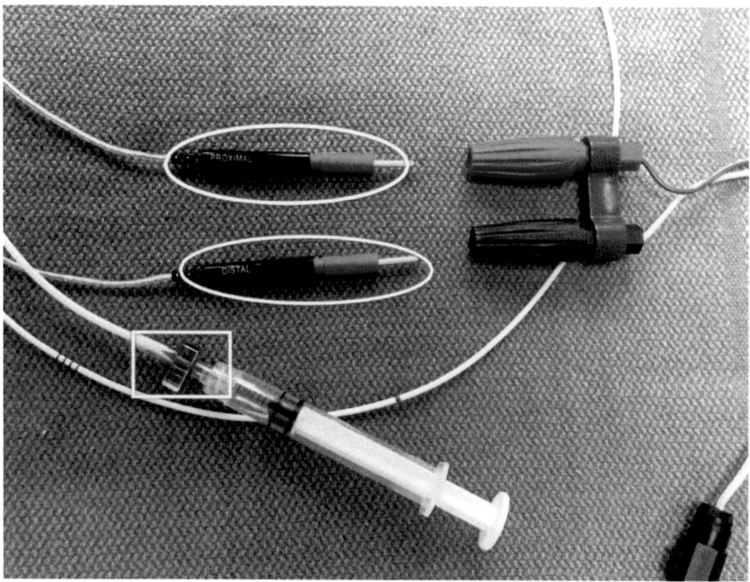

Fig. 16.3 Pacemaker leads with adapters (*circles*) and locking mechanism (*square*), pacing cable

or fall on the floor. In that event, leads can be inserted directly into the pulse generators in some models, but may be necessary to connect the cable to the pacing lead.

Catheters are either floating (balloon-tipped) or semirigid leads. Rigid catheters are used only with fluoroscopic control or with experienced operators using echo guidance. Temporary leads are bipolar and usually 90–100 cm long, with 10-cm markings similar to CVP catheters. Balloon-inflated catheters cannot be used in the absence of forward flow, e.g., asystolic cardiac arrest. In that scenario, insertion can be attempted without inflation. At least one company makes pulmonary artery catheters with separate pacing ports available, but these leads are not regarded as stable for the pacer-dependent patient.

The pacing leads are 3–5 Fr. in diameter and fit well in a 6 Fr. introducer. Using a much larger introducer (8–9 Fr.) may allow blood leakage at the proximal entry portion of the introducer and increase the risk of vascular complications. Use of previously placed larger sheath can be done if absolutely necessary, but contamination of the pacing lead coupled with the slow leakage of blood can quickly lead to infection and possible sepsis or endocarditis.

Temporary leads are bipolar with the distal tip of catheter (negative electrode) in direct contact with the heart. The distal or negative lead serves as the cathode that delivers the pacing stimulus to the heart. The *proximal* electrode is about 1 cm from the distal tip and is connected to the *positive* terminal of the pulse generator either directly or by bridging cable as shown in Fig. 16.3. The anode or positive electrode is multifunctional. It grounds or returns electrical stimulus to the pulse generator and is responsible for sensing inherent myopotentials. Bipolar leads as shown in Fig. 16.4a and b are much less sensitive to outside electrical mechanical interference or EMI in contrast to unipolar leads.

16.7 Pulse Generators |(External Pacemakers)

A number of pulse generators for external pacing are available, and two commonly used devices from Medtronic are shown below (Fig. 16.5). On the right is a single-chamber model and, on the left, a dual chamber model. The dual chamber model is frequently utilized in postoperative cardiac surgery patients with epicardial atrial and ventricular leads in place. The dual-chamber device can be used to pace either in the atrium, ventricle, or both chambers as in A–V sequential pacing. Dual-chamber pacing is not typically used in the emergency situation unless functioning wires have been previously positioned intraoperatively during cardiac surgery.

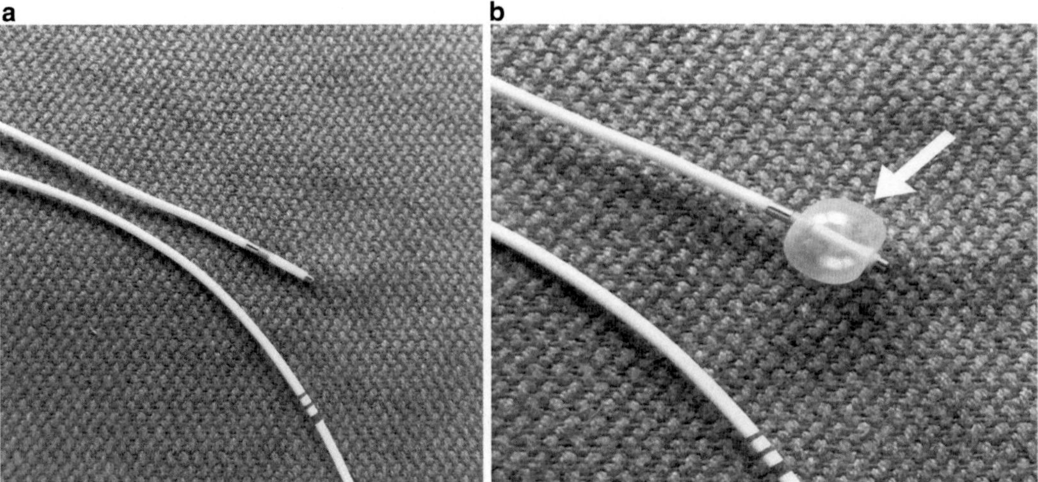

Fig. 16.4 (**a**) Bipolar lead tip deflated. (**b**) Bipolar tip with balloon inflated (*arrow*)

A dial controls the current or electrical output, measured in *milliamps* (mA), usually from 0.1 to 25 (max). A separate dial controls the *rate* and another to adjust the *sensitivity* that establishes the threshold based on the amplitude of the intrinsic R wave required to suppress the pacemaker from pacing in VVI mode. Sensitivity is measured in millivolts (mV) and determines the size of the cardiac signal that the generator will recognize. For urgent pacemaker insertion, the threshold is set to low to allow for *asynchronous* (VOO) or "fixed-rate" pacing. Some generators like the dual-chamber device (below left) have an "asynchronous" or "emergency" setting exclusively for this purpose.

With the sensitivity set high, the generator delivers a pulse only when there is no intrinsic ventricular depolarization at a set rate or R–R interval. This is *demand* (VVI) mode or synchronous pacing. In patients with intrinsic ventricular depolarization, this may be optimal after placement to prevent pacing in the vulnerable period or "R-on-T"-mediated VT or VF.

16.8 Insertion

Most providers are more comfortable with the "blind" or floating-balloon catheter technique in the emergency room or critical care unit. We will describe this technique as the preferred method as it is generally faster and less complex in the absence imaging.

Alternatively, five-lead electrocardiography (ECG) may be used to guide lead placement in the monitored patient. The ECG-guided technique uses sensing from the distal (negative) lead attached to a precordial lead on an ECG machine to give the operator feedback via waveform for catheter position. ECG-guided technique is feasible albeit somewhat more challenging [7, 8].

16.9 Typical Bedside Insertion

After placement of the introducer or sheath, the balloon on the pacing lead should be checked for leaks with inflation 1.5-ml air or saline prior to insertion. One can check for air leaks easily by submerging the catheter tip underwater and inflating looking for bubbles. When inflated, the balloon allows for flow-directed insertion and protects the myocardium by limiting the amount of exposed distal lead with the notion of limiting the risk of cardiac perforation.

The pacing catheter is connected either directly to the generator or optimally to the cable with pacemaker on at max (20–25 mA) output, with least sensitivity (*asynchronous* mode), and rate 80–100 or at least 10 bpm greater than

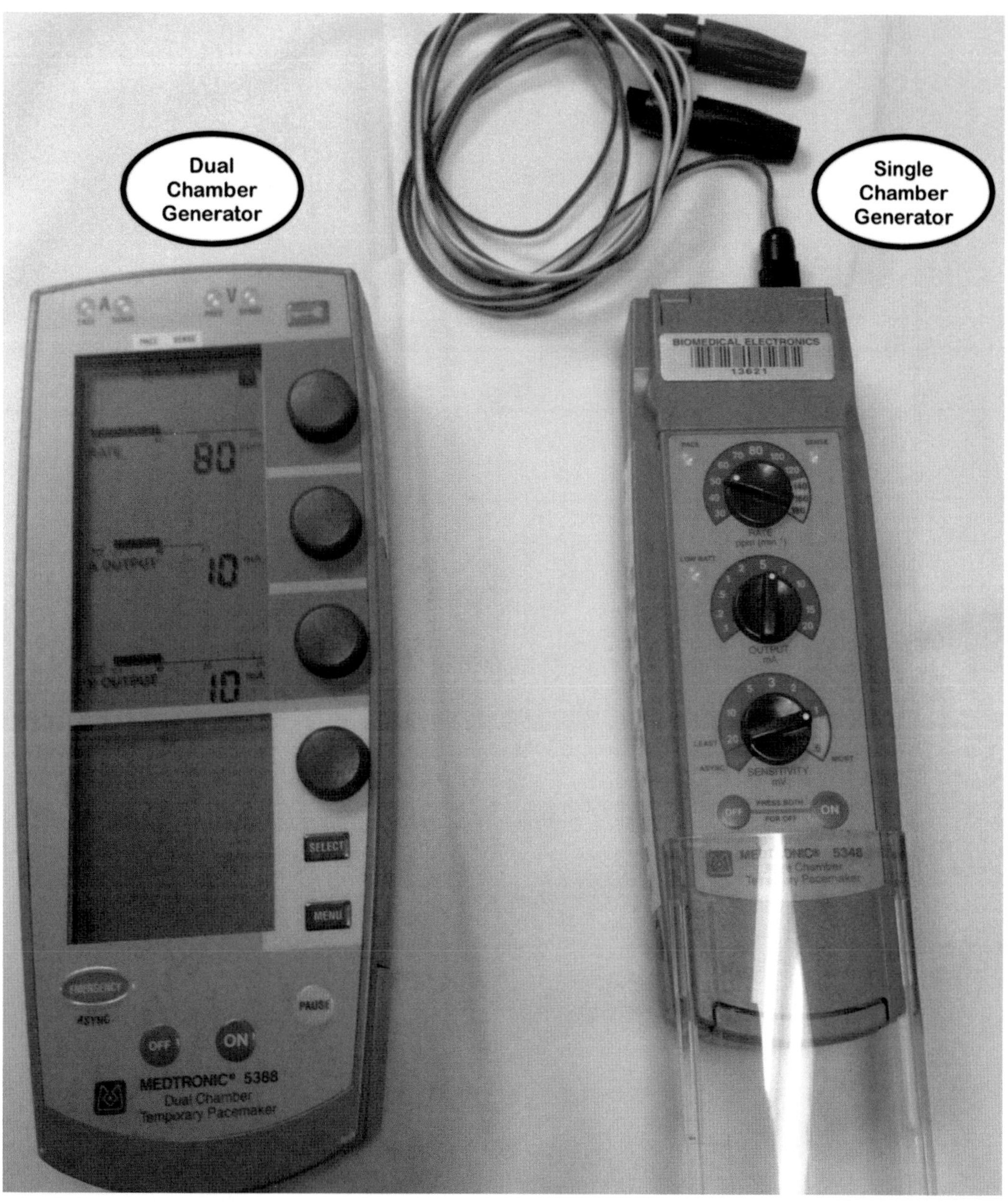

Fig. 16.5 Pacemaker generators. Dual chamber above *left*; single chamber, above *right*

intrinsic rhythm. All connections need to be secured prior to any manipulation.

With the balloon deflated, the catheter is advanced through the sheath to at least 15 cm and less than or equal to 20-cm mark on catheter and then inflated. The locking mechanism (Fig. 16.3 square) on the catheter hub is engaged by sliding in place to ensure balloon inflation throughout the passage of the catheter. Then advance the catheter slowly while the ECG monitor is watched for evidence of capture (Fig. 16.6, typical flow-directed pacing catheter). Pacer spikes will be apparent and ventricular capture will be achieved when catheter touches the endocardium. Pacer spikes are followed by a widened QRS. The balloon should be deflated immediately following capture

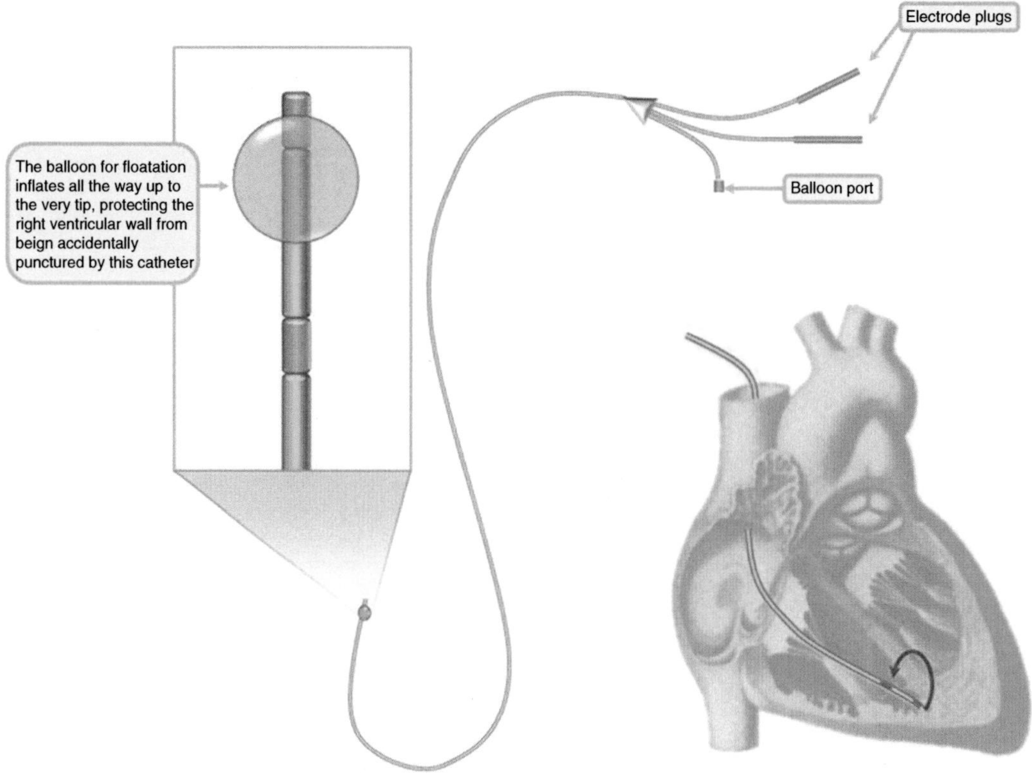

Fig. 16.6 Typical transvenous pacing catheter in RV

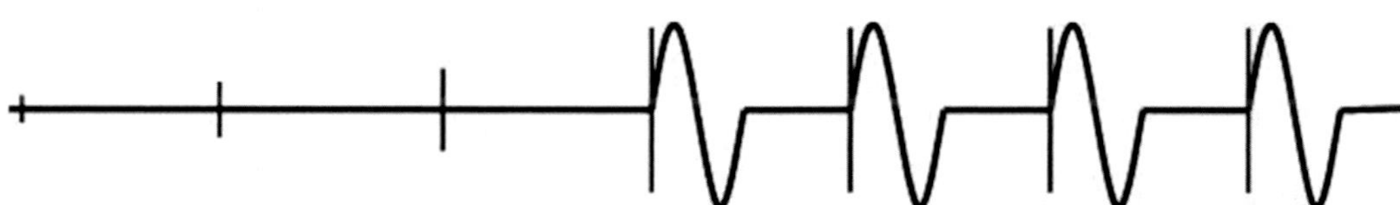

Fig. 16.7 Schematic of RV capture as lead contacts endocardium

to avoid transitioning into the pulmonary outflow tract. If fluoroscopic or continuous transthoracic echo available, deflate the balloon as soon as tricuspid valve transitioned or entry into RV seen. The wide QRS pattern will be similar to a left bundle branch block as the electrode contacts the anterior apical wall of the right ventricle (Fig. 16.7). On the 12-lead ECG, QRS should have LBBB morphology and a superior axis (i.e., a negative QRS complex in II, III, and AVF) (Fig. 16.8).

If pacer spikes are not seen or there is no ventricular capture evident on monitor, recheck all connections as well as battery and consider refloating catheter with balloon inflated as above. One clue indicating electrical failure as opposed to inadequate catheter placement may be the presence of reproducible PVCs, indicating catheter tip contact the right ventricular endocardium without capture. Catheter insertion should always be attempted with balloon inflated to prevent ventricular perforation. Only in asystole should one insert a semirigid lead or catheter with balloon deflated without fluoroscopy or continuous echographic visualization. Transthoracic echo (TTE) assessment can identify lead passage from

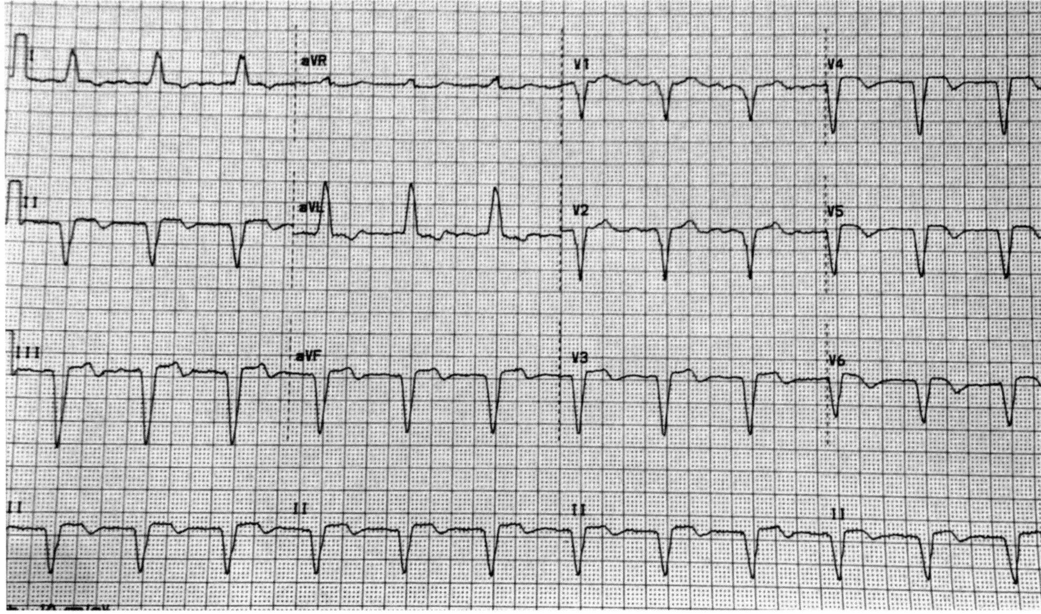

Fig. 16.8 12-lead ECG with right ventricular pacing

the RA to RV from either the superior or inferior vena cava via the subcostal or apical four-chamber view using the standard cardiac probe. In post-sternotomy patients with exiting chest tubes or mechanical assist devices, transesophageal (TEE) echo has successfully assisted and verified catheter tip placement in the RV apex. Use of echo also allows for diagnosis of potential complications such as perforation or impending tamponade related to the procedure [9, 10].

16.10 Placement with ECG Guidance

An alternative strategy to blind placement of the temporary pacemaker wire involves the use of ECG guidance. In this case, one can take advantage of the sensing capability of the wire and allow the physician to monitor the catheter progression as it moves toward the right ventricle. This technique involves connecting the distal (negative) electrode on the end of the catheter to one of the precordial leads of a 12-lead ECG via an alligator clip. In essence, this creates a unipolar intracardiac signal or intracardiac ECG. Moving through various chambers will create unique (polarity and magnitude) intracardiac signals for each chamber including the SVC, RA, RV, and IVC.

Starting at the SVC, the electrograms of both the atrium and ventricle are present with a negative polarity reflective of cardiac depolarization occurring in the opposite direction. Upon entering the right atrium, the atrial signal increases in amplitude and becomes larger than right ventricular activity. Furthermore, intracardiac activity demonstrates a positive deflection (amplitude) with further progression toward the IVC or tricuspid valve. Crossing into the right ventricle brings a dramatic increase in ventricular amplitude, while atrial signal becomes diminutive. Upon touching the endocardial surface, S–T segment elevation is noted. Testing for capture threshold and deflating the balloon would then follow.

Using ECG-guided wire placement can provide relevant information when blind placement proves to be unsuccessful, and fluoroscopy is not readily available. It can clearly give relative catheter tip position for challenging cases [7].

After verifying catheter position and achieving consistent capture, one should try to ascertain a pacing or capture threshold. This is done by slowly reducing the current until failure to capture is demonstrated. The minimum energy able to reduce defines capture threshold. Final settings should be greater than 2 times the threshold value to ensure continued capture. Of note, maintaining current output at maximum settings for extended periods can potentially lead to early inflammation and fibrosis at the lead tip, with eventual loss of capture. Ideal capture thresholds are typically less than 2 mA. If thresholds are excessively high, one may contemplate repositioning the catheter to a new location. This is particularly true if a prolonged period of temporary pacing is anticipated. High thresholds can be a reflection of poor endocardial contact, making loss of acute capture higher or contact with scarred portions of the right ventricle. Contemplation of catheter repositioning should be weighed with respect for the underlying rhythm. For patients presenting with complete heart block and a ventricular escape rhythm, acute pacing therapy often extinguishes any escape rhythm leaving asystole in the absence of pacing.

Following successful placement, the catheter and sheath should be secured with an external loop to prevent dislodgement. Silk or nonabsorbable braided suture may be used in at least two places with a loop to prevent dislodgement and loss of capture. If your institution has chlorhexidine sponges available for central lines, place it around sheath exit site and apply dressing accordingly. Chest X-ray (CXR) should be done and reviewed immediately following placement to identify lead and check for pneumothorax. Portable CXR should show catheter tip at the anterior-inferior aspect of the cardiac shadow, usually to the left of the thoracic spine. Bedside TTE or TEE ultrasound can be used to verify lead tip position which is optimally in anterior RV apex (Fig. 16.9, arrow pointing to lead tip in RV apex).

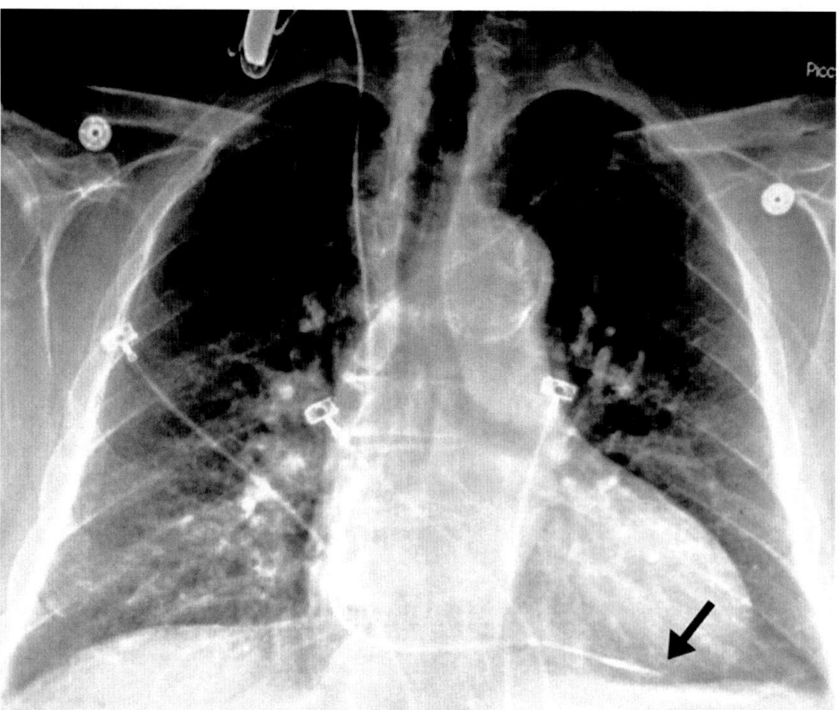

Fig. 16.9 TPM lead tip in RV apex (*arrow*)

16.11 Maintenance of Effective Pacing

Pacing can be configured in either *demand* (sensing) or *asynchronous* (nonsensing) mode. If demand (synchronous pacing) is desired, the ventricular *rate* can be set at or below the patient's intrinsic depolarization (heart rate) and *sensitivity* increased. Appropriate *sensing* can be verified by a flashing light on the generator. Note that if too high, a setting has the potential for inappropriate sensing of myopotentials from patient movement or other electrical stimuli. Occasionally, oversensing can occur from P waves or even large T waves. Catheter maintenance should include rechecking of the stimulation threshold as well as the sensitivity. The stimulation threshold is a minimal amount of current (mA) required to initiate ventricular capture or depolarization. This is accomplished by increasing the pacer rate over the patient's intrinsic rate approximately 10 bpm, as well as turning the sensitivity down. The lowest sensitivity effectively ignores any intrinsic signals. The EKG on the monitor should show 1:1 capture at the rate you have entered (VOO mode). Slowly reduce the amount of current or mA until 1:1 capture is transiently lost. The point at which capture is lost is the minimal pacing threshold. Then increase the mA at least two times the threshold for safety.

The sensing threshold checks the pacemaker ability to sense or recognize the patient's intrinsic heart rhythm or myopotentials. Appropriate sensing of each intrinsic depolarization can be verified by the sensing flashing light at the top of the generator. If the patient is asystolic or has an intrinsic rhythm below 30, continue VOO or asynchronous mode (which is the maximum sensitivity setting). Do not routinely check sensing in that situation as long as each pacing spike is followed by ventricular capture.

To check sensing threshold, turn the sensitivity dial counterclockwise toward a higher numerical setting. The sensing light at the top of the generator, which flashes when sensing, will stop. The pacemaker is now less sensitive to the patient's heartbeat. Then turn the sensitivity dial clockwise (down) until the sensing light starts flashing again. This is the sensitivity threshold. Set the sensitivity, measured in millivolts (mV), at half the sensitivity threshold value obtained.

Pacing threshold and sensitivity, as well as the catheter insertion length should be recorded every shift. When checking for return of any underlying rhythm, do not *pause* or suddenly stop pacing. Slowly "walk" or decrease rate to allow intrinsic sinus node or escape rhythm to return.

16.12 Complications

Complications can occur in over 20 % of patients treated with temporary transvenous pacemaker placement [11]. Complications are broadly divided into three main categories:

I. Venous access-related complications
II. Electrode catheter-related complications
III. Electrical device-related complications

I. Venous access-related complications: These include pneumothorax, hemothorax, and air embolism
   - Pneumothorax:

     The risk of pneumothorax is directly related to the operator experience, site of venous access (femoral < IJ access < subclavian access), and number of attempts. Most of the time, pneumothorax is small and is incidentally detected on chest x-ray. Use of non-rebreather oxygen mask helps in resolving the pneumothorax by displacing nonabsorbable nitrogen in the pneumothorax with absorbable oxygen. Operator must be able to perform a chest tube thoracostomy if needed. Tension pneumothorax should always be a differential if hypotension, hypoxemia, or pulseless electrical activity is noted during the insertion of transvenous pacemaker.
   - Hemothorax:

     Hemothorax results from the trauma to great vessels. Making sure that the coagulation profile (PT/PTT/INR/platelet count) is normal or near normal reduces the risk of hemothorax. Minimizing the number of attempts with appropriate use of guidance has also been shown to reduce the risk of hemothorax. The posterior approach for internal jugular vein can reduce both complication rates from pneumothorax and also inadvertent invasion of carotid artery.

- Air embolism:

  Air embolism during the venous access is rare but can be a fatal complication. Air embolism risk increases with the presence of preexisting pulmonary disease. Cough maneuver increases the risk of air embolism.

II. Electrode catheter-related complications: These include perforation, dislodgement, diaphragmatic stimulation, malpositioning, and catheter-induced arrhythmia [12, 13].

- Perforation: Though perforation of great vessels, right atrium, or right ventricle is rare, this complication can be fatal. Usually this complication can be tolerated by local auto-tamponade mechanism. It manifests clinically as failure to capture and failure to sense the pacemaker potential. Perforation should be suspected with sudden loss of capture, new chest or shoulder pain, development of pericardial friction rub, or rhythmic muscle spasm from diaphragmatic or chest wall stimulation [14, 15]. The most serious manifestation of cardiac perforation is cardiac tamponade. Initial suspicion of tamponade should occur by recognition of hemodynamic compromise in the bedside exam and is supported by chest radiography which shows enlarged cardiac border. Bedside echocardiogram is confirmatory. Treatment with emergent pericardiocentesis is warranted if signs of tamponade such as diastolic collapse are present. Very small effusions can sometimes be monitored with serial echo.
- Electrode catheter displacement: This usually occurs in first 24–48 h post-implantation and is seen in 2–5 % of implants. Electrode catheter displacement is manifested as intermittent undersensing or loss of capture on telemetry. This complication can be resolved by electrode catheter repositioning or replacement and properly securing the electrode catheter in place.
- Diaphragmatic stimulation: This complication occurs secondary to phrenic nerve irritation. Proper position of the electrode catheter resolves this complication. Decreasing the mA to appropriate levels may reduce stimulation.
- Electrode catheter malpositioning:

  This complication leads to unacceptable pacing and sensing thresholds. The presence of atrial or ventricular septal defects can allow for left heart malposition of the electrode catheters. Ventricular electrode catheters are more prone for the left heart malposition of the catheters. If a right bundle branch pattern is detected on telemetry, left-sided ventricular lead position should be excluded. Likewise, intended ventricular wire can fail to traverse the atrium or even enter the coronary sinus. In patients with previous tricuspid annuloplasty or repair, it may be impossible to place catheter without fluoroscopy. It's considered a relative contraindication to placement in those patients. Proper ECG-guided and fluoroscopy-guided electrode catheter repositioning may resolve this complication.
- Catheter-induced arrhythmia:

  Atrial and ventricular arrhythmias are rare complications and can be resolved by repositioning of the electrode catheters. An extremely irritable myocardium may be amenable to treatment with antiarrhythmic agents; however pacing thresholds may increase with drugs such as amiodarone. Sustained VT or ventricular fibrillation can occur, and external defibrillator should be immediately available. Transient atrial tachyarrhythmia or new right bundle branch block has been reported. Particular care should be used when placing a temporary pacemaker wire blindly in a patient with LBBB as manual pressure along the right bundle branch can cause marked asystole and recovery can be absent for hours.

III. Complications related to the electrical performance of the pacemaker electrode catheter and the generator: This complication usually manifests as failure to sense and failure to capture.
   - Failure to capture: Here the pacemaker stimulus is present, but the depolarization and resultant contraction of the atrium or ventricle is absent. Causes of failure to capture can be multifold. Poor endocardial contact, lack of functioning myocardium at electrode catheter contact site due to local myocardial necrosis, electrode catheter dislodgement and electrode catheter fracture, generator-lead connection problems, generator malfunction, and battery depletion are some of the causes of failure to capture. Hypoxia, acidosis, and electrolyte imbalances can cause and aggravate the problem of failure to capture. Correction of underlying derangement solves this complication.
   - Failure to sense: Failure of pacemaker circuit to sense intrinsic P or R waves leads to this complication. Generator and battery malfunction, electrode catheter displacement, electrode catheter fracture, and inadequate cardiac signal due to local myocardial necrosis manifest as failure to sense. Correction of underlying problem is vital for resolving this complication.

16.13 Summary

Our chapter is an overview of the bedside procedure associated with the insertion of a potentially lifesaving modality. It is by no means a complete background on identification of abnormal rhythms, pacing modes, or chronic pacemaker maintenance. It is extremely important for provider contemplating pacemaker insertion to familiarize oneself with the type of leads, pulse generators, and connectors available in each ICU and have a thorough background in venous access. It is not unreasonable to establish internal jugular or subclavian access with an appropriate-sized sheath in a controlled fashion preemptively to provide straightforward access should the need arise. As previously mentioned, correction of all possible reversible causes of heart block or bradycardia will be treated aggressively to prevent unnecessary exposure to potential complications. Immediate follow-up with chest radiographs following insertion, as well as access to bedside echo to evaluate for pericardial effusion, will ensure prompt treatment of problems associated with the procedure.

The provider should consider reviewing videos that are available as well as visit to the cardiac catheterization laboratory or electrophysiology lab to view pacemaker wire insertion in a controlled fashion [16, 17]. Finally, nurses in the postop cardiac ICU have extensive experience with temporary epicardial pacemakers, often managing and maintaining dual-chamber devices. It's highly recommended that you spend time with some nursing staff at the bedside and review temporary dual-chamber leads and the devices used in the perioperative surgical setting.

References

1. Parker J. Cleland JGF Choice of route for insertion of temporary pacing wires: recommendations of the medical practice committee and council of the British Cardiac Society. Br Heart J. 1993;70:294–6.
2. Tracy CM, Epstein AE, Darbar D, et al. 2012 ACCF/AHA/HRS focused update of the 2008 guidelines for device-based therapy of cardiac rhythm abnormalities: a report of the American College of Cardiology Foundation/American Heart Association Task Force on practice guidelines. J Am Coll Cardiol. 2012; 60(14):1297–313.
3. Koman E, Gupta A, Subzposh F et al. Outcomes of temporary active-fixation lead implantation after transvenous lead extraction in pacemaker dependent patients. J Am Coll Cardiol. 2015;65(10_S). doi:10.1016/S0735-1097(15)60324-2.
4. Francis GS, Williams SV, Achord JL, et al. Clinical competence in insertion of a temporary transvenous ventricular pacemaker. J Am Coll Cardiol. 1994; 23(5):1254–125.

5. Link MS, Atkins DL, Passman RS. Electrical therapies: automated external defibrillators, defibrillation, cardioversion, and pacing (Part 6). 2010 American Heart Association guidelines for cardiopulmonary resuscitation and emergency cardiovascular care. Circulation. 2010;122:S706–19.
6. Bernstein AD, Daubert JC, Fletcher R, et al. The revised NASPE/BPEG generic code for anti-bradycardia, adaptive-rate, and multisite pacing. PACE. 2002;25:260–4.
7. Harrigan RA, Chan TC, Moonblatt S. Temporary transvenous pacemaker placement in the emergency department. J Emerg Med. 2007;32:105–11.
8. Sovari AA, Kocheril AG. Transvenous cardiac pacing technique in medscape. http://emedicine.medscape.com/article/80659-technique. Accessed 1 Aug 2014.
9. Aguilera PA, Durham BA, Riley DA. Emergency transvenous cardiac pacing placement using ultrasound guidance. Ann Emerg Med. 2000;36:224–7.
10. Pinneri F, Frea S, Naid K, et al. Echocardiography-guided versus fluoroscopy-guided temporary pacing in the emergency setting: an observational study. J Cardiovasc Med. 2013;14(3):242–6.
11. Ayerbe JL, Sabate RV, Garcia CG, et al. Temporary pacemakers: current use and complications. Rev Esp Cardiol. 2004;57:1045–52.
12. Kossaify A. Temporary endocavitary pacemakers and their use and misuse: the least is better. Clin Med Insights Cardiol. 2014;8:9–11.
13. Lumia FJ, Rios JC. Temporary transvenous pacemaker therapy: an analysis of complications. Chest. 1973;64:604–8.
14. Austin JL, Preis LK, Crampton RS, et al. Analysis of pacemaker malfunction in the coronary care unit. Am J Cardiol. 1982;49:301–6.
15. Mahapatra S, Bybee KA, Bunch TJ, et al. Incidence and predictors of cardiac perforation after permanent pacemaker placement. Heart Rhythm. 2005;2:907–11.
16. Baer H et al. Insertion of transvenous pacemaker. http://youtu.be/5BiQQYjw6no. Accessed 1 Aug 2014.
17. Sacchetti A. Temporary transvenous pacemaker review. http://youtu.be/GPAXS7FyQHQ. Accessed 1 Aug 2014.

17 The Intra-aortic Balloon Pump

Gerardina Bueti and Kelly Watson

The intra-aortic balloon pump (IABP) has been widely used in critical care medicine for the management of intractable unstable angina and cardiogenic shock [1]. With continued advancements in the technology, the IABP is the most commonly used mechanical cardiac assist device in critically ill patients [2]. The National Center for Health Statistics data reveals that over 37,000 intra-aortic balloon pumps were placed in the United States in 2004 and had increased to more than 130,000 by 2010 [3].

17.1 Device Contents

The pump consists of a polyethylene balloon attached to a double lumen 8 Fr to 9.5 F catheter [1] (Fig. 17.1). Typically, a 34 cm^3 or 40 cm^3 balloon is used and is dependent on the patient's body surface area (BSA) [4]. The external lumen is the filling chamber, inflated with helium or CO_2 [1, 5]. The balloon diameter when fully expanded should not exceed 80–90 % of the patient's descending aorta [1]. The extracorporeal components include an electronically controlled pump with a valve in continuity with a pressurized gas source [6].

The catheter is connected to an external console (Fig. 17.2) and is synchronized to the heart using electrocardiogram (EKG) signals with the QRS phase or the central aortic pressure generated from a transducer at the tip of the balloon [7]. CO_2 is more soluble in blood which reduces the risk of embolism in the event of balloon rupture; helium is the most commonly used gas due to its decreased density allowing for more efficient filling and emptying times [8].

17.2 Principles of the IABP

Success of IABP therapy relies on augmentation with the systolic and diastolic phases to optimize the physiologic benefit of the cardiac support [6], synchronized by EKG or blood pressure [8]. Balloon inflation initiates with the onset of diastole which corresponds with the middle of the T wave; the peak of the R wave corresponds with the beginning of LV systole and the balloon deflates (Fig. 17.3) [1].

If cardiac arrhythmia such as atrial fibrillation occurs, the EKG may cause inconsistent balloon inflation (Fig. 17.4). The systemic arterial waveform may be used for augmentation: the IABP is adjusted to inflate after aortic valve closure correlating with the dichrotic notch and to deflate prior to the aortic valve opening, correlating with the systolic arterial upstroke (Fig. 17.5) [1].

G. Bueti, MHS, PA-C (✉)
Cardiothoracic Surgery Critical Care, Duke University Medical Center, 2301 Erwin Road, Durham, NC 27710, USA
e-mail: gerry.bueti@duke.edu

K. Watson, MS, PA-C
Cardiothoracic Surgery, Duke University Medical Center, Box 3864, Durham, NC 27710, USA

D.A. Taylor et al. (eds.), *Interventional Critical Care*, DOI 10.1007/978-3-319-25286-5_17

Table 17.1 Supplies needed for IABP removal

2 % chlorhexidine swab	Tegaderm
Sterile gloves and scissors	Appropriate PPI
Sterile gauze	Femoral artery pressure device (institution dependent)

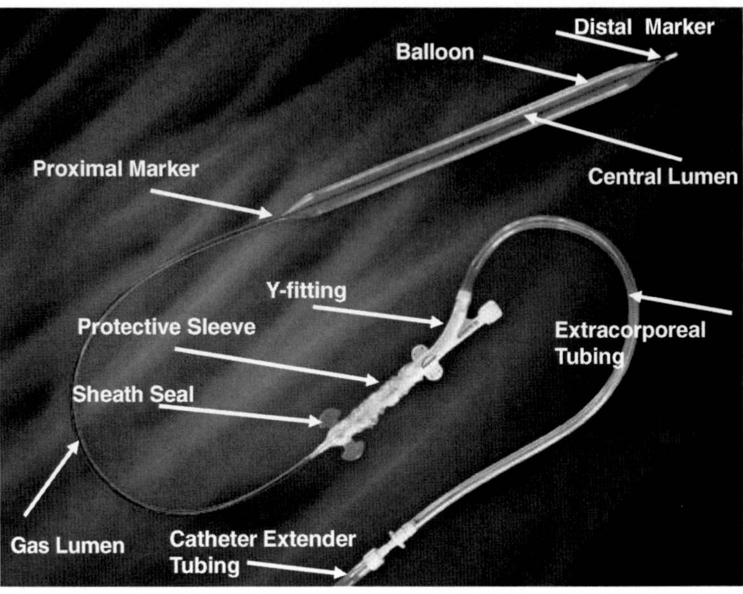

Fig. 17.1 Contents of the intra-aortic balloon pump kit (Courtesy of Maquet Holding B.V. & Co. KG, Rastatt, Germany)

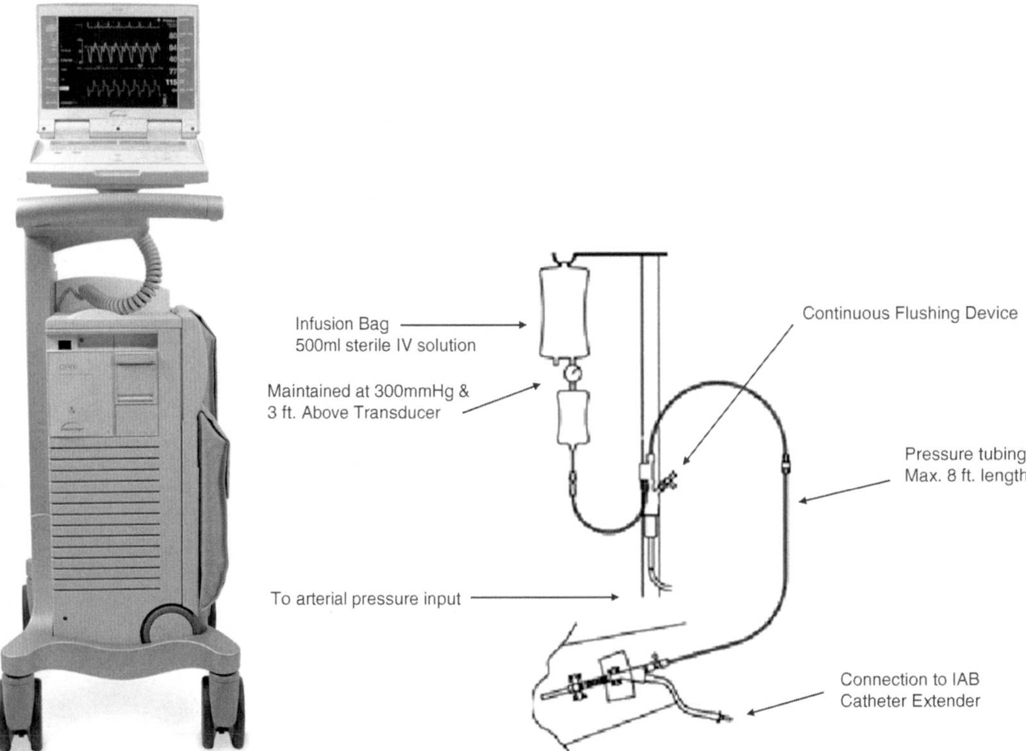

Fig. 17.2 The IABP console; the pressure system between the IABP and the Console. (Courtesy of Maquet Holding B.V. & Co. KG, Rastatt, Germany)

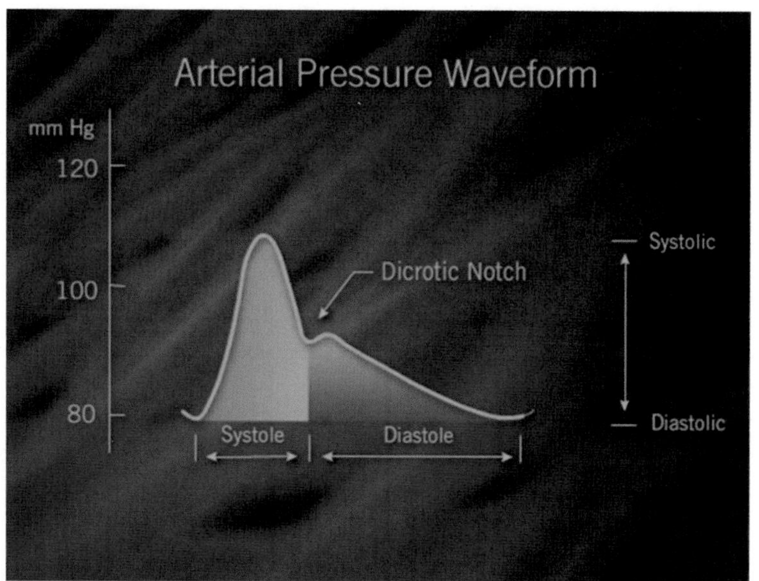

Fig. 17.3 Arterial pressure waveform as seen on the IABP monitor

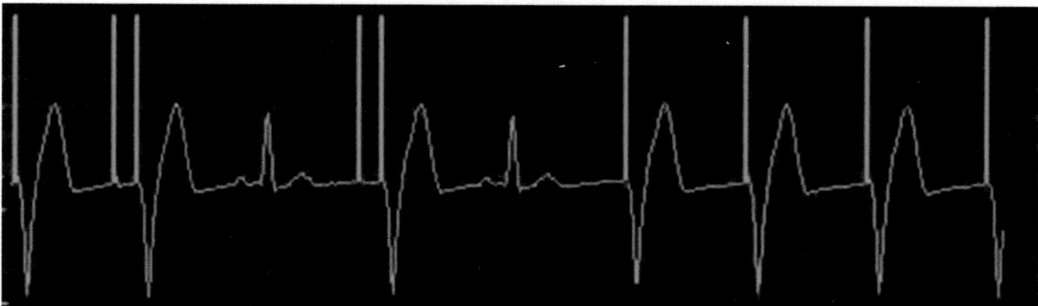

Fig. 17.4 Intra-aortic balloon pump dyssynchrony on EKG sensing [1]

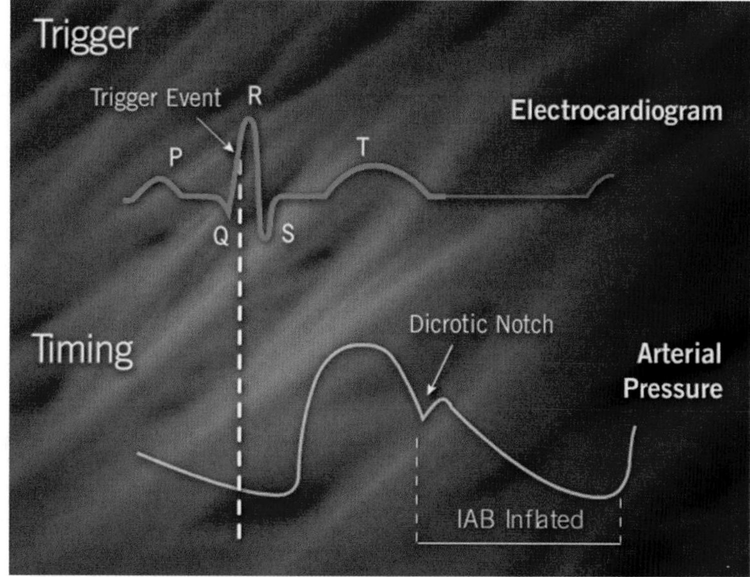

Fig. 17.5 Demonstration of IABP augmentation with EKG

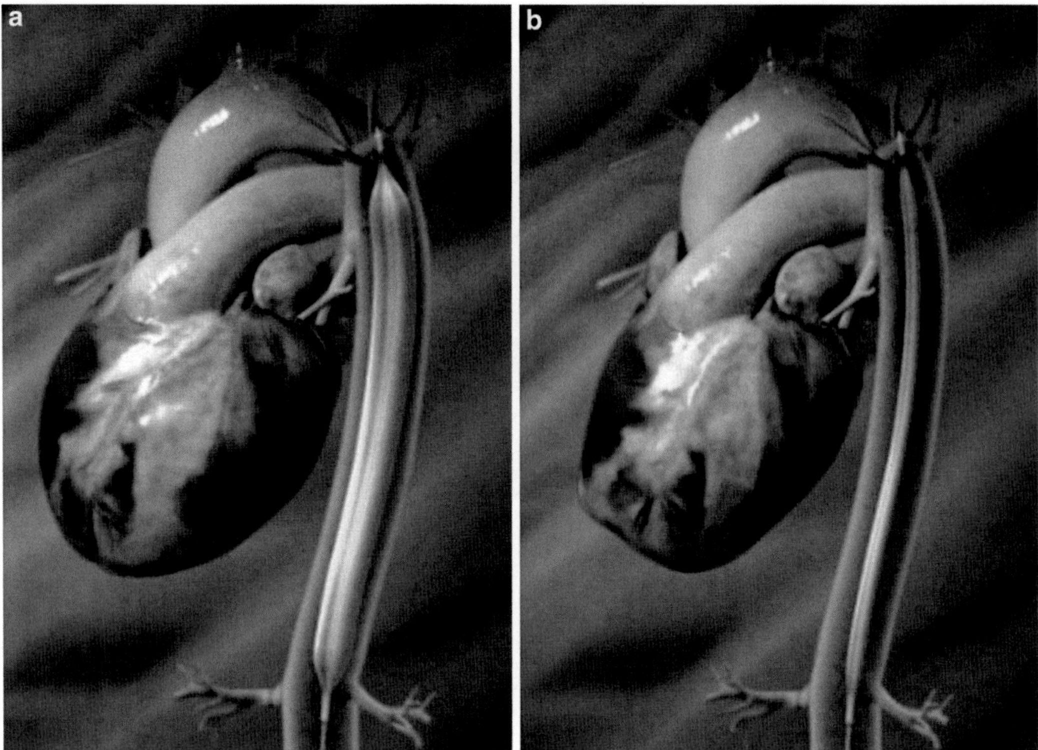

Fig. 17.6 (**a**) IABP inflation during diastole, (**b**) IABP deflation during systole

Physiologically, the early diastolic phase corresponds with the aortic valve closing to counterpulsate blood through the coronary arteries, increasing diastolic pressure [9]. This also allows for increased stroke volume and cardiac index, decreased pulmonary capillary wedge pressure and lower total pulmonary vascular resistance and left atrial and left ventricular end-diastolic pressure (LVEDP) [9]. During systole, the balloon deflates to generate a negative pressure to drive blood forward through the aorta. This function reduces afterload and augments the left ventricular (LV) function (Fig. 17.6).

Trigger and timing is managed from the central console (Fig. 17.7). Balloon inflation triggers can be set from blood pressure or EKG tracing with the function to change inflation to deflation ratios from 1:1 to 3:1 support depending on the patient's hemodynamic stability.

Perfusion is improved distal to the IABP into the mesentery and lower extremities. Ultimately, cardiac output is improved due to decreased systemic vascular resistance and reduction of the duration of isovolumetric contraction [8].

17.3 Indications and Contraindications

Approximately 10–15 % of patients undergoing cardiac surgery receive an IABP to reduce intraoperative risk or in the setting of complications coming of cardiopulmonary bypass (CBP) [5]. The use of IABP on patients undergoing high-risk cardiac surgery or IABPs is typically inserted in patients who fall into three different groups:

1. Increase diastolic coronary perfusion
2. Afterload reduction
3. Prophylaxis for hemodynamic stabilization

There are few contraindications for intra-aortic balloon pump where fatal outcomes may occur: known aortic dissection where instrumentation to

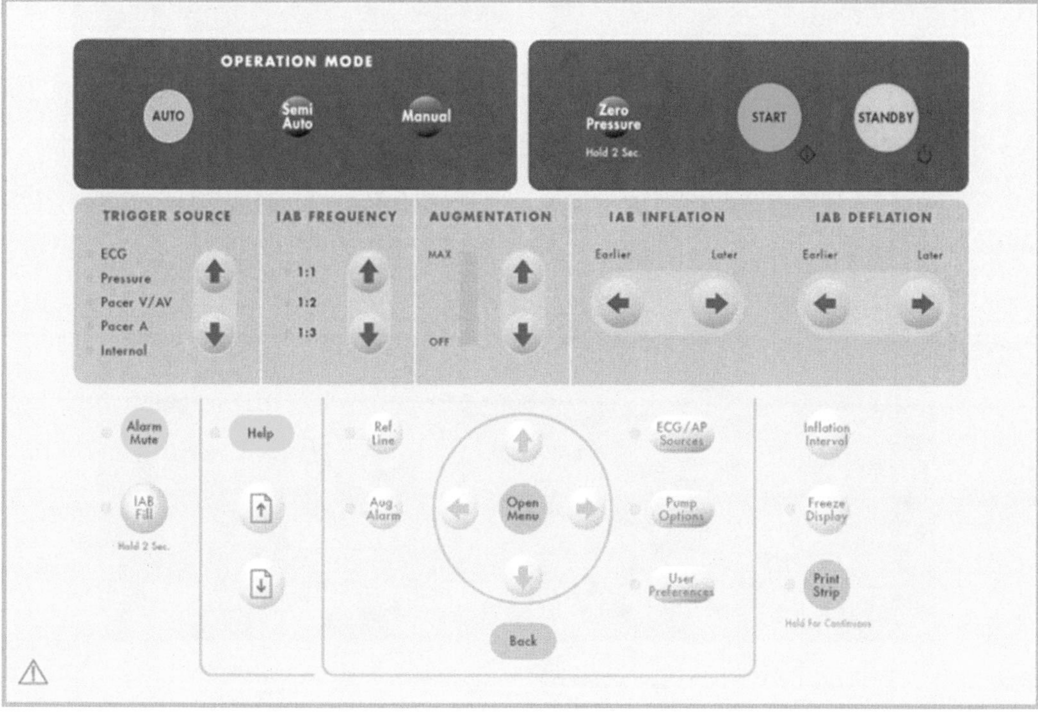

Fig. 17.7 The IABP main console

the lumen may cause exacerbation, aortic insufficiency, severe peripheral vascular calcification, or intolerance of anticoagulation [5].

17.4 Placement

Approximately two thirds of the IABP insertions in the United States occur in the cardiac catheterization lab using fluoroscopy guidance, one fourth are placed in the operating room, and the remaining are occurring at bedside in the Intensive Care Unit setting [10]. Placement of the IABP is most commonly achieved through the femoral artery via percutaneous Seldinger technique in the right femoral artery [3]. Ideally, pulses at the common femoral artery and distal throughout the leg should be assessed and recorded before balloon insertion. If there is concern for vascular compromise prior to balloon placement, alternate approaches should be considered (i.e., axillary artery). The femoral puncture site should be above the femoral bifurcation and below the inguinal ligament to avoid injury of the inferior epigastric artery and reduce the likelihood of retroperitoneal hemorrhage [10].

Steps to Insertion:

1. After the femoral pulse has been identified, the procedural area is prepped and draped.
2. An introducer needle or micropuncture needle is used to puncture the femoral artery. Ultrasound guidance may be used to identify the femoral artery if pulsation is weak or body habitus poses a challenge. If the patient has a palpable femoral pulse, the typical landmark for the femoral artery is one third the distance from the anterior superior ileac spine to the pubic symphysis.
3. Once arterial access has been identified (Fig. 17.8), evident by bright red pulsatile blood flow through the needle lumen (Fig. 17.9), a long guide wire is introduced. If a micropuncture kit is used, the smaller guide wire will introduce a small catheter (Fig. 17.10), to provide stability for

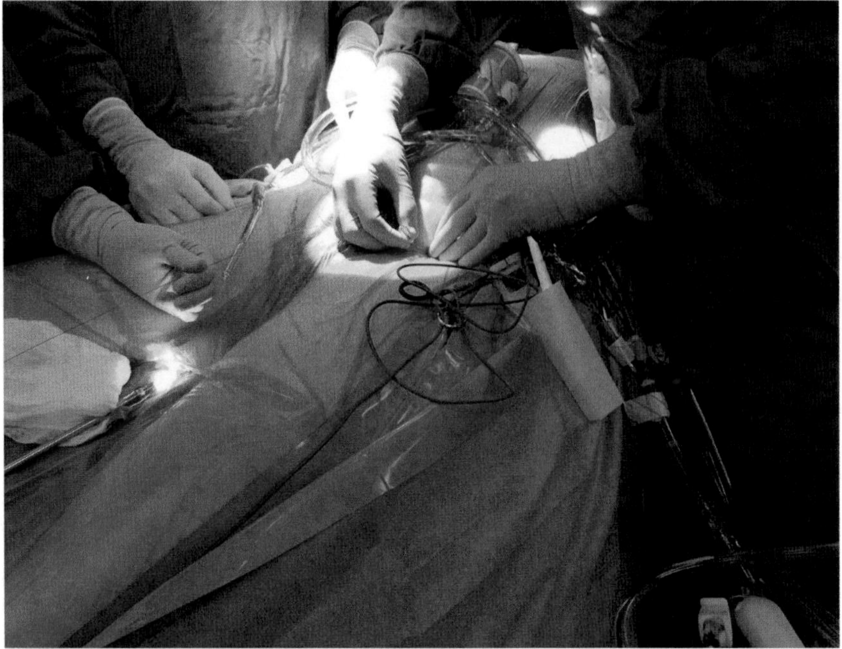

Fig. 17.8 Using the introducer needle to gain access to the femoral artery

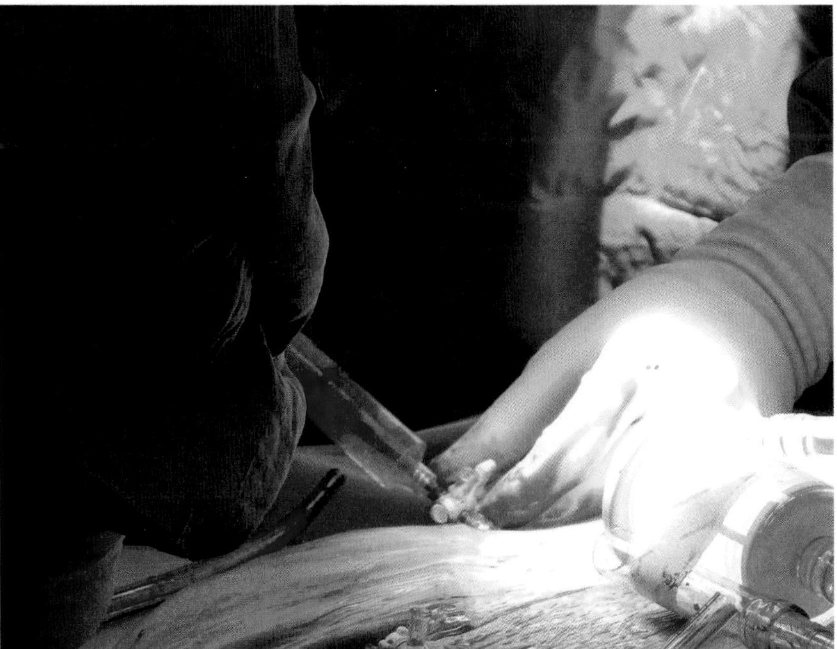

Fig. 17.9 Draw back from the femoral artery puncture site to confirm placement within the lumen

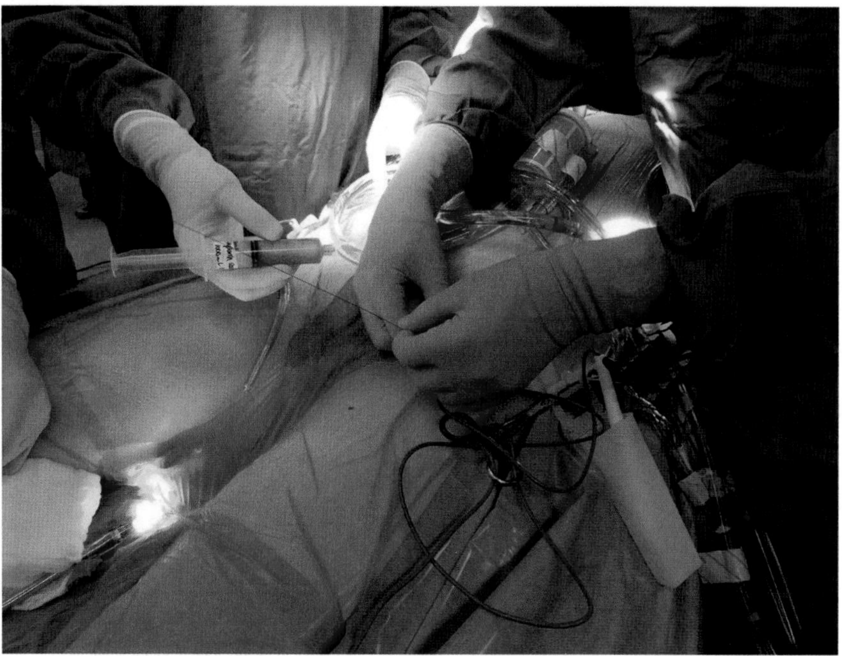

Fig. 17.10 Passing the first guide wire through the introducer needle into the femoral artery

introduction of the longer intra-aortic balloon pump guide wire.

4. Fluoroscopic guidance (cardiac catheterization lab) or transesophageal echocardiogram (TEE) is used to identify proper positioning of the guide wire distal to the left subclavian artery.
5. A small incision is made with the protractor blade at the guide wire exit site from the skin to allow for the introduction of the dilators into the tissue.
6. A series of 2–3 dilators are used to increase the diameter of the incision (Fig. 17.11a) and decrease the tissue resistance when advancing the flexible tip of the balloon pump catheter (Fig. 17.11b).
7. The catheter and polyethylene balloon are passed through the femoral artery lumen over the guide wire into the descending thoracic aorta with the intended positioning of 1–2 cm below the origin of the left subclavian artery (Fig. 17.12).
8. Proper positioning can be confirmed by direct visualization using fluoroscopy or transesophageal echocardiography. Radiographic confirmation of post-procedure position is common practice if placed in the ICU setting (Fig. 17.13).
9. The balloon tip should be identified distal to the aortic arch, approximately 1–2 cm inferior to the left subclavian artery (Fig. 17.14) [3].
10. The IABP is sutured into place. Once proper placement is achieved, the device should be sutured in place at the level of the skin with 2–0 or 3–0 vicryl or nylon suture. A sterile chlorhexidine dressing is placed at the incision site (Fig. 17.15).

After any reposition of the balloon, repeat radiographic confirmation of positioning should be obtained. The closer the balloon is positioned to the aortic valve, the greater increase in diastolic pressure; therefore, proper positioning can affect hemodynamics and balloon augmentation [11]. An IABP that is placed too distal can impair renal blood flow, leading to various other complications, including acute kidney injury, mesenteric ischemia, and lower extremity hypo perfusion injuries [12].

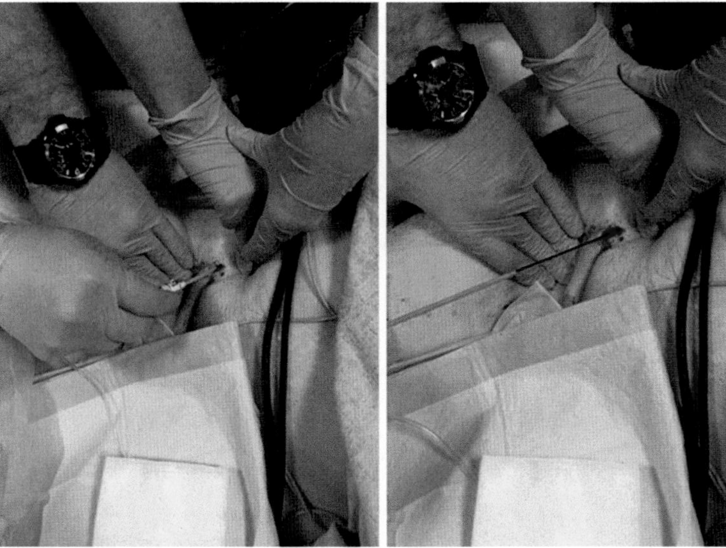

Fig. 17.11 Using Seldinger technique to sequentially dilate the skin and femoral artery (**a**) left (**b**) right

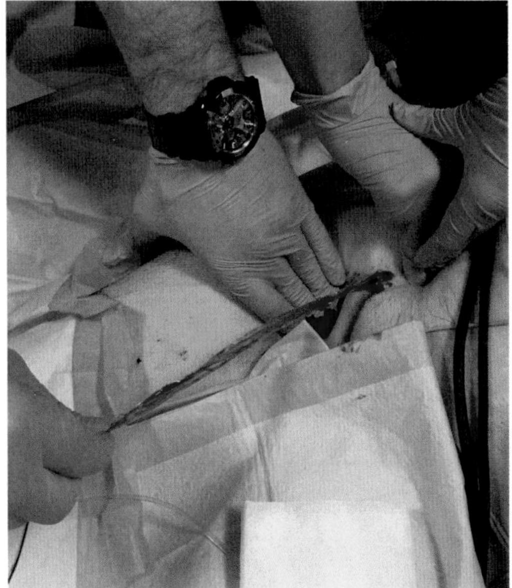

Fig. 17.12 Advancing the IABP over the guide wire into the descending aorta

17.5 Post-procedural Care

The patient is maintained in the supine position, to decrease dislodgement and intraluminal damage, which can prove challenging in patients who are alert and extubated. If the patient attempts to move their leg, intimal damage to the aorta may occur by the balloon tip. Digital ischemia is the most common complication of indwelling balloons and occurs in 10–15 % of patients [12]. Monitoring of distal pulses with manual palpation or Doppler (popliteal, dorsalis pedis, and posterior tibial arteries), skin color, temperature, and capillary refill should be performed on an hourly interval. Comparison with the opposing leg can provide insight of baseline temperature and skin turgor [12]. Additionally, the site should be monitored periodically for signs of infection, although this is rare. Among patients enrolled in the Benchmark Counterpulsation Outcomes Registry, the risk of surgical site infection in patients who underwent IABP placement for myocardial infarction (MI) was reported as 0.1 % [3].

17.5.1 Anticoagulation

Anticoagulation with unfractionated heparin is the current standard of care to decrease the risk of catheter-associated thrombosis. Monitoring of anticoagulation is achieved with interval measurement of activated partial thromboplastin times (APTT), with a goal of 50–70 s as the widely accepted range [1]. In order to reduce the risk of arterial thrombosis, it is important to ensure that balloon remains cycling to prevent hemostasis [13].

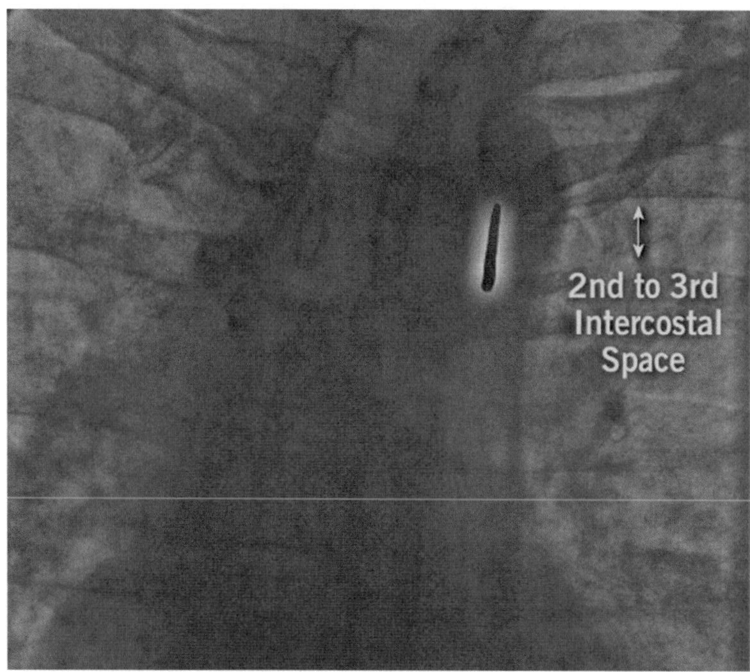

Fig. 17.13 The IABP tip properly positioned between the second and third intercostal spaces

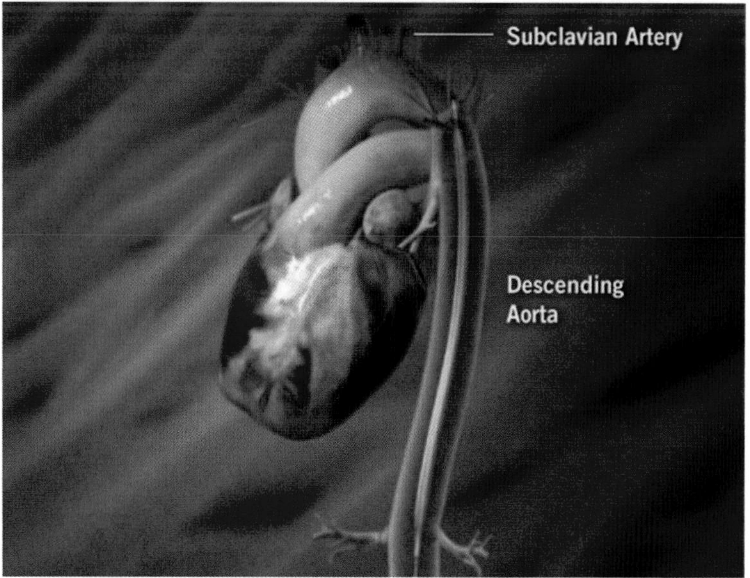

Fig. 17.14 Proper positioning of the balloon tip distal to the left subclavian artery

17.5.2 Pharmaceutical Support and Arrhythmia Management

As a mechanical circulatory assist device, the primary goal of the IABP is augmentation and cardiac output support. [3] The efficacy of the IABP depends on the extent of heart failure and native cardiac output, for this reason, the use of the balloon is concomitant with the use of inotropic and vasopressor support. [3, 14] Optimal hemodynamics can be achieved with the use of both α- and β-adrenergic agents. Simultaneous use

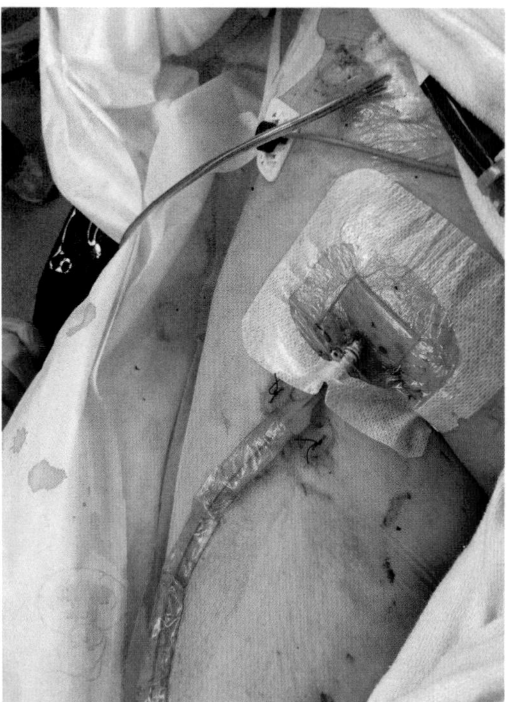

Fig. 17.15 The IABP sutured into place with an occlusive dressing over the access site

allows for additional support of mean arterial pressure in patients with heart failure and cardiogenic shock. Drugs that target α-agents may be especially beneficial because they improve blood pressure through peripheral vasoconstriction, affecting arterial compliance and increasing balloon effectiveness [14].

Arrhythmia management is imperative for optimal functioning of the IABP and cardiac function as arrhythmias affect balloon timing [14].

17.6 Troubleshooting

17.6.1 Timing Errors

To achieve maximal benefit of the IABP, it is essential that the balloon timing is properly functioning. Late inflation or early deflation can lead to suboptimal augmented stroke volume or decreased peak diastolic velocity [3], decreasing counterpulsation of blood through the coronary arteries and pulsation to the distal arteries. Issues with timing typically occur with arrhythmias or tachycardia, when the IABP is set to trigger in ECG mode with the descending slope of the T wave, marking the onset of diastole triggering balloon inflation.

17.6.2 Loss of Trigger

Loss of trigger occurs if the console cannot identify the R wave of the ECG tracing (Fig. 17.16). Troubleshooting includes:

1. Changing the ECG leads and cables
2. Adjusting the ECG gain or filter
3. Slaving the ECG tracing from the patient monitor
4. Using pressure triggering [13]

The IABP console has predetermined algorithms able to recognize pacemaker spikes that replace the QRS complexes of temporary or permanent pacing leads; however, the blood pressure triggering function should be used.

17.7 Complications Associated with IABPs

As a mechanical circulatory support device, the IABP has proven to provide temporary hemodynamic support when appropriate. As IABP is an invasive device, there can be potential complications including vascular, hematologic, and mechanical difficulties. Female gender, peripheral vascular disease, BSA (<1.65 m^2), and age ≥75 years old remain the most common independent predictors of serious adverse events [10].

17.7.1 Thrombocytopenia and Bleeding

The most frequently reported complication associated with IABP use is thrombocytopenia, defined by a serum platelet count below 150,000/mcl [150 x 109/L], or a 50 % or greater reduction in baseline platelet count, compared with labs

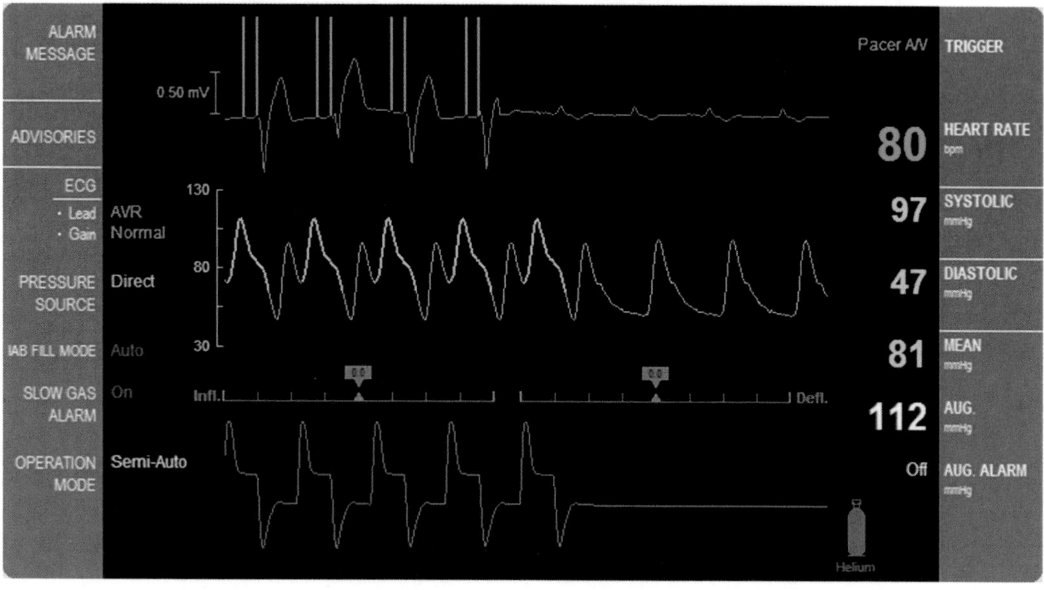

Fig. 17.16 Loss of IABP trigger and waveform on the main console monitor

prior to placement, occurring in 47–82 % of patients with the device [15]. Thrombocytopenia can lead to major bleeding and subsequent complications. The assumed cause of thrombocytopenia occurs as a result of the mechanical action of the device causing destruction of circulating platelets, in combination with routine use of heparin infusions [15]. As a result, it is important to check platelet counts at least daily or at increased intervals if there is clinical suspicion for bleeding. Although thrombocytopenia can lead to clinically significant bleeding, a large multicenter study has shown that thrombocytopenia was not an independent predictor of major bleeding or in hospital mortality [15].

17.7.2 Vascular

The most common complications relating to vascular issues include limb ischemia, arterial dissection, and thromboembolic complications [16]. Among patients enrolled in the benchmark intra-aortic balloon pump study, 2.9 % of patients had evidence of limb ischemia [10]. Overall complication rates were reported as 7 %, most commonly in females and diabetics due to smaller femoral arteries [3].

17.7.3 Balloon Leak

Given the design and function of the balloon, a potential but rare complication is an external luminal gas leak reported in about 1 % of patients [10]. IABP devices are programmed with gas leak alarms that will pause the device if a leak is suspected. Visible blood in the gas line also implies that there has been a balloon leak. If a leak has been suspected, the gas line should be clamped or disconnected, and the balloon should promptly be removed [13].

17.7.4 Removal of the IABP

Planned weaning and removal of IABP support can be initiated when the following variables are met:

1. Cardiac index (CI) is greater than 2.0 L/min/m^2.
2. A decrease in CI of less than 20 % when the IABP is weaned.
3. Inotropic support is minimal.
4. Urine output is great than 30 ml/h.
5. Heart rate is less than 100 beats/min.
6. Absence of angina.

7. Fewer than six ectopic ventricular beats/min.
8. No evidence of systemic hypoperfusion [12, 13].

Assuming that the patient does not have any urgent indications for removal, it is a common practice to wean the device by starting to wean the inflation ratio. Decreasing the frequency of IABP cycling allows for the observation of the performance patient's cardiac output. Typical weaning starts with 1:1, 2:1, and finally 3:1. Close monitoring occurs as the inflation ratio is decreased to determine if the patient can tolerate a lower inflation ratio without significant change in hemodynamics.

In elective removal, the therapeutic heparin should be held for greater or equal to 2 h prior to IABP removal [1]. Urgent removal is indicated when there is a concern for limb ischemia, for thrombosis, loss of peripheral pulses, or a balloon leak.

17.7.5 Removal

For Devices Placed Percutaneously

Most patients with an IABP had the device placed preoperatively via a percutaneous technique. These should be removed percutaneously with the removal process the same whether placed with or without introducer sheaths. Assuming that the patient has remained hemodynamically stable after the completion of the weaning trial, and the appropriate inotropes and vasopressors have been titrated, this is a relatively routine procedure in the Intensive Care Unit setting. Before the balloon is removed, it is essential to check coagulation studies and platelet count with the following coagulation parameters INR < 1.5, platelets > 50, 000.

The following supplies should be available for the removal of the IABP:

1. Ensure that all the supplies are in the room and the bedside nurse or another assistant are available to find additional supplies or assistance if required. Those involved in the procedure should wear proper personal protective equipment.
2. Removal with two people is adventitious as one person is able to hold distal pressure, while another can hold proximal pressure; however, this can be performed with an experienced single provider.
3. It is recommended that a time-out be performed to confirm patient identity and type of procedure to be performed.
4. If institutional guidelines recommend the use of a femoral artery pressure device, ensure that the "belt" has been placed under that patient before the balloon is removed so as not to disrupt manual pressure and hemostasis. The belt is positioned around the pelvis to allow the compression portion of the device is centered just above the skin insertion site (to place maximal pressure at the insertion site).
5. Transition the patient to the supine position, with all bedside monitoring devices on and positioned so that all members of the team are able to view the vital signs throughout the procedure.
6. Patient comfort should be assessed prior to the balloon pull with adequate parenteral or oral analgesia or sedation administered as needed. Local anesthetic use is variable.
7. Pressure should be applied to both proximal and distal points pertaining to the insertion site on the skin. A femoral pulse proximal and distal to the balloon site should be palpable. In obese and morbidly obese patients, the femoral pulse may be difficult to find. If a large pannus is occluding the insertion site or distorting normal anatomy, it can be adventitious to secure away from the procedural field using silk tape. If the pulse is still not palpable, use general anatomic landmark to estimate where the femoral artery courses. Pulses may not be palpable in patients with other mechanical circulatory device support such as a left ventricular assist device (LVAD) as native pulsatility may be poor due to a low ejection fraction and low cardiac output state.

8. The dressing should be removed from the insertion site and cleaned with a 2 % chlorhexidine solution (or equivalent), and any securing sutures are clipped and removed. Patients with an introducer sheath may have an additional stitch placed around the introducer catheter.
9. At the time of IABP removal, the device should be stopped, and the balloon catheter is disconnected from driveline.
10. The catheter should be removed slowly, until the proximal tip of the sheath is removed. Allow for a period of 1–2 s for arterial bleeding out of the insertion site, to evacuate any thrombi that have formed at the exit site.
11. Distal pressure should be applied, to decrease the risk of thrombi being displaced distally, followed by proximal manual pressure occluding arterial blood flow. Sterile gauze should be used to wipe the insertion site. This should be done periodically while pressure is being maintained to ensure hemostasis.
12. The distal pulses should also be frequently monitored for distal perfusion.
13. Pressure should be held for 30 min to ensure hemostasis. A sterile dressing is applied. If a compression device is planned, this should be placed over the dressing and secured. Use of a compression device varies among institutions.
14. The patient should be closely monitored after IABP removal. The patient should remain supine for 2 h and should be assessed periodically for hematoma formation, bleeding, and monitoring of distal perfusion, as 25 % of adverse events occur after the IABP has been removed [3].

17.7.6 Surgical Removal

When the IABP has been inserted intraoperatively via a femoral cutdown, or an arterial aneurysm or pseudoaneurysm is suspected, the IABP should be removed in an operating room setting with capabilities for open or percutaneous arterial repair. Surgical closure may be preferable in patients who are severely obese, have evidence of coagulopathy, or have prolonged IABP indwelling times [3].

References

1. Trost JC, David Hillis L. Intra-aortic balloon counterpulsation. Am J Cardiol. 2006;97:1391–8.
2. Baskett RJ, Ghali WA, Maitland A, Hirsch GM. The intraaortic balloon pump in cardiac surgery. Ann Thorac Surg. 2002;74:1276–87.
3. Zoltan G, Turi SKT. Intra-aortic balloon counterpulsation. http://clinicalgate.com/intra-aortic-balloon-counterpulsation/. Retrieved 26 May 2016.
4. Ben Bridgewater SYS. The intra-aortic balloon pump. Surgery. 2008;26:489–90.
5. Igor Gregoric CAB. Current types of devices for mechanical circulatory support. Elsevier Inc; New York, NY, USA 2012.
6. Jay K, Bhama RLK, Gleason TG. Mechanical support in cardiogenic shock. 6th ed. Philadelphia, PA: Saunders; 2011.
7. Stenz R. Intra-aortic counterpulsation. Anaesthesia Intensive Care Med. 2006;7:335–6.
8. Joseph L. Weidman, Michael G. Fitzsimons, FCCP. Circulatory assist devices. 5th ed. Elsevier Inc; 2013.
9. Igo SR, Hibbs CW, Trono R, et al. Intra-aortic balloon pumping: theory and practice. Experience with 325 patients. Artif Organs. 1978;2:249–56.
10. Ferguson III JJ, Cohen M, Freedman Jr RJ, et al. The current practice of intra-aortic balloon counterpulsation: results from the Benchmark Registry. J Am Coll Cardiol. 2001;38:1456–62.
11. Parissis H. Haemodynamic effects of the use of the intraaortic balloon pump. Hell J Cardiol HJC (Hellenike kardiologike epitheorese). 2007;48:346–51.
12. Bojar RM. Manual of perioperative care in adult cardiac surgery. 4th revised ed. Malden, MA: Wiley-Blackwell; 2004.
13. Beca J. Mechanical cardiac support. Cardiothoracic critical care. Amsterdam: Elsevier; 2007.
14. Papaioannou TG, Stefanadis C. Basic principles of the intraaortic balloon pump and mechanisms affecting its performance. ASAIO J. 2005;51:296–300.
15. Roy SK, Howard EW, Panza JA, Cooper HA. Clinical implications of thrombocytopenia among patients undergoing intra-aortic balloon pump counterpulsation in the coronary care unit. Clin Cardiol. 2010;33:30–5.
16. de Waha S, Desch S, Eitel I, et al. Intra-aortic balloon counterpulsation—basic principles and clinical evidence. Vascul Pharmacol. 2014;60:52–6.

Part IV

Thoracic Procedures

Thoracentesis

18

Brian K. Jefferson and Alan C. Heffner

18.1 Introduction

Pleural effusions accumulate due to an imbalance of production and absorption of pleural fluid. Thoracentesis serves to remove accumulated fluid from the pleural space via a needle or catheter. With approximately 173,000 procedures performed annually [1], thoracentesis may be divided into two categories based on the primary goal of the procedure. Diagnostic thoracentesis entails sampling of fluid for purposes of laboratory analysis. Therapeutic thoracentesis aims for larger fluid removal to achieve symptomatic and functional improvement. Thoracentesis most often serves both purposes simultaneously [2]. This chapter focuses on the indications, anatomy, technique, complications, and post-procedure management of needle or catheter-facilitated thoracentesis.

B.K. Jefferson, DNP, ACNP-BC, FCCM (✉)
Carolinas HealthCare System, Center for Advanced Practice, Charlotte, NC, USA
e-mail: brian.jefferson@carolinashealthcare.org

A.C. Heffner, MD
Pulmonary and Critical Care Consultants,
Carolinas HealthCare System, Charlotte, NC, USA

18.2 Indications

The primary goal of thoracentesis is the removal of fluid from the pleural space, which is typically diagnosed by chest radiograph, ultrasound, and/or computed tomography (Figs. 18.1 and 18.2). Diagnostic sampling enables characterization of the fluid to assist in determining the underlying disease process (Table 18.1). Therapeutic thoracentesis aims to improve cardiorespiratory function. Accumulating effusion compresses the affected lung with an impact on gas exchange and respiratory mechanics. Patient response varies with effusion size, rate of accumulation, and physiologic reserve. For patients on mechanical ventilation, worsening extrapulmonary compliance is manifested in elevated inspiratory pressures. Hemodynamic compromise is a late sign that may be associated with large pleural effusions. One final therapeutic indication for thoracentesis is infection source control in the context of parapneumonic effusion and empyema.

18.3 Contraindications

Necessity of an immediate alternative procedure such as open thoracostomy or thoracotomy is the only absolute contraindication to thoracentesis. However few relative contraindications warrant consideration, including clinically important coagulopathy. Clear thresholds of coagulopathy

D.A. Taylor et al. (eds.), *Interventional Critical Care*, DOI 10.1007/978-3-319-25286-5_18

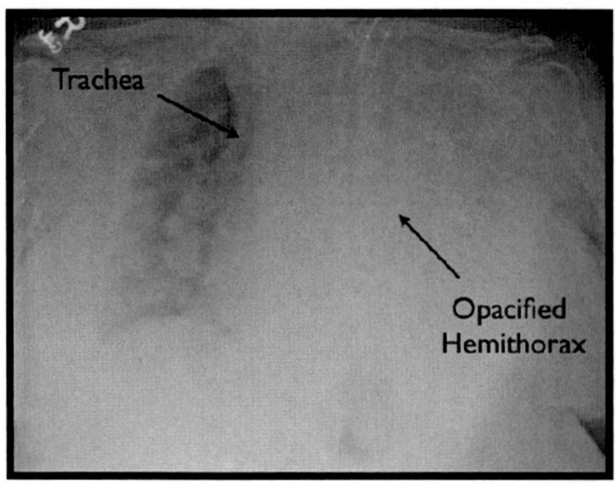

Fig. 18.1 Pleural effusion via chest radiograph

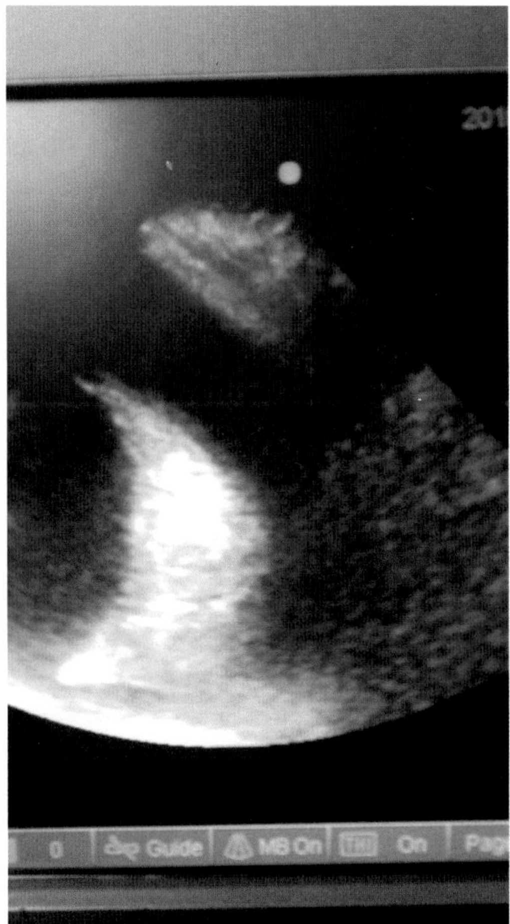

Fig. 18.2 Pleural effusion via ultrasound

Table 18.1 Etiology of pleural effusions

Transudative	Exudative
Congestive heart failure	Infections (bacterial, viral, fungal, TB)
Liver cirrhosis	Postsurgical effusions
Hypoalbuminemia	Pulmonary embolism
Nephrotic syndrome	Collagen vascular disease
Pericardial disease	Abdominal disease/ pathology
Myxedema	Chylothorax
Amyloidosis	Hemothorax
Atelectasis/trapped lung	

Thomas and Lee [20]

pertinent to thoracentesis bleeding risk remain undetermined. Similar to many minimally invasive procedures, bleeding risk is often overestimated, and we recommend against empiric coagulopathy reversal. Safe thoracentesis performed by experienced providers in patients with a protime INR > 1.5 and/or a platelet count <50 × 10^9/l is well documented [3]. Likewise it can be performed safely in patients undergoing antiplatelet therapy [4]. Brief discontinuation of systemic heparin anticoagulation should be based on the thrombotic risk associated with withholding anticoagulation but is generally recommended.

Increased risk of lung puncture in patients on mechanical ventilation is a common concern. However, there is no direct evidence that mechanical ventilation poses additional risk of pneumothorax [5].

18.4 Procedural Equipment

Equipment preparation is key to success. For diagnostic thoracentesis, a 3 cm, 21 gauge needle, 100 ml syringe, skin cleansing solution, and equipment for local anesthesia are essential supplies (Fig. 18.3). Spinal needles or longer procedure needles may be required to reach the pleural space in some patients. Therapeutic thoracentesis requires additional supplies (Table 18.2). Prefabricated commercial kits are also available with all necessary equipment.

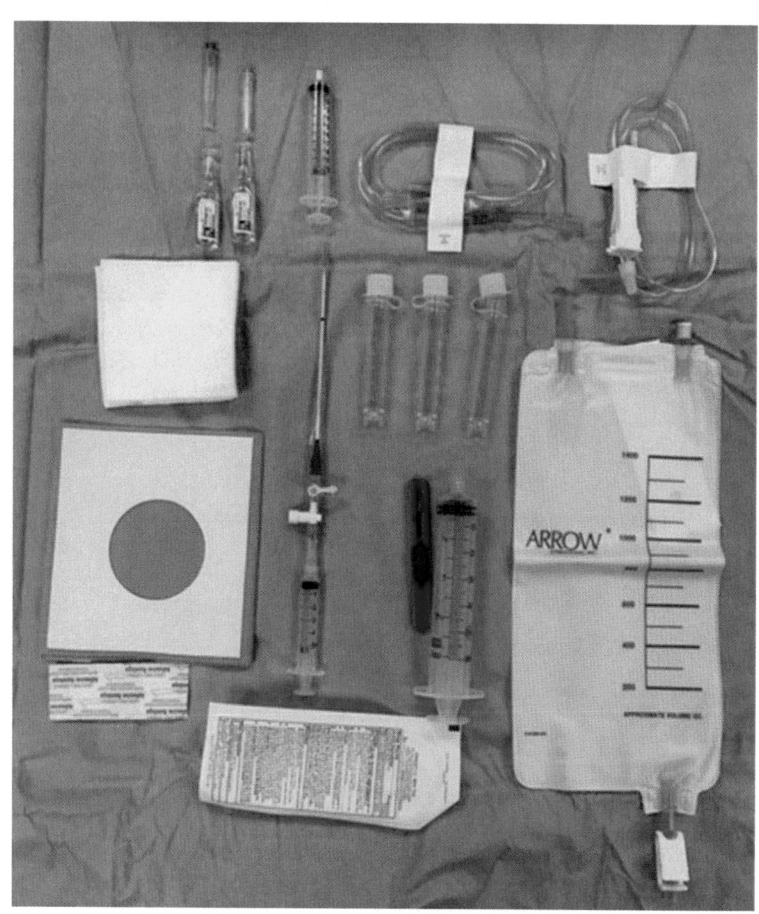

Fig. 18.3 Equipment for thoracentesis

Table 18.2 Equipment for thoracentesis

Sample equipment for diagnostic thoracentesis	
IV access	Marker for marking insertion point
Sterile gloves	Sterile towels and/or drape
Antiseptic solution (iodine, chloraprep, etc.)	Sterile 4×4 gauze pads
1 or 2 % lidocaine	Small needle for local anesthesia (23–25ga)
Catheter over needle assembly: 18 or 20 ga, 2 in. long	10 ml syringe for local anesthesia
Three way stopcock	Sterile 60 ml syringe
Pulse oximetry capability	Bedside table with pillow
CBC and chemistry tubes (two of each)	Anaerobic/aerobic culture bottles
Fungal and tuberculosis tubes	Emergency equipment available (ACLS, tube thoracostomy equipment)

Sample equipment for therapeutic thoracentesis (in addition to the above)	
18 gauge needle	Vacutainers or evacuated bottles (at least 1 l)
Drainage tubing for evacuated bottle	

Wiegand [21], Thomsen et al. [16]

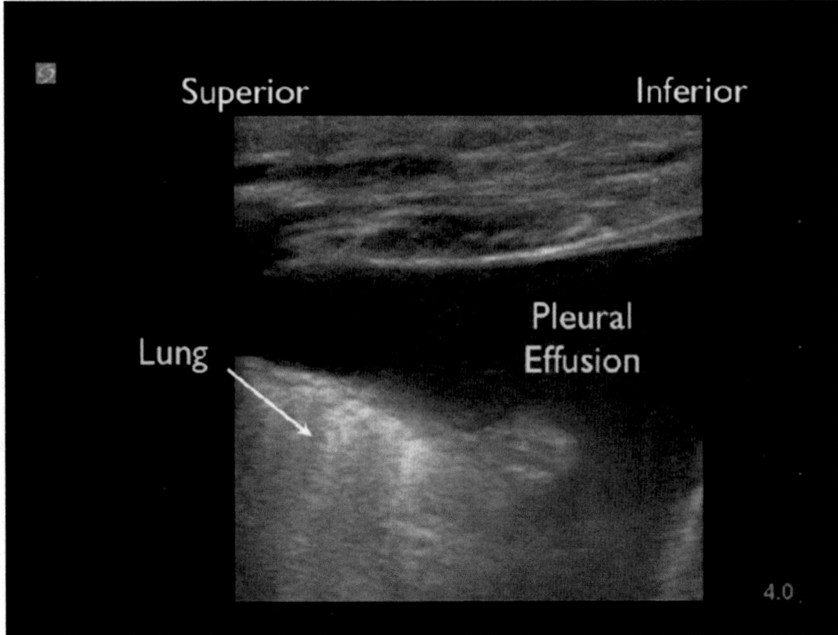

Fig. 18.4 Pleural effusion via ultrasound

Thoracic Ultrasound While thoracentesis has been practiced for a long time, ultrasound guidance has gained prominence to facilitate the procedure and assure safety. In fact Patel et al. [6] demonstrated that ultrasound-directed thoracentesis decreased the incidence of hemorrhage and pneumothorax from 38.7 % to 16.3 %, respectively. Studies clearly demonstrate the superiority of the ultrasound-guided versus traditional technique in decreasing complications [7, 8].

The evolution of a high-quality portable machine enables ultrasound-guided thoracentesis in the intensive care unit. The 3.5–5.0 MHz probe transducer is most appropriate for pleural ultrasound examination. Layered pleural fluid between the parietal and visceral pleura is identified as a hypoechoic collection deep to the thoracic wall (Figs. 18.2 and 18.4) [9]. Target pleural fluid pocket of at least 10 ml provides an appropriate buffer to avoid lung puncture [10].

18.5 Pertinent Anatomy

The pleura are composed of two membranes, which are serous in nature. The parietal pleura covers the inner wall of the thoracic cage via the costal, mediastinal, and diaphragmatic segments and attaches to the endothoracic fascia of the thoracic cage. The inner visceral pleura covers the lung surface [11]. A small amount of fluid is normally present to allow for frictionless movement of the lung with respect to the thoracic cage. From its most superior edge, the pleura lie approximately 2.5 cm above the medial third of the clavicle and inferior to the sternocleidomastoid muscle. Inferiorly, the pleura crosses the eighth rib at the midclavicular line, the tenth rib at the midaxillary line, and the twelfth rib at the lateral border of the erector spinae [12].

The scapula lies in the posterior thoracic cage and spans from the first to the seventh ribs. Of importance for thoracentesis, the most inferior scapular angle is at the level of the eighth rib and the T9 vertebral body [12].

The intercostal space (ICS) is primarily composed of muscle, fascia, and the neurovascular bundle. Intercostal muscle is comprised of three layers. The two outer layers include the external and internal intercostalis. The innermost layer of muscles is made up of the sternocostalis, intracostal, and the subcostal muscle layers. These muscles play a key role in respiration [13].

The neurovascular bundle is located within the subcostal groove of the superior rib. At the level of the first and second ICS, the intercostal artery (ICA) branches off from the superior ICA. For the third through eleventh ICS, the artery directly branches from the aorta. The posterior ICA courses with the ICS at the inferior rib margin where it is less protected by the subcostal groove more medially. As the ICA courses laterally, it assumes anatomic position within subcostal groove of the superior rib, at approximately 7 cm from the midline. This reference is a safe distance from the midline to perform the thoracentesis [14].

The ICAs become more tortuous with age. Current recommendation is to perform thoracentesis 9–10 cm lateral to the spine in elderly patients in an attempt to avoid iatrogenic injury [15]. The intercostal veins at each level drain directly into the azygos venous system [13].

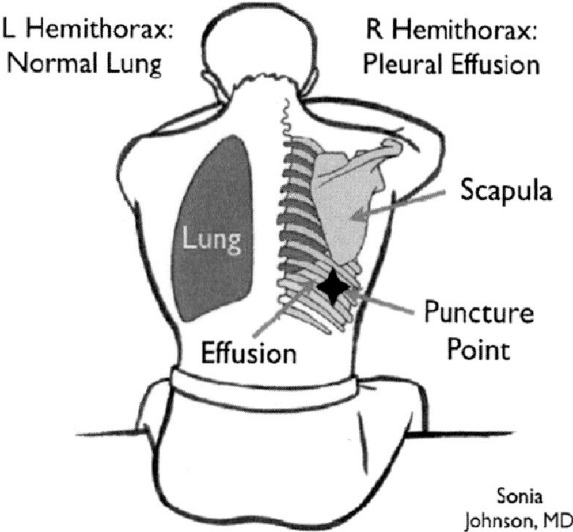

Fig. 18.5 Needle insertion in upright patient

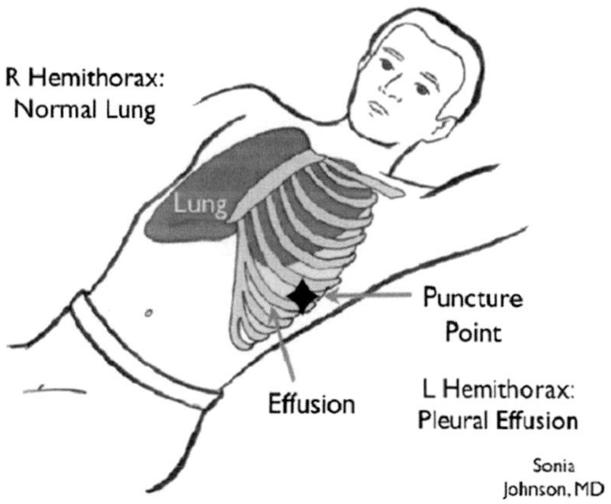

Fig. 18.6 Needle insertion in supine patient

18.6 Procedural Description

Following informed consent and patient and site confirmation, the patient and equipment are prepared. Patient positioning is critical for procedural success. Ideally, the patient will be placed in a sitting position on the side of the bed with the legs dangling off of the side (Fig. 18.5). For comfort, a bedside table with a pillow or linens should be placed in front of the patient to rest the arms. For patients who are unable to sit upright, the preferred position is on the side with the unaffected side down [2]. Once the patient is properly positioned, the location of the effusion and preferred site for needle entry are made with a marking pen.

The entry site can be located via two techniques. The top edge of the effusion can be identified via auscultation and percussion. Identifying this landmark, the needle/catheter insertion site is identified two intercostal spaces below the top edge of the effusion (Figs. 18.5 and 18.6). When available, ultrasound is the preferred method to identify the optimal target for effusion access. Localizing effusion depth >1.5 cm optimizes procedure safety. Ultrasound guidance also facilitates directional placement of the drain. As an example, placement of the drain one interspace above the diaphragm optimizes effusion drainage for patients who can assume an upright or semi-upright position. The latter is the preferred method of site selection as blind insertion can lead to inaccurate placement of the needle/catheter system [16]. The needle insertion point is 7–10 cm lateral to the spine [14, 15].

Once the insertion site is identified, the skin cleansing solution needs to be applied at and around the site followed by placement of a drape or surgical towels around the insertion site [17]. Local anesthesia with either 1 or 2 % lidocaine is instilled to anesthetize the skin, periosteum, and pleural membrane. After the skin wheal, the needle should be inserted to the superior edge of the inferior rib. At all times when the needle is in motion, the provider should be aspirating the syringe plunger. Lidocaine should be injected onto the rib periosteum as it is heavily innervated. Next the provider walks the needle over the rib, moving forward towards the pleural space once over the superior rib margin. As the provider is moving the needle forward to the pleural space, lidocaine should be injected intermittently to assure adequate tissue anesthesia. As the needle pierces into the pleural space, pleural fluid will enter into the syringe. The needle should be slightly withdrawn to inject lidocaine at the parietal pleura. As needle is removed, the proceduralist should take mental note of the insertion depth to reach the pleural space [17].

The needle or catheter-over-needle assembly attached to a 60 ml syringe is next inserted along the anesthetized path while maintaining the same vigilant orientation to the rib and neurovascular bundle (Fig. 18.7). Once fluid is aspirated, the needle should not be advanced further. The catheter is next advanced while maintaining strict control of the needle. With the patient holding his/her breath at end expiration, the needle is next removed with immediate covering of the catheter hub with the gloved hand. This is to prevent air entry in the catheter. Next the 3-way stopcock is attached with the off position towards the patient. Then the 60 ml syringe is attached to the stopcock, and the stopcock is turned so that it is open to the patient and syringe. The necessary amount of fluid is withdrawn for laboratory analysis. Finally the stopcock is turned to the off position towards the patient followed by the removal of the syringe [17].

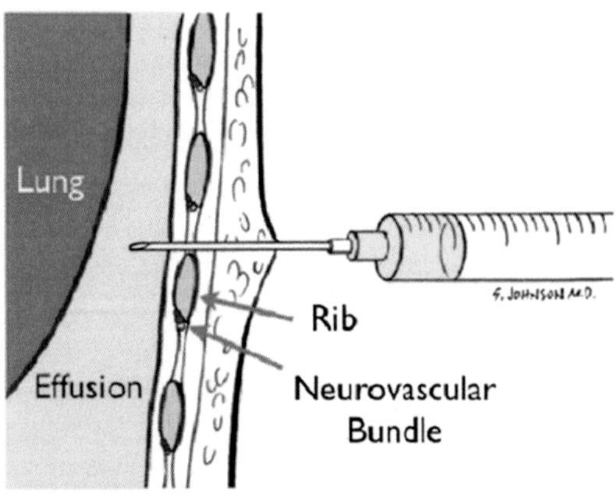

Fig. 18.7 Needle insertion above rib

Once this fluid is secured, additional fluid can be removed if necessary. The additional equipment necessary for this is drainage tubing, an 18 gauge needle, and a 1 l (or larger) drainage bottle or fluid collection bag. Another alternative option in the absence of a collection system is the continued use of a large syringe similar to that used for fluid removal for diagnostic testing [18]. One end of the drainage tubing is attached to the stopcock. A needle is attached to the other end and is then inserted into the vacutainer. Then the stopcock needs to be turned so that it is open between the patient and the vacutainer. Fluid will begin to collect into the container. The maximum amount of fluid to be drained during the procedure is 1.5 l, so as to prevent re-expansion pulmonary edema [17].

Once the necessary amount of fluid is removed, the stopcock is next turned off towards the patient. The catheter is removed during end expiration with the patient holding his breath to prevent air entry into the pleural space, causing an iatrogenic pneumothorax. Removal of the catheter is followed immediately by the placement of an occlusive dressing [17].

18.7 Post-Procedure Management Considerations

Post-procedure management involves patient monitoring for clinical response and potential complications (Table 18.3).

Table 18.3 Potential complications

Pneumothorax	Post-procedural pain
Hemorrhage	Re-expansion pulmonary edema
Visceral injury	Infection

Havelock et al. [16]

Post-procedure pain will depend on the effectiveness of local anesthesia during the procedure. Minimal discomfort is anticipated for most uncomplicated procedures. Thus the pain can often be treated with nonsteroidal antiinflammatory medications or narcotics as need for more intense pain.

A wide range of pneumothorax incidence (1–30 %) is described, depending on the experience level of the provider. Pneumothorax can occur in any of three different ways: direct injury to the lung parenchyma during needle insertion, air entrainment from the needle or catheter assembly, or visceral pleural injury stemming from rapid drop in pleural pressure during fluid evacuation with re-expansion of the lung causing a shear-type injury from the presence of visceral pleural adhesions. An immediate post-procedure chest radiograph is not necessary unless there is suspicion for pneumothorax [16].

When present, post-thoracentesis pneumothoraces may not require chest tube insertion. Those at highest risk for progressing to tension pneumothorax occur from direct injury to the lung parenchyma. Risk is increased for those patients on positive pressure ventilation.

Clinically significant hemorrhage is another potential complication with a documented incidence approximating <1 %. The best method to minimize the risk of hemorrhage is vigilance in assuring needle insertion over the superior edge of the inferior rib at the target ICS. Routine assessment of post-procedure hemoglobin is not standard [3, 4, 6]. Signs of hemorrhage can occur acutely or in delayed fashion. Clinical evidence of hemorrhage necessitates aggressive resuscitation and thoracostomy tube placement. In addition to supportive measures, cardiothoracic surgery or interventional radiology may be warranted to control cases of arterial hemorrhage [19].

Post-thoracentesis re-expansion pulmonary edema (RPE) is rare, impacting <1 % [19] but carries mortality as high as 20 % [1, 19]. RPE is thought to occur from either large pleural volume removal or a rapid drop in pleural pressure below −20 cmH_2O. Excessive negative intrapleural pressure causes rapid re-expansion of the lung which releases inflammatory mediators, leading to increased pulmonary capillary permeability. Reperfusion injury following expansion of atelectatic lung may also contribute. Prevention of RPE focuses on limiting volume removal to 1.5 l although this threshold is not based on strong evidence [9, 19]. RPE usually presents anytime within 24 h post-thoracentesis with complaints of chest pain, persistent cough (with or without frothy sputum), dyspnea, increased work of breathing, respiratory failure, and occasionally hemodynamic instability. Management strategies are primarily supportive including respiratory support with supplemental oxygen or positive pressure ventilation, depending on the severity. Other supportive therapies may include diuresis, steroids, and vasopressor and inotropic agents to support hemodynamics [9].

18.8 Summary Bullet Points

1. Thoracentesis is a core diagnostic and/or therapeutic critical care procedure for the evaluation and removal of pleural fluid.
2. Ultrasound guidance enhances safety by decreasing complications, improving procedural safety.
3. Coagulation thresholds for thoracentesis are ill defined, but moderate coagulopathy appears to pose low risk and empiric attempts to reverse coagulopathy prior to the procedure are not evidence based.
4. Post-procedure management includes monitoring for post-procedural pain, hemorrhage, pneumothorax, and RPE. Routine post-procedure chest radiograph is not warranted.

References

1. Daniels CE, Ryu JH. Improving the safety of thoracentesis. Curr Opin Pulm Med. 2011;17:232–6.
2. Sachdeva A, Shepherd RW, Lee HJ. Thoracentesis and thoracic ultrasound: state of the art in 2013. Clin Chest Med. 2013;34:1–9.
3. Hibbert RM, Atwell TD, Lekah A, Patel MD, Carter RE, McDonald JS, et al. Safety of ultrasound-guided thoracentesis in patients with abnormal preprocedural coagulation parameter. Chest. 2013;144(2):456–63.
4. Mahmood K, Shofer SL, Moser BK, Argento AC, Smathers EC, Wahidi MM. Hemorrhagic complications of thoracentesis and small bore chest tube placement in patients taking clopidrogel. Ann Am Thorac Soc. 2014;11(1):73–9.
5. Gordon CE, Feller-Kopman D, Balk EM, Smetana GW. Pneumothorax following thoracentesis: a systematic review and meta-analysis. Arch Intern Med. 2010;170(4):332–9.
6. Patel MD, Joshi SD. Abnormal preprocedural international normalized ratio and platelet counts are not associated with increased bleeding complications after ultrasound-guided thoracentesis. Am J Roentgenol. 2011;197:W164–8.
7. Cavanna L, Mordenti P, Berte R, Palladino MA, Biasini C, Anselmi E. Ultrasound guidance reduces pneumothorax rate and improves safety of thoracentesis in malignant pleural effusion: report on 445 consecutive patients with advanced cancer. World J Surg Oncol. 2014;12:139–44.
8. Patel PA, Ernst FR, Gunnarsson CL. Ultrasonography guidance reduces complications and costs associated with thoracentesis procedures. J Clin Ultrasound. 2012;40(3):135–41.
9. Feller-Kopman D, Berkowitz D, Boiselle P, Ernst A. Large-volume thoracentesis and the risk of reexpansion pulmonary edema. Ann Thorac Surg. 2007;84:1656–62.
10. Mayo PH, Hayden HR, Tafreshi M, Doelken P. Safety of ultrasound-guided thoracentesis in patients receiving mechanical ventilation. Chest. 2004;125(3):1059–62.
11. Liang C, Shuang L, Wei L, Bolduc JP, Deslauriers J. Correlative anatomy of the pleura and the pleural spaces. Thorac Surg Clin. 2011;21:177–82.
12. Sayeed RA, Darling GE. Surface anatomy and surface landmarks for thoracic surgery. Thorac Surg Clin. 2007;17:449–61.
13. Ellis H. The ribs and intercostal spaces. Anaesth Intensive Care Med. 2008;9(12):518–9.
14. Choi S, Trieu J, Ridley L. Radiological review of intercostal artery: anatomical considerations when performing procedures via intercostal space. J Med Imaging Radiat Oncol. 2010;54:302–6.
15. Yoneyama H, Arahata M, Temaru R, Ishizaka S, Minami S. Evaluation of the risk of intercostal artery laceration during thoracentesis in elderly patients using 3D-CT angiography. Intern Med. 2010;49:289–92.
16. Havelock T, Teoh R, Laws D, Gleeson F. Pleural procedures and thoracic ultrasound: British Thoracic Society pleural disease guideline 2010. Thorax. 2010;65 Suppl 2:ii61–76.
17. Thomsen TW, DeLaPena J, Setnik GS. Videos in clinical medicine. N Engl J Med. 2006. http://www.nejm.org.ahecproxy.ncahec.net/doi/full/10.1056/NEJMvcm053812. Retrieved 13 Sept 2014.
18. Hatch N, Wu TS. Advanced ultrasound procedures. Crit Care Clin. 2014;30:305–29.
19. Wrightson JM, Helm EJ, Rahman NM, Gleeson FV, Davies JO. Pleural procedures and pleuroscopy. Respirology. 2009;14:796–807.
20. Thomas R, Lee YC. Common benign pleural effusions. Thorac Surg Clin. 2013;23:25–42.
21. Wiegand DJ. AACN procedure manual for critical care. 6th ed. St. Louis, MS: Elsevier; 2011.

Needle Thoracostomy for decompression of Tension Pneumothorax

19

Cragin Greene and David W. Callaway

19.1 Introduction

This chapter will focus on the use of needle thoracostomy in the management of tension pneumothorax. Tension pneumothorax is a life-threatening condition that must be intervened upon immediately. The fastest and easiest way to relieve tension physiology is through needle thoracostomy. This procedure can be accomplished quickly and with limited resources, allowing more time for definitive management of the underlying processes leading to the development of the pneumothorax [1–3]. The presentation of tension physiology can vary in different patient populations, making it challenging to identify; however early recognition and intervention are necessary to prevent morbidity and mortality.

19.2 Indications

The indication for needle thoracostomy or thoracic needle decompression is tension pneumothorax. Early recognition of tension pneumothorax is essential in the management of this process. Needle decompression is performed to relieve tension physiology but does not necessarily correct the underlying pneumothorax. Tension pneumothorax is an imminently life-threatening condition that requires immediate intervention to prevent death [1–3]. Although in some instances needle decompression is definitive management, it is almost always performed as a temporizing measure to allow more time for chest tube placement and management of the precipitating event. Understanding of the transition from pneumothorax to tension pneumothorax is necessary to aid in early recognition.

19.3 Pathophysiology

A pneumothorax develops when air enters the pleural space separating the potential space that exists between the parietal and visceral pleura. Pneumothoraces are classified as spontaneous or nonspontaneous. A spontaneous pneumothorax occurs with no obvious underlying secondary cause. A nonspontaneous pneumothorax occurs as a result of injury to the pleura caused by blunt or penetrating trauma or iatrogenic sources (mechanical ventilation or invasive procedures) [1, 4, 5]. Air can continue to accumulate in the pleural space if the defect in the pleural lining acts as a one way valve. Negative intrathoracic pressures during inspiration will open the defect allowing air to enter the potential space; positive intrathoracic pressures created during exhalation close the defect not allowing the air to escape [1, 3–5]. With each respiratory cycle air continues

C. Greene, MHS, PA-C (✉) • D.W. Callaway, MD
Department of Emergency Medicine, Carolinas Medical Center, 1000 Blythe Blvd, Charlotte, NC 28203, USA
e-mail: cragin.greene@carolinashealthcare.org; David.Callaway@carolinashealthcare.org

D.A. Taylor et al. (eds.), *Interventional Critical Care*, DOI 10.1007/978-3-319-25286-5_19

to accumulate in the pleural space increasing intrapleural pressure. If this process continues eventually tension physiology will develop. The dynamics for patients on positive pressure ventilation are slightly different in that air is forced into the pleural space through the visceral pleura by the positive pressure generated by the ventilator. The air does not escape during exhalation, resulting in continued accumulation of intrapleural air.

Tension pneumothorax develops when increased intrapleural pressures results in complete collapse of the affected lung, mediastinal shift to the contralateral side, compression of the unaffected lung, and kinking of the great vessels. The altered respiratory dynamics and loss of lung volume cause profound hypoxia, while the disruption of blood flow through the great vessels causes circulatory collapse. The end result is obstructive shock and eventually death [1–3].

19.4 Identification

Signs and symptoms of tension pneumothorax in the awake and spontaneously breathing patient may include chest pain, respiratory distress, tachycardia, hypotension, tracheal deviation, jugular venous distension, diminished breath sounds, and hyperresonance to percussion. This constellation of findings is not present in all patients with tension physiology which can obscure the provider's early recognition of this life-threatening condition. It may be more difficult to identify tension pneumothorax in mechanically ventilated patients as many of the signs and symptoms are blunted or altered as a result of ventilator mechanics and patient status (sedated or comatose). Recognition of hypoxia, increased ventilator pressures, hypotension, and asymmetric lung sounds may be the only clues that tension physiology is developing [1, 3, 6].

19.5 Confirmatory Imaging

The diagnosis of tension pneumothorax is made on the basis of clinical findings, and confirmatory imaging is not necessary. Hemodynamically unstable patients where tension pneumothorax is the suspected cause should undergo immediate needle decompression to reverse tension physiology and shock [5, 7]. If tension pneumothorax is suspected and the patient is relatively stable, confirmatory imaging can be considered. The three main imaging modalities for the evaluation of pneumothorax are ultrasound, X-ray, and CT. There are pros and cons to each imaging modality. Ultrasound can be performed quickly and easily by the treating provider, it is readily available and easily portable. Real-time confirmation of a pneumothorax can be identified. Confirmation of decompression can be achieved at the bedside by the visualization of pleural sliding and comet tail artifact [3, 8]. The main con is that the provider must be trained and comfortable with the use of ultrasound. X-ray is usually readily available; thoracic structures are identified as reference points for evidence of tension. Cons to X-ray are that you must rely on additional ancillary staff to perform the X-ray which may result in a delay. It is the least sensitive of the three studies and may miss the presence of pneumothorax, especially in the supine position. CT is excellent at identifying pneumothorax and is the gold standard at identifying occult pneumothorax; however the patient must be transported to the CT scanner, resulting in a delay as well as a period of time without access to the patient while in the scanner [3, 8].

19.6 Site Selection

Traditionally the primary site for needle decompression has been the second intercostal space (ICS) in the midclavicular line (MCL). The eighth edition of adult trauma life support (ATLS) recommends using a 5 cm, 14 gauge needle-based catheter in the second ICS for needle decompression [5]. Due to high failure rates of successfully entering the pleural space decompressing intrapleural air, alternative sites have been studied. The appropriate length of the needle selected for decompression has also been evaluated in recent studies. The hypothesis regarding high failure rates included insufficient needle length to enter the pleural space, obstruction, user error, and excessive chest wall thickness (CWT) [9, 10]. Selecting the site for decompression may be influenced by factors such as overlying trauma, hematoma, subcutaneous air, or difficult access secondary to environmental factors or patient positioning [10]. Recent CT, ultrasound, and cadaveric studies have evaluated the fourth and fifth ICS at the midaxillary line (MAL) and anterior axillary line (AAL) with regard to CWT. Identifying a thinner area of chest wall would potentially increase success rates with the standard 5 cm needle. The chest wall at the fourth and fifth ICS AAL was decreased compared to the second ICS MCL in the range of 5–13 mm depending on the study reviewed [2, 9, 10]. It was also noted in all locations that CWT increased with increase in body mass index. The distance to vital structure (pericardium, aorta, pulmonary artery, inferior and superior vena cave, and pulmonary veins) was evaluated to determine the risk associated with increasing needle length. Measurements were taken at the left and right fourth AAL and second MCL at multiple angles of entry with respect to deep vital structures (DVS). 80 mm was the cutoff for distance to radiographic injury as an 8 cm 14 gauge needle was proposed as an alternate needle for decompression. Assuming appropriate angle of entry, radiographic decompression would be obtained with an 8 cm needle at all sites >96 % of the time compared to the 5 cm needle which would only achieve decompression at the second ICS MCL 66 % L and 76 % R [2]. The site with the greatest increase of risk for injuring DVS was at the left AAL. This risk was only significantly increased if the angle of entry was not perpendicular [2].

19.7 Anatomy

Understanding the anatomy of the chest wall is crucial in minimizing injury during this procedure. When approaching the second ICS MCL, the primary structures to avoid includes the neurovascular bundle that runs inferior to each rib, the internal mammary artery medial to the site of entry, thoracic great vessels medially, and the subclavian vessels superiorly. When approaching the fourth and fifth ICS at the AAL, the neurovascular bundle continues to run immediately inferior to each rib. Additional concerns include diaphragmatic injury, liver on the right, and cardiac injury on the left.

The second ICS MCL can be easily identified using the sternum as a landmark. Palpate the jugular/suprasternal notch at the superior aspect of the sternum. Immediately below the jugular notch is the manubrium of the sternum. Palpate inferiorly until a ridge is felt; this is the sternal angle and the location of articulation of the second costal cartilage with the sternum. Palpate laterally to identify the second rib [11, 12]. The space between the second and third rib is the second ICS. The MCL is the midpoint on the clavicle measured from the jugular notch to the distal clavicle or acromioclavicular joint. The intersection of the MCL and the second ICS is the location for needle decompression (see Figs. 19.1 and 19.2).

The fourth and fifth ICS AAL is best identified by having the patient lay supine with their arm abducted and extended behind the head to expose the axilla. Palpate and count the ribs in the axillary fossa to identify the fourth and fifth ribs. Alternatively the ribs can be counted by identifying the sternal angle to represent the second rib. Continue to palpate down the chest moving slightly laterally until you palpate the fourth and fifth ribs [11, 12]. The nipple is usually directly overlying the fourth rib which aligns with the midaxillary portion of the fifth rib; however this landmark can be unreliable in women and with varying body habitus [5, 11, 12]. Palpate along the fourth or fifth rib laterally to the AAL. The site for needle decompression will be in the triangle of safety. The triangle of safety (safe triangle) is outlined by the AAL medially, MAL laterally, and the fourth or fifth intercostal space inferiorly. The AAL runs along the lateral aspect of the pectoralis major. The MAL runs downward from the apex of the axilla [13] (see Figs. 19.3 and 19.4). Be aware that this site may be more superior than you expect and the spacing between the ribs in this location is narrower than at the second ICS MCL. There is also greater respiratory excursion as you move laterally on the chest wall.

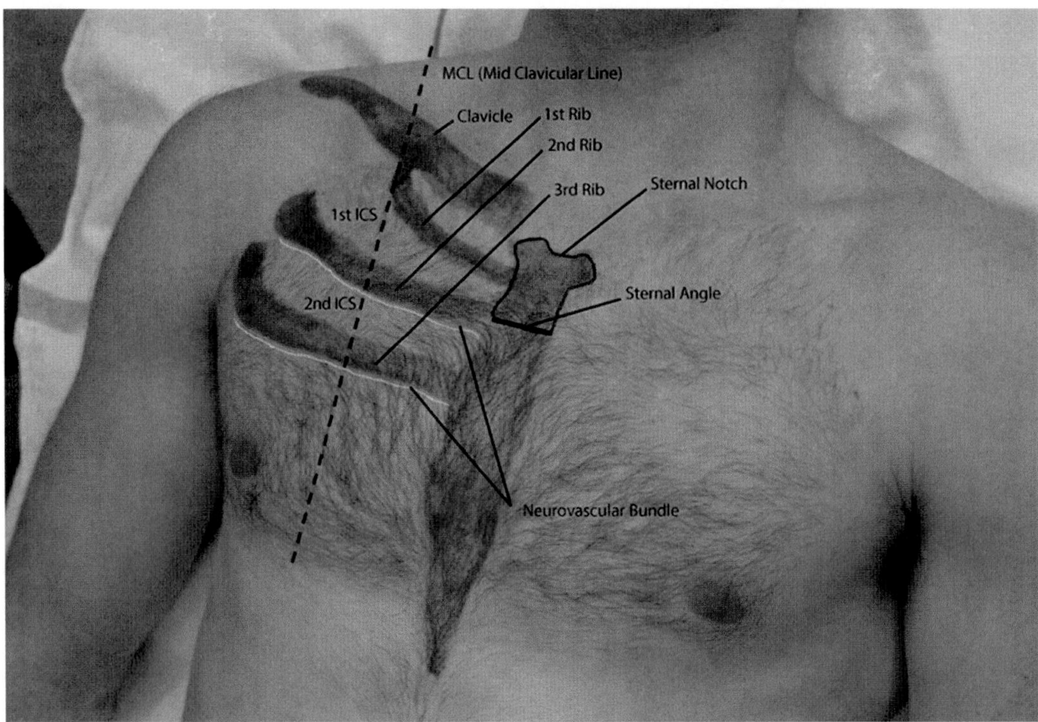

Fig. 19.1 Anterior chest wall landmarks

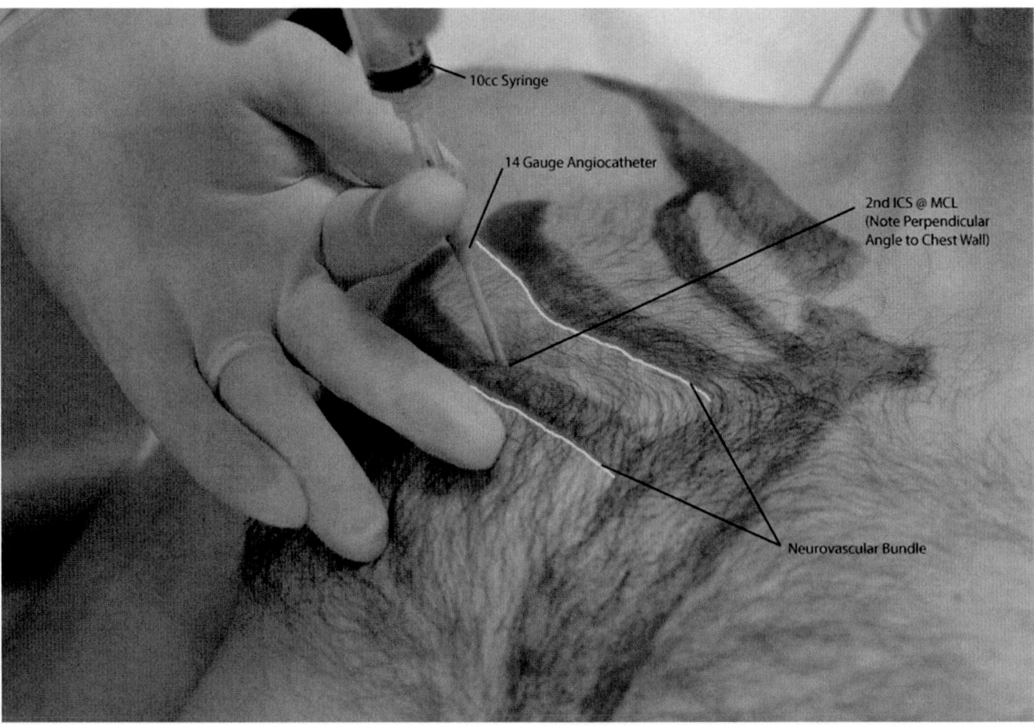

Fig. 19.2 Needle decompression second intercostal space

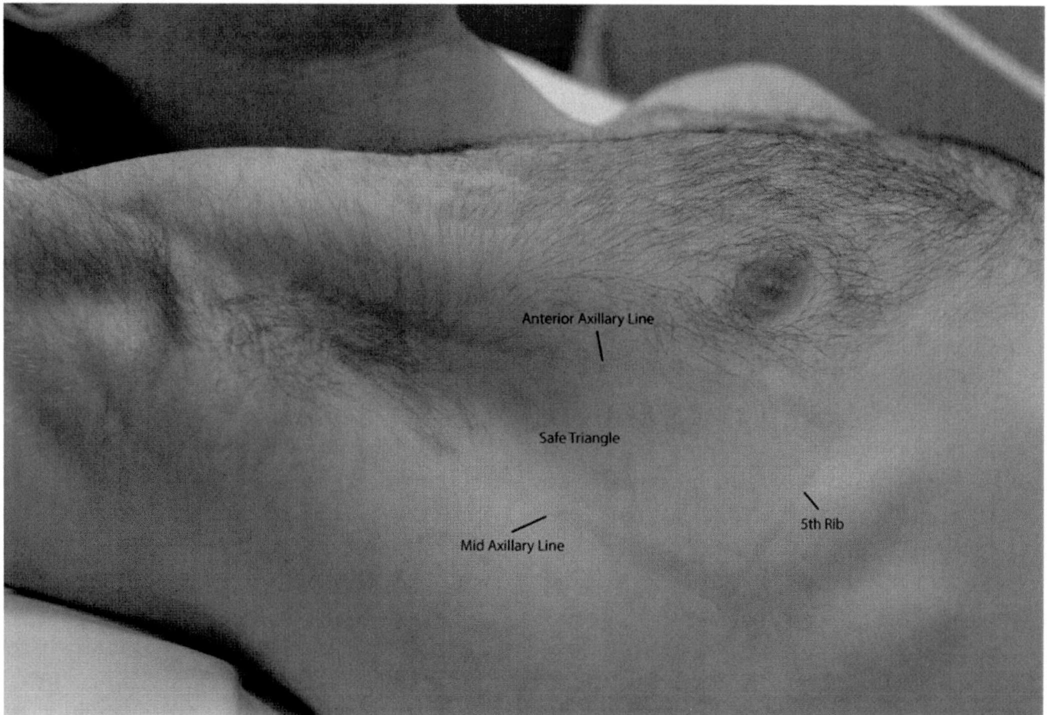

Fig. 19.3 Safe triangle

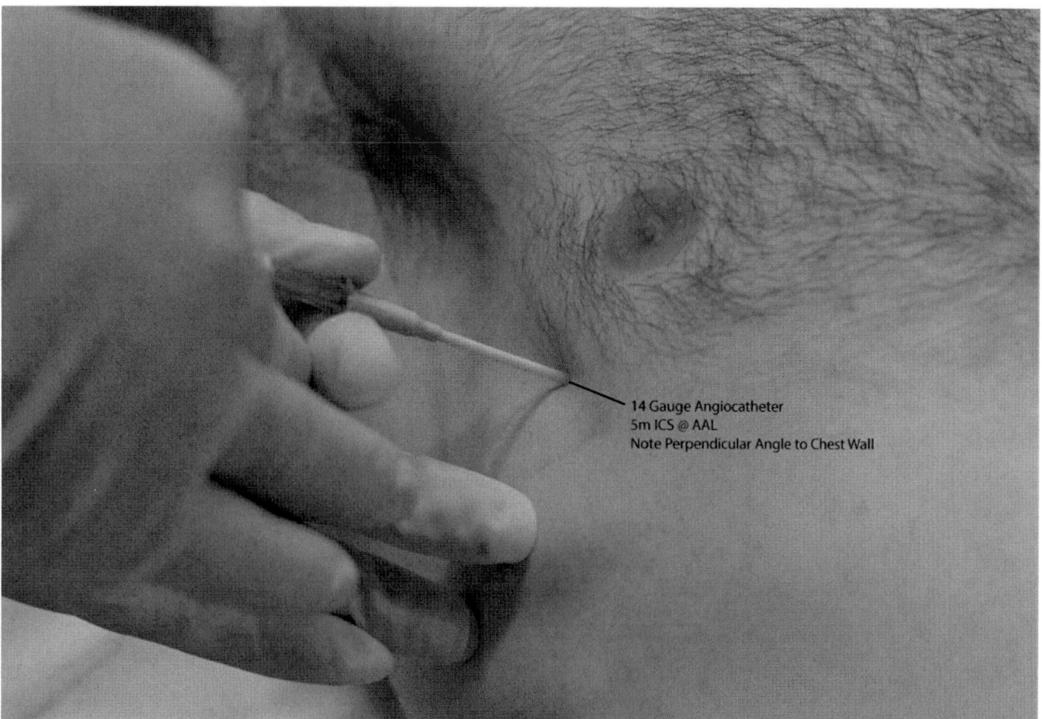

Fig. 19.4 Anterior axillary line approach

19.8 Equipment

This is a fairly simple procedure and does not require extensive setup or equipment. The main piece of equipment is a large bore 5–8 cm 14–16 gauge 5–8 cm over the needle catheter. The angio-catheter should not contain any safety devices such as an auto-retractor. These safety devices will take away the ability to appreciate air return when the pleural cavity is entered. It may be helpful to attach a 10 cc syringe to the angiocatheter to improve control of the needle as well as allow for aspiration during the procedure. The syringe will fill with air upon entering the pleural cavity. The patient should be placed on a cardiac monitor and have supplemental oxygen during the procedure. Additionally if the patient is stable and time allows, the decompression site can be anesthetized prior to decompression. If there is a potential delay in the placement of a chest tube, a three-way stopcock can be attached to the angiocatheter, allowing intermittent relief of air if intrapleural pressure re-accumulates [1, 5, 7] (see Fig. 19.5).

- 14–16 gauge 5–8 cm over the needle catheter (without retractable needle or other safety device that would impede recognition of air return).
- Antiseptic skin cleanser such as chlorhexidine or povidone-iodine.
- Cardiac monitor.
- Supplemental oxygen.

19.8.1 Optional

- Lidocaine with smaller needle and syringe for local infiltration.
- 10 cc syringe.
- 3 way stopcock.

19.9 Procedure

- Indication: tension pneumothorax.
- Contraindications: there are no absolute contraindications.
- Have additional personnel prepare for tube

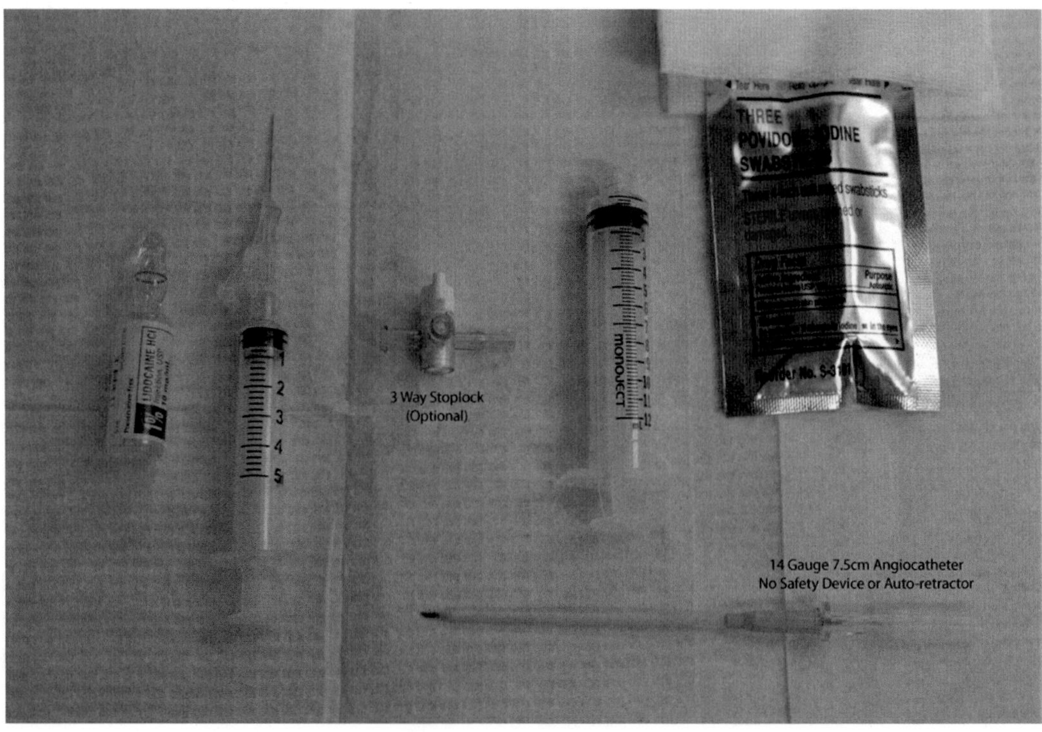

Fig. 19.5 Supplies

thoracostomy while performing needle decompression.

1. Obtain informed consent. This is not always possible as patients with tension pneumothorax may be unconscious or too unstable, and decompression should not be delayed.
2. Place the patient on a cardiac monitor and supplemental oxygen.
3. Place the patient in the supine position with the head of the bed elevated 30–40°. This will allow for the intrapleural air to rise to the superior portion of the lung increasing the distance from the parietal to visceral pleura decreasing the likelihood of penetrating the visceral pleura and lung parenchyma.
4. Identify and mark the site of decompression:
   (a) Second ICS MCL: palpate the sternal angle to identify the second rib; follow this laterally to the MCL. Palpate the third rib and place a mark or indentation just superior to the third rib in the MCL. It is important to enter the pleural space immediately above the third rib to avoid the neurovascular bundle that runs inferior to each rib.
   (b) Fourth or fifth ICS MAL-AAL: choose your preferred method of counting ribs either using the clavicle or sternum as a landmark or start counting in the axillary fossa. The site for decompression will be in the fourth or fifth ICS at or between the midaxillary and anterior axillary line. It is important to enter the pleural space immediately above the fifth or sixth rib to avoid the neurovascular bundle that runs inferior to each rib.
5. Apply antiseptic solution to the area (chlorhexidine or povidone-iodine).
6. If the patient is stable and time allows, anesthetize the area with lidocaine. Start by creating a superficial skin wheal and then infiltrate the deeper tissues for best effect.
7. Align the 14–16 gauge angiocatheter (plus or minus an attached 10 cc syringe) perpendicular to the skin at the site marked in step 4a or 4b. Penetrate the chest wall until a rush of air exits through the angiocatheter. If you are using a 10 cc syringe, you will need to aspirate the plunger of the syringe to allow for air to enter the syringe. Once air is identified stop advancing the needle of the angiocatheter. Advance the catheter over the needle until the hub of the catheter is touching the skin and the catheter is fully inserted.
8. If there is an anticipated delay in placing a chest tube, consider placing three-way stopcock to the hub of the catheter. The use of a three-way stop cock is sited in much of the prehospital and military literature where transport times and accessibility to tube thoracostomy can be delayed.

19.10 Complications

- Failure: if no rush of air is appreciated and there is no improvement in patient condition, consider immediate tube thoracostomy. If the time to prepare for tube thoracostomy may result in patient deterioration, consider repeating needle decompression with a longer angiocatheter.
- Re-accumulation: if the tension pneumothorax re-accumulates and tube thoracostomy cannot be performed immediately, needle decompression will need to be repeated. The small size of the catheter is prone to filling with debris and clot as well as kinking and dislodging. An occluded or dislodged catheter is ineffective and will need to be replaced.
- Bleeding: there is risk of hemorrhage at all sites of decompression. Injury to the thoracic great vessels or pericardium could cause catastrophic hemorrhage and pericardial tamponade.
- Diaphragmatic and solid organ injury can be seen with needle thoracostomy in the fourth and fifth ICS bilaterally.

References

1. Thomsen TW, Feller-Kopman D, Setnik GS. Needle thoracostomy. Procedures Consult, ClinicalKey Web site. 2012. Available at: https://www.clinicalkey.com/#!/ContentPlayerCtrl/doPlayContent/19-s2.0-mp_IM-007. Posted January 10, 2012. Accessed 22 Sept 2013.

2. Chang SJ, Ross SW, Kiefer DJ, Anderson WE, Rogers AT, Sing RF, Callaway DW. Evaluation of 8.0-cm needle at the fourth anterior axillary line for needle chest decompression of tension pneumothorax. J Trauma Acute Care Surg. 2014;76(4):1029–34. doi:10.1097/TA.0000000000000158.
3. Ball CG, Wyrzykowski AD, Kirkpatrick AW, Dente CJ, Nicholas JM, Salomone JP, Rozycki GS, Kortbeek JB, Feliciano DV. Thoracic needle decompression for tension pneumothorax: clinical correlation with catheter length. Can J Surg. 2010;53(3):184–8.
4. Shields TW, Ponn RB, Rusch VW. The lung, pleura, diaphragm, and chest wall, chapter 58—pneumothorax. In: Shields TW, LoCicero J, Ponn RB, Rusch VW, editors. General thoracic surgery. 6th ed. Baltimore, MD: Lippincott Williams & Wilkins; 2009. p. 739–52.
5. American College of Surgeons. 4 thoracic trauma. In: ATLS, advanced trauma life support for doctors. 8th ed. Chicago, IL: American College of Surgeons; 2008. p. 87–8, 108.
6. Leigh-Smith S, Davies G. Indications for thoracic needle decompression. J Trauma. 2007;63(6):1403–4. doi:10.1097/TA.0b013e31814279cb.
7. Pfenninger JL, Fowler GC. Pfenninger and Fowler's procedures for primary care, Chapter 121, tube thoracostomy and emergency needle decompression of tension pneumothorax. 3rd ed. Philadelphia, PA: Mosby Elsevier; 2011.
8. Omar HR, Abdelmalak H, Mangar D, Rashad R, Helal E, Camporesi EM. Occult pneumothorax, revisited. J Trauma Manag Outcomes. 2010;4:12. doi:10.1186/1752-2897-4-12.
9. Inaba K, Ives C, McClure K, Branco BC, Eckstein M, Shatz D, Martin MJ, Reddy S, Demetriades D. Radiologic evaluation of alternative sites for needle decompression of tension pneumothorax. Arch Surg. 2012;147(9):813–8. doi:10.1001/archsurg.2012.751.
10. Sanchez LD, Straszewski S, Saghir A, Khan A, Horn E, Fischer C, Khosa F, Camacho MA. Anterior vs lateral needle decompression of tension pneumothorax: comparison by computed tomography chest wall measurement. Acad Emerg Med. 2011;18(10):1022–6. doi:10.1111/j.1553-2712.2011.01159.x. Epub 2011 Sep 26.
11. https://www.inkling.com/read/bates-guide-physical-examination-and-history-taking-lynn-bickley-11th/chapter-8/chapter-8-overview
12. https://www.inkling.com/read/gray-anatomy-students-drake-vogl-mitchell-2nd/chapter-3/ch03-reader-sa-0
13. Laws D, Neville E, Duffy J, Pleural Diseases Group, Standards of Care Committee, British Thoracic Society. BTS guidelines for the insertion of a chest drain. Thorax. 2003;58:ii53–9. doi:10.1136/thx.58.suppl_2.ii53.

Tube Thoracostomy (Chest Tube) 20

Scott Suttles, Dennis A. Taylor, and Scott Sherry

20.1 Indications

Chest tube thoracostomy is a procedure in which a tube is placed into the chest for the removal or drainage of air, blood, or other fluids from the intrapleural or mediastinal space [1].

The thoracic cavity is a closed space; disruptions in the integrity of this closed space may result in a loss of the negative pressure within the intrapleural space. Air or fluid that accumulates within this space competes with the space occupied by the lung which causes a collapse of the lung. Conditions that cause collapse of the lung include trauma (blunt or penetrating), surgery, disease, or iatrogenic sources.

S. Suttles, MSN, APRN, ACNS-BC, CCRN-CSC (✉)
Pikeville Medical Center, Trauma Services,
Pikeville, KY, USA
e-mail: scott.suttles@pikevillehospital.org;
S_suttles@outlook.com

D.A. Taylor, DNP, ACNP-BC, FCCM
Carolinas HealthCare System, Charlotte,
NC 28232, USA
e-mail: Dennis.taylor@carolinashealthcare.org

S. Sherry, MS, PA-C, FCCM
Oregon Health & Science University, Portland,
OR 97239, USA
e-mail: sherrys@ohsu.edu

20.2 Patient Assessment

Approach the patient and begin assessing the airway, breathing, and circulatory status. Airway patency and air exchange may be impeded if the patient has developed a large accumulation of air and/or fluid within the chest cavity. Assess the breathing ability of the patient by first observing for rise and fall of the chest and then assess for the presence and absence of breath sounds bilaterally. Observe the trachea and neck veins to determine if there is enough pressure within the chest to displace the trachea or to cause distention of the jugular veins. Evaluate the circulatory status of the patient to determine if the pressure within the chest cavity is increased to the extent that it may impede the filling of the heart.

20.3 Pneumothorax (Closed or Open)

Closed Pneumothorax In closed pneumothorax, the chest wall remains intact; however, the pleural space is interrupted. As air enters into the pleural space, it cannot escape, therefore compressing the lung impeding oxygenation. A closed pneumothorax occurs without obvious injury and is often seen in patients with chronic lung conditions (cystic fibrosis, emphysema, tuberculosis) and blunt chest

D.A. Taylor et al. (eds.), *Interventional Critical Care*, DOI 10.1007/978-3-319-25286-5_20

trauma or from iatrogenic causes (mechanical ventilation with high amounts of positive end-expiratory pressure).

- *Assessment*: Patients with a closed pneumothorax may complain of chest pain, dyspnea, tachypnea, and diminished or absent breath sounds on the affected side.
- *Chest radiograph*: In most situations, the pulmonary vessels are not visible beyond the visceral pleural line. In an upright position with a patient that has a pneumothorax, most of the air accumulates in the apex of the lung.

Open Pneumothorax An open pneumothorax occurs when the chest wall and the pleural space have been penetrated, either from penetrating trauma, complications during invasive procedures (central venous catheter placement or needle thoracentesis), or during surgery (thoracotomy). This opening allows for air to enter into the pleural space on inspiration and cannot exit on exhalation compressing the lung. As the lung collapses, the alveoli become under ventilated resulting in hypoxemia and acute respiratory failure may develop.

- *Assessment*: In addition to the assessment findings of a closed pneumothorax, patients may also present with subcutaneous emphysema or a chest wound that creates a sucking sound on inspiration.

Tension Pneumothorax A tension pneumothorax develops as air enters into the pleural space and cannot escape. Air accumulates within the chest with each breath; the pressure inside the chest rises and causes the lung to collapse. As the pressure increases, the mediastinal structures (heart, vena cava, aorta, and trachea) are compressed and shift to the unaffected side. The result is a decrease in cardiac output from the diminished venous return to the heart and potential compression of the heart itself. Radiographically, a tension pneumothorax may show a distinctive shift of the mediastinum to the contralateral side and flattening or inversion of the ipsilateral hemidiaphragm.

In the presence of trauma, differentiation between tension pneumothorax and cardiac tamponade must be made. A clinical diagnosis can be made through assessment; absent breath sounds and hyperresonance over the affected hemithorax and a deviated trachea (a late sign) away from the affected hemithorax can be attributed to a tension pneumothorax.

- *Assessment*: Patients with tension pneumothorax may present with hypotension, tachycardia, dyspnea, or chest pain. Breath sounds may be diminished or absent on the affected side. Percussion of the chest wall may reveal a hyperresonant sound over the affected side. Tracheal deviation away from the affected side may be present in late cases of tension pneumothorax. The jugular veins may be distended from the increased pressure within the chest, impeding venous return to the heart; however, in the presence of trauma, this may not be evident if the patient has significant blood loss.

Hemothorax A hemothorax results from an accumulation of blood in a hemithorax. Hemothorax can be caused by blunt or penetrating thoracic trauma. Compression of the lung prevents adequate ventilation and the loss of circulating blood increases the likelihood of shock. A volume of 300 ml is needed for a hemothorax to be evident on an upright chest X-ray. A massive hemothorax is present if there is an accumulation of 1500 ml of blood in a hemithorax.

- *Assessment*: Patients that present with hemothorax may exhibit the same signs and symptoms of hypovolemic shock, hypotension, and tachycardia. The breath sounds may be diminished or absent over the affected hemithorax. Jugular vein distention is not usually present due to the amount of blood lost within the chest cavity. Percussion of the chest wall on the affected side may reveal a hyporesonant sound for patients with massive hemothorax.

20.4 Hemopneumothorax

Empyema: A collection of pus. Tube thoracostomy is the initial treatment and immediate drainage can improve septic physiology but frequently requires surgical intervention, i.e., video-assisted thoracic surgery (VATS).

Cholothorax: A collection of fluid containing bile. Usually occurs after a liver injury.

Hydrothorax: A collection of noninflammatory serous fluid.

Pleural effusion: An abnormal collection of pleural fluid within the chest cavity.

20.5 Preparation/Setup

Patient Preparation

- After the physical assessment is complete, review the patient's medical/surgical history or in the presence of trauma review the mechanism of injury. Review of pertinent history may help determine the etiology of the pneumothorax, pleural effusion, or empyema.
- Review any diagnostic results such as radiology exams or arterial blood gases to confirm the presence of fluid or air in the chest, hypoxemia, or respiratory demise.

Explanation

- Explain to the patient and family the risks and benefits of chest tube placement. Answer all questions and explain the pathophysiology behind the disease process that necessitates the insertion of a chest tube.

Consent

- Obtain informed consent prior to insertion of the chest tube from the patient or family member. In an emergent situation, consent may be implied if the patient or family member is not able to give informed consent.

Site Marking

- Correct site marking prior to insertion reduces the likelihood of improper placement of invasive devices. Insertion site may be determined by the type of chest drainage tube necessary to remove fluid or air from the chest cavity [2].

Size of Chest Tube

- Determine the appropriate size of chest drainage tube to be used. Removal of fluid from the chest requires a larger tube size than evacuation of air.

Positioning of the Patient

- Ensure that the patient is properly positioned to allow for adequate access to the insertion site.

Intravenous Access

- Confirm that the patient has adequate intravenous access available for administration of IV fluids, sedatives, or analgesics. A pre-insertion dose of an antibiotic may be recommended.

Analgesics/Sedatives

- Administer analgesics or sedatives to decrease the amount of discomfort experienced by the patient. Ensure that local and institutional procedures are followed when providing procedural sedation.

Cardiac Monitor

- Assessment of the patient's cardiac status should be monitored continuously during the insertion of the chest tube. A baseline assessment should be documented and trended during the procedure.

Continuous Pulse Oximetry

- Continuous pulse oximetry should be monitored to assess the patient's oxygenation status during chest tube insertion.

Assemble Supplies

- Ensure that the proper supplies are available and a sufficient quantity is on hand to reduce the time needed to complete the procedure.

20.6 Technical/Logistics/ Operationalize the Procedure

- Hand hygiene.
  - Perform hand hygiene to reduce the potential for transmission of microorganisms per institutional policy.

- Time out.
  - Perform a pre-procedure verification to ensure the correct procedure is being performed on the correct patient. Mark the insertion site with a surgical marking pen. Refer to institutional policy to time out verification procedure.
- Prepare equipment.
  - Obtain a bedside table or stand to place the equipment needed for tube placement. Open the outer wrapper of the insertion tray, remove the tray, and place it on the stand. Open the inner wrapper of the tray using sterile technique.
  - Chest tube insertion is a sterile procedure and requires sterile personal protective equipment unless the procedure is performed during a life-threatening situation. Don sterile attire per institutional policy.
  - Have an assistant during the preparation and insertion periods of the procedure to open needed equipment while sterility is maintained.
  - Have the assistant open and place the chest tube in the insertion tray using sterile technique.
- Site selection.
  - Identify the insertion site by locating the fifth and sixth intercostal space in the anterior axillary or midaxillary line. Use nipple as topical landmark unless patient has pendulous breasts (see Fig. 20.1).
- Site preparation and draping of the insertion site; PPE.
  - Prepare the skin around the insertion site with an antiseptic solution per institutional policy. Ensure that a large area is prepared surrounding the insertion site. Use sterile towels or surgical drapes to cover the area surrounding the insertion site. PPE include sterile gown, gloves, caps, and mask. Also eye protection is needed (see Figs. 20.2 and 20.3).
- Anesthetize the insertion site.
  - Using 1 % Lidocaine, anesthetize the skin, subcutaneous tissue, muscle, pleura, and periosteum surrounding the insertion site. This reduces sensation of pain and discomfort experienced by the patient during the insertion of the chest tube. When infiltrating the tissue with Lidocaine, withdraw

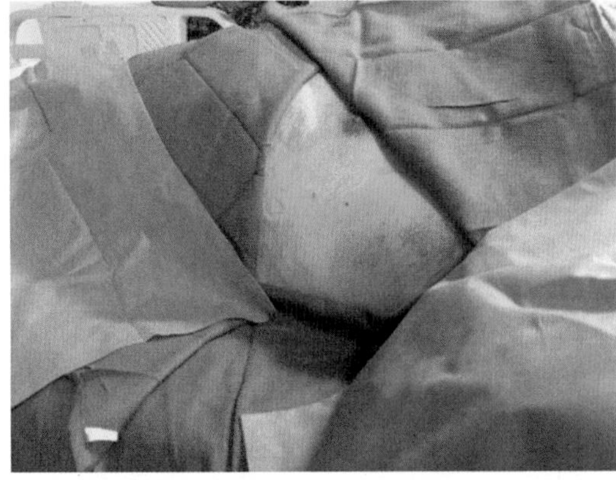

Fig. 20.2 Prep and drape

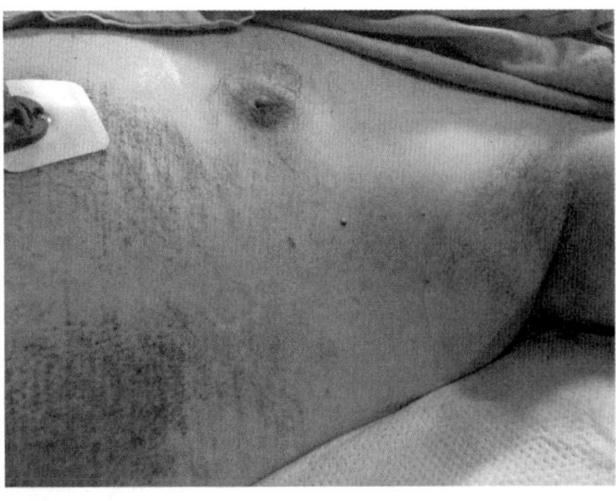

Fig. 20.1 Left chest wall

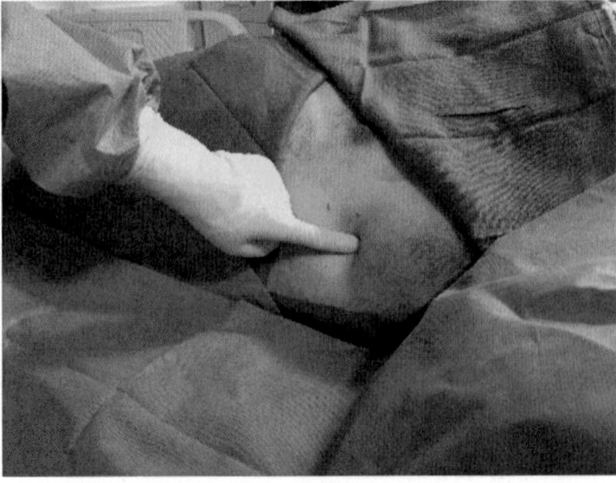

Fig. 20.3 Locate ribs

on the syringe periodically to assess for the presence of air. 30–40 ml of Lidocaine may be needed to anesthetize the area for insertion. Use a 25 gauge needle to inject the Lidocaine into the tissue and parietal pleura. Slowly withdraw the needle after an adequate depth has been reached to anesthetize the pleura. Use a generous amount of Lidocaine to infiltrate the underlying tissue; this ensures that a sufficient amount of anesthetic is delivered (see Fig. 20.4).

- Make the skin incision.
  - Using a no. 10 blade, make an incision parallel to the ribs that is 2–3 cm in length directly over the inferior surface of the rib in the area where the local anesthetic was injected. Ensure that the incision is deep enough to dissect the subcutaneous tissue underlying the skin (see Fig. 20.5).
  - The incision should be large enough to allow for a finger to be inserted (see Fig. 20.6).

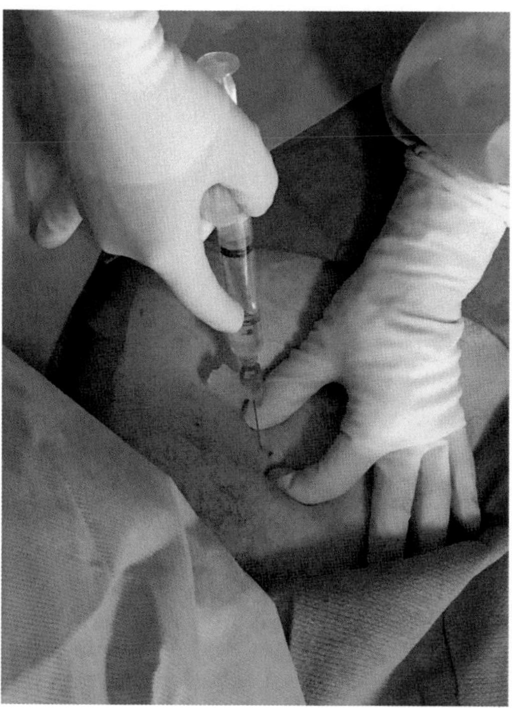

Fig. 20.4 Local anesthetic

- Introduce a curved clamp into the pleural space.
  - Ensure that the tips of the curved clamp are directed downward during insertion into the pleural space (see Fig. 20.7).
  - Insert the curved clamp into the incision made through the skin and subcutaneous tissue, aim toward the superior portion of the rib until the pleural space is reached.
  - Once the clamp has been advanced to the superior portion of the rib, continue to push with steady pressure until the clamp has entered the pleural space.
  - Hold the clamp with both hands, using the fingers of one hand to ensure that the clamp does not enter too deeply into the pleural space injuring the underlying lung tissue (see Fig. 20.8).

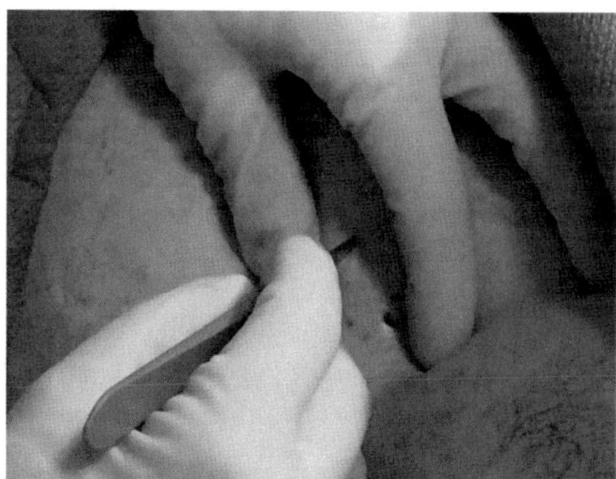

Fig. 20.5 Incision of skin

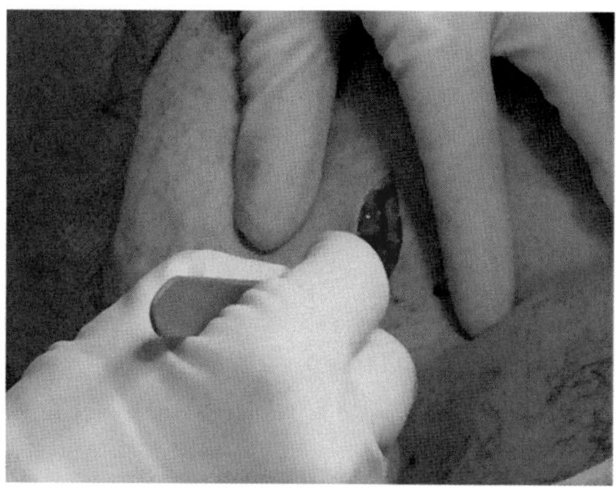

Fig. 20.6 Incision through subcutaneous tissue

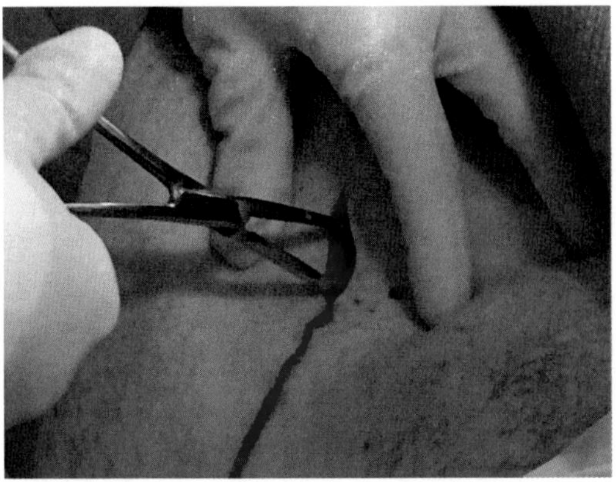

Fig. 20.7 Blunt dissection

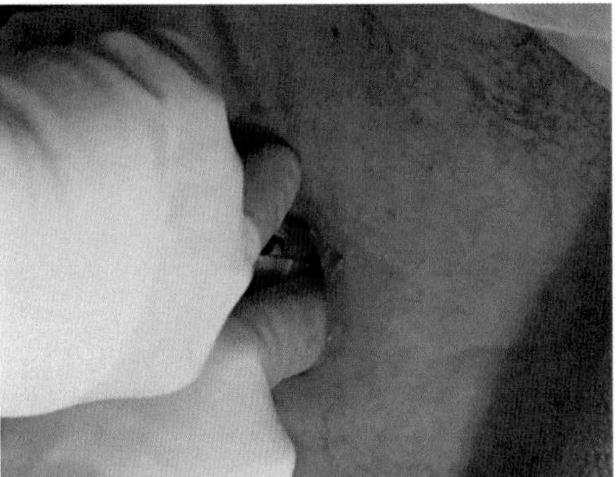

Fig. 20.8 Entering pleural space

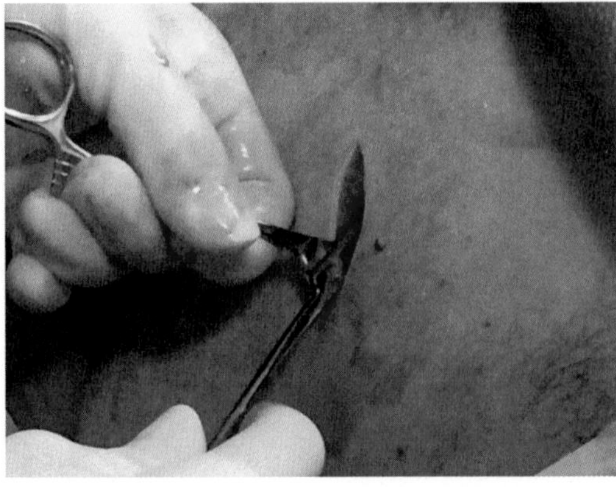

Fig. 20.9 Dilating space between ribs

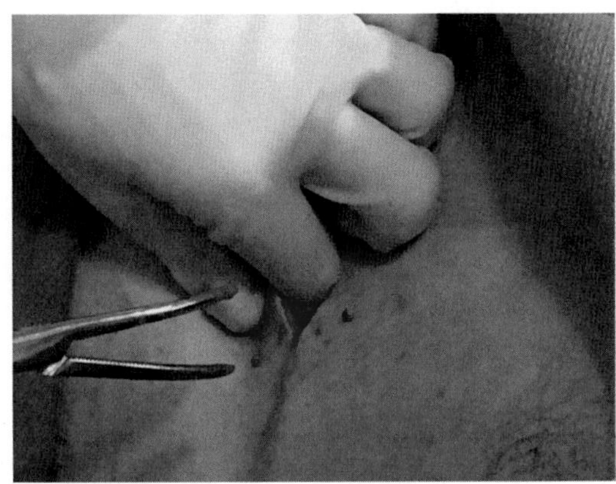

Fig. 20.10 Insert finger into pleural space

- Perform blunt dissection.
  - After the clamp has been inserted into the pleural space, spread the clamp to increase the size of the hole. As the clamp is retracted, close and open the clamp to increase the size of the hole (see Fig. 20.9).
- Dilate the insertion tract with the index finger.
  - Use the index finger to enter the insertion tract and enter the pleural space. Sweep the index finger inside the pleural space to ensure that adhesions and other obstructions such as blood clots are cleared from the insertion tract.
  - The lung should touch the index finger during inspiration (see Fig. 20.10).
- Insert the chest tube with a curved clamp.
  - Using the curved clamp, grasp the proximal end of the chest tube securely, and guide the tube through the insertion tract into the pleural space. Some tubes come with trocars. Trocars can be bent with the metal tip withdrawn into the tube which can allow it to be used as a "guide" like a stylette, but trocars should never be used to puncture into the chest (see Fig. 20.11).
  - For air within the chest cavity, aim the chest tube toward the posterior and superior region of the hemithorax. If the chest tube is inserted for fluid accumulation, ensure that it is directed toward the posterior and inferior portion of the hemithorax.

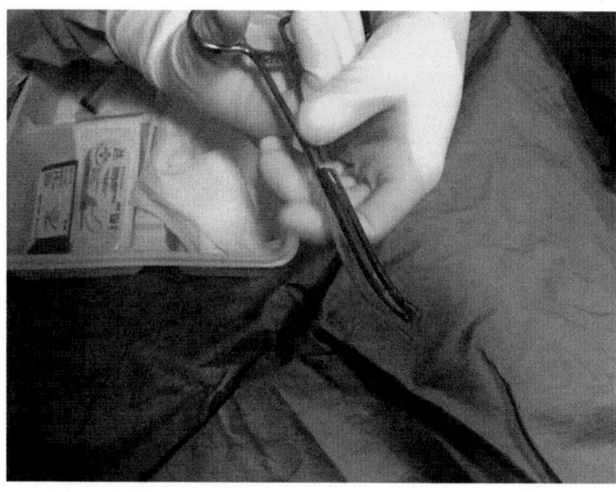

Fig. 20.11 Clamping chest tube

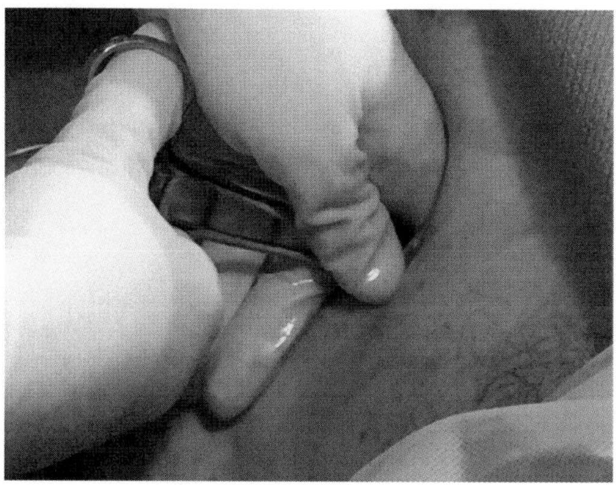

Fig. 20.12 Insertion of chest tube

  Tube advancement should be gentle. The lung is very fragile—never force the tube against significant resistance (see Fig. 20.12).

- Remove the clamp and guide the tube into the pleural space.
  - Advance the chest tube until the sentinel hole is inside of the pleural space.
  - Fluid or condensation may be noted within the tube (see Fig. 20.13).
- Connect the tube to the chest drainage collection system.
  - With the help of an assistant, connect the chest tube to the drainage system (see Fig. 20.14).
- Secure the tube to the chest wall with suture.
  - Using suture (#2 Ethibond), create a "stay" suture on the superior side of the incision site

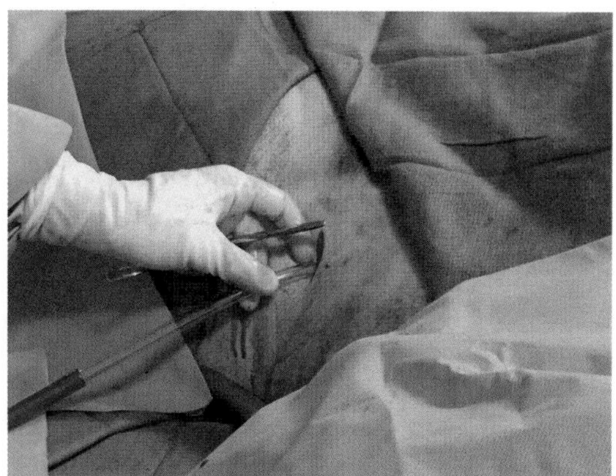

Fig. 20.13 Advancing chest tube

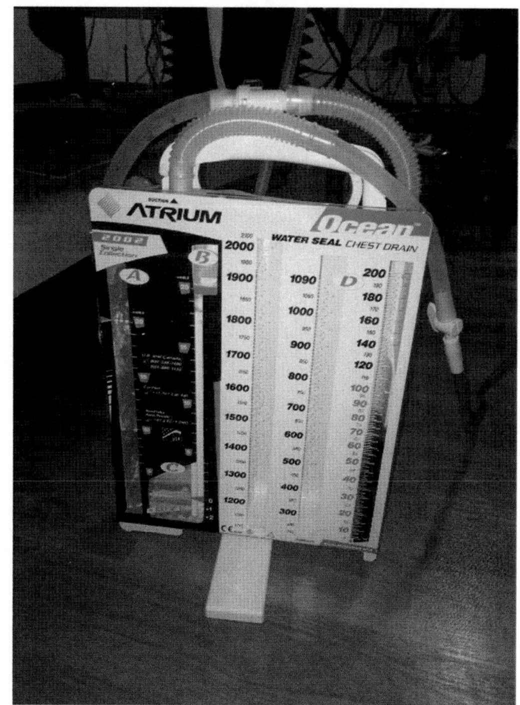

Fig. 20.14 Collection system

to close any skin and ensure that the hole size is decreased, minimizing the entrance of air into the surrounding subcutaneous tissue.

  - Wrap the ends around the chest tube twice and tie the loose ends tight enough to depress the tube slightly but not so tight that the suture collapses the tube. This is to ensure that the tube is secured adequately (see Figs. 20.15, 20.16, and 20.17).

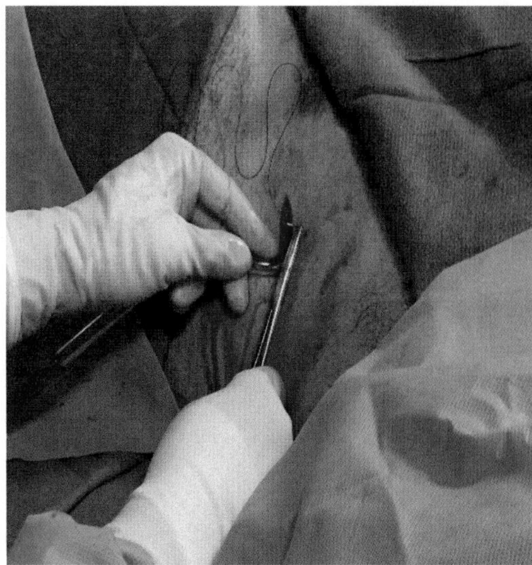

Fig. 20.15 Suturing CT into place

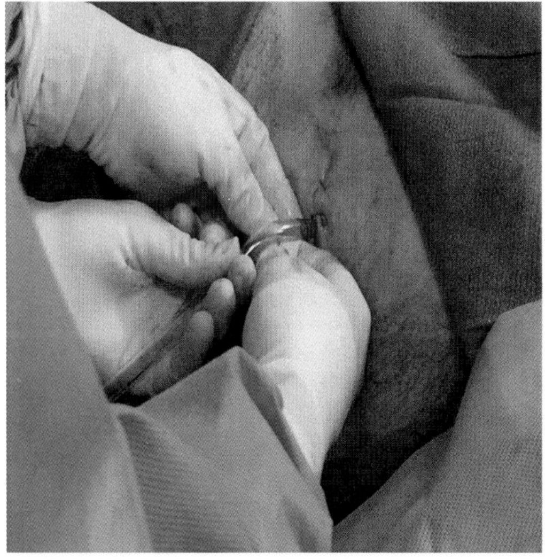

Fig. 20.16 Securing suture around CT

- Apply dressings over the insertion site and tube.
  - Apply petrolatum gauze dressing around the tube, this helps to provide an airtight seal around the chest tube at the insertion site (see Fig. 20.18).
  - Apply 4×4 gauze dressings over the insertion site and cover the entire dressing with tape.

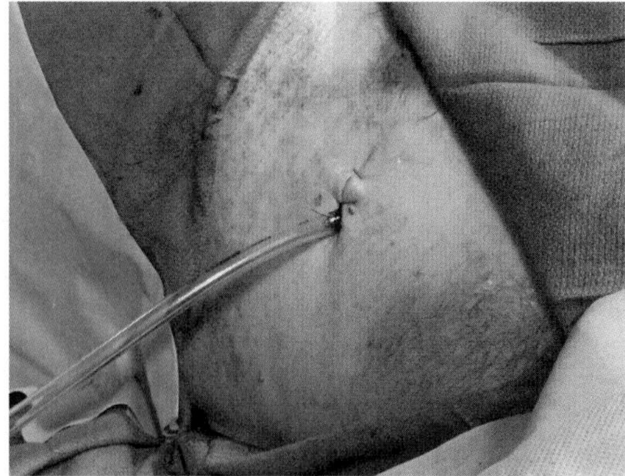

Fig. 20.17 Closing wound

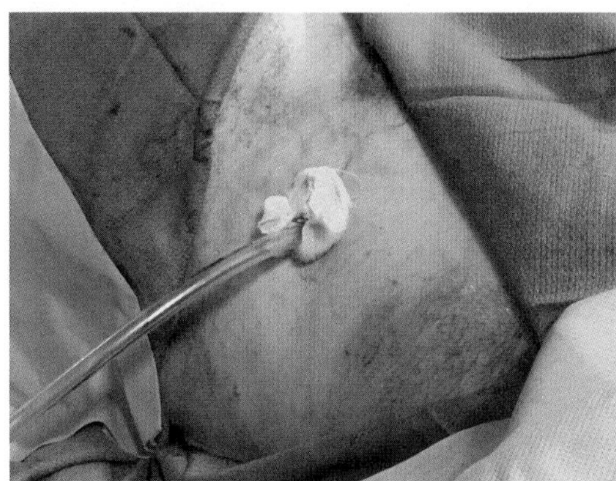

Fig. 20.18 Occlusive dressing

  - Secure the tube to the patient's skin with tape below the insertion site to prevent the tube from being dislodged.
- Secure all connections with tape.
  - This helps reduce the incidence of air leaks within the system. Check for air leaks and document at this time. If one is present, take a moment to check connections and insertion site.
- Obtain a radiograph of the chest.
  - Confirm placement of the tube with a chest radiograph. If the tube was placed for fluid accumulation, monitor for reduction of fluid within the chest cavity. If the tube was placed for air accumulation, confirm re-expansion of the lung.

  - Ensure that the break in the radiopaque marker on the tube is within the pleural space.
- Record in the patient's medical record.
  - Indications for insertion.
  - Insertion depth and size of the tube.
  - Vital signs before and after chest tube insertion.
  - The amount and consistency of fluid that drains from the chest.
  - Presence of air leak.
  - Complications.
  - How the patient tolerated the procedure.
  - FOCA is an acronym commonly used—fluctuation, output, color, air leak.

20.7 Complications/Pitfalls for the ICU

- Malposition.
  - The most common complication of tube thoracostomy is tube malposition. Chest tubes that are malpositioned represent a form of penetrating trauma and should be managed accordingly. A pulmonary or thoracic surgery service consult should be considered before manipulating a chest tube that is malpositioned in a stable patient.
- Organ injury.
  - The most common organ injury during tube thoracostomy is the lung. Perforation of the heart, liver spleen, and diaphragm are also potential injuries. Controlled entry into the pleural space can reduce the incidence of organ injury.
- Infection.
  - Increased duration of indwelling chest tubes can lead to potential for infection.
- Re-expansion pulmonary edema.
  - Rapid re-expansion of a large pneumothorax may cause re-expansion pulmonary edema. It also occurs with the drainage of large amounts of pleural fluid.

References

1. American College of Surgeons Committee on Trauma. Thoracic trauma, Chapter 4. In: Advanced trauma life support. 9th ed. pp. 94–112; 2013.
2. Benns M, et al. Does chest tube location matter? An analysis of chest tube position and the need for secondary interventions. J Trauma Acute Care Surg. 2015;78(2):386–90.

Pericardiocentesis

21

Liza Rieke and Brian Cmolik

21.1 Introduction

The pericardial sac consisting of two layers, an outer parietal pericardium and an inner visceral pericardium, can typically hold 15–50 ml of serous fluid [1]. Rapid accumulation of even a small amount of additional fluid can cause a patient to become symptomatic [2]. Cardiac tamponade occurs when enough fluid, in the form of serous fluid (hydropericardium), blood (hemopericardium), pus (purulent pericarditis), or gas (pneumopericardium), accumulates in the pericardium, exceeding the ability of the pericardium to distend, and causes symptoms.

The most common first symptom is dyspnea [3, 4]. Guberman and his colleagues found paradoxical pulse, dyspnea, tachypnea, and tachycardia to be the most frequent signs and symptoms [4]. Another classic clinical syndrome that can occur in some patients with acute cardiac tamponade is Beck's triad. Beck first described the acute cardiac compression triad in 1935 and defined it as falling arterial pressure, rising venous pressure, and a small quiet heart [5]. It is important to know that Beck's triad was in reference to surgical patients with acute tamponade from intrapericardial hemorrhage due to trauma or myocardial or aortic rupture, and medical patients who gradually develop a pericardial effusion may not display any of Beck's triad. Today's definition of Beck's triad includes hypotension, jugular venous distention, and distant heart sounds. Hypotension occurs as the pericardium is filled with fluid and is no longer able to distend, decreasing the ability of the right ventricle to fill, which in turn reduces stroke volume. This process reduces systolic blood pressure. The pressure of the fluid buildup in the pericardial sac reduces the diastolic filling of the right ventricle causing an increase in central venous pressure which is evidenced by distended jugular veins. The fluid-filled pericardium also muffles heart sounds [6]. Treatment should not be delayed if all components of Beck's triad are not present. The complete triad was present in only 41 % patients with cardiac tamponade in one trauma study [7]. Morbidity and possibly mortality are risks of waiting for the full complement before intervening.

L. Rieke, ACNP (✉)
8840 Belton Drive, North Ridgeville,
OH 44039, USA

US Department of Veterans Affairs, Louis Stoke
Cleveland VA Medical Center,
10701 East Blvd, Surgery 112 (W),
Cleveland, OH 44106, USA
e-mail: Liza.Rieke@VA.gov

B. Cmolik, MD
US Department of Veterans Affairs, Louis Stoke
Cleveland VA Medical Center,
10701 East Blvd, Surgery 112 (W),
Cleveland, OH 44106, USA
e-mail: Brian.Cmolik@VA.gov

D.A. Taylor et al. (eds.), *Interventional Critical Care*, DOI 10.1007/978-3-319-25286-5_21

Another common symptom of pericardial tamponade is pulsus paradoxus in which the systolic blood pressure drops more than 10 mmHg with inspiration during normal breathing [2, 6]. Adolf Kussmaul first described pulsus paradoxus in 1873 as a palpable diminution of the radial pulse on inspiration in patients with cardiac tamponade [1]. The pathophysiology of pulsus paradoxus is explained by the significantly reduced intrathoracic pressure during inspiration that allows more venous return to right ventricle. On the next cardiac cycle, the pulmonary vascular beds are filled and exceed the output of the right ventricle. In turn, the blood return to the left ventricle is reduced and the atrial and ventricular pressures drop during inspiration. This is demonstrated by a >10 mmHg drop in systolic blood pressure during inspiration [8]. Some coexisting conditions can mask the presence of pulsus paradoxus. Extreme hypotension, pericardial adhesions, right ventricular hypertrophy without pulmonary hypertension, severe aortic regurgitation, and atrial septal defects [9]. Sometimes pulsus paradoxus exists without the presence of cardiac tamponade in conditions such as massive pulmonary embolism, profound hypotension, and obstructive lung disease [9].

Once a symptomatic pericardial effusion is identified, a method of draining the fluid to release the pressure must be implemented to restore hemodynamic stability. The first successful pericardiotomy was performed in 1815 by Romero and was an open procedure involving an incision through the chest wall and into the pericardium under direct vision [10]. The first successful closed technique was documented in 1840 by Franz Schuh; it was a blind technique of inserting a trochar, without incision, to the fourth intercostal space [10]. Since that time, medicine has evolved to the point in which echocardiography-guided pericardiocentesis has become the gold standard [11]. Ideally this procedure should take place with ultrasound guidance and under sterile conditions. During a cardiac arrest in which pericardial tamponade is suspected, a blind technique may still be used if no imaging equipment is available. Pericardiocentesis may only provide a temporary solution until a more definitive intervention can take place. An emergent surgical consultation should be obtained to evaluate the need for definitive drainage. In trauma patients, pericardiocentesis is a temporizing maneuver when thoracotomy is not an available option. However, when a qualified surgeon is present, ATLS emphasizes immediate thoracotomy as definitive management [12].

21.2 Causes

Patients at highest risk for pericardial tamponade include those with acute or chronic pericarditis, malignancy, end-stage renal disease, recent cardiac surgery, infection, and trauma to the chest. The most common cause of pericardial tamponade is intrapericardial hemorrhage [5]. Sources of intrapericardial hemorrhage are penetrating wounds to the heart, myocardial infarction, cardiac contusion, auricle rupture, coronary or aortic aneurysm rupture, rupture of the base of sclerotic aorta, neoplasms, scurvy, tuberculosis of the pericardium, and purpura [5]. One large review of pericardial effusions found that the most common diagnosis was acute idiopathic pericarditis (20 %), followed by iatrogenic effusion (16 %), malignancy (13 %), chronic idiopathic effusion (9 %), acute myocardial infarction (8 %), end-stage renal disease (6 %), congestive heart failure (5 %), collagen vascular disease (5 %), and infection (4 %) [13].

21.3 Indications

First and foremost, cardiac tamponade is a clinical diagnosis. It is important to maintain a high degree of suspicion of cardiac tamponade in patients with appropriate clinical signs and symptoms. The most common symptoms of cardiac tamponade include [6, 11, 14]:

Symptoms

Dyspnea.
Anxiety.
Chest pain.
Cold, moist skin.
Weak or imperceptible pulse.
Nausea.
Dysphagia.

Signs

Beck's triad (jugular venous distention, distant heart sounds, and hypotension).

Pulsus paradoxus (a drop in SBP of more than 10 mmHg with inspiration during normal breathing [2]).
Electrical alternans—alternating high and low voltage QRS complexes.
Kussmaul's sign—rise in jugular venous pressure (JVP) on inspiration.
Cough.
Unconsciousness.
Pericardial friction rub.
Tachypnea.
Low-voltage QRS.
Cardiomegaly on CXR.
Right-side heart collapse on echocardiography.

Once a patient presents with any of the above signs and symptoms and cardiac tamponade is suspected, a bedside cardiac ultrasound should be obtained by a skilled practitioner. The FAST exam includes two different cardiac views to determine if there is cardiac tamponade. The first view is the subxiphoid view in which the ultrasound probe is placed in the subxiphoid region with the marker dot toward the patient's right shoulder. The probe is then angled toward the left shoulder and allows the right ventricle to be viewed adjacent to the left lobe of the liver. In this view, a pericardial effusion can be recognized between the liver and the heart while having the patient take a deep breath with enhance the image [15]. The second ultrasound view to evaluate for cardiac tamponade is the parasternal view in which the ultrasound probe is placed just left of the sternum at the fourth and fifth intercostal space directly over the center of the heart with the maker dot facing 4 o'clock. This view shows the anterior and posterior pericardium [15]. Common echocardiogram findings consistent with cardiac tamponade include presence of pericardiac fluid and diastolic collapse of the right atrium or ventricle [11, 14].

21.4 Contraindications

In an emergency situation in which a patient is unstable, life is threatened, or no other immediate intervention is available, there is no absolute contraindication to pericardiocentesis. According to the European Society of Cardiology guidelines, aortic dissection is a major contraindication to pericardiocentesis [2].

There are a few relative contraindications for a stable patient with cardiac tamponade which include coagulopathy, anticoagulant therapy, thrombocytopenia, small effusions, loculated effusions, and posteriorly located effusions [2]. Traumatic pericardial effusion, myocardial rupture, and aortic dissection are surgical emergencies and should not be delayed by a pericardiocentesis procedure [14].

21.5 Preparation

21.5.1 Equipment

In ideal circumstances, this procedure should take place in an emergency department, intensive care unit, or cardiac catheterization lab. A pericardiocentesis kit that has all the necessary equipment and a procedure cart with sterile equipment is optimal for promptness in this clinical emergency. If neither is available to you, the essential equipment is listed below:

Sterile gown.
Sterile gloves.
Facemask with shield or protective eyewear.
Cap.
Chlorhexidine-based skin preparation solution.
18-gauge spinal needle.
Three-way stopcock.
20-ml or larger syringe.
20–25 gauge needle for local anesthetic infiltration.
Local anesthetic (1 or 2 % lidocaine).
Nasogastric tube.
Wire with alligator clips on each end (for non-ultrasound procedures) (Figs. 21.1 and 21.2).

21.6 Positioning

Ideal positioning of a patient is semirecumbent with the head of bed at 30–45° angle as it brings the pericardium closer to the anterior chest. Supine positioning is also acceptable (Fig. 21.3).

21.6.1 Monitoring

Ensure continuous ECG and hemodynamic monitoring. Obtain adequate IV access. Provide airway

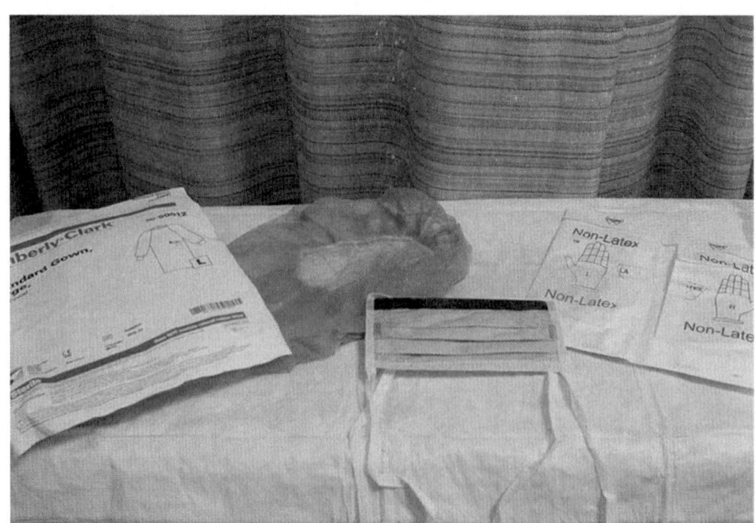

Fig. 21.1 Sterile attire

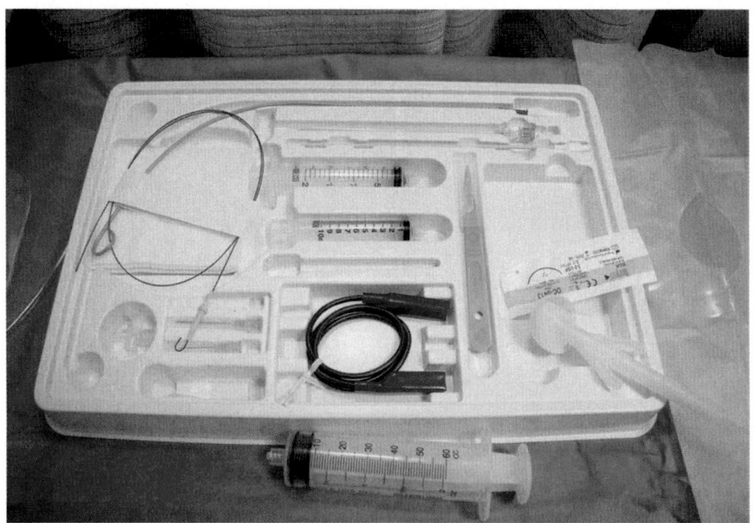

Fig. 21.2 Sterile pericardiocentesis tray

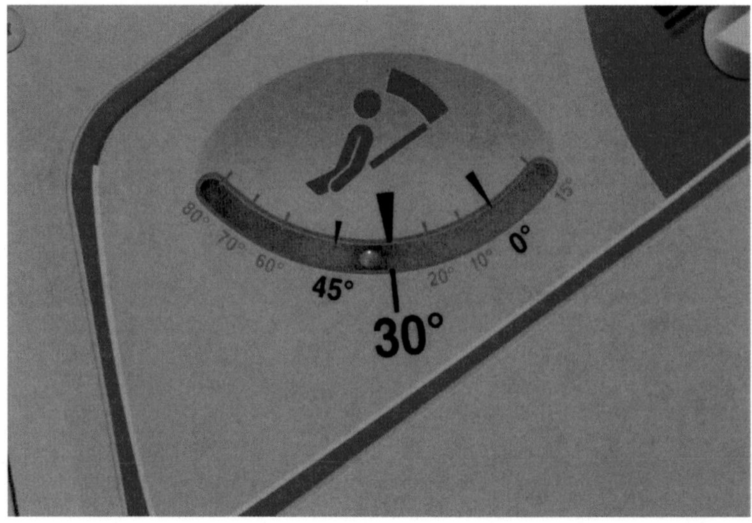

Fig. 21.3 Head of bed at least 30°

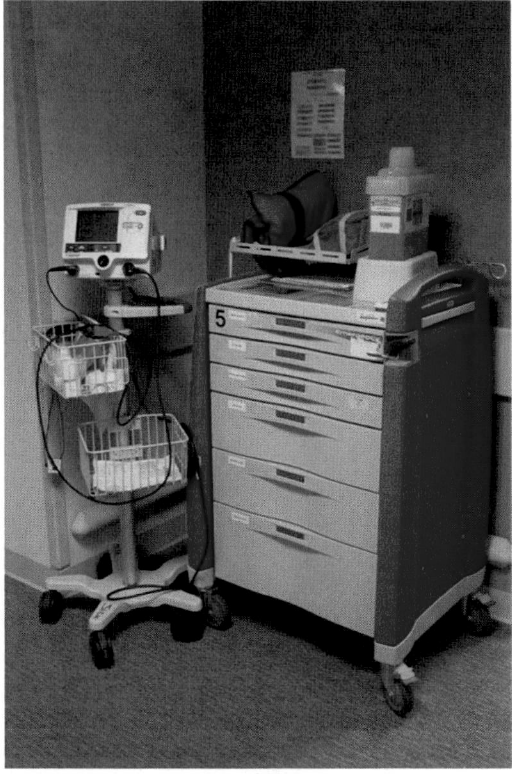

Fig. 21.4 Code cart and defibrillator

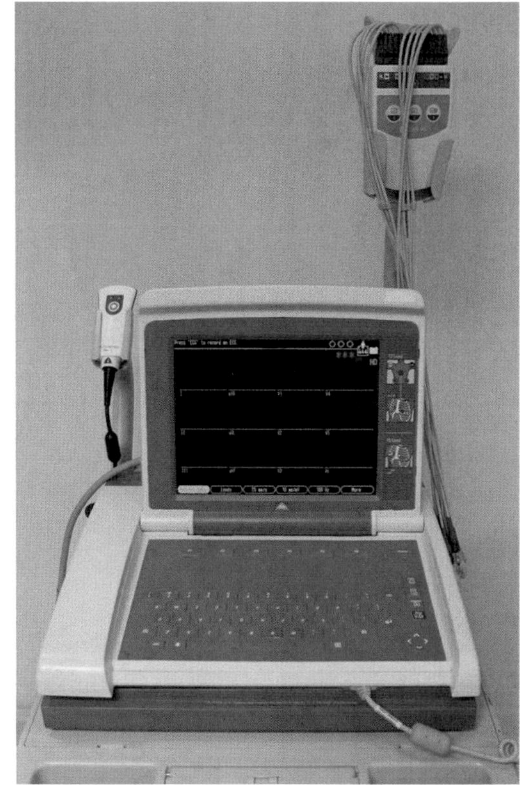

Fig. 21.5 ECG machine

and respiratory support as necessary. Have code cart and defibrillator nearby (Figs. 21.4 and 21.5).

21.7 Techniques

With each technique, preparation is similar:

- Prepare the equipment and patient as rapidly as possible as this is an emergent procedure for an unstable situation.
- If time permits, place nasogastric tube to decompress the stomach and reduce risk of gastric perforation.
- Position patient in semirecumbent position.
- Utilize ultrasound to determine point of maximal effusion closest to the skin and furthest from any other surrounding structures.
- Prepare chest and upper abdominal area with chlorhexidine-based skin preparation solution.
- Utilize local anesthetic if time permits.
- Drape the area surrounding target site with sterile towels.
- Don sterile attire.
- Place ultrasound probe in sterile sleeve.
- If available, using continuous echography guidance, find your target location; insert the needle, while continuously aspirating; and advance the needle into the fluid collection.
- Confirm placement of the needle in the pericardial effusion by flushing 5 ml of agitated normal saline to form a microbubble contrast into the space to confirm on ultrasound.
- Remove needle and allow catheter to remain in pericardial effusion.
- Withdraw fluid until effusion no longer present and patient is hemodynamically stable.
- Remove catheter and place dressing over insertion site.
- Send fluid for diagnostic testing.
- Obtain CXR.
- Obtain formal echocardiogram.
- Consult surgery for possible surgical intervention (Figs. 21.6, 21.7, 21.8 and 21.9).

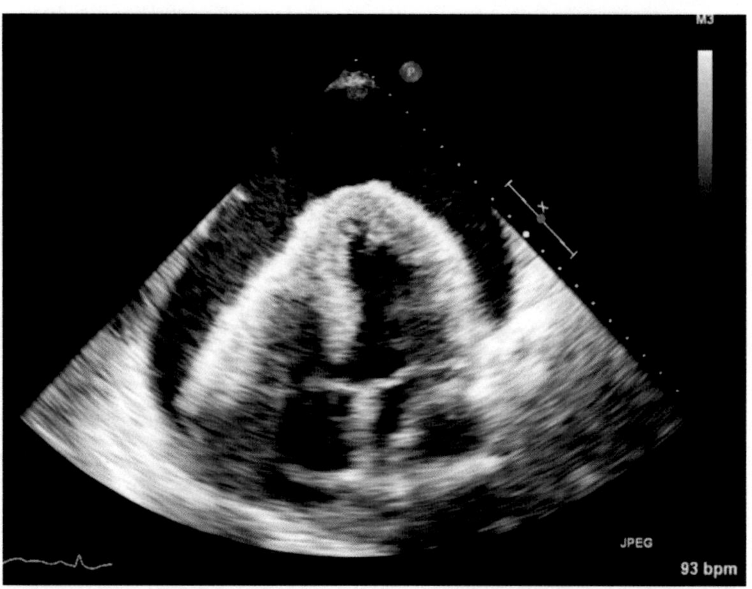

Fig. 21.6 Pericardial effusion

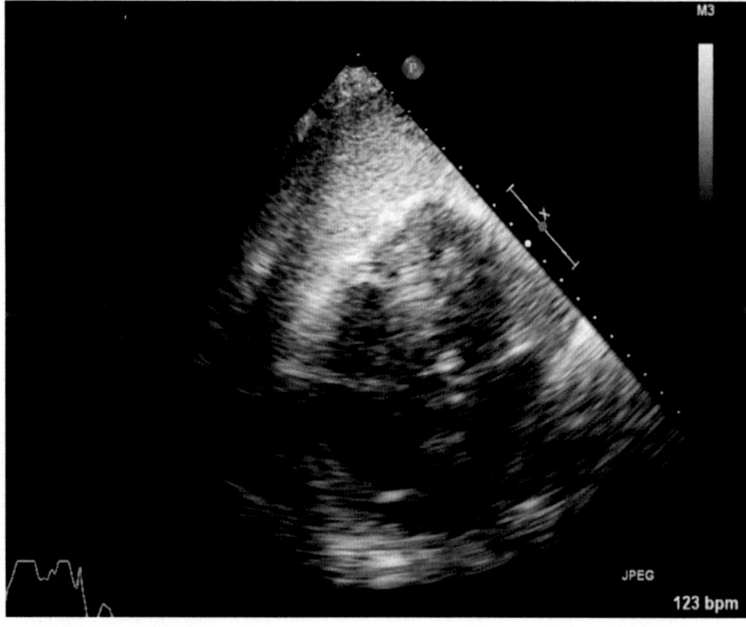

Fig. 21.7 Agitated saline contrast

Ultrasound-Guided Subxiphoid Approach Find target location just below the xiphoid process and the left costal margin. Insert the spinal needle with the stylet or a steel core with polytef-sheathed needle; once the needle has punctured the skin, remove the stylet and attach a three-way stopcock and a 20-ml syringe. With continuous aspiration, advance the needle toward the left shoulder. Using ultrasound, guide the needle toward the largest fluid collection. Empty the fluid from the syringe by attaching tubing to three-way stopcock. Remove fluid until hemodynamic stability is reached or no further fluid is available (Figs. 21.10 and 21.11).

Ultrasound-Guided Parasternal Approach Find target location in the fifth intercostal space just lateral to the sternum. Use ultrasound to locate the largest fluid collection and guide the needle perpendicularly into the pericardial sac to aspirate (Figs. 21.12 and 21.13).

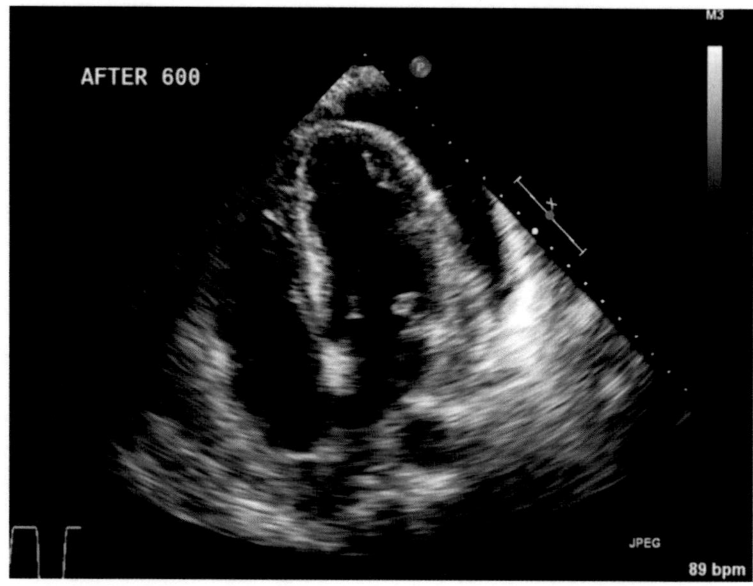

Fig. 21.8 Drainage of 600-ml pericardial fluid

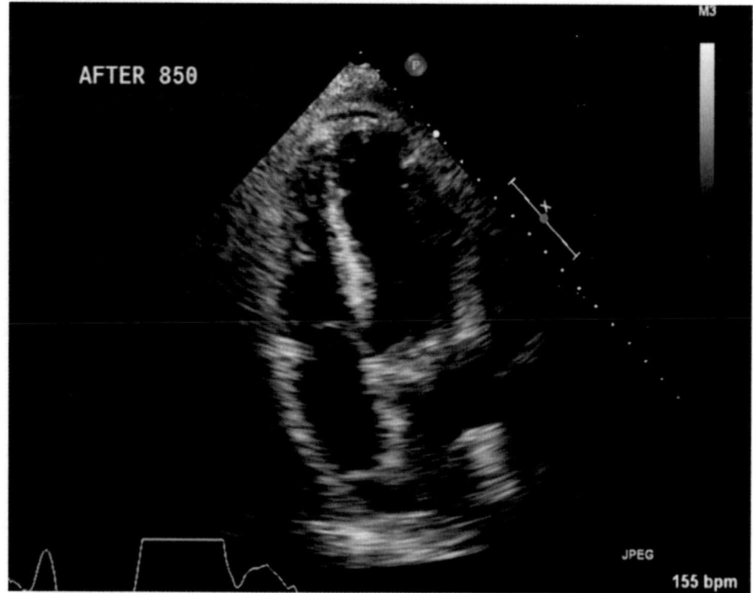

Fig. 21.9 Drainage of 850-ml pericardial fluid with resolution of pericardial effusion

Ultrasound-Guided Apical Approach Find target location in the intercostal space below and 1 cm lateral to the apical beat. Use ultrasound to locate the largest fluid collection and insert needle, aim toward right shoulder, and aspirate (Figs. 21.14 and 21.15).

Electrocardiographic Approach Note that guidelines state that ECG injury monitoring is not an adequate safeguard [2]. When ultrasound is not available, attach a sterile alligator clip and wire to the spinal needed and connect the other end of the wire to a precordial lead (i.e., V1) on a continuous ECG monitor. As you advance the needle (using any above approaches), monitor the ECG for ST elevation. If ST elevation occurs, the needle is advanced too far and in contact with the myocardial surface. If this occurs, withdraw the needle until the ST elevation resolves and then redirect the needle and aspirate fluid (Fig. 21.16).

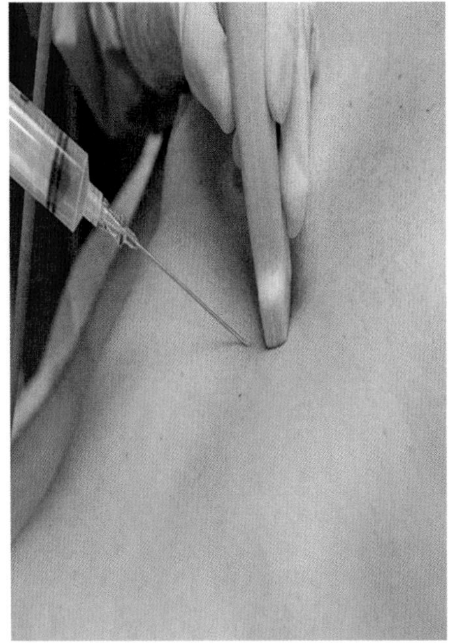

Fig. 21.10 Ultrasound-guided subxiphoid approach

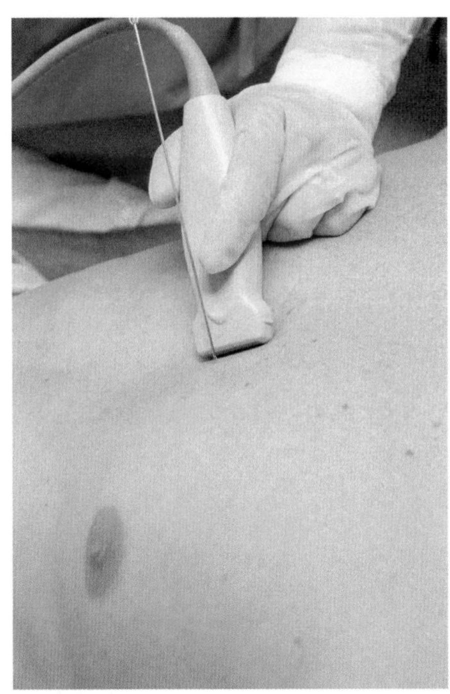

Fig. 21.12 Ultrasound-guided parasternal approach

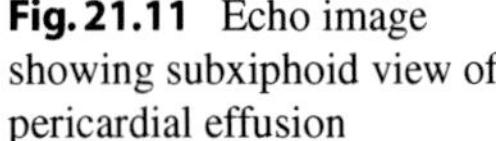

Fig. 21.11 Echo image showing subxiphoid view of pericardial effusion

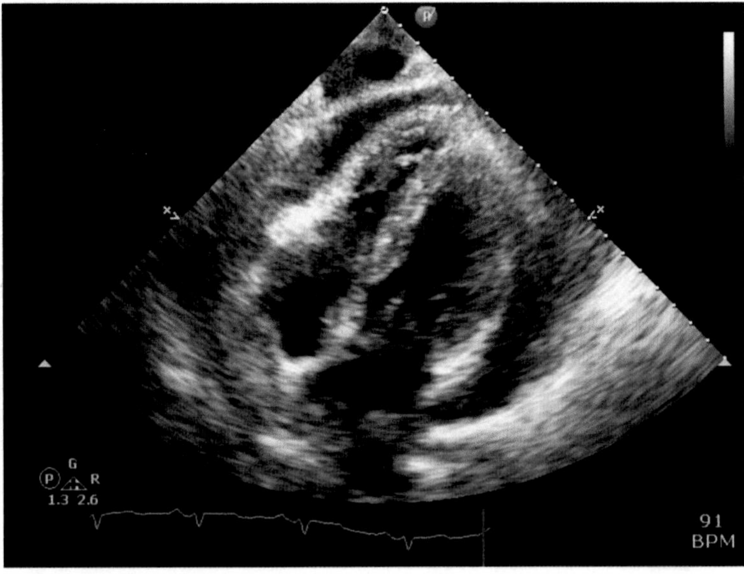

Blind Approach Use only with true emergency and when neither ultrasound nor electrocardiographic monitoring is available. Find target just below xiphoid process and left costal margin. Insert needle at 45° angle and advance toward left shoulder with continuous aspiration until a fluid return is obtained. Obtain ultrasound and CXR as soon as immediately available. This technique has the highest risk of damage to adjacent structures as the liver, lung, diaphragm, and GI tract are all within the vicinity (Fig. 21.17).

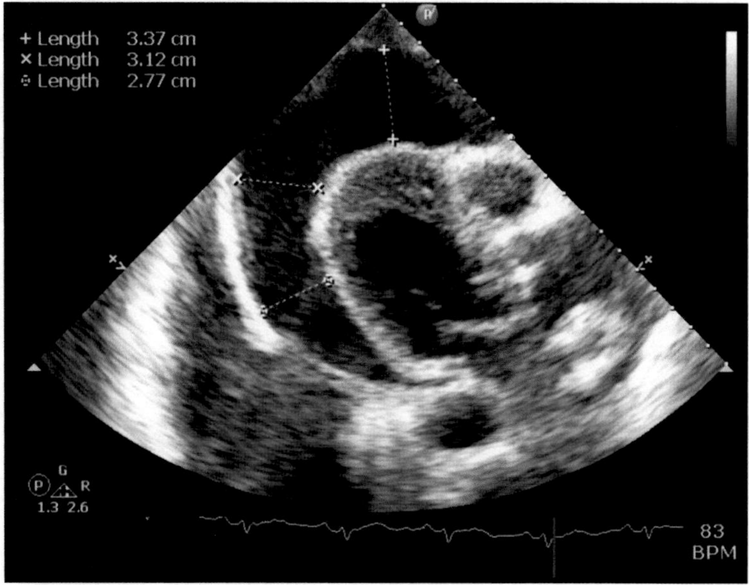

Fig. 21.13 Echo image showing parasternal view of pericardial effusion

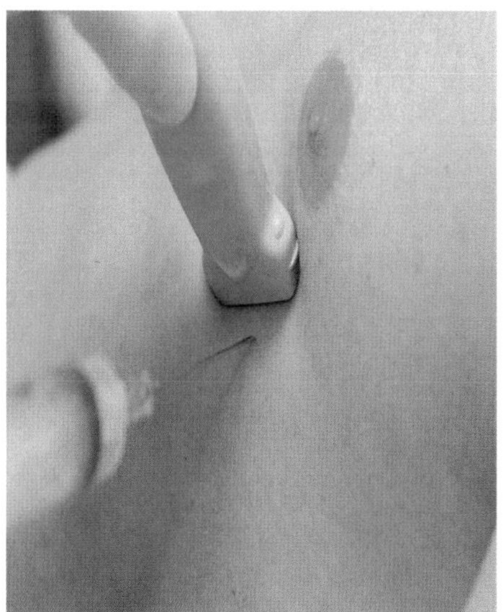

Fig. 21.14 Ultrasound-guided apical approach

21.8 Post-Procedure Care

Once the pericardiocentesis is completed, remove the catheter and place a dry sterile dressing over the insertion site. Ensure that the patient is hemodynamically stable. Obtain a formal ultrasound to ensure completion of drainage, adequate cardiac function, and no complications. A CXR should also be obtained to evaluate for a pneumothorax. An ECG should be obtained to evaluate for arrhythmias. Cardiology and surgery consults should be obtained to determine if definitive treatment is necessary. Aspirated fluid can be sent for analysis, gram stain, and culture to determine cause of pericardial effusion.

21.9 Complications

The complications associated with emergent pericardiocentesis for cardiac tamponade have significantly decreased with the introduction of M-mode echocardiography-assisted pericardiocentesis in 1978 [16]. Callahan and his group had no deaths in a series of 610 consecutive pericardiocentesis procedures guided by 2-D echocardiography [17]. The latest reported incidence of major complications is 1.3–1.6 % [2]. The most serious and common complications are laceration and perforation of the myocardium and coronary vessels [2].

Other complications include rhythm disturbances, pneumothorax, and infection [2]. Bastian and his colleagues found no adverse events in patients undergoing primary pericardiocentesis via subxiphoid approach after pericardial effusion was confirmed on echocardiography with resolution of the pericardial effusion in 81 % of patients. However, patients requiring a second

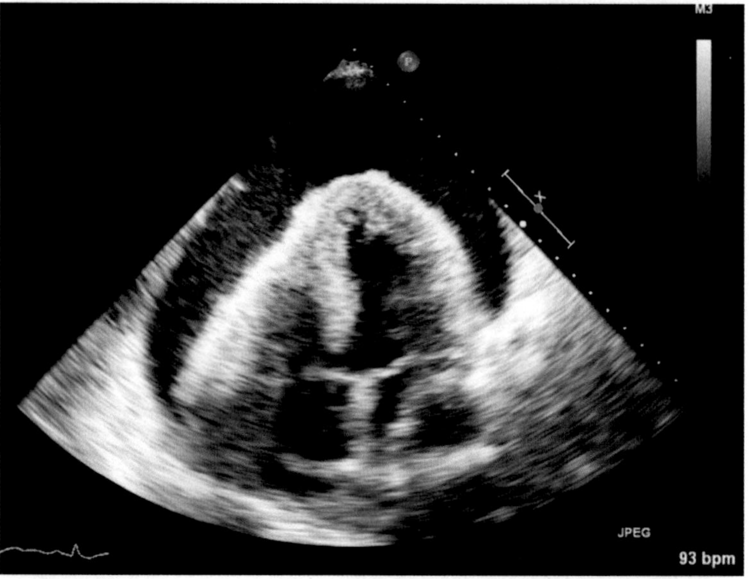

Fig. 21.15 Echo showing apical view of pericardial effusion

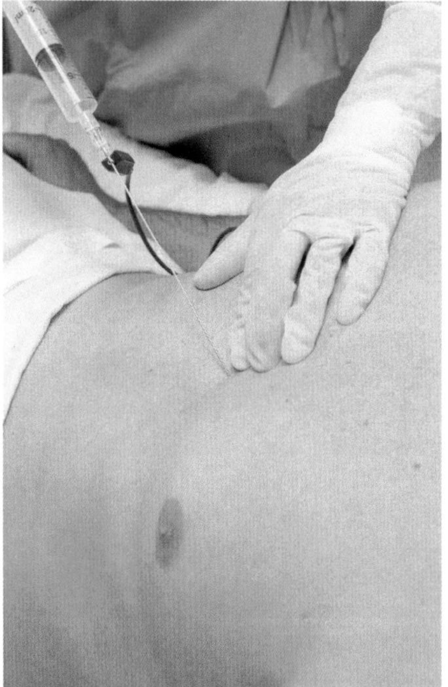

Fig. 21.16 ECG guided pericardiocentesis

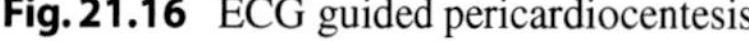

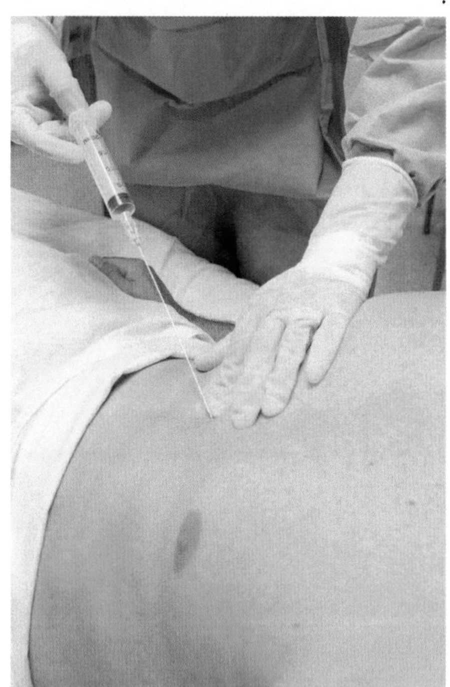

Fig. 21.17 Blind subxiphoid approach for pericardiocentesis

pericardiocentesis had a much higher complication rates and suboptimal results [18]. Callahan's group performed 132 consecutive pericardiocentesis procedures in 117 patients. The subcostal approach was used in 25 % and chest wall puncture (majority in anterior axillary fifth–seventh intercostal) was used in 64 % of patients. They used echocardiogram to choose site that is closest to the skin where the needle track will most effectively avoid any vital structures, but the actual procedure was done without continuous echocardiographic visualization. Callahan's group had no deaths, one pneumothorax, and only three minor complications [19].

21.10 Summary

Cardiac tamponade is a clinical diagnosis. Once tamponade is suspected, if drainage is indicated, it is best done in elective or semi-elective fashion if possible. Cardiac echography is the standard of care for guiding the procedure. However, if the cardiac tamponade is life-threatening and imaging modalities are not available, the techniques are described for safe non-image-guided drainage of the pericardial space. Cardiac tamponade is a rare emergency that quickly leads to cardiac arrest and requires prompt clinical diagnosis and intervention.

Special Acknowledgments Fred Carpenter and FRC Photography for all of the photographs included in this chapter.

Jose Ortiz, MD, for providing the ultrasound images included in this chapter.

References

1. Roy CL, Minor MA, Brookhart MA, Chourdhry NK. Does this patient with a pericardial effusion have cardiac tamponade? JAMA. 2007;297:1810–8.
2. Maisch B, Seferovic PM, Ristic AD, Erbel R, Rienmuller R, Adler Y, et al. Guidelines on the diagnosis and management of pericardial diseases executive summary; the task force of the diagnosis and management of pericardial diseases of the European society of cardiology. Eur Heart J. 2004;25:587–610.
3. Gandhi S, Schneider A, Mohiuddin S, Han H, Patel AR, Pandian NG, et al. Has the clinical presentation and clinician's index of suspicion of cardiac tamponade changed over the past decade? Echocardiography. 2008;25:237–41.
4. Guberman BA, Fowler NO, Engel PJ, Gueron M, Allen JM. Cardiac tamponade in medical patients. Circulation. 1981;64:633–40.
5. Beck CS. Two cardiac compression triads. JAMA. 1935;104:714–6.
6. Beck CS, Cushing EH. Circulatory stasis of intrapericardial origin; the clinical and surgical aspects of the pick syndrome. JAMA. 1934;102:1543–9.
7. Wilson RF, Bassett JS. Penetrating wounds of the pericardium or its contents. JAMA. 1966;195:105–10.
8. Synovitz CK, Brown EJ. Pericardiocentesis. In: Tintinalli JE, editor. Tintinalli's emergency medicine: a comprehensive study guide. 7th ed. New York, NY: McGraw-Hill; 2011.
9. Spodick DH. Acute cardiac tamponade. N Engl J Med. 2003;349:684–90.
10. Kilpatrick ZM, Chapman CB. On pericardiocentesis. Am J Cardiol. 1965;16:722–8.
11. Mallin MP, Butts C. Emergency cardiac ultrasound: evaluation for pericardial effusion and cardiac activity. In: Adams JG, editor. Emergency medicine. Philadelphia: Saunders; 2013. p. 43–9.
12. American College of Surgeons. ATLS: advanced trauma life support for doctors (student course manual). 9th ed. Chicago, IL: American College of Surgeons; 2012.
13. Sagrista-Sauleda J, Merce J, Permanyer-Miralda G, Soler-Soler J. Clinical clues to the causes of large pericardial effusion. Am J Med. 2000;109:95–101.
14. Fitch MT, Nicks BA, Pariyadath M, McGinnis HD, Manthey DE. Emergency pericardiocentesis. N Engl J Med. 2012;366:e17.
15. Reardon R. Ultrasound in trauma—the FAST exam: focused assessment with sonography in trauma. In: Hoffmann B, editor. Ultrasound guide for emergency physicians: an introduction. updated 2008 [cited 2014 June 23]. Available from: http://www.sonoguide.com/FAST.html.
16. Martin RP, Rakowski H, French J, Popp RL. Localization of pericardial effusion with wide angle phased array echocardiography. Am J Cardiol. 1978;42:904–12.
17. Callahan JA, Seward JB. Pericardiocentesis guided by two-dimensional echocardiography. Echocardiography. 1997;14:497–504.
18. Bastian A, MeiBner A, Lins M, Siegel EG, Moller F, Simon R. Pericardiocentesis: differential aspects of a common procedure. Intensive Care Med. 2000;26:572–6.
19. Callahan JA, Seward JB, Nishimura RA, Miller FA, Reeder GS, Shub C, et al. Two-dimensional echocardiographically guided pericardiocentesis: experience in 117 consecutive patients. Am J Cardiol. 1985;55:476–9.

Part V

Neurological Procedures

22 Intracranial Pressure Monitoring

Danny Lizano and Rani Nasser

22.1 Introduction

Intracranial hypertension (IC-HTN) is a common neurologic complication in critically ill patients as it is the common pathway in the presentation of many neurologic and non-neurologic disorders [1]. Normal intracranial pressure (ICP) is 10–15 mmHg in the adult patient. ICH is an important predictive factor that affects patient mortality [2, 3]. Intractable IC-HTN (persistently above 20–25 mmHg) can lead to death or severe neurologic damage by either reducing cerebral perfusion pressure (CPP) thus causing cerebral ischemia or by physically compressing the brain or other vital structures. Rapid identification of elevated ICP is needed in order to intervene appropriately to avoid the aforementioned negative effects of elevated ICP. ICP monitoring provides this important data for patients with intracranial hypertension or at an increased risk of high ICP, which can guide treatment. Treatments such as hyperosmolar therapy may be titrated on the basis of ICP. Moreover, the pattern as well as response to certain therapies helps provide clinicians insight into prognostication.

Intracranial pressure measurements were first performed by Guillaume and Janny in 1951 [4]. In 1960, Lundberg reported the first continuous monitoring of ICP using an intraventricular catheter in a series of 130 patients [5]. These landmark advances in neurological medicine gave clinicians a vital tool to care for patients with elevated ICP or the potential to develop elevated ICP. ICP monitoring is now a standard procedure for the management of various etiologies, head trauma being the most common and well described. Given the importance of this potentially lifesaving procedure, which was initially only placed by neurosurgeons, the demand for ICP monitor placement has exceeded the supply of surgeons in some institutions. Given this need, non-neurosurgeons including intensivists and Advanced Practice Providers (i.e., physician assistants and nurse practitioners) have shown to be appropriate candidates to place these monitors [6–8]. With appropriate training, placement of ICP monitors by Advanced Practice Providers (APPs) have the same complication rate of neurosurgeons, thus being a viable option for institutions [8]. This may provide a higher standard of care to institutions in which access to neurosurgeons is limited.

D. Lizano, MSHS, PA-C, FCCM (✉)
Division of Critical Care Medicine, Department of Medicine, Montefiore Medical Center, Bronx, NY, USA
e-mail: dlizanopa@gmail.com

R. Nasser, MD
Department of Neurosurgery, Montefiore Medical Center, Albert Einstein College of Medicine, Bronx, NY, USA
e-mail: Rani.nasser@gmail.com

D.A. Taylor et al. (eds.), *Interventional Critical Care*, DOI 10.1007/978-3-319-25286-5_22

22.2 Indications

In the setting of severe brain injury, regardless of the etiology, the patient will often have a poor neurologic exam and require mechanical ventilation. For patients that fall into this category, the neurologic exam may not be a reliable indicator of ongoing brain injury secondary to intractable ICP. Patients on mechanical ventilation are oftentimes started on sedation (usually short acting) for ventilator synchrony. In other scenarios for neuroprotective reasons, a patient may be started on sedatives and paralytics, foregoing a neurologic exam all together for long periods of time [9]. For this reason, any comatose patient (even if medically induced) with any pathology that can cause IC-HTN requires ICP monitoring. ICP monitoring can better characterize the nature of intracranial hypertension. These are best characterized by Lundberg waves [10]. The P1 (percussion wave) represents arterial pulsation during the ICP waveform. The P2 wave (tidal wave) is representative of intracranial compliance. The P3 wave (dicrotic wave) is seen during aortic valve closure (Fig. 22.1). Interpreting these waves may give the clinician insight into the patterns of pressure as well as the integrity of the ICP monitoring system. Moreover, if telemetric transduction is not possible, ICPs may be measured manually if an external ventricular drain is placed. The fluid column may be raised at the level of the external auditory meatus to characterize a manual pressure reading.

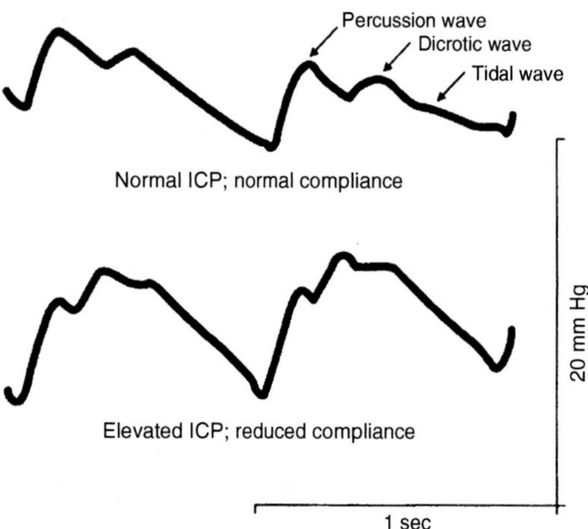

Fig. 22.1 Intracranial pressure waveform in conditions of normal (*top*) and abnormal (*bottom*) intracranial compliance. Reprinted with permission from Elsevier [11]

While considering whether a patient is a candidate for ICP monitoring, the clinician must also consider the type of ICP monitor to place. The most obvious difference between monitors is the ability to evacuate CSF in addition to measuring ICP which offers a therapeutic benefit if needed. ICP monitors such as the Codman® or Camino® systems which are placed below the dura into the cerebral parenchyma do not allow for CSF drainage. These types of catheters are some of the most accurate ways of measuring ICP compared to monitors placed in the subarachnoid, subdural, or epidural space [12]. External ventricular drainage (EVD) systems contain a catheter that goes through the frontal cortex into the ventricular system and allows for the measurement of ICP as well as diversion of CSF. Although being the most invasive of ICP monitors, EVDs are still considered the gold standard for ICP measurement [13–14]. This treatment modality is required in patients with hydrocephalus, large amounts of intraventricular blood, and IC-HTN, which would benefit from CSF evacuation. The benefits of placement must be weighed against its greater risk of bleeding and injury to the brain.

The most common indication for the placement of an ICP monitor would be patients with traumatic brain injury (TBI). Any patient who presents with a closed head injury (as evidenced by an abnormal head CT) with a Glasgow Coma Scale (GCS) score of 8 T or below requires the placement of an ICP monitoring device [12, 15]. In addition, patients with a normal head CT with two or more of the following risk factors require continuous ICP monitoring: age > 40, systolic blood pressure (SBP) <90, decerebrate or decorticate posturing on motor exam (unilateral or bilateral). Those with a higher GCS score who do not require sedation and have a reliable and stable neurologic exam generally do not require placement of an ICP monitor [15]. It would be reasonable to follow the patient closely without continuous ICP monitoring in the aforementioned scenario. This is often complicated in pediatric scenarios where the child is too young or developmentally delayed. In these circumstances, following a neurologic exam becomes challenging, and the need for invasive pressure monitoring may be needed to monitor ICPs.

Other common indications for placement of ICP monitors include intracranial hemorrhages such as subarachnoid hemorrhage (SAH) with intraventricular blood and acute hydrocephalus. It is also indicated in SAH patients with no radiographic signs of hydrocephalus but with significant amount of intraventricular blood, as they are at such a high risk of developing hydrocephalus. In patients with Hunt and Hess Grade 3 or greater SAH without obvious hydrocephalus may also benefit from prophylactic ICP monitoring (EVDs in particular). Intracranial hemorrhages, specifically intraventricular hemorrhages, also require the placement of ICP monitors, for similar reasons as SAHs.

Large ischemic hemispheric strokes are not indications for ICP monitoring. The deteriorating neurologic exam of these patients is usually due to the displacement of midline structures such as the thalamus and the brain stem than of a mechanism of globally increased ICP; therefore ICP monitoring will be of little benefit [16]. On the other hand, ischemic cerebellar strokes with postinfarction edema causing obstructive hydrocephalus is an indication for the placement of an ICP monitor. Specifically an EVD would be most appropriate in this situation. However, this should be quickly followed by a decompressive hemicraniectomy. There is a theoretical risk of upward herniation in circumstances where CSF diversion causes the cerebellum to herniate superiorly towards the tentorium.

Cerebral edema is the leading cause of death in patients with fulminant hepatic failure. Cerebral edema occurs in up to 80 % of patients with patients presenting with Grade 4 hepatic encephalopathy [17]. As a result it is recommended to place an ICP monitor to this group of patients as it can help guide treatment as well as help allocate organs to patients with better neurologic prognosis [18] (please refer to Table 22.1 for a complete list of indications for ICP monitoring).

Table 22.1 ICP insertion: indications and contraindications

Indications	Contraindications
Common	*Relative*
Traumatic brain injury with GCS < 8 (or >8 if on sedation)	Coagulopathy
Subarachnoid hemorrhage	Known bleeding disorder
Intracranial hemorrhage (ICH)	Anticoagulation therapy
Hydrocephalus	Platelet inhibitor use
Fulminant hepatic failure	Scalp infection
Space occupying lesions: epidural and subdural hematomas, tumors, abscesses	Lack of specialized personnel
Uncommon	Collapsed cerebral ventricles (for EVD)
Reye syndrome	CNS infections
Hypertensive crisis with encephalopathy	Severe midline shift causing displacement of ventricle
Lead ingestion with encephalopathy	
Meningitis/encephalitis leading to malapsorption of CSF	

22.3 Contraindications

There are few contraindications for ICP monitoring. Coagulopathy must be corrected before an attempt at placement of ICP monitor, as to limit iatrogenic intracerebral bleeding from the procedure. The recommended coagulation profile should be as follows:

- Platelets >100,000/mcl.
- INR <1.5.
- PT and PTT < 1.5 times normal.
- Platelet inhibition with antiplatelet agents such as aspirin/clopidogrel or from uremia must be also be ruled out.

Patients with thrombocytopenia must be transfused to a goal platelet count of greater than 100,000/mcl. In patients unresponsive to platelet therapy, the clinician can consider the infusion of platelets during the procedure to minimize bleeding. In the setting of platelet dysfunction from

Aspirin (ASA), it is recommended to transfuse 1–2 units of platelets, preferably during the procedure. Patients on antiplatelet agents such as clopidogrel that cannot be reversed with platelet transfusion, the risk of placing such a drain must be weighed against its potential benefits. For other causes of platelet dysfunction such as uremia (as noted by a high BUN) or alcohol abuse, the injection of DDAVP 0.3 mcg/kg before the procedure is reasonable.

Patients with elevated international normalized ratio (INR) (>1.5) should be corrected with the transfusion of fresh frozen plasma (FFP), if rapid correction is necessary. Depending on the initial INR, FFP should be given based on the patients weight given more units of FFP if the initial INR is higher, to a goal of <1.5 [19–21]. The following is a potential guideline the clinician may refer to based on the initial INR [19]:

- INR 1.6–1.9: 10–15 ml/kg
- INR 2–3: 21 ml/kg
- INR 3–4: 29 ml/kg
- INR 4–5: 36 ml/kg
- INR 5–6: 43 ml/kg
- INR 6 or greater: 50 ml/kg

The effect of FFP usually lasts for 2–6 h, so it is best to perform the procedure within that time frame, preferably within 2 h. The clinician must also be aware of the possible side effects of FFP transfusion. The most common is fluid overload, especially in patients who have a significant cardiac history with a predisposition to heart failure. Transfusion related acute lung injury (TRALI) has also been identified as a complication of FFP transfusion [22]. In patients whom transfusion of FFP may be problematic given the volume load, four-factor prothrombin complex concentrate (Kcentra by CSL Behring LLC) may be given to temporarily reverse the effect of Coumadin [23–25].

- INR 2–<4: 25 units/kg, not to exceed 2500 units
- INR 4–6: 35 units/kg, not to exceed 3500 units
- INR >6: 50 units/kg, not to exceed 5000 units

The injection of 5–10 mg IV or PO of vitamin K is also prudent to provide long-term reversal of coagulopathy from Coumadin (SC or IM routes have variable absorption). Vitamin K does not take effect until approximately 6 h after the dose is given.

Recombinant activated factor VIIa (rFVIIa, NovoSeven, Novo Nordis A/S, Bagsvaerd, Denmark) given as a 40 mcg/kg or 2.4 mg IV injection can immediately correct coagulopathy due to warfarin use, liver failure, or patients unresponsive to FFP [26, 27]. It has been shown to safely expedite the emergent placement of intracranial monitors in cases where it would be a lifesaving procedure [28].

In the setting of a large intracranial hemorrhage where the etiology of the bleeding has not been identified, the clinician must be careful not to place the catheter in the hemorrhagic collection to avoid possible disruption or rupture of an underlying mass, aneurysm, or arteriovenous malformation [28]. Placement of an ICP monitor within a blood clot will result in unreliable values as well as clot the system in the case of an EVD, rendering the monitor/drain ineffective. In instances where there is IC-HTN and the ventricles are collapsed, the benefit of placing an EVD will not outweigh its risk and therefore is not recommended. In circumstances with slit ventricles, using an intraparenchymal intracranial pressure monitor may be more optimal, as there is no immediate need for CSF diversion.

22.4 Complications

After placing an ICP monitor or EVD, a CT scan of the head should be obtained to rule out some complications that can occur during placement (Table 22.2). Malposition and malfunctioning of ICP monitors or EVDs are the most common complications associated with this procedure

Table 22.2 Complications

Common	Uncommon
Malpositioning	Infection
Erroneous values	Intracerebral hemorrhage
Erroneous zeroing	Overdrainage of CSF causing subdural hematoma
	Air leakage in to ventricle or subarachnoid space

with and incidence of 12–17 % versus 7–22 %, respectively [29, 30]. Malposition is most commonly seen with intraventricular devices, where the catheter either misses the ventricle or is inserted too far into the ventricle. Malfunctioning occurs in different ways for different types of monitors. If too much CSF is drained, the ventricles collapse around the EVD, blocking the catheter. Parenchymal catheters can have a major problem of a drifting zero point as most cannot be re-zeroed like EVDs, resulting in greater inaccuracy with length of monitoring. This inaccuracy can lead to treatment decisions based on inaccurate clinical data. Catheters can also be dislodged or damaged making the monitor obsolete.

A CT scan may also diagnose hemorrhagic complications such as intraparenchymal, subdural, and, in the case of EVDs, intraventricular bleeding. Recent studies have shown that catheter-related hemorrhages are more common for EVDs versus intraparenchymal monitors with the range being 1–33 % versus <1–2.8 %, with the risk of significant hematoma requiring surgical evacuation being 0.5 % [12, 31, 32]. If a small hemorrhage is found, serial CT scans of the head should be performed to make sure the blood clot does not expand. Whenever evidence of a large or expanding hemorrhage is identified, the device should be removed without delay.

Infection, such as local skin infection, osteomyelitis, meningitis, ventriculitis, encephalitis, can occur with the use of ICP monitors. The reported infection rates range from 0 to 27 % [32, 33]. Factors that have been found to increase the risk of infection in ICP monitors are increased duration of monitoring, steroid use, and associated trauma patients with open depressed fractures. Symptoms suggestive of infection should prompt CSF analysis for cell count and culture along with antibiotic therapy, as appropriate. Practices that can help reduce the incidence of infection are the use of aseptic technique during placement, limiting manipulation of ICP monitors for sampling or flushing (if using an EVD), and administration of antibiotics during placement. Continuing prophylactic antibiotics for ICP monitors remains a controversial topic (please refer to your specific institutional protocol) [34]. The routine removal and replacement of ICP monitors after 5 days is not recommended as it has not shown to reduce infection rates and actually increases the risk of infection [35].

22.5 Procedure

Before starting this procedure, informed consent from the patient or appropriate surrogate is paramount. However, given the acuity of neurological illness, it may be necessary to obtain administrative consent.

22.5.1 Anesthesia

Care must be taken to avoid any movement by the patient during this procedure, be it voluntary or involuntary. Adequate sedation and analgesia must be given in order to achieve this goal. Depending on the patient's neurologic status before the procedure, they may or may not be intubated. The decision must be made in order to prophylactically intubate the patient for airway protection prior to starting the procedure. This may be a safer option for patients with an already borderline neurologic exam as they will receive medications that can further alter their consciousness, thus compromising their airway. For those who are already in a comatose state, the clinician must avoid involuntary movements from the patient. A GABA receptor agonist should suffice in preventing these movements, typically a bolus of propofol 50–100 mg IV can be used. Alternatively a midazolam 2–4 mg bolus can be given for this purpose. It should be reminded that propofol does have an advantage of being shorter acting as compared to benzodiazepines such as midazolam. The use of any sedative can also have some cardiovascular effects such as hypotension and bradycardia (more common with propofol). The clinician must be aware of this and have fluids easily accessible as well as a vasopressor (ie., Neo-Synephrine or norepinephrine) if required for resuscitation. The skin incision is the most painful part of ICP placement, and usually a subcutaneous inoculation of local anesthetic around the incision site and extending down to the periosteum should suffice. If a tunneling technique is to be used then the local anesthetic should be injected along this area as well. If further analgesia is required, then a fentanyl 25–50 mcg bolus can be given.

If the ICP monitor will be placed on a patient who is conscious and adequately protecting their airway and can cooperate with the practitioner, then it would be reasonable to proceed with conscious sedation. Please refer to your institution's policies and guidelines regarding providing conscious sedation. In general, care must be taken to provide supplemental oxygen via a facemask, keeping a close observation of the patient's oxygenation and breathing patterns. If at any point, the patient's respiratory status is compromised, the procedure should be suspended, and the airway should be protected via endotracheal intubation (assuming that the benefits of ICP monitor placement outweigh the risk of intubation).

22.5.2 Materials

A typical intracranial access kit will have the following components: (Fig. 22.2)

A. Shaver
B. Drape
C. Ruler
D. Marker
E. Lidocaine
F. Sutures
G. Small sterile towel
H. Large sterile towel
I. Lidocaine
J. Ruler
K. Marker

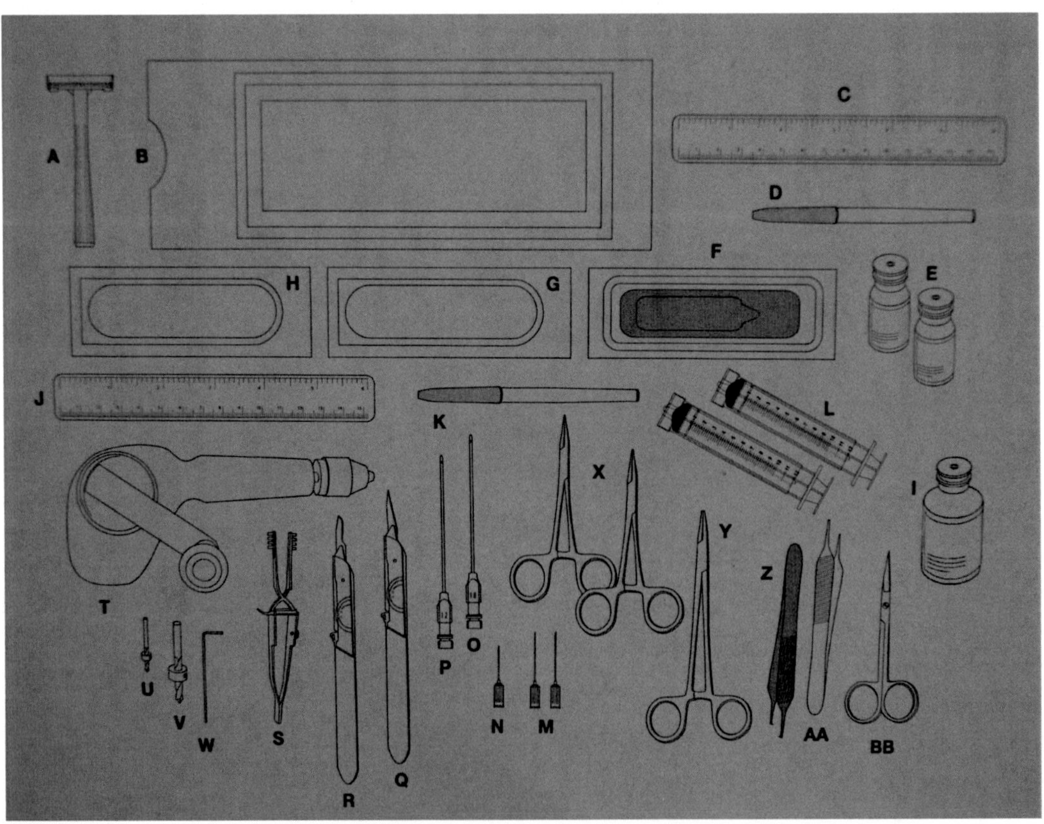

Fig. 22.2 Materials include in a typical cranial access kit

L. 10 ml syringe × 2
M. Small angiocatheter
N. Large angiocatheter
O. Small spinal needle
P. Large spinal needle
Q. 11 blade
R. 15 blade
S. Retractor
T. Drill
U. Small drill bit
V. Drill bit
W. Hex key
X. Hemostat
Y. Needle Driver
Z. Toothed forceps
AA. Toothless forceps
BB. Suture scissors

22.5.3 Insertion Techniques

22.5.3.1 Tunneled Intraparenchymal ICP Monitor (Codman®)

Additional items needed:

- Codman® box with cables and ICP wire
- Tunneling device
- Sterile saline
- Sterile dressing

1. Keep the head elevated at 30° with the neck straight. This will ensure that the venous drainage from the head will help naturally lower ICPs.
2. Identify Kocher's point (located 10 cm from the glabella and 3 cm from the midline). This can be confirmed by drawing an intersection from the mid-pupillary line as well as a line 1 cm anterior to the coronal suture. This is similar to the site of an external ventricular drain (Fig. 22.3). This site can be converted from an ICP monitor to an EVD if CSF diversion is desired.
3. Shave and prep the area thoroughly.
4. Incise the skin (0.5–1 cm length) down to the pericranium over Kocher's point and place a small self-retaining retractor.
5. Drill the bone through the outer cortical layer, inner cancellous layer, and inner table.
6. Create a tunnel before opening the dura. Within the sterile field at an appropriate location away from Kocher's point, make skin incision towards the direction of Kocher's point.
7. Use the tunneling device with the stylet in to create the tunnel towards Kocher's

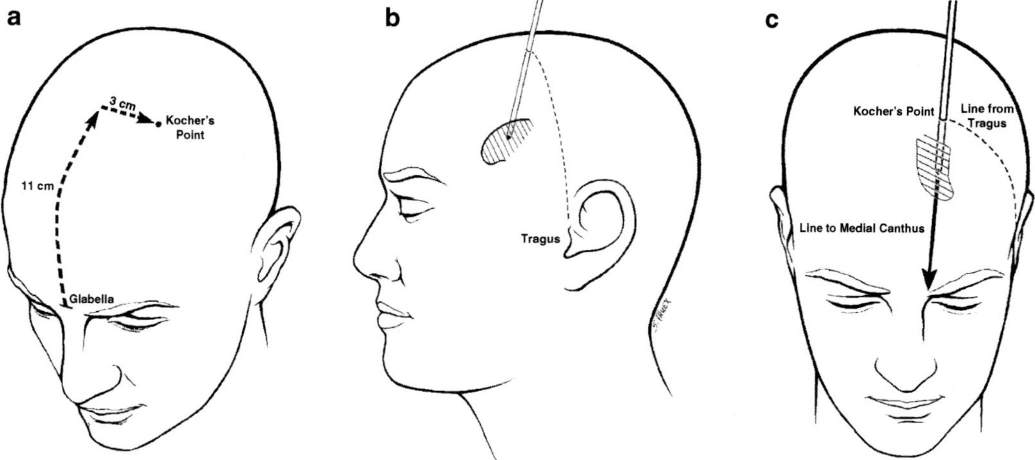

Fig. 22.3 Depiction of ideal ICP monitor placement at Kocher's point: (1–2 cm anterior to the coronal suture in mid-pupillary line or 11 cm posterior from the glabella and 3 cm lateral from midline). The ideal trajectory is toward the ipsilateral medial canthus with the catheter maintained in the same coronal plane as the tragus. Reprinted with permission from Springer [28]

point. Then remove the stylet, leaving the sheath in place. Feed the ICP catheter from the incision site and through the sheath. Remove the sheath.

8. Zero the device by handing the distal portion of the wire to the bedside nurse/assistant who will connect this to the cable of the Codman box. Make sure to maintain sterility of the proximal portion during this step. Place the tip of the ICP catheter under sterile saline. The assistant should then turn on the Codman box and select the calibrate screen. Record the calibration number and label it on the box.
9. Open the dura with a spinal needle or number 11 blade.
10. Place the ICP monitor 1–1.5 cm deep from the dura and confirm placement with a waveform or an ICP number.
11. Close the skin incision at Kocher's point in standard fashion. Place a "U-stitch" around the catheter where it exits the skin. For added security, create a redundant loop of wire and anchor it to the skin with suture.
12. Make sure to confirm a waveform at the end of the procedure.
13. Removal of this device is accomplished by pulling the catheter from the exit site and closing the tunnel site with a stitch.

22.5.3.2 Intraparenchymal ICP Bolt (Camino®)

Additional items needed:

- Camino® box with cables, including drill bit specific to the kit.
- Petroleum gauze.

1. Follow the steps 1–4 mentioned previously (may consider using a site slightly anterior to Kocher's point, leaving the option for placing and EVD with minimal complications).
2. Attach drill bit that is included in the monitoring device kit to be inserted. Cranial access kits include additional drill bits, which will create an inappropriate burr hole that is not compatible with the bolt.
3. Drill the bone through the outer cortical layer, inner cancellous layer, and inner table.
4. Open the dura with a spinal needle or number 11 blade.
5. Pass ICP catheter through the bolt prior to insertion to measure the depth to which the catheter is to be inserted. Keep note of the catheter markings from the extracranial portion of the catheter (as it exits the bolt) as this will be the depth you will be inserting the catheter when bolt is in place. For adults, this distance is usually 6.25 cm from the top of the cap which is then pulled back to around 6 cm.
6. Place the bolt into the burr hole perpendicular to the scull. Screw in the bolt clockwise with your hand to finger tight. The bolt can enter the skull at different depths. This is especially true for different age group. A spacer can be used to offset the Camino® bolt (to keep the distance consistent).
   a. Neonates: 2–3 mm spacer
   b. Pediatrics: 3–5 mm spacer
   c. Adults: 0.5–1 cm spacer
7. Place stylet into the bolt before zeroing the ICP monitor to ensure the dura has been opened and then remove. The ICP catheter must be zeroed to ambient air prior to insertion.
8. Pass the ICP catheter through the bolt, securing it at the desired depth by tightening the compression cap (until snug). Gently pull back on the ICP catheter to make sure it is secured.
9. Suture the skin around the bolt using a "U-Stitch". Close any remaining portion of the skin incision with simple interrupted stitches.
10. Wrap the base of the bolt with petroleum gauze.
11. For added security, create a redundant loop of the ICP catheter and anchor it to the skin with suture.

22.6 Pearls

- Preferable to place ICP monitor over region of suspected increased pressure.
- Place ICP monitor with consideration for possible surgical intervention.

  - Try to avoid the region of an intraparenchymal hemorrhage, stroke, or underlying mass.
- Hold the drill perpendicular to the skull to prevent slipping of drill while drilling. Be careful not to use too much pressure to avoid inadvertently drilling too deep and puncturing the dura.
- It is important to re-zero ICP monitor (under sterile saline) if it does not correlate with the arterial line (some devices are not capable of re-zeroing after the procedure is finished).
- If an error occurs during initial calibration:
  - Reset the Codman box and make sure all connections are secure.
  - If resetting does not work, then change the box/cable.
  - Inspect for a defect in the ICP wire. Retunnel another wire if necessary.
- Prophylactic antibiotic coverage for the ICP monitor may prevent cerebritis.
- Confirmatory imaging may be acquired stereotactically in the event of external drain conversion for CSF diversion.
- Children with a fontanel may serve as a natural ICP monitor. Can also use this as a site for monitor placement so that drilling through the skull can be avoided.

22.7 Pitfalls

- Going too deep with the ICP monitor may cause hemorrhage.
- Caution introducing bone fragments into the parenchyma during burr hole drilling.
- Constant surveillance of waveform to ensure accuracy and consistency of ICP monitor. Following inaccurate information may lead to treatment errors.

22.8 Conclusion

ICP monitoring has proven to be effective and is the standard technique for accessing ICP in patients with various etiologies of brain injury. Given the demand for placement of ICP monitors, non-neurosurgeons including intensivists, physician assistants, and nurse practitioners have been shown to place these monitors at the bedside with similar results as neurosurgeons. These clinicians must remain familiar with the technical aspects of placing these monitoring devices. If performed correctly, these devices can be placed efficiently and safely in the ICU. This provides the severely brain injured patient the appropriate care they need in a timely fashion.

References

1. Miller JD, Butterworth JF, Gudeman SK, et al. Further experience in the management of severe head injury. J Neurosurg. 1981;54(3):289–99.
2. Stocchetti N, Penny KI, Dearden M, et al. Intensive care management of head-injured patients in Europe: a survey from the European brain injury consortium. Intensive Care Med. 2001;27:400–6.
3. Vik A, Nag T, Fredriksli OA, et al. Relationship of "dose" of intracranial hypertension to outcome in severe traumatic brain injury. J Neurosurg. 2008;109:678–84.
4. Guillaume J, Janny P. Monometrie intracranienne continue: Interet de la methode et premiers resultats. Rev Neurol (Paris). 1951;84:131–42.
5. Lundberg N. Continuous recording and control of ventricular fluid pressure in neurosurgical practice. Acta Psychiatr Scand Suppl. 1960;149:1–193.
6. Barber M, Helmer S, Morgan J, et al. Placement of intracranial pressure monitors by non-neurosurgeons: excellent outcomes can be achieved. J Trauma Acute Care Surg. 2012;73(3):558–63.
7. Ekeh A, Ilyas S, Saxe J, et al. Successful placement of intracranial pressure monitors by trauma surgeons. J Trauma Acute Care Surg. 2013;76(2):286–91.
8. Young PJ, Bowling WM. Midlevel practitioners can safely place intracranial pressure monitors. J Trauma Acute Care Surg. 2012;73(2):431–4.
9. Eisenber HM, Frankowski RF, Contant CF, et al. High-dose barbiturate control of elevated intracranial pressure in patients with severe head injury. J Neurosurg. 1988;69:15–23.
10. Lescot T, Naccache L, Bonnet MP, et al. The relationship of intracranial pressure Lundberg waves to electroencephalograph fluctuations in patients with severe head trauma. Acta Neurochir (Wien). 2005;147(2):125–9. discussion 129.
11. Chesnut RM, Marshall LF. Management of head injury. Treatment of abnormal intracranial pressure. Neurosurg Clin N Am. 1991;2(2):267–84.
12. Polvlisock JT, Bullock R. Guidelines for the management of severe head injury 3rd edition. Brain Trauma Foundation. J Neurotrauma. 2007;24 Suppl 1:37–54.
13. Miller JD. Measuring ICP, in patients—its value now and in the future. In: Hoff JT, Betz AL, editors. Intracranial pressure. Berlin: Springer; 1989. p. 5–15.

14. Wartenberg KE, Schmidt JM, Mayer SA. Multimodality monitoring in neurocritical care. Crit Care Clin. 2007;23(3):507–38.
15. Narayan RK, Kishore PR, Becker DP, et al. Intracranial pressure: to monitor or not to monitor? A review of our experience with severe head injury. J Neurosurg. 1982;56:650–9.
16. Wijdicks EF, Sheth KN, Carter B, et al. Recommendations for the management of cerebral and cerebellar infarction with swelling. Stroke. 2014;45:1222–38.
17. Keays RT, Alexander GJ, Williams R. The safety and value of extradural intracranial pressure monitors in fulminant hepatic failure. J Hepatol. 1993;18:205–9.
18. Vaquero J, Fontana RJ, Larson AM, et al. Complications and use of intracranial pressure monitoring in patients with acute liver failure and severe encephalopathy. Liver Transpl. 2005;11:1581–9.
19. Holland LL, Brooks JP. Toward rational fresh frozen plasma transfusion: the effect of plasma transfusion on coagulation test results. Am J Clin Pathol. 2006;126:133–9.
20. O'Shaughnessy DF, Atterbury C, Bolton Maggs P, et al. British Committee for standards in haematology, blood transfusion task force: guidelines for the use of fresh-frozen plasma, cryoprecipitate and cryosupernatant. Br J Haematol. 2004;126:11–28.
21. Chowdhury P, Saayman AG, Paulus U, Findlay GP, Collins PW. Efficacy of standard dose and 30 ml/kg fresh frozen plasma in correcting laboratory parameters of haemostasis in critically ill patients. Br J Haematol. 2004;125:69–73.
22. Kleinman S, Caulfield T, Chan P, et al. Toward an understanding of transfusion-related acute lung injury: statement of a consensus panel. Transfusion. 2004;44:1774–89.
23. Chapman SA, Irwin ED, Beal AL, et al. Prothrombin complex concentrate versus standard therapies for INR reversal in trauma patients receiving warfarin. Ann Pharmacother. 2011;45:869–75.
24. Ferreira J, DeLos Santos M. The clinical use of prothrombin complex concentrate. J Emerg Med. 2013;44(6):1201–20.
25. Van Aart L, Eijkhout HW, Kamphuis JS, et al. Individualized dosing regimen for prothrombin complex concentrate more effective than standard treatment in the reversal of oral anticoagulation therapy: an open, prospective randomized controlled trial. Thromb Res. 2006;118:313–20.
26. Shami VM, Caldwell SH, Hespenheide EE, et al. Recombinant activated factor VII for coagulopathy in fulminant hepatic failure compared to conventional therapy. Liver Transpl. 2003;9:138–43.
27. Park P, Fewel ME, Garton HJ, et al. Recombinant activated factor vii for the rapid correction of coagulopathy in nonhemophilic neurosurgical patients. Neurosurgery. 2003;53:34–8.
28. Stuart RM, Madden C, Lee A, et al. Intracranial monitoring. In: Frankel HL, DeBoisblanc BP, editors. Bedside procedures for the intensivist. New York: Springer; 2010. p. p307–22.
29. Gelabert-Gonzalez M, Ginesta-Galan V, Sernamito-Garcia R, et al. The camino intracranial pressure device in clinical practice. Assessment in 1000 cases. Acta Neurochir (Wien). 2006;148(4):435–41.
30. Karkala UK, Kim LJ, Chang SW, et al. Safety and accuracy of bedside external ventricular drain placement. Neurosurgery. 2008;63 Suppl 1:162–6.
31. Narayan RK, Kishore PR, Becker DP, et al. Intracranial pressure: to monitor or not to monitor? A review of our experience with severe head injury. J Neurosurg. 1982;56(5):650–9.
32. Bekar A, Dogan S, Abas S, et al. Risk factors and complication of ICP monitoring with a fiberoptic device. J Clin Neurosci. 2009;16:236–40.
33. Beer R, Lackner P, Pfausler B, et al. Nosocomial ventriculitis and meningitis in neurocritical care patients. J Neurol. 2008;255:1617–24.
34. Prabhu VC, Kaufman HH, Voelker JL, et al. Prophylactic antibiotics with intracranial pressure monitors and external ventricular drains: a review of the evidence. Surg Neurol. 1999;52:226–37.
35. Arabi Y, Memish ZA, Balkhy HH, et al. Ventriculostomy-associated infections: incidence and risk factors. Am J Infect Control. 2005;33(3):137–43.

Extraventricular Drains and Ventriculostomy

23

Senthil Radhakrishnan and Eric Butler

An external ventricular drain (EVD), as the name implies, is a system used to drain cerebrospinal fluid (CSF) from the ventricles of the brain into an external collection chamber via a sterile closed system. The system has four distinct parts: the ventricular catheter, the intracranial pressure (ICP) transducer, the manometer, and the drainage bag.

Also referred to as the extraventricular drain or ventriculostomy, it allows the temporary drainage of CSF from the lateral ventricles of the brain and serves as a diagnostic tool to monitor ICP or a therapeutic tool to drain excess CSF and intraventricular hemorrhage (IVH) and reduce ICP in the preoperative, intraoperative, or postoperative setting. The system employs a combination of gravity and the ICP to serve its purpose.

A retrospective epidemiology study done in 2008 revealed that more than 24,000 EVDs are placed each year in the United States alone [1]. Even though it is one of the most commonly performed procedures in neurosurgery, it requires frequent revision. Another retrospective study revealed that approximately 23 % of all EVDs placed had to be revised after initial placement. The study revealed that only 6 % of EVDs were replaced due to improper initial placement. Catheter occlusion accounted for 8 %, while 7 % were due to accidental removal or disruption of the EVD [2].

23.1 Cerebrospinal Fluid and the Ventricles

The human ventricular system is composed of four CSF-filled spaces that are normally in communication with each other (Fig. 23.1). CSF flows from the two lateral ventricles located in the two cerebral hemispheres into the third ventricle that is located inferior to the lateral ventricles and in between the thalamus and hypothalamus through the foramen of Monro. From the third ventricle, flow is directly through the cerebral aqueduct of Sylvius into the fourth ventricle located in the brain stem and encased by the pons and medulla anteriorly and the cerebellum posteriorly. From the fourth ventricle, the CSF flows through the foramen of Magendie and Luschka into the central canal of the spinal cord. As the CSF flows into the central canal, some of the CSF flows into the cisterns of the subarachnoid space and around the dural venous sinuses and eventually reabsorbed into the venous system via arachnoid villi and restored back in to the blood circulation [3].

The two lateral ventricles are larger in volume when compared to the third and fourth ventricles. Each lateral ventricles can be anatomically divided

S. Radhakrishnan, MS, PA-C (✉) • E. Butler, MPAS, PA-C
Division of Neurosurgery, Duke University Medical Center, Durham, NC, USA
e-mail: Senthil.radhakrishnan@duke.edu; Eric.butler@duke.edu

D.A. Taylor et al. (eds.), *Interventional Critical Care*, DOI 10.1007/978-3-319-25286-5_23

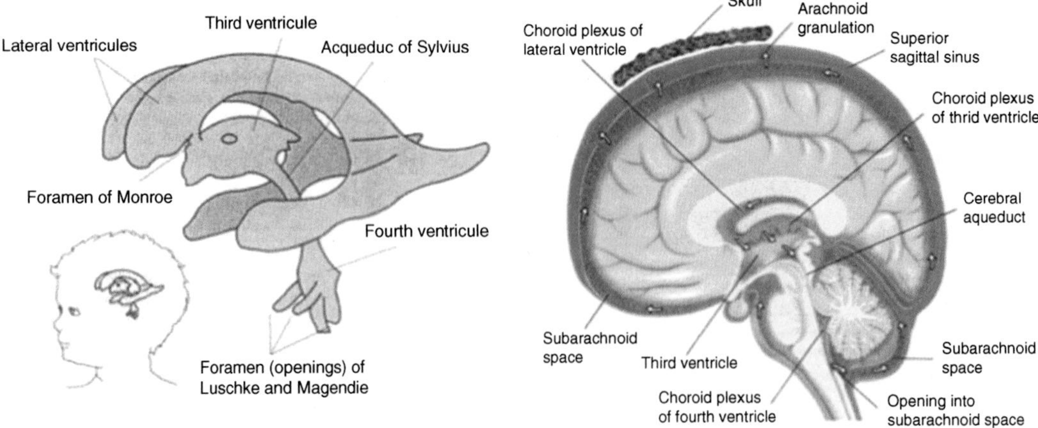

Fig. 23.1 Cerebral ventricular system

into a body, frontal horn (anterior), occipital horn (posterior), and temporal horn (inferior).

CSF is produced by the highly vascular and specialized choroid plexus located in the ventricles at a rate of approximately 20–25 ml/h averaging approximately 500 ml/day. The ventricles and subarachnoid space contain about 100–150 ml of CSF at any given time. CSF plays an important role in providing buoyancy to protect the brain and spinal cord from shock and trauma as well as maintaining a constant extracellular fluid chemical environment for neuronal activity, transport of essential nutrients, and acid–base regulation.

23.2 Intracranial Pressure

ICP is the pressure inside the cranium and is measured in the same unit as blood pressure: mmHg. The normal ICP in adults ranges <10–15 mmHg [4]. According to the Monro–Kellie doctrine, the pressure within the skull translates to the pressure within the brain tissue and CSF. Also since the volume within the cranium is anatomically fixed, the doctrine states that the sum of the pressures of the contents, namely, brain tissue, CSF, and blood, should remain constant at any given time. Hence in any pathological state, the increase in pressure in one of the components must be negated by a decrease in one or the other two components to keep the ICP normal [5].

Sustained elevation of ICP is associated with increased mortality and morbidity. Blood flow to the brain is affected by fluctuations in the ICP. Cerebral perfusion is dependent upon the mean arterial pressure (MAP) and the ICP. Cerebral perfusion pressure (CPP) = MAP − ICP. Regardless of where the pathology is, be it in the brain tissue or CSF or intracranial blood, the resultant increased ICP results in decreased CPP. When there is an increase in ICP, autoregulation raises systolic blood pressure (SBP), vasodilates intracranial blood vessels, and increases MAP. This autoregulation attempts to restore CPP but does not always do so perfectly. Autoregulation can only take place in a fixed range, and beyond this range, the small arterioles cannot make changes at systolic pressures outside of 60–160 mmHg [6].

When increases in ICP overwhelm the body's compensatory mechanisms, there is decreased cerebral blood flow. At critically low levels, alterations in neuroglial metabolism result in ischemia and eventually infarction of brain tissue. In the most serious of instances, this can lead to herniation and death [4, 7].

23.3 Indications for an External Ventricular Drain [3, 4, 8]

There are a myriad of conditions that can cause intracranial hypertension where placement of an EVD may be considered. Examples include space-occupying lesions, intracranial hemorrhage (ICH) secondary to trauma, vascular malformation or coagulopathy, infection of the central nervous system (CNS), and polytrauma requiring heavily sedating medications where monitoring of a patient's neurological examination is not possible. An ICP monitor, such as an EVD, is usually not warranted in a patient who can localize noxious stimuli or follow commands consistently. These patients can often be followed with serial and reproducible neurological examination. However, regardless of the mechanism of insult, the two most important inclusion criteria for insertion of an EVD are a Glasgow Coma Scale (GCS) ≤8 and either an abnormal CT brain or a normal CT brain with ≥2 of the following risk factors [4]:

Age >40 years.
SBP <90 mmHg.
Unilateral or bilateral decerebrate or decorticate posturing on motor exam.

Specific conditions that have been cited as the potential cause for placement of an EVD are as follows [3, 9]:

1. Subarachnoid hemorrhage (SAH) Hunt and Hess grade ≥3 due to rupture of any aneurysm or arteriovenous malformation (AVM), arteriovenous fistula (AVF), cavernous malformation, or trauma.
2. Intracranial mass lesions causing vasogenic and/or cytotoxic edema, midline shift, and/or signs of herniation.
3. Infection: meningitis, cerebral abscess, epidural abscess, subdural empyema, and cryptococcal.
4. Traumatic or atraumatic intracranial hemorrhage (ICH): epidural hematoma (EDH), subdural hematoma (SDH), intracerebral or intraparenchymal hemorrhage (ICH/IPH), hypertensive hemorrhage, and IVH.
5. Traumatic brain injury (TBI) including diffuse axonal shear injury (DAI) and contusions.
6. Penetrating injury: gunshot wounds and open skull fractures.
7. Hydrocephalus due to either increased CSF production (rare), obstruction of CSF flow pathway, or decreased reabsorption. EVD catheter placement usually is the same for either communicating hydrocephalus caused by poor reabsorption in the subarachnoid villi or noncommunicating hydrocephalus due to obstruction anywhere within the four ventricles. EVD placement may change if there is a trapped ventricle requiring selective placement to drain that ventricle or placement of two even up to three EVD catheters.
8. Chiari malformation causing obstruction of CSF outflow due to the downward displacement of the posterior fossa structures.
9. Idiopathic intracranial hypertension also known as benign intracranial hypertension or pseudotumor cerebri.
10. Elective intraoperative placement to facilitate brain relaxation/prevent tight brain or herniation of brain through craniotomy site. Note: CSF should be drained only after the dura is opened to prevent intraoperative rupture of aneurysm [4].

23.4 Contraindications for Placement of EVD

If there is a need to monitor intracranial pressures, other than a patient with a GCS ≥8 and or following commands with a reliable neurological exam to follow [4], the contraindications for an EVD placement are generally relative, meaning they can be modified or treated to make the situation more favorable.

1. Coagulopathy.
2. Anticoagulation.
3. Thrombocytopenia.
4. Active infection at or near potential insertion site on the scalp, over osteomyelitis in the cranial vault or trajectory traversing epidural abscess or subdural empyema.
5. Lack of facility and personnel to monitor the EVD.

Patients on anticoagulant or antiplatelet therapy pose an additional risk of procedure-related bleeding or expansion of an already existing intracranial hemorrhage. A good history, current coagulation panel, and proper reversal of these medications are crucial prior to insertion of an EVD. It is relatively easy to reverse the effect of warfarin with fresh frozen plasma (FFP), vitamin K, and prothrombin complex (PCC). Correcting the INR to ≤1.3 before insertion of EVD decreases risk of bleeding/expansion of intracranial bleed [10]. In contrast, while the new class of anticoagulants such as dabigatran (direct thrombin inhibitor), rivaroxaban, and apixaban (factor Xa inhibitors) are gaining popularity due to their anticoagulation properties with more reliable dose–response relationships without the need for blood-level monitoring [11], there is a lack of proven antidote for reliably reversing their effects in the event of an intracranial hemorrhage or prior to an EVD insertion [12].

Rapid reversal of anticoagulation prior to EVD insertion can be achieved by FFP or recombinant factor VIIa (rVIIa) or PCC. Situations requiring multiple doses of FFP may cause volume overload and take valuable time and critically delay the procedure. Due to its rapid reversal capacity, rVIIa has a propensity to cause increased thrombotic complications like myocardial infarction and venous thromboembolisms [12]. PCC is the newest arsenal to combat the effects of anticoagulants and is comprised of either three factors (factor II, IX, and X) or four factors (factor II, VII, IX, and X). These are being used more often for its rapid reversal properties and low-volume requirements preventing volume overload and reportedly being superior to FFP [13, 14].

Thrombocytopenia is a relative contraindication that can be corrected with platelet transfusion. The American Association of Hematology recommends a platelet count >100,000/μl prior to a neurosurgical procedure. Platelet count in patients who have received antiplatelet therapy such as aspirin and clopidogrel is irrelevant as the platelets are dysfunctional and are usually treated with a unit of platelets before neurosurgical procedure [15].

The table below matches the anticoagulant with its appropriate antidote.

Anticoagulant	Emergent reversal agents
Unfractionated heparin	Protamine sulfate (within 4 h)
Enoxaparin	Protamine sulfate (within 8 h), rVIIa
Fondaparinux	Consider rVIIa but no specific antidote
Lepirudin	Consider FFP and cryoprecipitate but no specific antidote
Argatroban	Consider FFP and cryoprecipitate but no specific antidote
Warfarin	FFP and vitamin K or PCC (3 or 4 factor)
Dabigatran	Limited data to consider FFP, rVIIa, and PCC. Dialysis may be needed
Rivaroxaban	PCC (3 or 4 factor), FFP, rVIIa
Apixaban	PCC (3 or 4 factor), FFP, rVIIa

Intraparenchymal fiberoptic monitors, subarachnoid bolts, and epidural sensors are sometimes used as less invasive monitoring systems for measuring intracranial pressures, but they cannot drain CSF. These are employed when an EVD is technically impossible or if the goal is just to measure ICP and there is no indication for therapeutic drainage of CSF.

23.5 Monitoring Intracranial Pressure Waveform

Even with the advent of modern less invasive microtransducers for ICP monitoring, the EVD with an external pressure transducer is still used to monitor ICP because they provide an added advantage as a conduit to egress CSF and thereby decrease ICP. In other words, an EVD can be both diagnostic and therapeutic. When an EVD is attached to an external pressure transducer, it can be used to obtain accurate ICP and this can be displayed as a waveform on the monitor. It is imperative to understand the basic component of ICP waveform.

Understanding ICP waveforms can help identify patients at risk for developing decreased cerebral perfusion due to increased ICP and decreased compliance of the brain which in turn aids in timely intervention [9]. The ICP waveform bears some correlation with the cardiac cycle and is a triphasic wave with three distinct peaks. From an ascending to descending amplitude they are P1, P2, and P3, where P1 is the tallest and P3 the shortest (Fig. 23.2). Any change in the amplitude from this norm is a reflection of changes in the CPP and compliance of the brain [16].

Also known as the "percussive" wave, the tallest first peak P1 is the result of arterial pressure transmitted from the choroid plexus. "Tidal" wave, the second peak P2, signifies brain compliance and the last peak P3 is referred to as the "dicrotic" wave and is the result of the aortic valve closure. As the ICP increases, the amplitudes of these waves increase, and if it goes unchecked, P2 may not only become taller than P1 but may also displace it (Fig. 23.3). Changes in waveform amplitudes, especially increase in P2, precede actual increase in ICP. Since ICP waveform correlate with arterial pressure waveforms, rise and fall of systemic blood pressure results in similar rise and fall in ICP [17].

Decrease in brain compliance also results in pathological waves that are best visualized when plotted against time and was originally described by Lundberg. Lundberg A waves are pathological and warrant immediate intervention. The "A" waves reflect acute and abrupt increase in ICP lasting approximately 5–10 min followed by a rapid decrease caused by early herniation of the brain. Lundberg B waves fall and rise intermittently at a frequency of 0.5–2 waves/min and are associated with an unstable ICP and are often associated with vasospasm in cerebral blood vessels [16].

23.6 EVD Insertion Sites

EVD insertion is a common bedside procedure performed based on a sound understanding of surface anatomy and relationship of anatomical landmarks. Even though it is a free-hand bedside

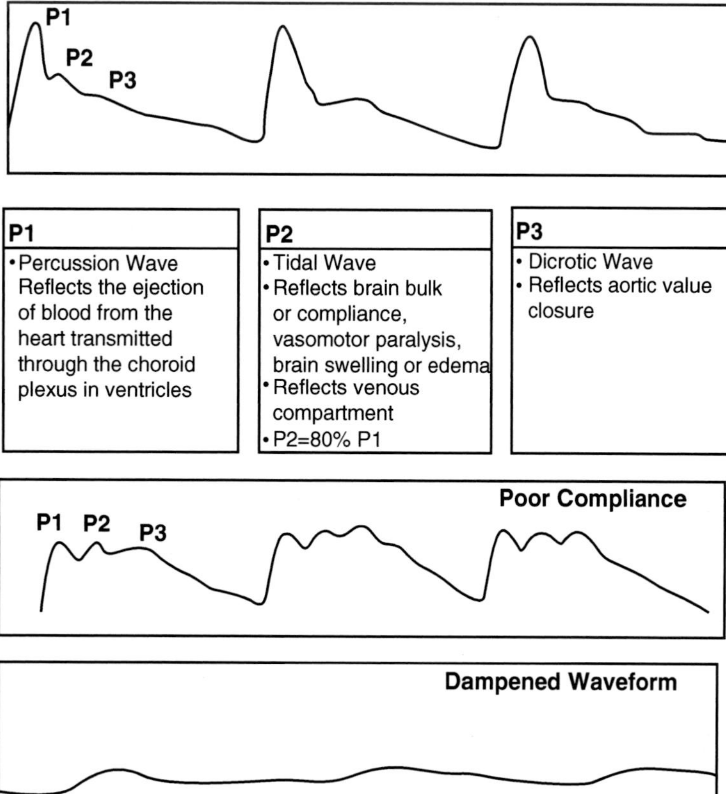

Fig. 23.2 Intracranial pressure waveforms

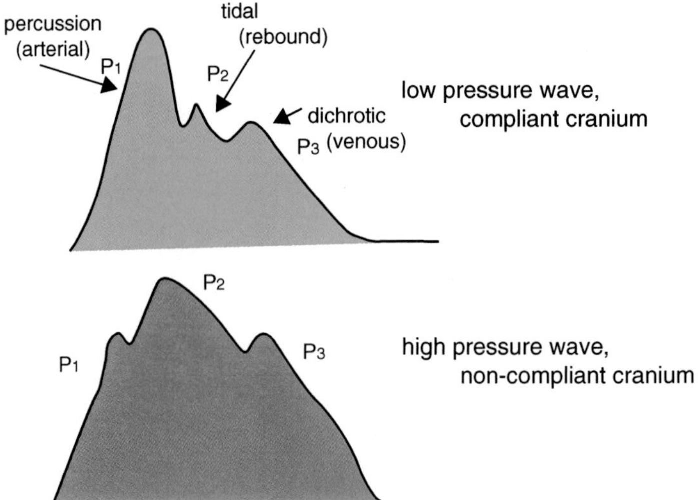

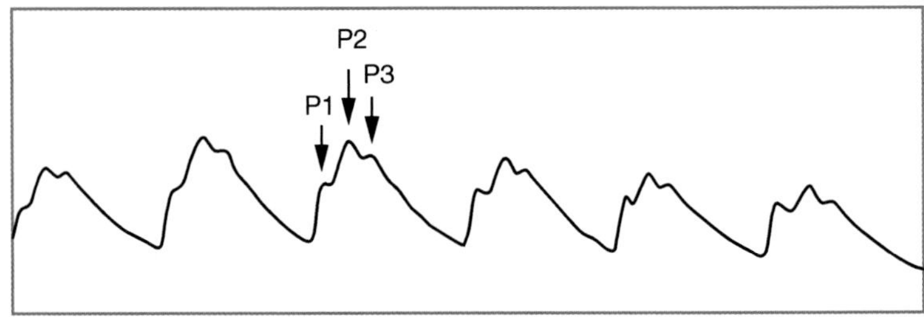

Fig. 23.3 ICP Waveform analysis

procedure and done outside the operating room, it must be done with utmost sterile technique and aseptic precautions with careful attention to detail. A recent CT scan of the brain usually precedes an EVD insertion to facilitate decision on the entry and trajectory of the EVD catheter. The common sites of insertion of the EVD catheter are:

23.7 Kocher's Point

Cranial location: frontal.

Landmarks: 10–11 cm posterior to the nasion and 3 cm lateral to the midline which correlates to the mid-pupillary line. It is 1 cm anterior to coronal suture (Fig. 23.4).

Trajectory: perpendicular to the skull with trajectory in the coronal plane, toward the medial canthus of the ipsilateral eye.

Placement: frontal horn of the lateral ventricle close to the foramen of Monro.

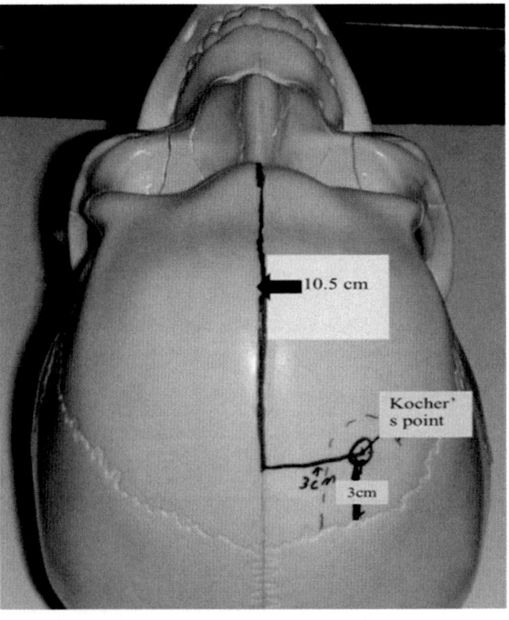

Fig. 23.4 Anatomic location of Kocher point

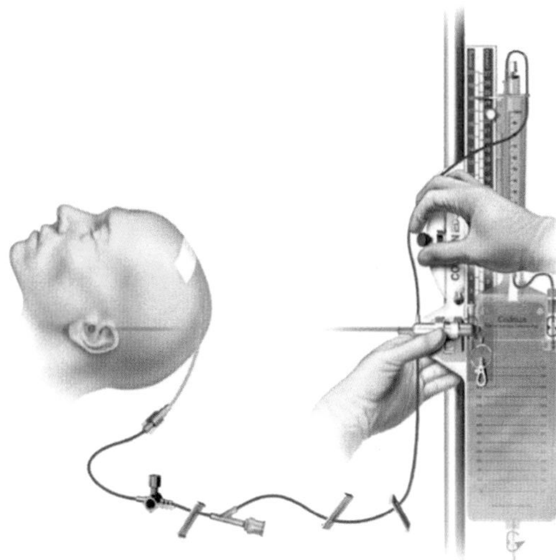

Fig. 23.5 Leveling of transducer

Depth: <5–7 cm from the outer table of the skull [4].

Notes: predominantly placed in the right side as it is the nondominant side in majority of the patients, lies anterior to the motor strip and lateral to the superior sagittal sinus [18].

23.8 Frazier's Point

Cranial location: parieto-occipital.

Landmarks: 6–7 cm superior to inion and 3–4 cm lateral to midline which is 1 cm anterior to the lambdoid suture.

Trajectory: perpendicular to the skull toward the glabella or medial canthus in the sagittal plane [4] or contralateral medial canthus [19].

Placement: traverses the length of the lateral ventricle with the tip in the frontal horn beyond the foramen of Monro.

Depth: after passing 5 cm, the stylet should be held and the rest of the catheter soft passed further up to 10 cm from the outer table of the skull [18].

Notes: inherently carries increased risk for misplacement of the catheter with increased morbidity [19].

23.9 Keen's Point

Cranial location: posterior parietal.

Landmarks: 2.5–3 cm superior and 2.5–3 cm posterior to the ear.

Trajectory: perpendicular to the cortex.

Placement: frontal horn of the lateral ventricle.

Depth: 4–5 cm [20].

23.10 Dandy's Point

Cranial location: occipital.

Landmarks: 3 cm above the inion and 2 cm lateral to midline.

Trajectory: perpendicular to the cortex and slightly cephalic [20].

Placement: frontal horn of the lateral ventricle.

Depth: 4–5 cm.

Note: more common in infants than adults where it coincides with the lambdoidal suture and mid-pupillary line. The trajectory carries a risk of damage to visual pathways [4].

23.11 Paine's Point

Paine's and modified Paine's points are done intraoperatively after craniotomy to induce brain relaxation while performing pterional craniotomy and transsylvian craniotomy approaches for repair of unruptured intracranial aneurysms [21] and are beyond the scope of this chapter and expertise of the authors (Image 23.1).

Kocher's point at the right frontal area is the most widely used approach due to its ease of placement compared to others and more forgiving secondary to approaching via the nondominant hemisphere. The most preferred location of the tip of the catheter is for it to terminate in the frontal horn of the lateral ventricle just anterior to the foramen of Monro as it is free of choroid plexus and prevents clogging. Patient can remain supine with the EVD out of the way of other monitors. Additionally, the patient may be positioned to accommodate any other injuries (Images 23.2 and 23.3).

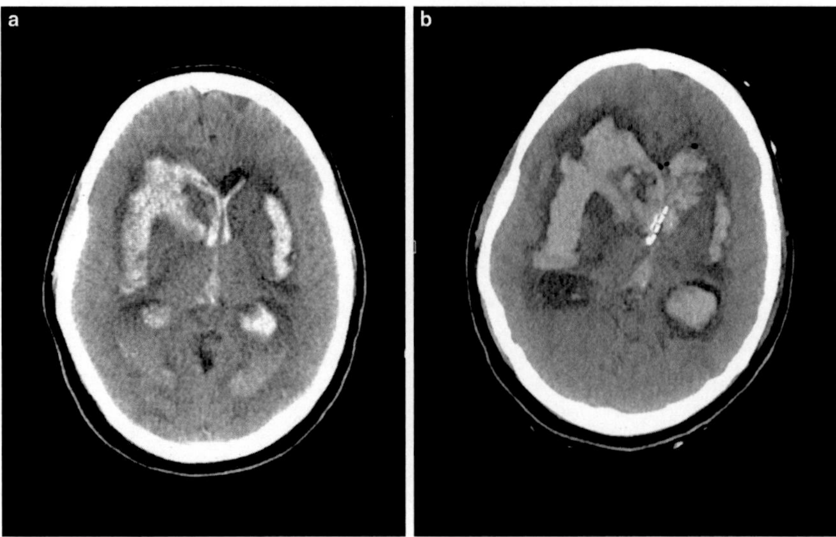

Image 23.1 (**a**) Massive intraventricular hemorrhage. (**b**) External ventricular drain terminating at third ventricle

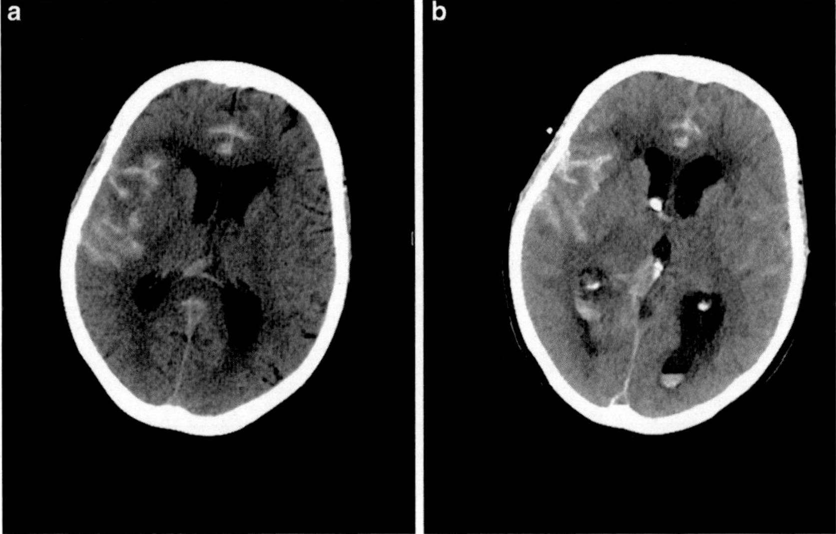

Image 23.2 (**a**) Subarachnoid hemorrhage. (**b**) External ventricular drain terminating in the inferior aspect of the right frontal horn just superior to the foramen of Monroe

23.12 Procedure

Since EVD insertion on the right side at the Kocher's point is the most commonly employed procedure for ICP monitoring and CSF drainage at the authors' institution, it is explained in detail with step-by-step procedures. A single dose of broad spectrum IV antibiotic such as cefazolin or in case of penicillin allergy vancomycin is recommended prior to incision. The adaptation and attention to aseptic precautions cannot be overemphasized. Furthermore several studies have documented that antimicrobial-impregnated catheters decrease the rate of CSF infections and their use is encouraged. A recent large meta-analysis and systematic review concluded that the overall rate of infection in the antimicrobial-impregnated EVD

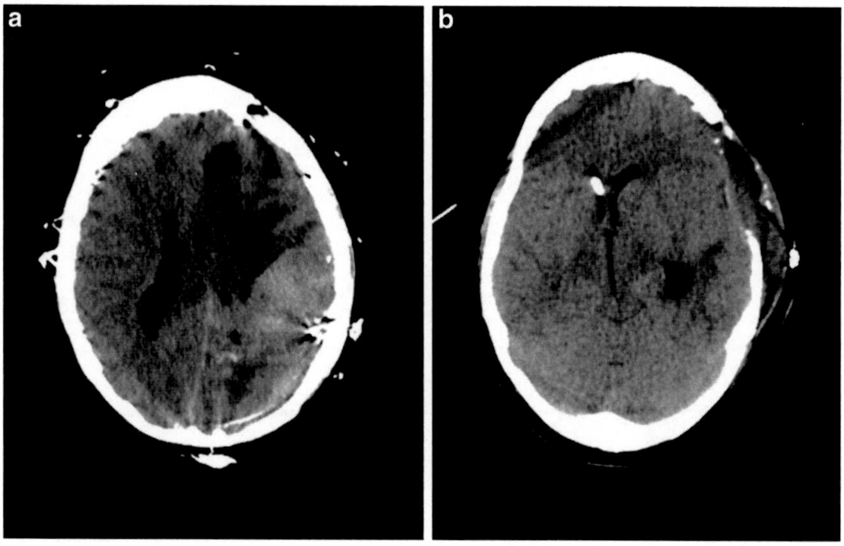

Image 23.3 (**a**) Left parietal intraparenchymal hemorrhage. (**b**) External ventricular drain terminating in the right frontal horn and patient is s/p left hemicraniectomy

Table 23.1 Interpretation of ICP changes

Conditions that increase ICP	Waveform changes
Increased mass lesion	Increase waveform amplitude (P2)
Increased CSF volume	Increase/decrease waveform amplitude: little change in waveform components
Increased blood pressure	Increase waveform amplitude (P1)
Increased venous volume Hypoventilation Venous compression	Increase waveform amplitude (P2) Rounding of ICP waveform due to increase in later waveform components

With permission from Codman

catheters was 3.6 % compared to 13.7 % in the standard EVD catheters along with a significant decrease in the rate of bacterial colonization of the catheter [22].

The key to a successful procedure even when done under an emergent situation is being thoroughly prepared and have all necessary things readily available. Having a second pair of hands to help in the authors' experience can reduce time and help adherence to sterile technique (Table 23.1).

23.13 EVD Placement

1. View the appropriate studies (CT/MRI) to assess the pathology and determine the necessary trajectory.
2. Consent the patient when appropriate or surrogate in accordance with your institutional guidelines.
3. Check coagulation parameters and platelets. Correct if necessary.
4. Order preprocedural antibiotics in accordance with your institutions' protocols.
5. Gather your supplies and prepare your work area. See Table 23.2.
6. Kocker's point on the right side is the most commonly used placement point and will be the focus of this section.
7. Using a tape measure, map out Kocker's point. At this point, you can place an empty EKG lead at the nasion and tragus in order to make them easier to find after you drape.
8. Using electric hair clippers, remove the hair over an area adequate to place the EVD, tunnel approximately 3–4 cm away from the site, and place an occlusive dressing.

Table 23.2 Preparation for procedure

Equipment						Extras
Cranial access kit	Sterile gown × 2	25 Ga needle	Sterile marking pen × 2	Sterile gauze boat	CSF culture tubes × 2	Needle driver
EVD catheter kit	Sterile gloves × 2	18 Ga needle	Preservative free normal saline flush	Chlorhexidine scrub kit/swabs	3/0 nylon suture × 3	Bone wax if not in kit
EVD drainage system	Surgical cap and mask × 2	10 cc sterile syringe	Electric hair shaver	Chlorhexidine BIO patch/coated Tegaderm patch	Benzoin swabs/ mastisol swabs	Spinal needle if not in cranial access kit
Sterile no flush transducer	Sterile drape sheet × 2 and/or sterile clear cranial drape	5 cc sterile syringe	EKG leads × 2	Sterile package towels (4 total)		Bipolar cautery if available

9. Place the patient in supine position with the neck neutral and the nose directly up. Using a surgical marking pen, draw out the midline and the coronal suture as well as your line coming off midline to Kocker's point (Fig. 23.4).
10. Ensure that all of your supplies are placed in an easily accessible location and put on a mask, surgical cap, and a pair of sterile gloves.
11. Prep the entire shaved area with iodine or chlorhexidine (CHG)-based prep according to your institutions' protocols. Prep widely and allow the prep to dry. While the prep dries, use this time to put on your sterile gown and new sterile gloves.
12. Use sterile towels to drape out the work area and remark your lines if you have scrubbed them off. Place the sterile cranial drape over the work area. It is highly recommended to obtain clear cranial drapes so that you can still see the relevant surface anatomy.
13. Using lidocaine with epinephrine and a 25 gauge needle, raise a large weal over Kocker's point. You can also inject over the planned exit site of your tunneled catheter at this point.
14. Ensure that your pt. is appropriately anesthetized for their level of consciousness
15. Make your incision thru the skin, down to bone. It is preferred to use an inverted J incision so that it may be used for future shunt placement; however it is acceptable to use a 3 cm linear incision as well.
16. Place a small retractor into the incision and spread it apart so that you can visualize the bone. At this point you should scrape the periosteum to either side of the incision away from where you are going to be drill. Also ensure at this point that you are not drilling on or posterior to the coronal suture.
17. You are ready to drill the hole that will be used for placement of the catheter. You should begin to assess your trajectory. Ideally this will be in a plane perpendicular to the skull. Your target is an intersection of two planes. One in sagittal plane moving posterior from the ipsilateral medial canthus and one in coronal plane moving medial from just in front of the ipsilateral tragus. Where these planes meet 4.5–5.5 cm below the inner table of the skull is your target. There are several commercially available guides or stereotactic systems available for clinicians that may be helpful for those that do not place these catheters on a regular basis.
18. Once you have decided on your trajectory, set the depth stop on the drill that you are using.

Keep in mind that the drill stop is not intended to stop the drill from plunging if you push hard. It is there as a visual guide. You do not want to plunge the drill bit into the brain and create a new hemorrhage. Apply light pressure and begin to spin the drill bit faster. Allow the drill bit to do the work; you do not have to push the drill bit thru the bone. You will feel a distinctive change in resistance when you penetrate the outer table of the skull and enter the cancellous bone which is softer. The same is true when you leave the cancellous bone and enter the inner table. At this point check your depth stop to ensure that you do not have more than approximately 2–4 mm to go. As you exit the inner table, there will be a complete loss resistance; stop turning the drill bit at this point; you do not want to tear any vessels on the surface of the dura. Remove the drill and clear any bone chips away with sterile saline and some pickups. If heavy bleeding is encounter in the bone, use bone wax to stop the bleeding before proceeding any further.

19. Now it is time to puncture the dura. It is important to inspect the dura for vessels before this is done to ensure that bleeding is minimized. Use a spinal needle to make a small puncture in the dura that can then be enlarged; using the tip of the needle, enlarge the hole in the shape of a cross until it is large enough to pass the catheter.
20. After wetting the ventricular catheter with sterile saline, using two hands to steady the catheter, assume the same trajectory that was used to drill the skull. Ensure that the stylet is to the tip of the catheter but not beyond. Begin advancing the catheter slowly through the parenchymal tissue. At approximately a depth of 4–5 cm, you should feel a distinctive change in resistant; this is what is termed as "feeling the pop." This is actually the catheter penetrating the wall of the ventricle and entering the fluid-filled space of the ventricle. If you feel this, stop and withdraw the stylet to see if you have CSF return. *If* you do not feel this by 6 cm, *stop* anyhow and withdraw the stylet to see if you have CSF return.
21. If you have return of CSF from the catheter, leave the stylet out and soft pass the catheter to a maximum distance of 6–7 cm at the skull surface. You are now ready to tunnel the catheter and begin suturing it in place.
22. If you have not gotten CSF return, you need to gently replace the stylet and remove the catheter. Clean the tip of the catheter to remove any tissue clogging the holes. Reassess your trajectory and try again. You should not make more than three passes at maximum without CSF return. If you do not get CSF return on your third pass, it is recommended to leave that catheter in place and secure it like you would a successful pass and get a CT scan to assess the placement of the catheter.
23. Once the catheter is in place and you have CSF return, you should keep the tip of the catheter clamped to ensure that overdrainage doesn't occur. At this time you use the manometer to measure the opening pressure and collect 3 ml of CSF into two separate collection tubes for CSF analysis.
24. Using the trocar provided with the EVD kit, tunnel the catheter away from the incision area for at least 3–4 cm. Keep in mind future planning of shunt trajectory so that your tunnel misses where the shunt would need to be. Where the EVD exits the skin, use a 3–0 nylon suture to secure this tightly to the skin without restricting flow. The EVD should lay flat against the bone in the incision when it has been successfully tunneled and sutured in place.
25. Cut the trocar off the catheter and place the provided luer lock on the catheter and secure with a 3–0 silk tie.
26. Using 2–0 or 3–0 Vicryl suture, you can attempt to close the galea, but do no sew through the drain. Then use 3–0 nylon to close the skin, again taking great care not to puncture the catheter. The best practice here is to throw all the sutures first and then tie them, that way you have the best visualization of the entire wound when you put a needle in it.
27. After the skin is closed, wrap the catheter in a coil on the head and use the 3–0 nylon suture to secure it to the scalp at three separate locations.

Again, this needs to be tight to keep the catheter from being pulled out, but not so tight as to restrict flow of CSF. Using tincture of benzoin to outline the area of the dressing, place an occlusive dressing over the coiled catheter. It is recommended to use a CHG eluding patch or coated Tegaderm type dressing.

28. After making sure that the drainage system is completely flushed, attach the distal end of the ventricular catheter to the drainage system. Ensure that there is appropriate flow of CSF at the drip chamber and level the drainage system to the patients' tragus (Fig. 23.5). This corresponds to the foramen of Monro. The appropriate drainage level will be determined by the opening pressure, the pathology present, and the desired treatment effect.
29. It is worth mentioning here that having a second skilled and experienced individual help with these procedures is always very helpful and recommended. Have a second pair of hands to help get into sterile gown, to hold the head still while you drill, and to have an extra pair of eyes to look at the trajectory that you are using. Always use all the help available to you.

References

1. Sekula RF, Cohen DB, Patek PM, Jannetta PJ, Oh MY. Epidemiology of ventriculostomy in the United States from 1997 to 2001. Br J Neurosurg. 2008;22(2):213–8.
2. Philips SB, Varela PN, Abdelhak T, Cory JJ, Krishnamurthy S. External ventricular catheter position, malfunction, and replacement. Why do EVDs fail? Neurocrit Care. 2010;13:S169.
3. Blumenfeld H. Neuroanatomy through clinical cases. Sunderland, MA: Sinauer Associates; 2002.
4. Greenberg MS. Handbook of neurosurgery. 7th ed. Florida: Thieme; 2006.
5. Mokri B. The Monro–Kellie hypothesis: applications in CSF volume depletion. Neurology. 2001;56(12):121746–8.
6. Jull N, Morris GF, Marshall SB, Marshall LF. Intracranial hypertension and cerebral perfusion pressure: influence on neurological deterioration and outcomes in severe head injury. The executive committee of the International Selfotel Trial. J Neurosurg. 2000;92:1–6.
7. McCance KL, Huether SE, Brashers VL, Rote NS. Pathophysiology: the basis for disease in adults and children. 6th ed. Philadelphia, PA: Mosby Elsevier; 2010.
8. Bratton SL, Chestnut RM, Ghajar J, Connell Hammond FF, Harris OA, Hartl R, et al. Guidelines for the management of sever traumatic brain injury. VI. Indications for intracranial pressure monitoring. J Neurotrauma. 2007;24 Suppl 1:S37–44.
9. Czosnyka M, Pickard JD. Monitoring and interpretation of intracranial pressure. J Neurol Neurosurg Psychiatry. 2004;75:813–21.
10. Hunter HB, Schellinger PD, Hartmann M, Kohrmann M, Juettler E, Wikner J, et al. Hematoma growth and outcome in treated neurocritical care patients with intracerebral hemorrhage related to oral anticoagulant therapy: comparison of acute treatment strategies using vitamin K, fresh frozen plasma, and prothrombin complex concentrates. Stroke. 2006;37:1465–70.
11. Cervera A, Amaro S, Chamorro A. Oral anticoagulant associated intracerebral hemorrhage. J Neurol. 2012;259:21–224.
12. James RF, Palys V, Lomboy JR, Lamm Jr JR, Simon SD. The role of anticoagulants, antiplatelet agents, and their reversal strategies in the management of intracerebral hemorrhage. Neurosurg Focus. 2013;34(5):E6.
13. Pabinger I, Brenner B, Kalina U, Knaub S, Nagy A, Ostermann H. Prothrombin complex concentrate (Beriplex P/N) for emergency anticoagulation reversal: a prospective multi-national clinical trial. J Thromb Haemost. 2008;6:622–31.
14. Van Aart L, Eijkhout HW, Kamphuis JS, Dam M, Schattenkerk ME, Schouten TJ, et al. Individualized dosing regimen for prothrombin complex concentrate more effective than standard treatment in the reversal of oral anticoagulant therapy: an open, prospective randomized controlled trial. Thromb Res. 2006;118:313–20.
15. Campbell PG, Sen A, Yadla S, Jabbour P, Jallo J. Emergency reversal of antiplatelet agents in patients presenting with an intracranial hemorrhage: a clinical review. In: Department of Neurosurgery Faculty Papers. Paper 11. 2010. http://jdc.jefferson.edu/neurosurgeryfp/11
16. Ravi R, Morgan RJ. Intracranial pressure monitoring. Curr Anaesth Critical Care. 2003;14:229–35.
17. Kirkness CJ, Mitchell PH, Burr RL, March KS, Newell DW. Intracranial pressure waveform analysis: clinical and research implications. J Neurosci Nurs. 2000;32:271–7.
18. Connolly Jr ES, McKhann II GM, Huang J, Choudhri TF, Komotar RJ, Mocco J. Fundamentals of operative techniques in neurosurgery. 2nd ed. New York: Thieme; 2010.
19. Lee CK, Tay LL, Ng WH, Ng I, Ang BT. Optimization of ventricular catheter placement via posterior approaches: a virtual reality simulation study. Surg Neurol. 2008;70(3):274–7.
20. The ISPN Guide to Pediatric Neurosurgery. 2010. http://guide.ispneurosurgery.org/
21. Park J, Hamm I-S. Revision of Paine's technique for intraoperative ventricular puncture. Surg Neurol. 2008;70:503–8.
22. Wang X, Dong Y, Qi XQ, Li YM, Huang CG, Hou LJ. Clinical review: efficacy of antimicrobial-impregnated catheters in external ventricular drainage—a systematic review and meta-analysis. Crit Care. 2013;17(4):234 [Epub ahead of print].

24 Lumbar Puncture and Drainage

Christian J. Schulz and Andrew W. Asimos

24.1 Introduction

This chapter will discuss the commonly seen indications, contraindications, anatomy, procedural performance, and complications of lumbar puncture (LP) or "spinal tap" in the emergent setting. LP is performed as a diagnostic intervention to evaluate cerebrospinal fluid (CSF) or as a therapeutic intervention for many neurologic conditions. While the procedure can be technically challenging, clinician success readily improves with knowledge and experience performing the procedure. CSF is collected by utilizing a hollow bore needle to access the lumbar cistern. In patients being evaluated for meningitis or encephalitis, antibiotic administration should not be delayed by either computed tomography (CT) imaging or completion of LP. While most complications are benign and self-limited, the clinician should be aware of rare, but serious, complications that may result in disability or death.

C.J. Schulz, PA-C (✉) • A.W. Asimos, MD
Department of Emergency Medicine, Carolinas Medical Center-Main, 1000 Blythe Boulevard, Charlotte, NC 28203, USA
e-mail: Christian.schulz@carolinashealthcare.org; Andrew.Asimos@carolinashealthcare.org

24.2 Indications

Lumbar puncture (LP) is a minimally invasive procedure performed for both diagnostic and therapeutic evaluation. In the emergency medicine and critical care settings, it is most often used to evaluate for meningitis or encephalitis [1], specifically in patients presenting with headache and fever without a source and certainly in the setting of recent travel. While it has been reported that modern third generation CT of the head is extremely sensitive in identifying subarachnoid hemorrhage (SAH) within the first 6 h of symptom onset [2], LP may be pursued in patients with a negative CT for SAH who have a concerning clinical presentation (e.g., thunder-clap onset or "worst ever" headache) or in those who have negative CT imaging with symptom onset of >6 h. In non-emergent settings, LP is more often used in the evaluation of unexplained neurologic symptoms after neuroimaging to diagnose and treat pseudotumor cerebri, degenerative neurologic diseases, Guillain–Barré syndrome, neurosyphilis, tuberculosis, metastatic disease, or as a route of delivery for medications, specifically for spinal anesthesia, intrathecal administration of antibiotics, and chemotherapeutic agents, or to perform myelography.

D.A. Taylor et al. (eds.), *Interventional Critical Care*, DOI 10.1007/978-3-319-25286-5_24

24.3 Contraindications

LP should not be performed in patients with intracranial mass or abscess as a sudden decrease in intracranial pressure may cause cerebral herniation. It should also be avoided in any patient with epidural abscess or overlying skin infection as this may spread or introduce bacteria into the subarachnoid space [3]. Caution should be used in performing LPs on patients with coagulopathy or underlying bleeding disorders as this may result in epidural hematoma formation. If LP is indicated in the latter case, however, it may be necessary to reverse the coagulopathy, infuse clotting factors, or administer fresh frozen plasma prior to performing the procedure [4].

24.4 Anatomy

The brain floats in a thin layer of CSF that circulates within the ventricular system and extends to the subarachnoid space of the brain and spinal cord. While the choroid plexus may produce up to 500 ml of CSF each day, about 150 ml is present at any given time [5]. CSF provides protection from injury and filters cellular waste from brain tissue. In its natural state, the fluid is a clear and colorless substance that consists primarily of water and is measured as mm H_2O.

The brain and spinal cord are protected by three meningeal layers—the dura mater, arachnoid mater, and pia mater. The dura mater, or "tough mother," is the strong and dense outermost meningeal layer that contains and protects the underlying structures. This area also contains the venous blood vessels that carry blood from the brain to the heart. The arachnoid mater, or "spider mother," forms the middle layer. It consists of a thin layer that attaches to the dura mater with web-like collections of fibers that extend through the subarachnoid space attaching to the pia mater. CSF circulates within this subarachnoid space and is constantly being reabsorbed into the bloodstream by the arachnoid villi. The pia mater, or "tender mother," is the thin and delicate innermost meningeal layer that envelops the brain and spinal cord. This layer contains blood vessels that allow for blood exchange, but the layer is essentially non-permeable and is the structure most responsible for maintaining the blood–brain barrier.

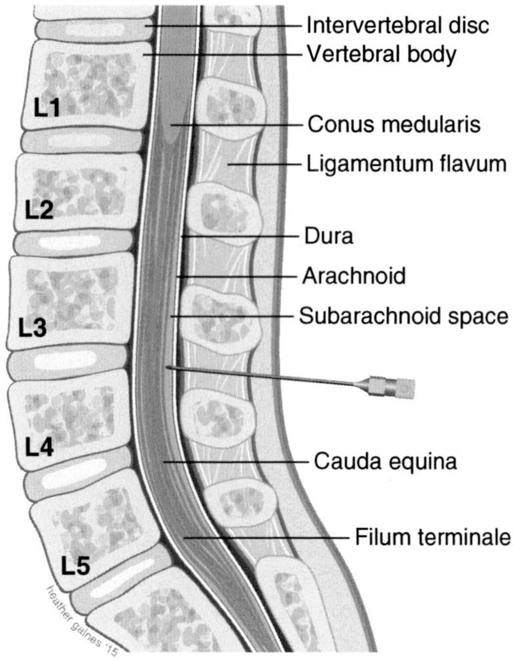

Fig. 24.1 Lumbar spine and cistern anatomy

The spinal cord originates from the medulla oblongata and terminates in the lumbar spine at the L3 level at birth. Although there may be some variation during growth to adulthood, the spinal cord eventually terminates at about the L1 level. This terminal end is called the conus medullaris. Fibrous terminal threads, called filum terminale, proceed distally to the level of the sacrum and provide longitudinal support to the spinal cord. Surrounding these threads is a bundle of spinal nerves which make up the cauda equina, or "horse's tail," which terminate at the S2 level. As the spinal cord terminates, the subarachnoid space becomes more prominent. This area is known as the lumbar cistern and is the area in which lumbar puncture is performed (Fig. 24.1).

24.5 Pre-Procedure

1. Antibiotic administration should not be delayed by neuroimaging, completion of LP, or in awaiting test results when the clinical suspicion of meningitis or encephalitis is likely. If a delay is anticipated, blood cultures should be obtained and empiric antibiotics should be administered. Antibiotics administered even up to 2 h prior to the procedure will not decrease CSF culture results due to the interval delay for the medication to cross the blood–brain barrier [4, 6].
2. CT of the head should be considered in all patients of advanced age, those who are immunocompromised or have a seizure history, and in patients who have papilledema or any focal neurologic symptoms prior to performing LP.
3. When possible, consent should be obtained which discusses the risks and benefits of performing the procedure. Explaining the steps of the procedure to the patient and family may help alleviate anxiety, but it will also provide the patient pertinent information regarding procedural expectations. Parents or significant others may feel more comfortable stepping out of the room during the procedure, but they may also be seated in front of the patient to provide emotional support and comfort.
4. Consider the use of conscious sedation, inhalant anesthetics, anxiolytic medications, local anesthetic injections, needle—free injections or topical anesthetic creams prior to the procedure on a case-by-case basis. The use of needle-free jet injection of 1 % lidocaine in infants seems to reduce pain before LP [7]. The use of topical anesthetic cream is also beneficial and may allow for lower dosage need of intravenous analgesic agents especially in the pediatric population [8]. Topical anesthetic creams, however, must be applied 30–60 min prior to the procedure and may not be practical to use in the emergency setting. In infants who require LP emergently, as little as 0.1 ml of oral sucrose on a pacifier provides pain relief in those <2–6 months of age, but local anesthetic infiltration will likely still be required to anesthetize the deep tissues in infants >3 months of age [9].
5. Ensure that adequate ancillary staff is available to assist with patient holding or equipment needs during the procedure.
6. Lumbar puncture tray (Fig. 24.2) and other equipment should be readily available at the bedside.
7. Ideally, the patient should be placed in the lateral recumbent position which will allow for opening pressure measurements. The patient should be instructed to lie in the fetal position

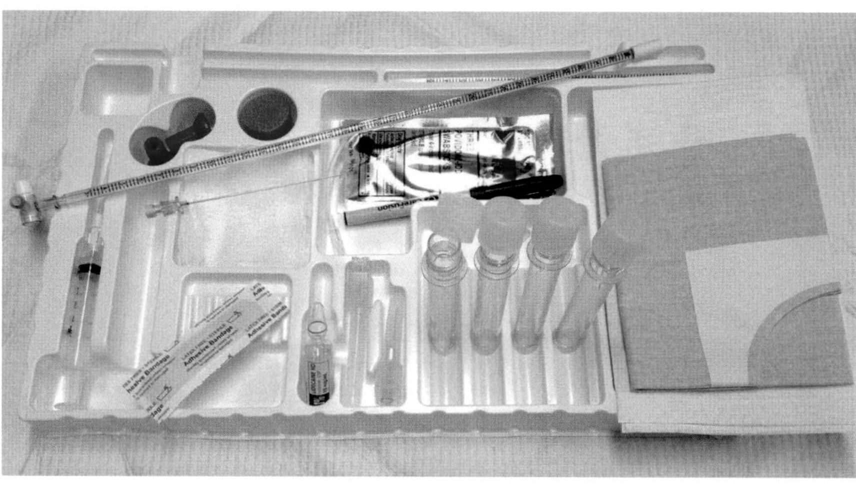

Fig. 24.2 Lumbar puncture tray

near the edge of the bed, with the shoulders and pelvis squared on the bed, chin tucked and knees flexed to the chest while maintaining alignment of the spine. Suggesting that the patient anteriorly flex the pelvis while simultaneously arching the low back will help flex the lumbar spine, thus opening the interspaces as opposed to protruding the sacrum which will close the interspaces.

8. Infants and obese patients may be placed in the upright position; however, opening pressure measurements are unable to be accurately obtained in this position. In newborns, optimal performance can be achieved by sitting the infant with hips flexed with spinal needle trajectory angled 65–70° and with proper spinal needle depth calculated as 2.5 × weight in kilograms + 6 mm [10]. Infant pulse oximetry should be monitored during the procedure as over flexion of the head can lead to hypoxia and respiratory arrest. Adults may be placed sitting upright on the examination bed while leaning over a tray stand to flex the lumbar spine.
9. The level of the iliac crest lies at the L4 spinous process (Fig. 24.3). The interspace cephalad to this is L3–L4 which is the ideal interspace for subarachnoid access in adults and older children. An additional interspace cephalad is L2–L3 which would also provide adequate subarachnoid access. The subarachnoid space narrows significantly, however, caudal to L3–L4 which makes subarachnoid access in these interspaces much less successful. The L1–L2 interspace should be avoided to ensure that the conus medullaris is not injured. The interspace caudal to the L4 spinous process is L4–L5 which is the ideal LP site in infants and younger children.
10. While palpating the spine of the iliac crest, locate the L4 spinous process. The sulcus cephalad to the L4 spinous process and caudal to the L3 spinous process is the L3–L4 interspace (Fig. 24.4). Using the thumbnail, an "X" can be impressed onto the skin overlying this area to identify the site at which lumbar puncture will be performed. This should be made at the midpoint between and at the midline level of the spinous processes (Fig. 24.5). It may help to remind the patient to flex the hips and arch the low back during the impression. Evaluating the L2–L3 interspace at this point is appropriate especially if the L3–L4 interspace does not adequately flex or is difficult to identify. Alternatively, a sterile skin marker can be used to create cross-hairs overlying this area. While there may be no advantage to utilizing bedside ultrasound guidance in routine LPs, it may be a valuable tool in identifying spinal landmarks, reducing complications, and improving efficiency particularly in obese and pediatric patients [11–14].

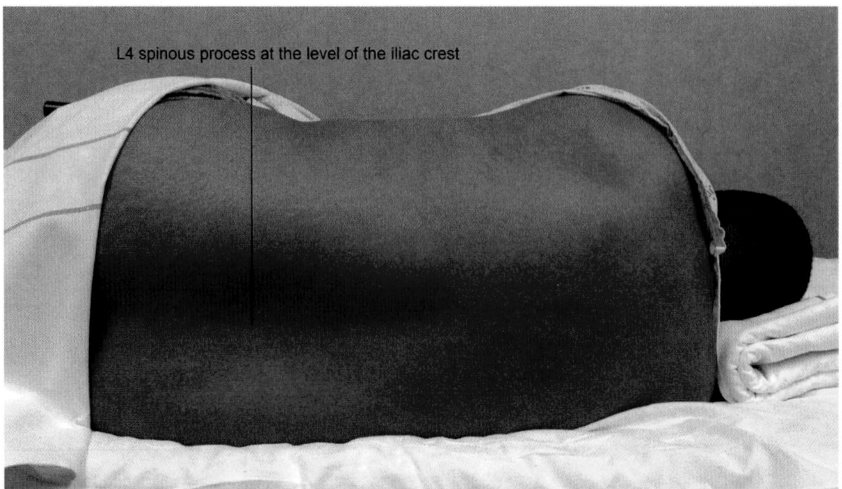

Fig. 24.3 Anatomic landmark to identify L4 spinous process

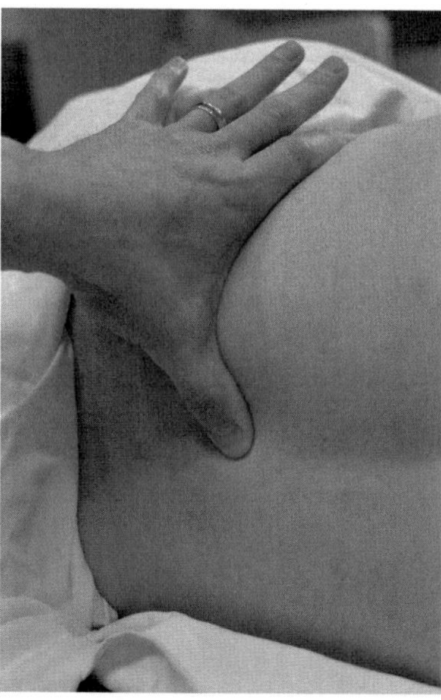

Fig. 24.4 Identifying the L3–L4 interspace

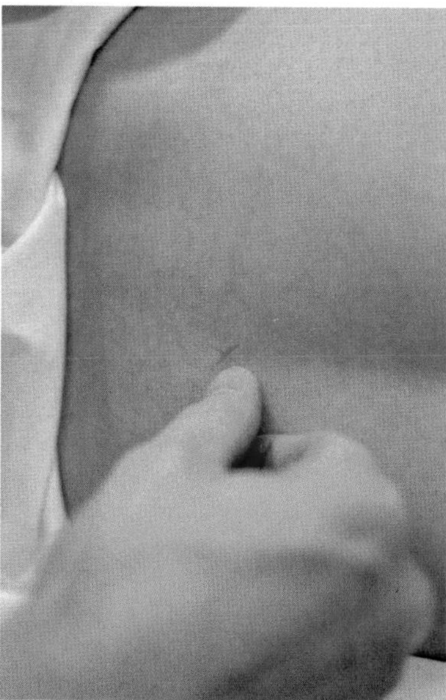

Fig. 24.5 Thumbnail impression marking the site of lumbar puncture

24.6 Procedure

1. Ensure that the LP tray is opened in a sterile manner. Don face mask, gown, and other personal protective equipment if needed.
2. Apply sterile gloves and inspect that all needed equipment is included in the LP tray.
3. A sterile drape may be placed on the surface of the bed. With sterile-gloved hands between a 1/3 fold of the sterile drape, carefully tuck it under the patient's flank.
4. Open the povidone-iodine swabs or use povidone-iodine and sterile gauze to prepare the skin in sterile fashion. If the patient has a povidone-iodine allergy, chlorhexidine may be used. At the site of the impressed "X" or cross-hairs, begin sterile preparation in small circles moving peripherally to create an approximate 10 cm area of povidone-iodine coverage. Three sterile cleansing passes should be performed while each time working from the central point to the periphery.
5. The paper backing strips on the fenestrated drape should be removed and the drape should be carefully applied over the patient's iliac crest with the "X" impression or cross-hairs in the open center portion of the fenestration. There should be no visible areas of non-cleansed skin within the fenestration. The povidone-iodine should be allowed to dry; however, any excess povidone-iodine can be wiped with sterile gauze. While maintaining sterile field, it may be judicious at this point to reidentify the L3–L4 interspace and perform a repeat "X" impression with the thumbnail so that the site can be confirmed.
6. Using the filter straw, aspirate the lidocaine 1 % into a 5 cc syringe. Remove the filter straw and affix a 25 gauge needle to the syringe. At the center point of the "X" impression or cross-hairs, inject a small amount of lidocaine forming a wheal. The needle can be withdrawn slightly and can be redirected toward the umbilicus in the trajectory that the spinal needle will follow so that a small amount of lidocaine can be injected deeper into the subcutaneous tissue. Next, affix a 22 gauge needle to the syringe, and with the remainder of the lidocaine 1 %, inject this deeper into the tissue following the same trajectory. Providing infiltration bilaterally may offer additional anesthetic benefit. Additional lidocaine may be required in larger-sized or obese patients to provide adequate local anesthesia.
7. While again suggesting that the patient anteriorly flex the pelvis and simultaneously arch

the low back, place the 20 gauge spinal needle bevel up to the L3–L4 interspace. The sulcus will likely be difficult to appreciate at this point as the injected lidocaine may skew landmarks, and so entering the skin at the site of the lidocaine injection is most practical. While 22 gauge spinal needles can be used in children of all ages, smaller spinal needle size can be considered given the clinical scenario. Non-stylet needles or "butterfly needles" increase the risk of subarachnoid cyst evolution and should not be used. Also consider that a 5 in. spinal needle may be required to successfully complete LP in obese patients.

8. It is important to maintain the spinal needle level in the midline of the interspace, but angled slightly toward the umbilicus. While stabilizing your hand with the index and middle fingers against the patient's back, brace the spinal needle with the thumb and index finger. With the opposite hand, hold the spinal needle hub between your thumb and index and middle fingers and slowly advance through the tissues (Fig. 24.6). If bone is encountered, simply withdraw slightly and redirect the spinal needle. It is not uncommon for the patient to feel pain down one leg during this procedure, but the patient should be encouraged to remain as still as possible until the procedure is completed.
9. Experienced providers will often feel the "pop" as the needle enters the dura, but this may not be readily identified in those less experienced in performing the procedure. Advance the spinal needle slightly and remove the stylet. It should be noted that a similar "pop" sensation may be felt with penetration of the ligamentum flavum; however, with the needle tip in this location, CSF drainage will not be seen with removal of the stylet.
10. If the dural "pop" is not appreciated after the spinal needle has been advanced 3 cm, it is good practice to remove the stylet and assess for fluid. If there is no CSF drainage, replace the stylet, advance 1–2 mm, and reassess until subarachnoid space access has been achieved. The CSF should appear clear or should clear as it is collected (Fig. 24.7). Xanthochromia, or the yellowish discoloration of CSF when compared against a white background, suggests SAH and may be seen within 2 h of symptom onset. If the fluid appears clotted, lumbar puncture should be repeated at an alternate level as this is likely a "traumatic tap" or inadvertent venous plexus puncture. Remember that it is not normal for blood to be in the subarachnoid space.
11. Once access has been confirmed, attach the stopcock onto the spinal needle and secure the manometer to assess opening pressure.

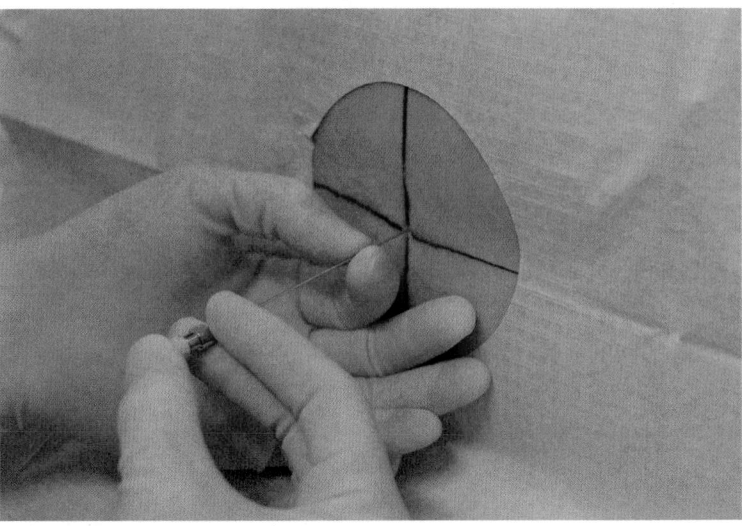

Fig. 24.6 Hand position when advancing the spinal needle

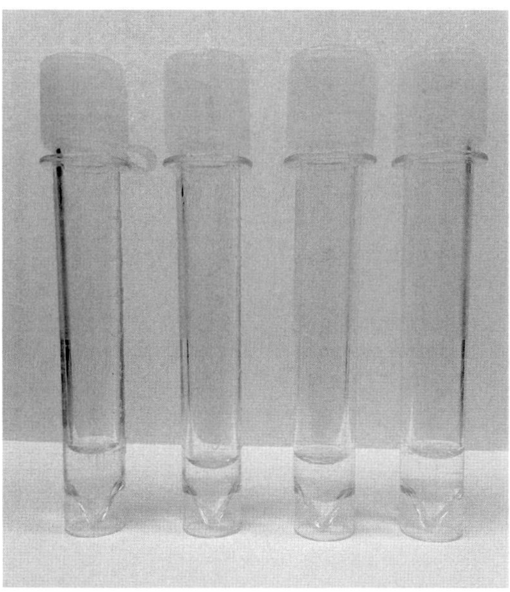

Fig. 24.7 CSF demonstrating blood-tinged clearing in the order of collection

It is important to maintain control, and placement of the spinal needle during this as the manometer can be cumbersome to attach and remove from the spinal needle. The opening pressure should be noted while the patient relaxes and slightly extends the lower extremities; however, there will be variation in the pressure with cough or respiration. An opening pressure range of 80–200 mm H_2O is normal in adults, while 50–100 mm H_2O is normal in children. In patients with elevated opening pressures consistent with pseudotumor cerebri, an appropriate amount of CSF should be drained to normalize pressure.

12. After obtaining the opening pressure, empty this fluid into CSF tube #1. Close the stopcock and remove the manometer. Next, collect CSF in tubes #2–4, ensuring that a minimum of 1 ml is obtained in each tube. Depending on the patient's clinical indication for LP, additional CSF may be required and this can be placed in tube #4. A total of 4–8 ml should be obtained considering tests needed. Ensure that the tubes are labeled in the order of collection or placed in sequential order to be labeled after the procedure.
13. Replace the stylet and withdraw the needle. Hold gentle pressure with a sterile gauze to the area and place a sterile dressing or adhesive bandage over the puncture site.

24.7 Post-Procedure

1. All sharps should be accounted for and disposed of properly.
2. Previous teaching has suggested that the patient be placed supine for 1–24 h post-procedure as it had been postulated that this position may limit occurrence of post-LP headache. While there is evidence that using atraumatic or blunt spinal needles may decrease occurrence of post-LP headache, there is no consensus that rest, intravenous fluids, patient position, or even spinal needle size prevents or limits occurrences of post-LP headache [15–18].
3. Antibiotics should be administered when indicated if not completed prior to performing LP.
4. Analgesic or antiemetic medications should be provided if needed.
5. CSF collection tubes should be labeled appropriately and hand carried to the facility laboratory.

24.8 CSF Tests

Generally, tube #1 should evaluate cell count with differential, tube #2 protein and glucose, and tube #3 gram stain and culture. A second cell count and differential as well as any additional tests can be evaluated via CSF collected in tube #4. Comparing the results from tube #1 and tube #4, the clinician should note stabilized or decreased CSF red blood cell (RBC) count which would suggest inadvertent venous plexus puncture, or a "traumatic tap."

The degree of CSF white blood cell count (WBC) pleocytosis can be calculated using the following corrective calculation:

$$\text{True CSF} = (\text{measured CSF WBC}) \times \frac{(\text{CSF RBC} \times \text{blood WBC})}{\text{blood RBC}}$$

or by calculating a CSF RBC to CSF WBC ratio of about 700:1 when peripheral cell counts are normal [19]. An RBC count of >10,000 in the final collection tube significantly increases the odds of SAH [20]. If SAH is suspected after review of test results, CT angiography of the head and neck should be performed. In children, "traumatic tap" may be suggested if for every 1000 cell increase in CSF RBCs, CSF protein increases by 1.1 mg/dl [21]; however, elevation in CSF RBCs is also a common finding of HSV infection which should be considered in the setting of "traumatic taps."

Elevation in the CSF WBC (>5) is suggestive of meningitis; however, CSF WBC count alone does not distinguish between viral and bacterial cases. In bacterial meningitis, cell counts are often markedly elevated and associated with an elevation in CSF protein and a decrease in CSF glucose, but normal cell counts may be seen especially in patients pretreated with antibiotics. Gram stain demonstrating polymorphonuclear cells and organisms further suggests bacterial meningitis, whereas CSF culture will confirm the diagnosis.

Additional studies such as Venereal Disease Research Laboratory (VDRL), India Ink, herpes simplex virus (HSV), *Cryptococcus*, cytology, oligoclonal bands, arbovirus antibodies, and immune complexes may be considered depending on patient age, comorbidities, and clinical presentation.

24.9 Complications

While LP is widely considered to be a safe procedure, it is not risk-free. The most widely reported complication is post-LP headache which may occur in 25 % of patients. Presumed to be a result of intracranial hypotension, this headache is generally described as positional, specifically worse with sitting upright or standing and better with lying supine. It is a self-limiting complication that may be treated with analgesic medications, caffeine, or by blood patch wherein venous blood is injected into the lumbar cistern via a second LP [22]. While platelet aggregation may be the mechanism by which headache resolves, it is likely that the effect of increasing CSF pressure during the injection is responsible for immediate resolution of the headache [23–25].

As the spinal needle penetrates several layers of tissue, minor bruising around or bleeding from the LP site may occur. Back pain at the site of LP is common and may persist for several days and in rare cases for several months, but this should be self-limited and may be treated with NSAIDS or other analgesic medications. It is possible that transient paresthesia or radiculopathic complaints occur during the procedure or shortly thereafter; however, rarely do patients experience radiculopathic complaints beyond this. Patients may find that back rest in the days immediately after the procedure may shorten the course of localized back pain; however, bed rest should generally not be recommended.

Subarachnoid cyst formation may occur as a complication of penetration into the subarachnoid space, but neurosurgical intervention is infrequently required. LP site infection, epidural abscess, and meningitis are serious complications, but are rarely reported. Patients presenting with these complications may be significantly ill or septic, and prompt identification and management is essential. Epidural hematoma is a potential complication caused from venous plexus injury during the procedure. Patients may complain of pain and have focal neurologic findings which may be a significant complication if cord compression leads to central cord ischemia. The condition is usually diagnosed by magnetic resonance imaging (MRI) of the lumbar spine and may require neurosurgical intervention.

One of the more concerning complications is that of cerebral herniation which is catastrophic and often fatal. Herniation usually occurs within the first 12 h after the procedure, most often in patients with previously unidentified brain mass or with significantly elevated intracranial pressure. The mechanism of herniation is thought to be due to a sudden drop in pressure as a result of the procedure and may occur in up to 5 % of patients undergoing LP who have bacterial meningitis [26, 27], although it may occur in patients with other neurologic conditions as well. Cerebral herniation can occur in patients with normal head

CT and this alone does not infer that LP is safe to perform. Clinical findings suggestive of impending herniation include deteriorating level of consciousness, Cheyne–Stokes respiration, posturing, or seizures. LP should be avoided in these patients and interventions to control intracranial pressure should be the priority followed by emergent CT evaluation [27, 28].

References

1. Johnson KS, Sexton DJ. Lumbar puncture: technique, indications, contraindications and complications in adults. In: Post TW, editor. UpToDate. Waltham, MA: UpToDate; 2015.
2. Perry JJ, Stiell IG, Sivilotti ML, Bullard MJ, Emond M, Symington C, Sutherland J, et al. Sensitivity of computed tomography performed within 6 hours of onset of headache for diagnosis of subarachnoid haemorrhage: prospective cohort study. BMJ. 2011;343:d4277.
3. Reihsaus E, Waldbaur H, Seeling W. Spinal epidural abscess: a meta-analysis of 915 patients. Neurosurg Rev. 2000;4(23):175–204.
4. Loring KE, Tintinalli JE. Central nervous system and spinal infections. In: Tintinalli JE, Stapczynski JS, Ma OJ, Cline DM, Cydulka RK, Meckler GD, editors. Tintinalli's emergency medicine: a comprehensive study guide. 7th ed. New York, NY: McGraw-Hill; 2011.
5. German JA, O'Brien J. Lumbar puncture. In: Pfenninger JL, Fowler GC, editors. Pfenninger and Fowler's procedures for primary care. 3rd ed. Philadelphia, PA: Elsevier Mosby; 2010.
6. Nau R, Sörgel F, Eiffert H. Penetration of drugs through the blood-cerebrospinal/blood-brain barrier for treatment of central nervous system infections. Clin Microbiol. 2010;23(4):858–83.
7. Ferayorni A, Yniquez R, Bryson M, Bulloch B. Needle-free jet injection of lidocaine for local anesthesia during lumbar puncture: a randomized controlled trial. Pediatr Emerg Care. 2012;28(7):687–90.
8. Whitlow PG, Saboda K, Roe DJ, Bazzell, Wilson C. Topical analgesia treats pain and decreases propofol use during lumbar punctures in a randomized pediatric leukemia trial. Pediatr Blood Cancer. 2015;62(1):85–90.
9. Baxter AL, Cohen LL. Pain management. In: Strange GR, Ahrens WR, Schafermeyer RW, Wiebe R, editors. Pediatric emergency medicine. 3rd ed. New York, NY: McGraw-Hill; 2009.
10. Oulego-Erroz I, Mora-Matilla M, Alonso-Quintela P, Rodriguez-Blanco, Mata-Zubillaga D, de Armentia SL. Ultrasound evaluation of lumbar spine anatomy in newborn infants: implications for optimal performance of lumbar puncture. J Pediatr. 2014;165(4):862–5.
11. Peterson MA, Pisupti D, Heyming TW, Abele JA, Lewis RJ. Ultrasound for routine lumbar puncture. Acad Emerg Med. 2014;21(2):130–6.
12. Mofidi M, Mohammadi M, Saidi H, Kianmehr N, Ghasemi A, Hafezimoghadam P, Rezai M. Ultrasound guided lumbar puncture in emergency department: time saving and less complications. J Res Med Sci. 2013;18(4):303–7.
13. Kim S, Adler DK. Ultrasound-assisted lumbar puncture in pediatric emergency medicine. J Emerg Med. 2014;47(1):59–64.
14. Shaikh F, Brzezinski J, Alexander S, Arzola C, Carvalho JC, Beyenne J, Sung L. Ultrasound imaging for lumbar puncture and epidural catheterisations; systemic review and meta-analysis. BMJ. 2013; 346:f1720.
15. Waise S, Gannon D. Reducing the incidence of post-dural puncture headache. Clin Med. 2013;13(1):32–4.
16. Jacobus CH. Does bed rest prevent post-lumbar puncture headache? Ann Emerg Med. 2012;59(2):139–40.
17. Crock C, Orsini F, Lee KJ, Phillips RJ. Headache after lumbar puncture: randomised crossover trial of 22-gauge versus 25 gauge needles. Arch Dis Child. 2014;99(3):203–7.
18. Møller A, Afshari A, Bjerrum OW. Diagnostic and therapeutic puncture performed safely and efficiently with a thin blunt needle. Dan Med J. 2013;60(9):A4684.
19. Meurer WJ. Central nervous system infections. In: Marx JA, Hockberger RS, Walls RM, editors. Rosen's emergency medicine: concepts and clinical practice. 8th ed. Philadelphia, PA: Elsevier Saunders; 2014.
20. Czuczman AD, Thomas LE, Boulanger AB, Peak DA, Senecal EL, Brown DF, Marill KA. Interpreting red blood cells in lumbar puncture: distinguishing true subarachnoid hemorrhage from traumatic tap. Acad Emerg Med. 2013;20(3):247–56.
21. Nigrovic LE, Shah SS, Neuman MI. Correction of cerebrospinal fluid protein for the presence of red blood cells in children with a traumatic lumbar puncture. J Pediatr. 2011;159(1):158–9.
22. Basurto OX, Martinez GL, Bonfill CX. Drug therapy for treating post-dural puncture headache. Cochrane Database Syst Rev. 2011;8:CD007887.
23. Kiki I, Gundogdu M, Alici HA, Yildirim R, Bilici M. A simple, safe and effective approach to prevent postdural puncture headache: epidural saline injection. Eurasion J Med. 2009;41(3):175–9.
24. Charsley MM, Abram SE. The injection of intrathecal normal saline reduces the severity of postdural puncture headache. Reg Anesth Pain Med. 2001;26(4): 301–5.
25. Turnbull DK, Shepherd DB. Post-dural puncture headache: pathogenesis, prevention and treatment. Br J Anaesth. 2003;91(5):718–29.
26. Rennick G, Shann F, de Campo J. Cerebral herniation during bacterial meningitis in children. BMJ. 1993;306(6883):953–5.
27. Joffe AR. Lumbar puncture and brain herniation in acute bacterial meningitis: a review. J Intensive Care Med. 2007;22(4):194–207.
28. Kwong KL, Chiu WK. Potential risk of fatal cerebral herniation after lumbar puncture in suspected CNS infection. HK J Paediatr. 2009;14:22–8.

Part VI

Maxofacial Procedures

Drainage of the Maxillary Sinus

25

Sarah A. Allen, Ronald F. Sing, and Matthew B. Dellinger

25.1 Introduction

Sinusitis is a recognized infectious complication in the critically ill patient. If left untreated, it can lead to serious complications, such as brain abscess formation, meningitis, postorbital cellulitis, and pneumonia. Patients that are at highest risk for developing sinusitis are those receiving ventilatory support via a nasotracheal tube; those with nasal colonization of gram-negative bacteria, facial trauma, nasogastric tubes, and nasoenteric tubes; or who have received antibiotic therapy.

The maxillary sinus is the most commonly affected. Diagnosis is often made with specific imaging studies (i.e., CT scan) as the classic signs for sinusitis (facial pain, malaise, fever, purulent nasal discharge) are often unobtainable because the patient is usually intubated, has other sources of infection, and is receiving analgesics and antipyretics [1]. The CT scan will usually demonstrate thickened mucosa as well as opacification of the sinus or an air-fluid level (Figs. 25.1 and 25.2).

Once the diagnosis of sinusitis is made (or suspected), nasal tubes are removed, decongestant is administered, and antibiotic therapy targeting the two most common organisms, *Staphylococcus aureus* and *Pseudomonas* species, is given [1].

Failure of medical therapy (i.e., nasal decongestants such as oxymetazoline or saline sprays) will often lead to surgical drainage of the involved sinus.

25.2 Anatomy

Within the maxillary bones lie the maxillary sinuses, which are the largest of the four sinuses. They are surrounded on all four sides by bony walls (Fig. 25.3).

Superior to the canine tooth is a bulge of thick bone in the anterior maxilla known as the canine eminence, and lateral to this is a depression called the canine fossa [2]. Take note that the infraorbital nerve lies just above this fossa approximately 1 cm below the orbital rim.

The ideal site for puncture is at the buccal gingival junction using the intersection of a line from the midpupillary axis, which intersects with a line at the level of the nasal vestibule [2].

25.3 Indications

*Symptomatic relief of acute maxillary sinusitis.
*Obtaining culture to guide in the choice of antibiotic therapy (usually in the ICU setting or in immunocompromised patients).

S.A. Allen, PA-C (✉) • R.F. Sing, DO, FACS, FCCM • M.B. Dellinger, MD
Carolinas Medical Center, Charlotte, NC, USA
e-mail: sarah.allen@carolinashealthcare.org

D.A. Taylor et al. (eds.), *Interventional Critical Care*, DOI 10.1007/978-3-319-25286-5_25

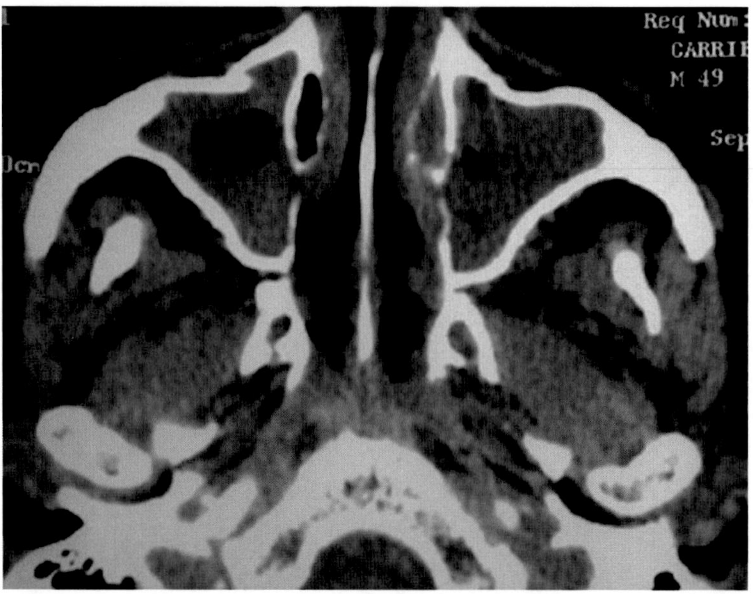

Fig. 25.1 Computed tomography of the maxillary sinuses showing air-fluid levels

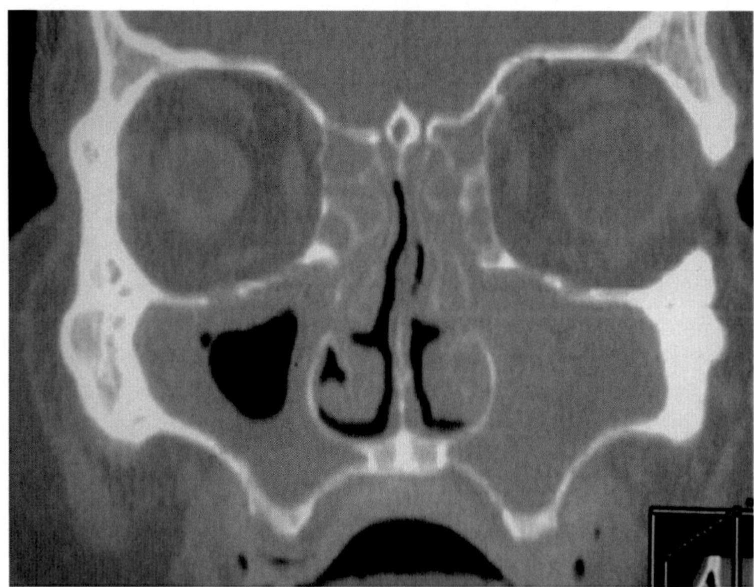

Fig. 25.2 Computed tomography of the maxillary sinuses showing thickened mucosa and air-fluid levels

25.4 Contraindications

*Careful consideration in patient with severe facial trauma. Otherwise no absolute contraindications.

25.5 Preparation/Materials

- 18G needle.
- 10 cc syringe.
- Local anesthetic (1 % or 2 % Xylocaine).
- Saline or antibiotic solution (if performing lavage).

25.6 Procedure/Technique

This procedure can be accomplished under local anesthesia via two approaches: either via the canine fossa or the inferior meatus (Fig. 25.4). This chapter will describe the canine fossa approach (Fig. 25.5).

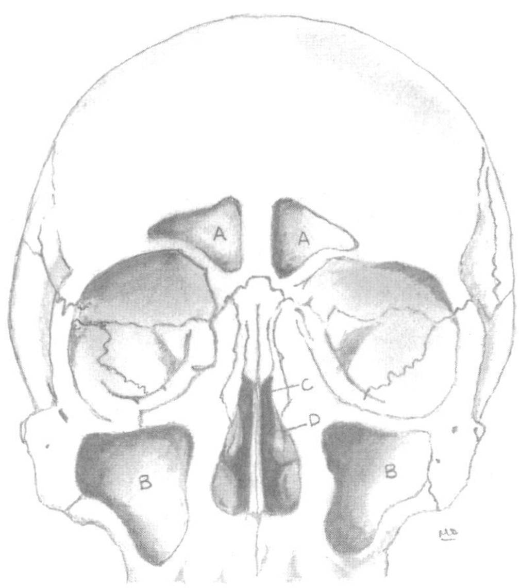

Fig. 25.3 Anatomy of the sinuses. (**a**) Frontal sinuses; (**b**) maxillary sinuses; (**c**) ethmoid sinuses; (**d**) sphenoid sinuses

- Identify the buccal gingival junction using the intersection of a line from the midpupillary axis, which intersects with a line at the level of the nasal vestibule [2].
- After application of adequate local anesthetic, insert the 18G needle at the aforementioned landmark. Use a slow and steady pressure while screwing the needle clockwise and counterclockwise at a 90° angle to the front of the maxilla [2].
- Use your nondominant hand to support entry to avoid slipping and penetrating the posterior wall of the sinus.
- Once entered, the maxillary sinus can be aspirated and/or lavaged with saline or an antibiotic-containing solution.

25.7 Complications

1. Posterior sinus wall puncture: this can be avoided by using the nondominant hand to support entry into the sinus to avoid the needle slipping and penetrating the posterior wall of the sinus.
2. Orbital puncture: injury can lead to retro-orbital hematoma, diplopia, subcutaneous orbital emphysema, or blindness [3]. Patients must be monitored closely for signs of elevated intraocular pressure.
3. Infraorbital nerve injury: using the nondominant hand for guidance of the needle can restrict the needle from gliding superiorly along the face of the maxilla and injuring the infraorbital nerve or orbit.
4. Bleeding: although rare, it is treated with nasal packing.

25.8 Conclusion

Sinusitis in the ICU patient can become a significant complication if left untreated. Drainage of the sinus (maxillary being most common) can be used to guide appropriate treatment modalities in patients affected with this type of infection.

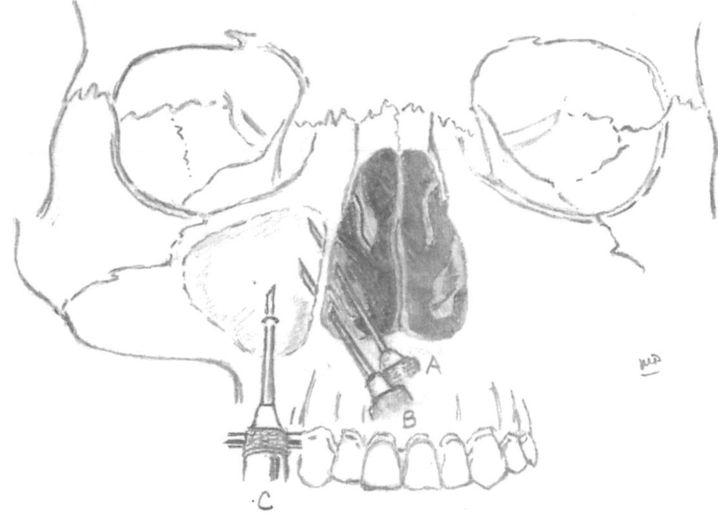

Fig. 25.4 Techniques for antral lavage. (**a**) Via the natural ostium; (**b**) via the inferior meatus; (**c**) via the canine fossa

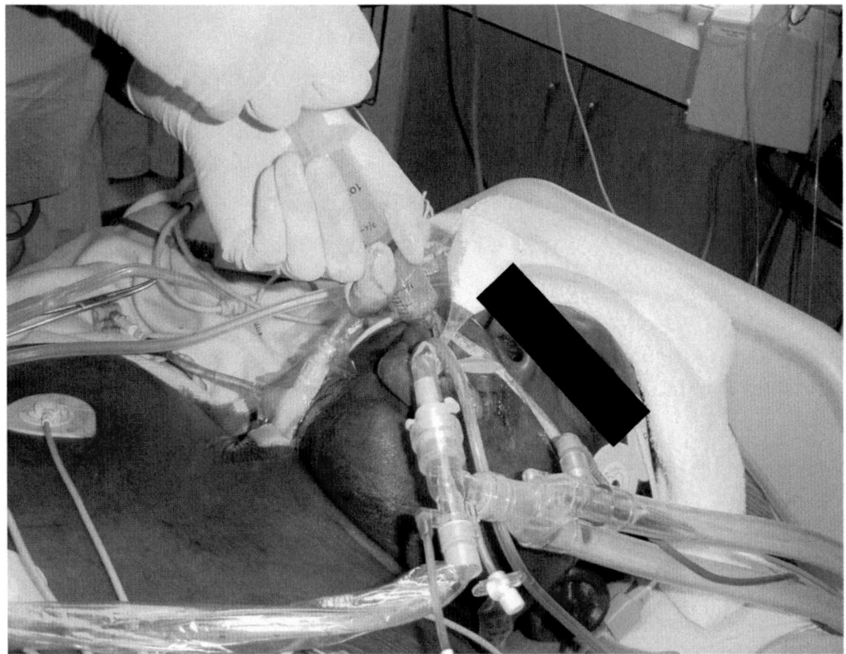

Fig. 25.5 Antral lavage via the canine fossa approach showing purulent aspirate from the maxillary sinus

References

1. Townsend Jr C, Beauchamp RD, Evers BM, Mattox KM. Sabiston textbook of surgery: the biological basis of modern surgical practice. 18th ed. Philadelphia: Saunders; 2008. p. 367. Chapter 15, surgical complications.
2. Schaitkin B. Canine fossa puncture: safe visualization of the recesses of the maxillary sinus. Oper Tech Otolaryngol Head Neck Surg. 2010;21(3): 160–62.
3. Lewis D, Busaba NY. Surgical management. In: Brook I, editor. Sinusitis: from microbiology to management. New York, NY: Taylor & Francis Group; 2006. p. 233–68.

26 Nasal Packing for Epistaxis

Jennifer J. Marrero and Ronald F. Sing

26.1 Introduction

Epistaxis is an acute hemorrhage or bleeding from the nostrils, nasal cavity, or nasopharynx. Epistaxis is a common occurrence in the general public with over half of the population likely to experience an event. Of this group approximately 6 % will seek medical attention and approximately 1.6 in 10,000 will require hospitalization [1]. There appears to be a bimodal distribution of occurrence with peaks in children and young adults and the older adult [2].

There are a myriad of causes for epistaxis which include trauma, foreign bodies, tumors, dry air, and most common cause of nose picking. Systemic factors include genetic clotting disorders such as von Willebrand's disease and medications such as warfarin (or other platelet inhibitors). However many episodes of epistaxis are idiopathic.

Many aspects of the treatment paradigm for epistaxis have not been evaluated in randomized trials. Nasal packing has been recognized as primary treatment for moderately severe epistaxis since it was first documented by Hippocrates in the fifth century BC (Singer et al. 2005) [12]. Commercially designed nasal tampons or epistaxis balloons were created as alternatives to ribbon gauze and are easier for less experience providers. Nasal tampons have shown effectiveness in 85 % of cases with no difference between the success rates of when compared to traditional ribbon gauze [2]. Other management options including cautery, embolization balloons, embolization, and fibrin glue exist although their use is variable. In a more recent randomized control trial involving 216 patients, Zahed et al. (2013) [13] demonstrated decreased rebleeding rates and increased patient satisfaction. There has been much debate, particularly as it is related to posterior epistaxis if surgery should be a primary treatment. A 2002 retrospective chart review and cost analysis determined that surgical intervention, which included embolization and ligation, carried a higher success rate, less hospitalization time, lower costs, and improved patient comfort than the traditional anterior/posterior packing [3]. Regardless of the treatment chosen, the use of stepwise management plans should limit complications and decrease the need for admission [2].

J.J. Marrero, MSN, ACNP-BC (✉)
Department of Trauma and Surgical Critical Care, Carolinas Medical Center, 1000 Blythe Blvd, Charlotte, NC 28203, USA

Carolinas HealthCare System/Carolinas Medical Center, Charlotte, NC 28232, USA
e-mail: Jennifer.marerro@carolinashealthcare.org

R.F. Sing, DO, FACS, FCCM
Carolinas HealthCare System/Carolinas Medical Center, Charlotte, NC 28232, USA
e-mail: Ronald.sing@carolinashealthcare.org

D.A. Taylor et al. (eds.), *Interventional Critical Care*, DOI 10.1007/978-3-319-25286-5_26

Prophylactic antibiotics for patients with nasal packing are controversial. There has been concern that patients with nasal packing were at risk for toxic shock syndrome as there has been a rate of 16.5 cases per 100,000 that was reported among patients with nasal packing from nasal surgery [4]. However it is unclear if this is related strictly to the packing or the surgery as patients who have sinonasal surgery with no nasal packing have had documented incidences of toxic shock syndrome [4]. A prospective study in the United Kingdom examined patients with nasal packing who received prophylactic antibiotics and compared them to patients who did not receive any antibiotics and determined there were no infectious processes that occurred in either group [5].

26.1.1 Indications

Bleeding sources are identified anatomically and have different treatment modalities. *Anterior bleeds*, which account for 90 % of epistaxis cases, are typically self-limiting and respond to conservative measures such as direct pressure. This location of bleeding is easily accessible as it originates at the Kiesselbach plexus or Little's area. This is the region in the anteroinferior part of the nasal septum where the anterior ethmoidal, sphenopalatine, greater palatine, and septal branch of the superior labial artery anastomose to form the vascular plexus [6]. Direct pressure should be applied to the cartilaginous part of the nose for approximately 20 min. If epistaxis continues, more invasive measures will need to be initiated.

Posterior bleeds are less common but can be life threatening and difficult to visualize and control. The sphenopalatine artery, the terminal branch of the maxillary artery, provides blood supply to the lateral nasal wall below the middle turbinates and is responsible for most cases of posterior epistaxis [6]. Direct pressure is not effective and difficult given the boniness of the nasal vault posteriorly. Posterior bleeds typically require packing.

26.2 Preparation and Setup

The advanced care practitioner (ACP) should explain the procedure to the patient. The explanation should include the possibility of discomfort and potential complications including difficulty breathing and continued hemorrhage.

The ACP should determine if premedication such as analgesia or an anxiolytic is warranted for the patient. Place patient in an upright position unless hemodynamic instability prevents this from occurring. Supplemental oxygen and emergency equipment including intubation supplies should be available. Adequate lighting and utilization of a headlamp will ease with examination. Gowns, gloves, mask, and eye protection for the ACP and other healthcare workers should be utilized and available. Additional supplies would include:

1. A commercially produced topical nasal decongestant or a mix of 2 % lidocaine and 1:1000 epinephrine-soaked cotton balls that are fashioned into a torpedo shape.
2. Nasal speculum.
3. Silver nitrate sticks.
4. Nasal tampons such as those made of polyvinyl alcohol sponge material, epistaxis balloons, or other packing materials (see Fig. 26.1).

A focused history and physical exam should aid the ACP in managing the acutely bleeding patient and include the following questions:

(a) Which side is bleeding?
(b) Are there any signs of trauma?
(c) Do medications include aspirin, warfarin, and platelet inhibitors?
(d) Do signs of hypovolemia or hypoxia include tachycardia, hypotension, and increased work of breathing?

Consider airway, breathing, and circulation (ABC) and stabilize the patient as needed before continuing. Consider correction of any anticoagulant medications if unable to control locally. Profuse bleeding may require airway control.

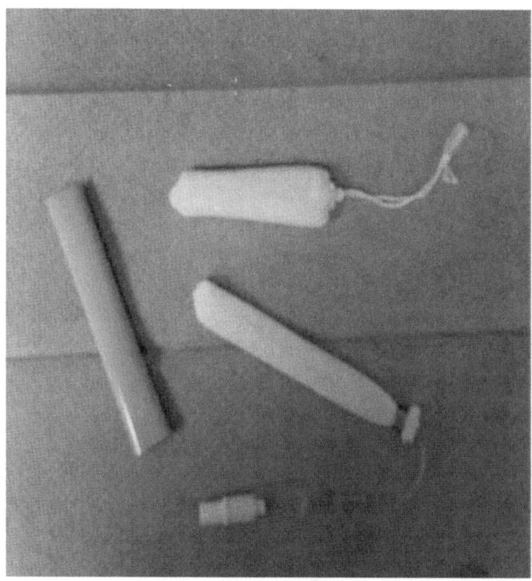

Fig. 26.1 Prefabricated nasal tampons are available with different options. One is compressed foam polymer that expands with water swelling and filling the nasal cavity applying pressure. The other has a balloon that is inflated with air to provide pressure. Apply surgical lubricant to the tampon and insert gently to maximum achievable depth and advance the tampon almost horizontally, along the floor of the nasal cavity. After application wetting the tampon with a small amount of topical vasoconstrictor such as pseudoephedrine may hasten its effectiveness. If using a tampon with a balloon, inflate the balloon with the amount of air recommended by the manufacturer

26.3 Procedure

1. Complete a focused history and physical examination if feasible. If unable to complete due to patient condition, any information obtained can be helpful.
2. Explain procedure to patient.
3. Prepare the nares with either:
   (a) Anesthetic-soaked cotton balls followed by dry cotton balls at the external nares.
   (b) Commercially produced decongestant such as pseudoephedrine nasal spray into nares followed by cotton balls and direct pressure for 10 min.
   (c) Additional option of utilizing ¼ or ½ inch packing gauze soaked with topical anesthetic and decongestant spray which will not leave any cotton fragments behind

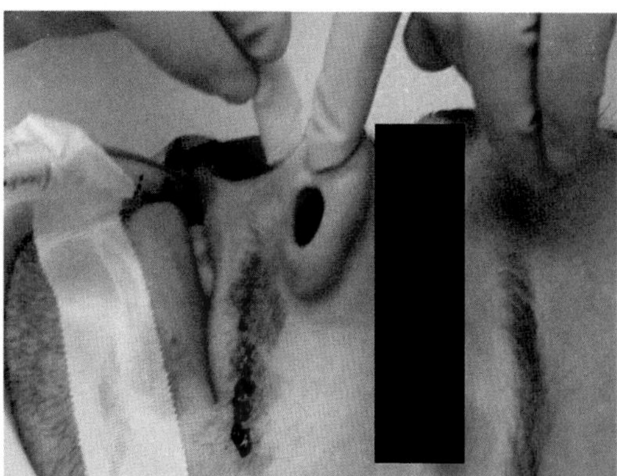

Fig. 26.2 Anterior packing using a prefabricated nasal tampon. Apply topical decongestant such as pseudoephedrine to nares prior to insertion. Apply surgical lubricant to the tampon and insert gently to maximum achievable depth and advance the tampon almost horizontally, along the floor of the nasal cavity straight back into maxillary sinus(es) below the inferior turbinates. Tape the strings or balloon to the side of face to keep in place

4. Remove the cotton balls/gauze and evacuate clots by suction or have patient blow gently.
5. Using a headlamp and speculum, examine nares for definitive source of bleeding.
6. If a vessel is visibly oozing, an attempt to chemically cauterize can be made. Apply silver nitrate stick for 5–10 s then to surrounding vessels for 5–10 s. An antibiotic ointment can be applied, and the patient will need to be observed for rebleeding.

Anterior Nasal Packing

If the bleeding does not stop with the above measures or a bleeding vessel is not easily identified, nasal packing will need to be considered.

1. Apply a generous amount of surgical lubricant to the prefabricated nasal tampon. If using epistaxis balloons, soak in sterile water for 30 s (see Fig. 26.2).
2. Insert into the nasal cavity along the septal floor and parallel to the hard palate until it is well within the nares.
3. Using a 20 ml syringe, inflate the device with air until the pilot cuff becomes rounded and feels firm when squeezed.
4. Tape the strings or the pilot cuff to the patient's cheek.

5. Consider adding topical hemostatic products such as oxidized regenerated cellulose (Surgiseal) and even fibrin glue.

Posterior Packing

If hemorrhage continues, it is likely a posterior bleed is present and posterior packing should be considered.

Posterior pharyngeal packing:

1. Cover cotton gauze roll with antibiotic ointment.
2. A lighted laryngoscope is used to retract the tongue and to allow exposure. Take care to avoid the endotracheal tube (see Fig. 26.3).
3. Utilize Magill forceps to place packing posterior and superior to the uvula. Do not use 4×4 but a long gauze packing as it is easy to leave one behind once the packing becomes bloody and compacted.
4. The packing that remains should be secured to the side of the patient's face with tape.
5. Generally anterior packing will need to be placed.

Additional options include the use of a sterile Foley catheter:

1. Remove the anterior pack and reexamine the nasal cavity. Suction and spray with anesthetic again.

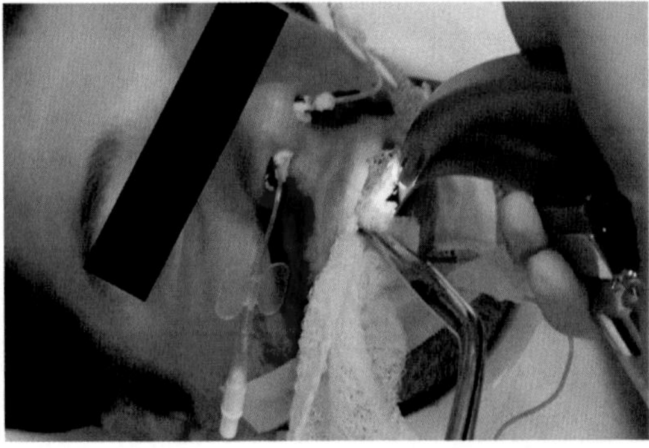

Fig. 26.3 Posterior packing with cotton gauze roll for continued bleeding. A lighted laryngoscope is used to retract the tongue and to allow exposure. Take care to avoid the endotracheal tube. Utilize Magill forceps to place packing posterior and superior to the uvula. Do not use 4×4 but a long gauze packing as it is easy to leave one behind once the packing becomes bloody and compacted

2. Apply mupirocin nasal ointment 2 % to Foley catheter.
3. Insert the catheter into the nostril.
4. Visualize the catheter tip in the back of the throat.
5. Inflate the balloon with up to 10 ml of sterile water.
6. Gently pull on the catheter toward you until you feel resistance and it seats posteriorly.
7. Secure with a clip to prevent dislodgement. Ensure the catheter is not pressing on the nose as alar necrosis could occur.
8. Consider repacking anteriorly.

26.4 Complications/Pitfalls in the ICU

Patients with posterior packing should be admitted for observation. Due to their risk of airway compromise and risk for bradydysrhythmias related to gagging/vageling due to stimulation of the deep oral pharynx with posterior packing, they should at a minimum be monitored with continuous pulse oximetry and telemetry. The ACP should plan ahead and anticipate the potential airway compromise and have equipment available to intubate. The ACP should be able to identify the signs of worsening respiratory status that would include increased work of breathing, tachycardia, and hypoxia. Some of these patients may require intubation.

Ongoing bleeding and dislodgement of packs are a risk and should be assessed with frequency. Initial laboratory evaluation should include a complete blood count, a serum chemistry, coagulation profile, and type and cross match for blood. An arterial blood gas may need to be obtained if there is concern for developing hypoxia or issues with ventilation in a patient.

Caution should be used with patients that have facial fractures particularly in the nasal bone and cribriform plate fractures. Maxillofacial fractures can present with profuse bleeding from the nose. Control of this massive nasal bleeding during the early stages can improve morbidity associated with severe exsanguination [7]. When common treatment modalities such as pressure, packing, and correction of coagulopathy fail to control hemorrhage, transcatheter arterial embolization by interventional radiology offers a safe alternative to surgical control [8].

Special consideration should be given to patients who receive anticoagulants such as warfarin or other platelet inhibitors and patients with acquired coagulopathies due to renal, liver disease, or genetic disorders such as hemophilia. They are at risk for life-threatening hemorrhage and need to be closely monitored. A prospective study performed in Zurich evaluated the need for blood transfusions in 591 epistaxis patients [9]. The study identified patients with hematologic disorders, trauma-related nosebleeds, and bleeds that were posterior in origin had a much higher rate of transfusion [9]. If bleeding continues, the ACP should consider initiation of fresh frozen plasma, vitamin K, and prothrombin complex concentrate or tranexamic acid administration.

Patients should be adequately resuscitated as indicated and undergo correction of coagulation abnormalities and electrolyte imbalances. Frequent assessment of patient's mental status, vital sign trends, and hourly urine output provides clues to the ACP about the end organ perfusion of the patient. Subtle changes can be missed and a diagnosis of shock can be overlooked. This can lead to detrimental effects on the patient including a prolonged hospitalization and even death.

If hemorrhage continues despite all previous measures, consideration for more invasive options should be considered. Consult with an otolaryngologist as indicated. Other options such as embolization and surgical ligation are available and both carry a success rate of 71–94 % [10]. However, they also have a risk of stroke, necrosis, and blindness [10, 11]. The decision between surgery and embolization should be based on the individual's comorbidities, anatomical setting, and availability of adequate interventional radiology and surgical specialty services [10].

Packing should be removed in 2–3 days. After packing is removed, nares should be moistened with bacitracin ointment twice a day along with Saline spray several times a day.

References

1. Viehweg TL, Roberson JB, Hudson JW. Epistaxis: diagnosis and treatment. J Oral Maxillofac Surg. 2006;64:511–8.
2. Pope LE, Hobbs CG. Epistaxis: an update on current 300 management. Postgrad Med J. 2004;81:309–14.
3. Klotz D, Winkle M, Richmon J, Hengerer A. Surgical management of posterior epistaxis: a changing paradigm. Laryngoscope. 2002;112:1577–82.
4. Schlosser R. Epistaxis N Engl J Med. 2009;360: 784–9.
5. Pepper C, Lo S, Toma A. Prospective study of risk of not using prophylactic antibiotics in nasal packing for epistaxis. J Laryngol Otol. 2012;126(3):257–9.
6. Douglas R, Wormald P. Update on epistaxis. Curr Opin Otolaryngol Head Neck Surg. 2007;15:180–3.
7. Shimoyama T, Kaneko T, Horie N. Initial management of massive oral bleeding after the midfacial fracture. J Trauma. 2003;54(2):332.
8. Bynoe RP, Kerwin AJ, Parker 3rd HH, Nottingham JM, Bell RM, Yost MJ, Close TC, Hudson ER, Sheridan DJ, Wade MD. Maxillofacial injuries and life-threatening hemorrhage: treatment with transcatheter arterial embolization. J Trauma. 2003;55(1):74.
9. Murer K, Nader A, Roth B, Holzmann D, Soyka M. THREAT helps to identify epistaxis patients requiring blood transfusions. J Otolaryngol Head Neck Surg. 2013;42(1):4.
10. Krajina A, Chrobok V. Radiological diagnosis and management of epistaxis. Cardiovasc Intervent Radiol. 2013;37:26–36.
11. Varshney S, Saxena R. Epistaxis: a retrospective clinical study. Indian J Otolaryngol Head Neck Surg. 2005;57(2):125–9.
12. Singer AJ, Blanda M, Cronin K. Comparison of nasal tampons for the treatment of epistaxis in the emergency department: a randomized controlled trial. Ann Emerg Med. 2005;45(2):134–9.
13. Zahed R, Moharamzadeh P, AlizadehArasi S, Ghasemi A, Saecdi M. A new and rapid method for epistaxis treatment using injectable form of tranexamic acid topically: a randomized controlled trial. Am J Emerg Med. 2013;31(9):1389–92.

Part VII

Gastrointestinal and Urologic Procedures

Enteral Access

27

Kate D. Bingham and John W. Mah

27.1 Introduction

Access to the upper gastrointestinal tract is often required in critically ill patients, and the placement of a nasoenteric or oroenteric tube frequently serves a dual purpose. Decompression and drainage of gastric secretions provide for comfort and safety in patients with abnormal forward motility due to ileus, outlet obstruction, or hypersecretion. The presence of an enteric tube also allows for administration of medications and nutritional support in patients incapable of swallowing once forward motility returns. While placement of a temporary enteric tube such as a Salem sump or small-bore silicone feeding tube is commonplace, there are techniques that enhance likelihood of successful placement in the location desired while minimizing the risk of complications [1].

K.D. Bingham, MS, PA-C, FCCM (✉)
Department of Quality and Patient Safety, Crozer-Keystone Health System, Healthplex Pavilion II Suite 225, 100 West Sproul Road, Springfield, PA 19064, USA
e-mail: katherine.bingham@crozer.org; kdbingham@msn.com

J.W. Mah, MD
Department of Surgery, Hartford Hospital, 80 Seymour Street, Hartford, CT 06102, USA
e-mail: John.mah@hhchealth.org

27.2 Indications

Decompression and drainage of the upper GI tract are best accomplished with a dual-lumen tube such as a Salem sump. The primary lumen serves as the drainage tube for air and liquid and is generally connected to low wall suction. The secondary lumen (often colored blue) allows entry of air necessary for the sump function and prevents the tube from adhering to the gastric wall and potentially causing mucosal erosion [2]. Suction should be kept at the lowest level that aids drainage, and tubes are best maintained on intermittent suction after initial evacuation of accumulated contents. Routine flushing of the secondary lumen with a small bolus (30–60 ml) of air helps maintain patency and sump function. Any occlusion of the secondary lumen by fluid or clamping/knotting prevents the tube from functioning as a drainage device; flushing or adjustment of suction to reestablish sump function should resolve any backup of fluid into the secondary lumen.

When decompression and drainage are no longer required, a Salem sump may be utilized as a short-term enteral access device for medications and tube feeding. However, the rigid nature of these PVC tubes and larger bore size creates discomfort, increases the risk of sinusitis, and impairs sinus drainage into the upper respiratory tract.

D.A. Taylor et al. (eds.), *Interventional Critical Care*, DOI 10.1007/978-3-319-25286-5_27

Enteral feeding tubes made of silicone are softer, more flexible, and of smaller bore size which enhances patient comfort and tolerance and minimizes sinus irritation and occlusion. They are well suited for tube feeding and administration of medications but do not allow aspiration of gastric contents given the collapse of soft walls. Commercial brands typically include a weighted tip to aid placement; the radiopaque tip and markings facilitate visualization on confirmatory radiographs. Some brands also contain a magnetized tip that can be externally manipulated with a magnet to aid placement.

Surgical or endoscopic placement of a feeding tube such as a gastrostomy or jejunostomy is an option for patients who require longer-term enteral access. The timing of placement of such tubes is controversial; however, placement of a more permanent feeding tube should be considered when complications of a temporary feeding tube are encountered and dysphagia is not resolving or when the need for permanent enteral access is determined.

27.3 Placement of Enteric Tubes

Prior to placing a nasoenteric tube of any kind, consideration must be given to the following:

- Relative and absolute contraindications for placement.
- Reason for placement and optimal tube type.
- Patient comfort and ability to follow directions during placement.
- Techniques to optimize final position.

27.4 Contraindications

Traumatic injury to the basilar skull or facial bones communicating with the nasal airway precludes placement of an enteric tube via the nasal route due to risk of inadvertent intracranial placement [3, 4]. Placement via the oral route is recommended in this circumstance. While most patients with such injuries will be intubated, an orogastric tube is rarely tolerated well in non-intubated patients, and only more rigid PVC tubes should be employed as thinner silicone feeding tubes are easily severed by chewing.

Esophageal and gastric anatomic abnormalities such as strictures, diverticuli, varices, and prior gastric or esophageal surgery (such as banding, gastric bypass, and esophagectomy) all raise concerns of complications with enteric tube placement, with strictures being most immediately concerning for risk of esophageal perforation. Placement in the setting of other esophageal and gastric abnormalities should be carefully weighed against the risks and avoided whenever possible; if deemed necessary, gentle placement by experienced hands is prudent.

Other systemic conditions should be considered as well. Coagulopathy and thrombocytopenia can lead to significant bleeding with even minor mucosal injury during placement, and placement of enteric tubes should be deferred if possible until the underlying diathesis is corrected.

Patient comfort and level of consciousness are critical in the successful placement of enteric tubes. Clear explanation for a responsive patient and simple directions can greatly facilitate placement. In unconscious or sedated patients, placement is more difficult and malposition not as easily recognized due to impaired communication.

27.5 Placing a Tube for Decompression

For conscious, cooperative, non-intubated patients—nasogastric:

1. Obtain necessary equipment and explain procedure to patient. For adult patients, a 14 or 16 French Salem sump tube is most commonly used.
2. Determine appropriate insertion length for tube: commonly the distance from tip of nose to tip of ear to tip of xiphoid is used to estimate length for placement.
3. Position patient sitting upright as much as possible and flex the head forward with chin toward the sternum.

4. Stretch out the tube to reduce coil memory and chance of looping on insertion. Lubricate the tube with surgical lubricant or topical anesthetic jelly. Consider spraying the posterior oropharynx with local anesthetic spray for comfort.
5. Insert the tube in either naris with tube in horizontal position (aiming for base of skull) and advance slowly. If the tube fails to pass easily, attempt in the other naris.
6. Advance tube to posterior oropharynx at which point the patient may gag. Encourage the patient to swallow as the tube is advanced more rapidly; sipping water via a straw may help. Stop and withdraw the tube if the patient cannot speak, begins coughing, or has ongoing gagging.
7. Advance tube to predetermined distance and auscultate an air bolus injected via the drainage port. Then aspirate on the drainage port; return of gastric contents is confirmation of positioning in the stomach or distal esophagus.
8. Connect to wall suction to evacuate gastric content. Secure the tube to the patient's nose with adhesive tape, taking care to avoid direct contact of the tube against the nares as pressure ulceration may result [5]. Use the markings on the tube as reference for the position of the tube at this point.
9. Radiographic confirmation of position is recommended prior to instillation of medications or tube feeding and serves to ensure the tube has not kinked or looped in the esophagus and the tip is intragastric and not esophageal or post-pyloric.

For intubated/tracheotomy patients—nasogastric or orogastric:

1. Obtain necessary equipment and explain procedure to patient, if responsive. For adult patients, a 14 or 16 French Salem sump tube is most commonly used.
2. Determine appropriate insertion length for tube:
   NG: distance from tip of nose to tip of ear to tip of xiphoid
   OG: lip to tip of ear to tip of xiphoid.
3. Position patient with head of bed elevated (if able) as much as possible.
4. Stretch out the tube to reduce coil memory and chance of looping on insertion.
   NG: lubricate the tube with surgical lubricant or lidocaine jelly.
   OG: lubrication may not be needed if oral secretions are present.
5. NG: insert the tube in either naris with tube in horizontal position (aiming for base of skull) and advance slowly. If the tube fails to pass easily, attempt in the other naris.
   OG: insert tube at corner of mouth between teeth and buccal mucosa and advance slowly. If the tube fails to pass easily, try opposite side of mouth or digital guidance.
6. Continue advancing the tube. Stop and withdraw the tube if the patient begins coughing; despite the presence of an endotracheal or tracheotomy tube with an inflated cuff, tubes can transit past the cuff.
   NG: lifting/flexing the patients' head forward may aid placement.
7. If resistance or looping occurs, consider utilizing direct laryngoscopy to visualize the tube and guide it into the proximal esophagus. Alternatively, in unresponsive or edentulous patients, digital guidance of the tube in the oropharynx may be utilized.
8. Advance tube to predetermined distance and auscultate an air bolus injected via the drainage port. Then aspirate on the drainage port; return of gastric contents is confirmation of positioning in the stomach or distal esophagus.
9. Connect to wall suction to evacuate gastric contents.
   NG: secure the tube to the patient's nose with adhesive tape, taking care to avoid direct contact of the tube against the nares as pressure ulceration may result.
   OG: secure the tube to the patients' endotracheal tube or tube holder.
   Use the markings on the tube as reference for the position of the tube at this point.
10. Radiographic confirmation of position is recommended prior to instillation of medications or tube feeding and serves to ensure the tube has not kinked or looped in the esophagus and the tip is intragastric and not esophageal or post-pyloric.

27.6 Temporary Feeding Tubes

The use of temporary feeding tubes is common in critical care, particularly in intubated, mechanically-ventilated patients requiring enteral nutritional support during resolution of their acute respiratory failure. While many patients tolerated gastric feeding, the theoretical benefit of a second barrier to reflux (the pylorus) in addition to the lower esophageal sphincter often leads to effort to position the tube as distally as possible. It is often possible to achieve this position at the bedside with attentive placement technique, thereby negating the need for fluoroscopy or travel to interventional radiology with their corresponding risks, inconvenience, and expense.

Supplies for Feeding Tube Placement
Feeding tube
60 cc luer-lock syringe
Cup of water
Lubricant or topical anesthetic jelly
Tape
Gloves
Stethoscope
Promotilant (optional)

27.7 Placing a Feeding Tube

1. Obtain necessary equipment and explain procedure to patient, if responsive. For adult patients, a 10 or 12 French silicone feeding tube (Dobhoff type) is most commonly used.
2. Position patient with head of bed elevated (if able) as much as possible and head in neutral or slightly flexed position.
3. Consider administration of promotilant (metoclopramide 10 mg IV within a few minutes of placement) to aid distal placement.
4. Remove wire stylet from feeding tube, lubricate with surgical lubricant, and then replace in feeding tube (aids later removal of stylet without displacement of tube). Close the side access port if present and ensure stylet connector is securely seated into tube. Generously lubricate the tip of the tube with surgical lubricant or topical anesthetic jelly. Consider spraying the posterior oropharynx with local anesthetic spray for comfort.
5. Insert the tube in either naris with tube in horizontal position (aiming for base of skull) and advance slowly. If the tube fails to pass easily, attempt in the other naris.
6. Advance tube to posterior oropharynx at which point the patient may gag. Encourage the patient to swallow as the tube is advanced. If resistance is met, pull the tube back a few centimeters, rotate, and reinsert. Stop and withdraw the tube if the patient cannot speak (non-intubated), begins coughing, or has ongoing gagging. Despite the presence of an endotracheal tube with an inflated cuff, tubes can transit past the cuff.
7. Continue advancing the tube to the 25 cm mark and stop. When the patient exhales (spontaneously breathing) or ventilator breath is initiated, briefly dip the hub of the tube into a cup of water. If bubbling occurs, the tube is likely in the airway; pull back the tube to the posterior oropharynx and reattempt advancement. If no bubbling occurs, the tube is likely in the esophagus and can continue advancement to 50 cm.
8. When at 50 cm, auscultate 20–30 cc air boluses at the LUQ, RUQ, and epigastrium. The loudest sound should be at the LUQ if the tube is in the stomach. While the tube could be used in this position, we recommend advancing the tube to the most distal position achievable.
9. To advance distally for duodenal placement, lower the head of the bed to 15° and position the patient right side down as able.
10. Insufflate the stomach with 500–1000 cc of air as rapidly as possible to stimulate peristalsis.
11. Slowly advance the feeding tube in 2–4 cm increments, rotating it slowly as you advance (to prevent looping). If any resistance is met, retract a 2–4 cm, rotate, instill a 10 cc air bolus, and readvance.
12. Continue advancing the tube until unable to overcome resistance with the above maneuvers or the tube is maximally inserted to the hub.

13. Do not remove the stylet! The stylet needs to stay in place until tube position is confirmed radiographically, as once removed it cannot be safely reinserted due to risk of tube and potential intestinal perforation. Secure the tube to the patient's nose with adhesive tape, taking care to avoid direct contact of the tube against the nares as pressure ulceration may result.
14. Radiographic confirmation is required for all feeding tubes prior to use. Use the markings on the tube as reference for the position of the tube at this point, which facilitates future assessment as to whether the tube has moved from the original radiographically confirmed position. Optimal position is depicted in Fig. 27.1, with the tube following the lesser curve of the stomach, crossing midline as it transits the pylorus, and following the C curve of the duodenum. A malpositioned tube, such as the example in Fig. 27.2, should be removed immediately.
15. Once radiographic confirmation is obtained, the stylet can be removed. If any resistance is felt with removal of the stylet, repeat radiographic assessment may be needed to ensure the tube did not retract during stylet removal.

27.8 Special Conditions: Suturing and Bridling

Other means of securing nasogastric and feeding tubes may be employed in patients with increased risk for dislodging the tube and requiring replacement or when frequent replacement is required in patients prone to repeatedly displacing or removing them due to agitation, delirium, or noncooperation. Suturing to the nasal septum is not recommended as tissue damage and loss can be cosmetically catastrophic. The use of a bridle that serves as an irritant when traction is applied to the tube is a safer alternative when other means of securing tubes are exhausted. Commercial magnetized bridle products are available, or a simple technique using pediatric suction catheters can be utilized to serve as a bridle [6].

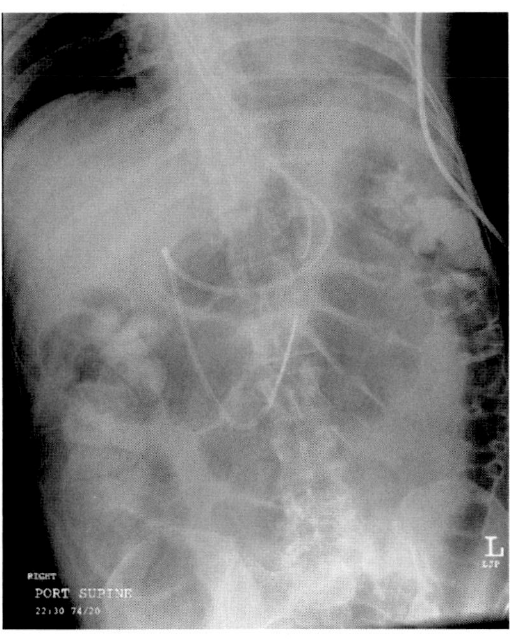

Fig. 27.1 Correctly positioned post-pyloric feeding tube with tip in distal duodenum

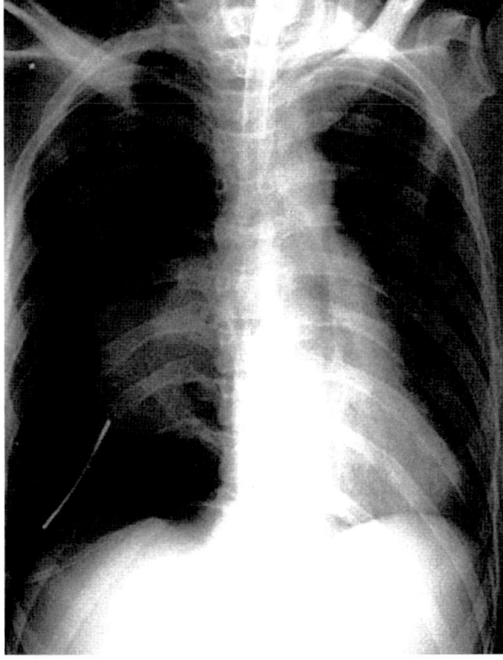

Fig. 27.2 Malpositioned feeding tube in right main stem bronchus

Bridling:

1. Obtain two pediatric suction catheters, McGill or other long forceps/clamp, and 2–0 or 3–0 silk suture.
2. Insert one pediatric suction catheter in each naris as you would an NG tube until the tips are visible in the oropharynx.
3. Pull the tips out through the mouth and secure/suture to each other using the silk suture. Suturing through the plastic tubing is most effective.
4. Pull back on the hubs of the suction catheters at the nares, returning the now connected suction catheters to the posterior nasopharynx.
5. Attach the feeding tube to the two suction catheters externally at the nares by braiding them together then taping securely.

27.9 Complications

The pulmonary complication associated with nasoenteric feeding tube placement carries significant morbidity. Placement of a tube into the airway can cause perforation of the trachea or bronchi, resulting in pneumothorax, empyema, or mediastinitis. Inadvertent administration of tube feedings, contrast, or medications can result in aspiration pneumonitis/pneumonia, pulmonary abscess, and empyema. Less morbid but still problematic is reflux from stenting by a nasoenteric tube, particularly rigid decompression tubes, lead to an increased risk of aspiration pneumonia.

The gastrointestinal complications associated with nasoenteric tubes include reflux esophagitis related to tube stenting the lower esophageal sphincter. Esophageal, gastric, or duodenal perforation may occur on insertion or due to mucosal ulceration over time. Narrow-bore feeding tubes are prone to clogging if close attention is not paid to routine flushing and appropriate administration of medications; liquid formulas are preferred over crushed meds whenever available. Osmotic diarrhea associated with tube feed formulas and many enteral liquid medication formulas (particularly those containing sorbitol) is also common.

Other complications include sinusitis from impaired sinus drainage due to tube occlusion. Epistaxis may occur on insertion or at a later point in time due to local mucosal irritation. Skin breakdown pressure necrosis at the nares or nasal septum may occur with subsequent cosmetic disfigurement [5, 7].

27.10 Conclusion

Thoughtful tube selection and knowledgeable placement are essential for optimizing tube function while minimizing complications and patient discomfort. The simple techniques described can improve successful placement with fewer attempts, less resource utilization, and potentially earlier initiation of tube feeding.

References

1. Lee JM, et al. Web-based teaching module improves success rates of postpyloric positioning of nasoenteric feeding tubes. JPEN. 2012;36:323.
2. Metheny NA, Meert KL, Clouse RE. Complications related to feeding tube placement. Curr Opin Gastroenterol. 2007;23:178.
3. Ferreras J, Junquera LM, Garcia-Consuegra L. Intracranial placement of a nasogastric tube after severe craniofacial trauma. Oral Surg Oral Med Oral Pathol Oral Radiol Endod. 2000;90:564.
4. Baskaya MK. Inadvertent intracranial placement of a nasogastric tube in patients with head injuries. Surg Neurol. 1999;52:426.
5. Banerjee TS, Schneider HJ. Recommended method of attachment of nasogastric tubes. Ann R Coll Surg Engl. 2007;89:529.
6. della Faille D, Schmelzer B, Hartoko T, et al. Securing nasogastric tubes in non-cooperative patients. Acta Otorhinolaryngol Belg. 1996;50:195.
7. Lai PB, Pang PC, Chan SK, Lau WY. Necrosis of the nasal ala after improper taping of a nasogastric tube. Int J Clin Pract. 2001;55:145.

Placement of Difficult Nasogastric Tube

28

Tracy R. Land

28.1 Indications

- Gastric decompression
- Short- to medium-term enteral nutrition (up to 6 weeks) [1]
- Short- to medium-term enteral medication administration

28.2 Contraindications

- Acute skull base fracture or surgery
- Acute facial fracture or surgery
- Acute nasal fractures or surgery

Orogastric tubes can be considered in these patients if they have an orotracheal tube in place.

- Esophageal varices
- Acute esophageal perforation
- Moderate to severe esophageal stricture
- Known tracheoesophageal fistula

If nasogastric (NG) or orogastric (OG) access is required, consider placement with direct endoscopic visualization only and expert consultation.

T.R. Land, MSN, ACNP-BC, CVNP-B (✉)
Department of Intensivist, Cardiac ICU, East Carolina Heart Institute at Vidant Medical Center, 115 Heart Drive, Greenville, NC 27834, USA
e-mail: Ceric_tracy_land@hotmail.com

If there has been any work on the plumbing, i.e., gastric bypass, gastric banding, and Nissan fundoplication, the placement of gastric tubes should be done with caution, and expert consultation should be considered.

28.3 Literature Review

There are very few current resources addressing difficult NG tube placement. The techniques fall into three categories: tube pliability, direct and indirect visualization, and patient position. Techniques for tube pliability include preshaping a tube by placing the tip of the tube in an oral airway and submersing the combination into ice water for approximately 20 min [2], filling an NG/OG tube with distilled water, and keeping the syringe in place [2]. If the tube is still not rigid enough, they recommend filling an NG/OG tube with distilled water and freezing [3]. These techniques are concerning because of the risk of aspiration. Other references recommend warming up the tube to make it more flexible [4]. Several articles suggest a stylet technique utilizing a ureteral guidewire [5], a 6-Fr angiography catheter [6], a guitar string as a guidewire [6], and an esophageal spring-tipped guidewire [7]. These techniques need to be used with great caution as they greatly increase the risk of perforation or in the instance of inadvertent tracheal intubation, a pneumothorax. It may be safest to leave the guitar string on the guitar and utilize it to serenade the

D.A. Taylor et al. (eds.), *Interventional Critical Care*, DOI 10.1007/978-3-319-25286-5_28

patient into a state of calm before placing the NG tube. One article recommended a pseudo stylet by securing a "Rusch" intubation stylet to the outside of the NG tube utilizing a 70 cm 3-0 silk suture tied with a quick release knot such as a Draw Hitch [8]. Although the article did not report any complications again, there is concern that utilizing an intubation stylet can increase the risk of esophageal perforation. Also this particular stylet and a 70 cm length suture are more likely to be available in the operating room than in the intensive care unit (ICU). Other studies recommend a Seldinger technique utilizing an endotracheal (ET) tube (#6.5–7.0) split longitudinally [2, 5]. This section also includes the recommendation of utilizing forceps or gloved fingers [5, 7]. This technique is limited by the size of the patient's mouth, the length of the provider's fingers, and quite frankly the provider's bravery. If gloved fingers are going to be utilized to help pass the NG/OG tube through the oropharynx, it is recommended that the patient be sedated and possibly paralyzed; absence of dentition would be a bonus.

Direct visualization techniques include the use of a nasendoscope or bronchoscope [9, 10], videolaryngoscope [2], or laryngoscope [3, 9]. Endoscopic use will allow for direct visualization of the tube from the oropharynx through the pyloris and into the duodenum. Patients with esophageal pathology should have any NG or OG tube placed with the assistance of endoscopy. The availability of equipment and trained personnel will most often require consultation of a specialty service. Covidien has recently come out with the Kangaroo™ feeding tube with IRIS Technology. This is a disposable feeding tube with a 3 mm camera in the distal tip, with LED lighting that allows the user to directly visualize placement via a proprietary monitor [11].

Indirect visualization can be accomplished with fluoroscopy and external magnet and monitor-assisted equipment such as the CORTRAK®2 Enteral Access System (EAS™).

Patient position is the least invasive of all techniques and the most effective. Positioning recommendations include neck extension, neck flexion, lateral neck pressure, lateral deviation of the thyroid cartilage and cricoid cartilage, and upward deviation of the thyroid cartilage or cricoid cartilage [2–6]. A simple recommendation was from an article in the British Medical Journal in 1981. They recommend that once the NG tube is past the nasopharynx, rotate the tube 180° allowing the tube to track along the posterior aspect of the oropharynx [4]. A study done by Ozer and Benumof published in Anesthesiology in 1999 best demonstrates why patient position is essential in the placement of an NG or OG tube in an orotracheally intubated and sedated patient. They took six patients who were orotracheally intubated and under general anesthesia and directly observed the passing of an NG tube and an OG tube via a fibrotic scope that was passed through each patients left naris. They found that passage of the NG or OG tube is most commonly blocked by the arytenoid cartilage and ipsilateral piriform sinus and that lateral neck compression or anterior deviation of the thyroid cartilage facilitated tube passage into the esophagus [10]. One very small study found that they have an 80 % first pass success rate with lateral positioning of the head compared to 40 % with a neutral head position. They believe that simply turning the patients head in the lateral position provides the same benefit of lateral neck compression or anterior deviation of the thyroid cartilage but with a slightly simpler technique [12].

28.4 Complications

Although placement of an NG or OG tube has become a routine procedure in the critical care setting, it is not without risk of serious complications (Figs. 28.1, 28.2, and 28.3).

- Intracranial placement can occur in the setting of basal skull injury or surgery, facial fracture, or nasal fracture.
- Esophageal perforation
- Tracheal intubation
- Pneumothorax
- Aspiration
- Knotted tube

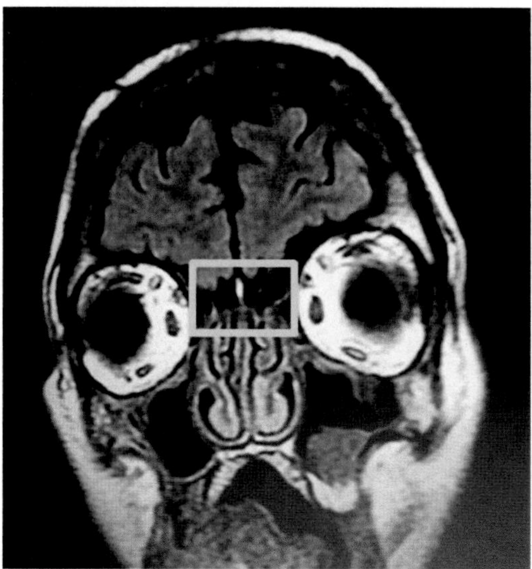

Fig. 28.1 MRI shows the close proximity of the nasal cavity to the brain. Photo by Tracy R. Land ACNP-BC, CVNP-BC

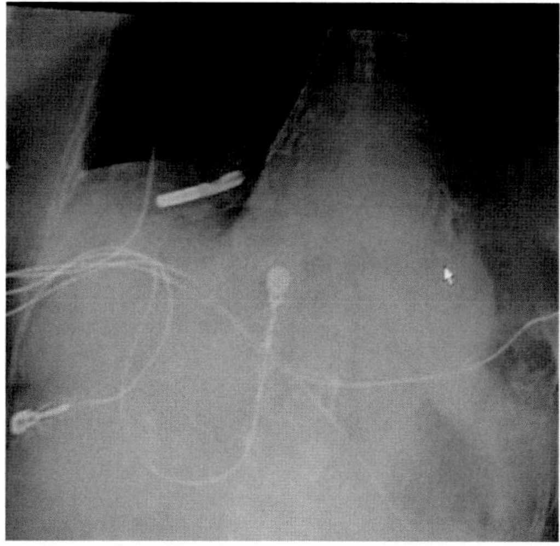

Fig. 28.2 Chest X-ray showing placement of a weighted feeding tube into the right mainstem bronchus. Photo by Tracy R. Land ACNP-BC, CVNP-BC

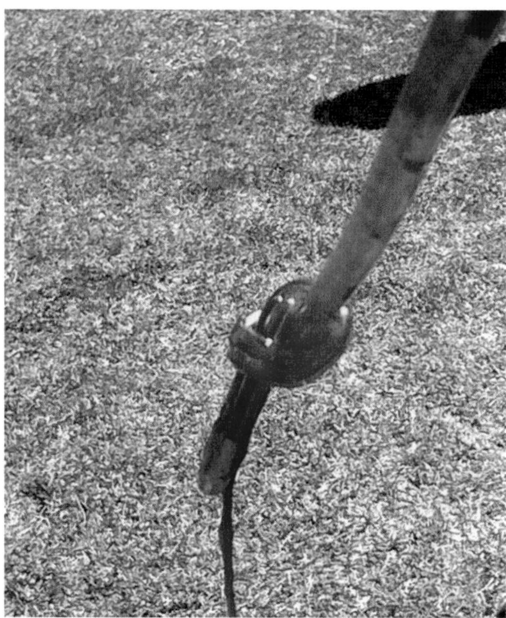

Fig. 28.3 Image of an NG tube right after removal. The tube was placed much deeper than the external measurement indicated; when the provider went to remove the tube he met resistance but ultimately pulled the tube out. The patient had epistaxis for approximately 20 min and mild sinusitis for a few days. Fortunately the patient did not suffer any long term effects. Photo by Richard Wiegert B.S., NREMT-P

28.5 Procedures

Measuring the required depth of the NG tube is usually performed by anchoring the distal tip of the NG tube at the tip of the nose, extending it to the ear and down to the xiphoid process. This is known as nose–ear–xiphoid (NEX) [13, 14]. Chen et al. performed a retrospective study of 31 patients who had NG tubes placed utilizing NEX and evaluated CT scans to identify the location of all the side holes on the NG tube. They found that only one out of 31 patients had all side holes placed beyond the esophagogastric junction. Another measurement technique is xiphoid–ear–nose (XEN) that was also inadequate in assuring that all side holes are beyond the esophagogastric junction [14]. Based on this information, the recommendation is to use NEX plus an additional 10 cm (Table 28.1).

Lateral Head Position NG:

1. Gather the standard equipment for tube placement.
2. Measure required depth for insertion beyond the esophagogastric junction utilizing NEX + 10 cm and mark your tube.
3. Once the naris is selected, turn the patient's head to the ipsilateral side if there are no contraindications, i.e., right naris = head turned to the right.

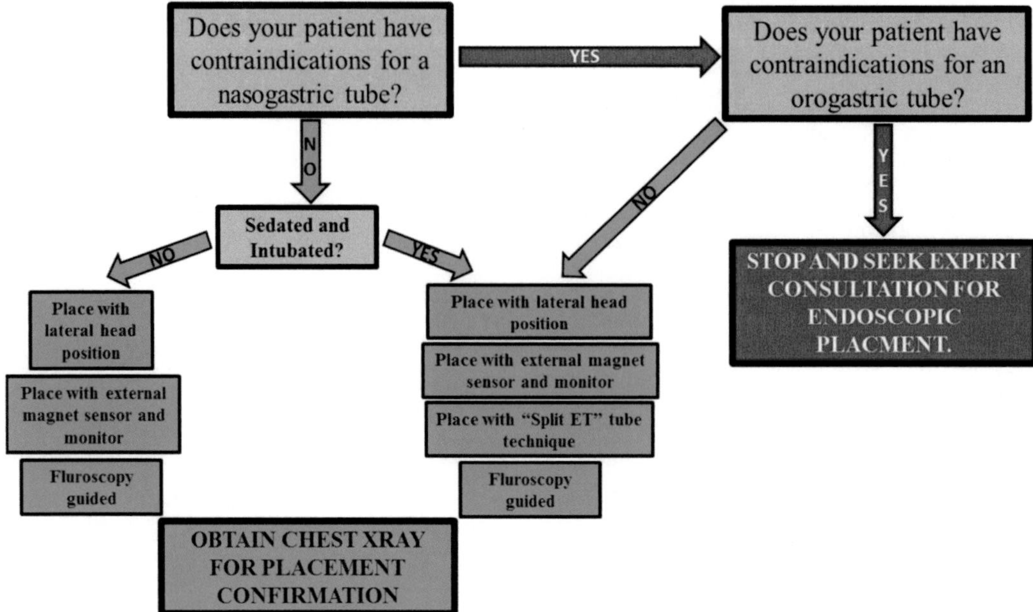

Table 28.1 NG/OG Tube Decision Matrix

4. Pass a pre-lubricated tube through the naris beyond the nasopharynx.
5. Rotate the tube 180° and advance until the tube reaches NEX + 10 cm mark.
6. Auscultate over the left upper quadrant while injecting a 20 ml air bolus.
7. If gurgling is heard, secure the tube to the naris and get a chest X-ray to confirm placement.
8. If gurgling is not heard, continue to advance up to an additional 10 cm, secure the tube at the naris, and get a chest X-ray to identify the tube position.
9. If at any time the patient has coughing, wheezing, oxygen desaturation, or difficulty ventilating, immediately remove the tube.
10. If the tube becomes difficult to pass at the gastroesophageal junction (NEX) or pyloric junction, a 5–10 ml bolus of air while advancing the tube will often facilitate passage of the tube beyond the sphincter.
11. Always confirm placement with a chest X-ray.

Lateral Head Position OG: This should only be performed in an orotracheally intubated patient.

1. Gather the standard equipment for tube placement.
2. Measure required depth for insertion beyond the esophagogastric junction utilizing NEX + 10 cm and mark your tube.
3. If there are no contraindications, rotate the patient's head to either the right or left.
4. Pass a tube through the mouth with the curve tracing down along the back of the oropharynx.
5. Once the tube is beyond the oropharynx, rotate it 180° to allow the tube to track along the posterior wall of the esophagus, and then advance the tube until NEX + 10 cm mark is reached. Lubrication is optional as saliva is generally sufficient for lubrication.
6. Auscultate over the left upper quadrant while injecting a 20 ml air bolus.
7. If gurgling is heard, secure the tube to the ET tube and get a chest X-ray to confirm placement.
8. If gurgling is not heard, continue to advance up to an additional 10 cm, secure the tube to the ET tube, and get a chest X-ray to identify the tube position.

9. If at any time the patient has coughing, wheezing, oxygen desaturation, or difficulty ventilating immediately, remove the tube.
10. If the tube becomes difficult to pass at the gastroesophageal junction (NEX) or pyloric junction, a 5–10 ml bolus of air while advancing the tube will often facilitate passage of the tube beyond the sphincter.
11. Always confirm placement with a chest X-ray.

Fluoroscopic-assisted placement:

1. Gather the standard equipment for tube placement.
2. Measure required depth for insertion beyond the esophagogastric junction utilizing NEX + 10 cm as a reference point.
3. Before initiating fluoroscopy make certain everyone in the room is wearing appropriate protective equipment.
4. Place a metal hemostat over the xiphoid process and acquaint yourself with your location and the patient's anatomy under fluoroscopy.
5. Pass a pre-lubricated tube through the naris beyond the nasopharynx.
6. Rotate the tube 180° and advance under fluoroscopic guidance until the tube reaches the desired location either in the gastric body or beyond the pylorus and NEX + 10 cm.
7. Secure the tube to the naris.
8. If at any time the patient has coughing, wheezing, oxygen desaturation, or difficulty ventilating immediately, remove the tube.
9. If the tube becomes difficult to pass at the gastroesophageal junction (NEX) or pyloric junction, a 5–10 ml bolus of air while advancing the tube will often facilitate passage of the tube beyond the sphincter.
10. A chest X-ray is not required to confirm placement if the tube was placed under fluoroscopic guidance.

Split ET tube-assisted placement: This should only be performed on an orotracheally intubated and sedated patient.

1. Gather the standard equipment for tube placement, a #6.5–7.0 ET tube, a scalpel, scissors, and a Magill forceps (Fig. 28.4).
2. Remove ET tube end cap (Fig. 28.5).

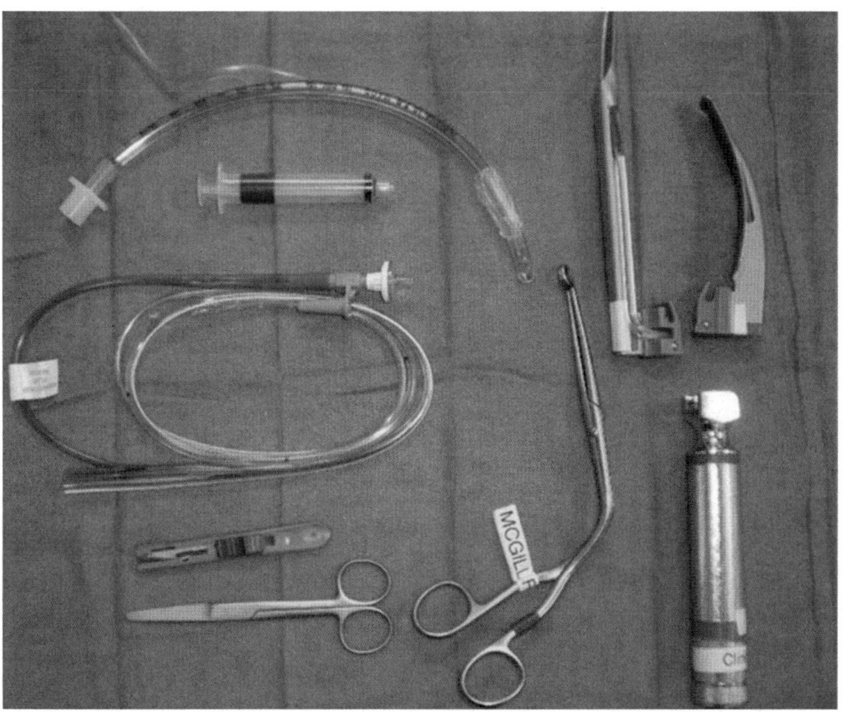

Fig. 28.4 Materials for split ET tube-assisted placement. Photo by Tracy R. Land, ACNP-BC, CVNP-BC

3. Using the scalpel make a longitudinal cut down the length of the ET tube. Scissors can also be utilized to assist in splitting the ET tube. Pull the cut open and work the ET tube to loosen up the cut (Figs. 28.6, 28.7, and 28.8).
4. Measure required depth for insertion beyond the esophagogastric junction utilizing NEX + 10 cm and mark your tube.
5. Once the naris is selected, pass a pre-lubricated tube through the selected naris beyond the nasopharynx until the tube can be visualized in the oropharynx (Fig. 28.9).
6. Utilizing the Magill forceps, grasp the distal portion of the tube, and pull it out of the mouth until the proximal portion of the tube is approximately 10 cm from the naris (Figs. 28.10 and 28.11).

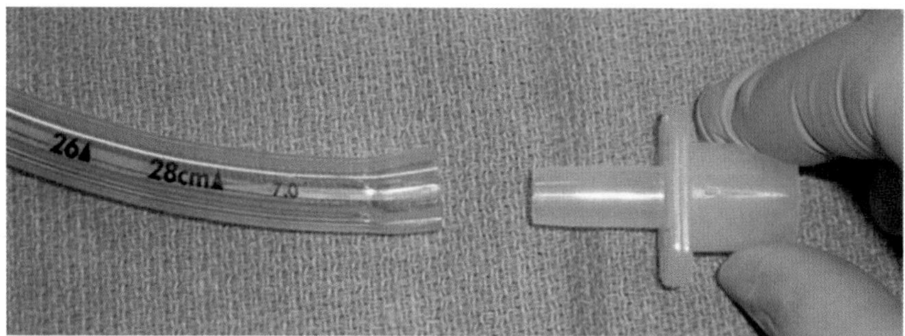

Fig. 28.5 Removal of the ET end cap in the split ET tube-assisted placement technique. Photo by Tracy R. Land ACNP-BC, CVNP-BC

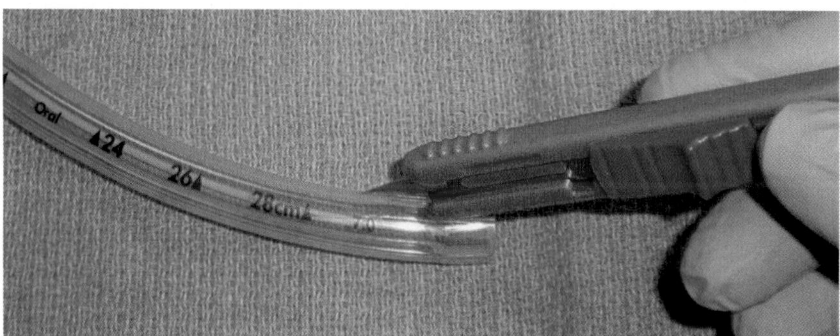

Fig. 28.6 Making an incision to the ET tube in the split ET tube-assisted placement technique. Photo by Tracy R. Land, ACNP-BC, CVNP-BC

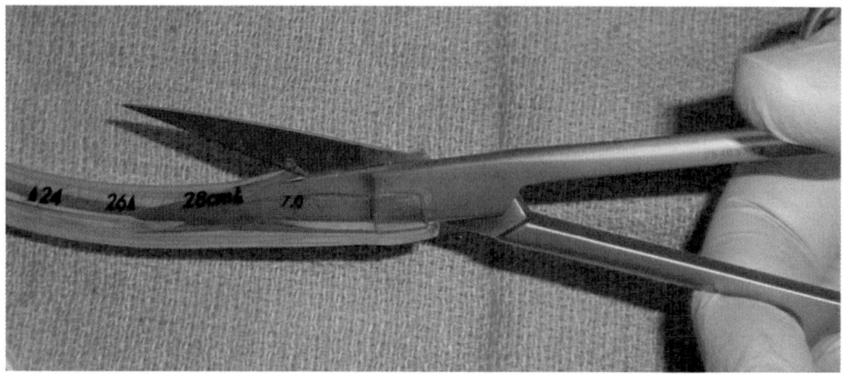

Fig. 28.7 Using scissors in cutting the ET tube in the split ET tube-assisted placement technique. Photo by Tracy R. Land, ACNP-BC, CVNP- BC

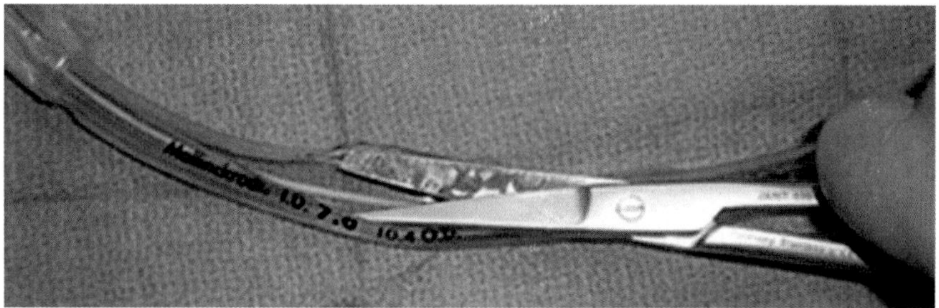

Fig. 28.8 Using scissors in cutting the ET tube in the split ET tube-assisted placement technique. Photo by Tracy R. Land, ACNP-BC, CVNP- BC

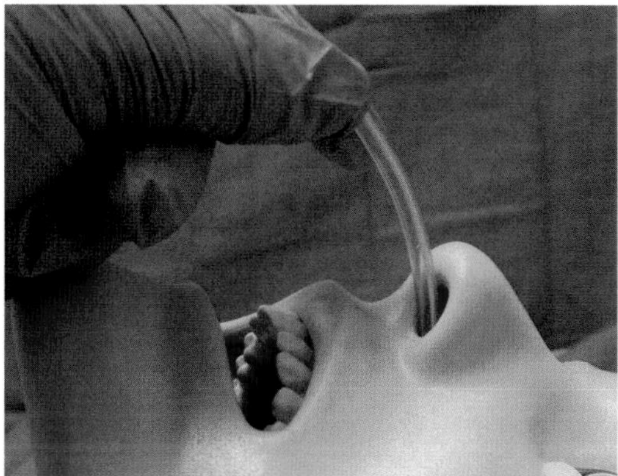

Fig. 28.9 Inserting the tube in the nares. Photo by Tracy R. Land, ACNP-BC, CVNP-BC

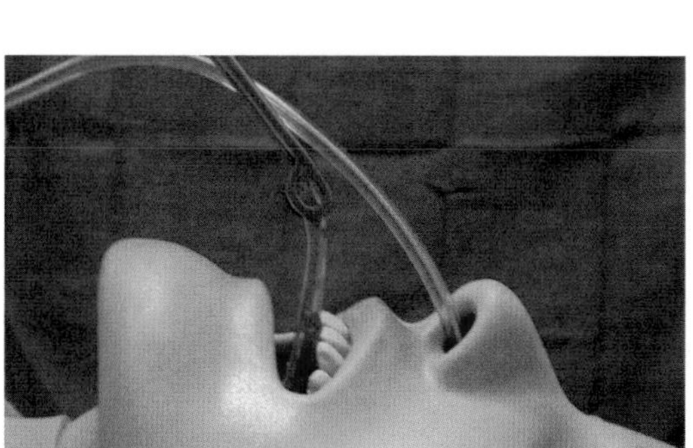

Fig. 28.10 Removal of the tube with Magill forceps via the oropharynx. Photo by Tracy R. Land, ACNP-BC, CVNP-BC

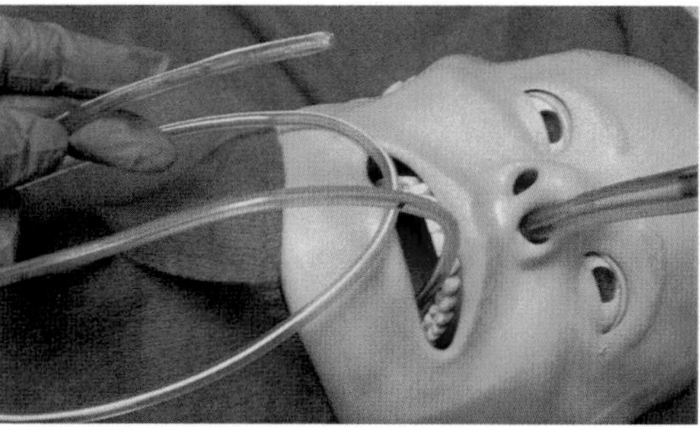

Fig. 28.11 Proper positioning of the tube in the nares. Photo by Tracy R. Land, ACNP-BC, CVNP-BC

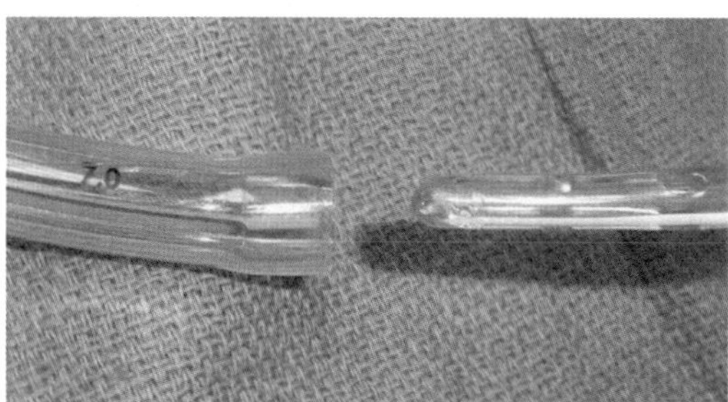

Fig. 28.12 Preparing placement of the NG tube into the ETT. Photo by Tracy R. Land, ACNP-BC, CVNP-BC

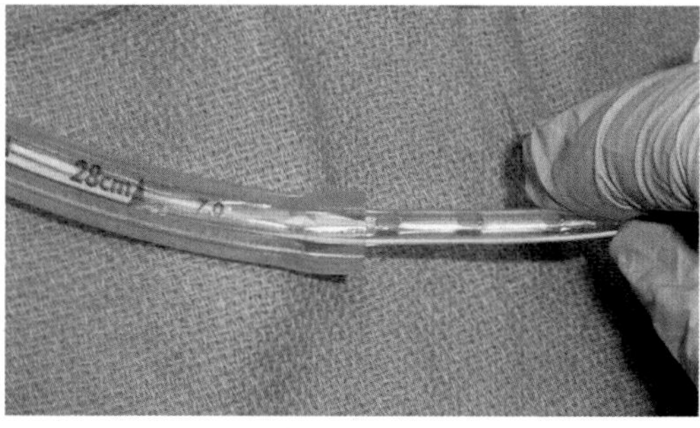

Fig. 28.13 Placement of the NG tube into the ET tube. Photo by Tracy R. Land ACNP-BC, CVNP-BC

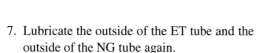

7. Lubricate the outside of the ET tube and the outside of the NG tube again.
8. Place the NG tube into the ET tube keeping the tip of the NG tube just inside the ET tube (Figs. 28.12 and 28.13).
9. Advance the ET tube blindly into the esophagus to approximately 18 cm and hold

securely in place. If you are having difficulty advancing the ET tube into the esophagus, you can utilize the lateral head maneuver or perform this under direct visualization with a laryngoscope or a videolaryngoscope (Fig. 28.14).

10. Advance the NG tube through the ET tube until you reach your NEX + 10 cm mark (Fig. 28.15).

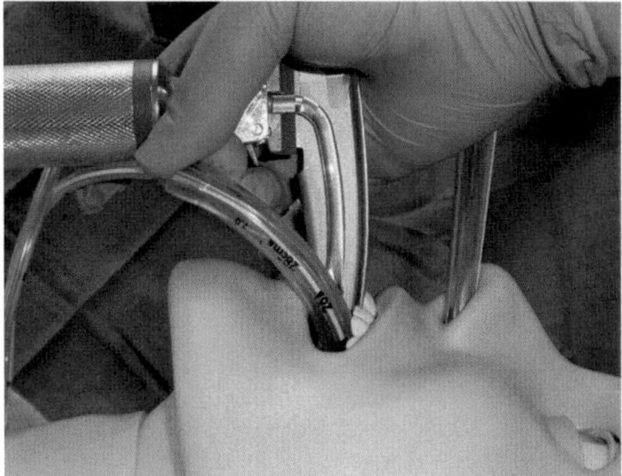

Fig. 28.14 Using the laryngoscope to assist insertion the NT tube into the esophagus. Photo by Tracy R. Land ACNP-BC, CVNP-BC

11. Gently peel the ET tube off of the NG tube (Fig. 28.16).
12. Remove ET tube completely from the patient's mouth and discard (Fig. 28.17).
13. Back the NG tube out of the naris until your NEX + 10 cm mark is at the naris (Figs. 28.18 and 28.19).
14. Auscultate over the left upper quadrant while injecting a 20 ml air bolus.
15. If gurgling is heard, secure the tube to the naris and get a chest X-ray to confirm placement.
16. If gurgling is not heard, continue to advance up to an additional 10 cm, secure the tube at the naris, and get a chest X-ray to identify the tube position (Fig. 28.20).
17. If at any time the patient has coughing, wheezing, oxygen desaturation, or difficulty ventilating, immediately remove the tube.
18. If the tube becomes difficult to pass at the gastroesophageal junction (NEX) or pyloric junction, a 5–10 ml bolus of air while advancing the tube will often facilitate passage of the tube beyond the sphincter.
19. Always confirm placement with a chest X-ray.

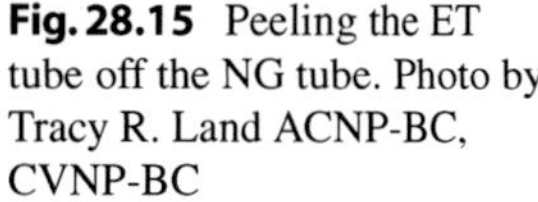

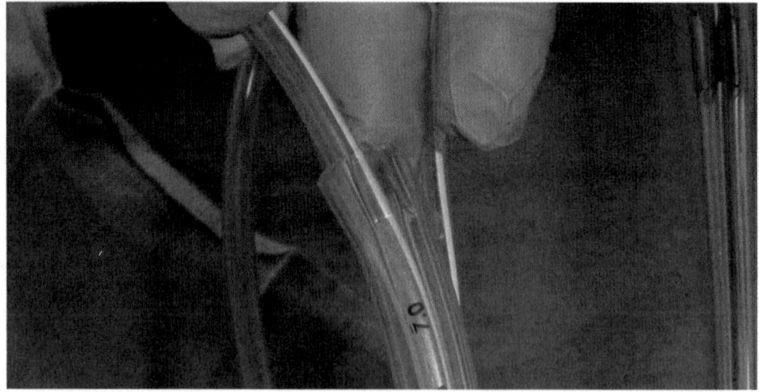

Fig. 28.15 Peeling the ET tube off the NG tube. Photo by Tracy R. Land ACNP-BC, CVNP-BC

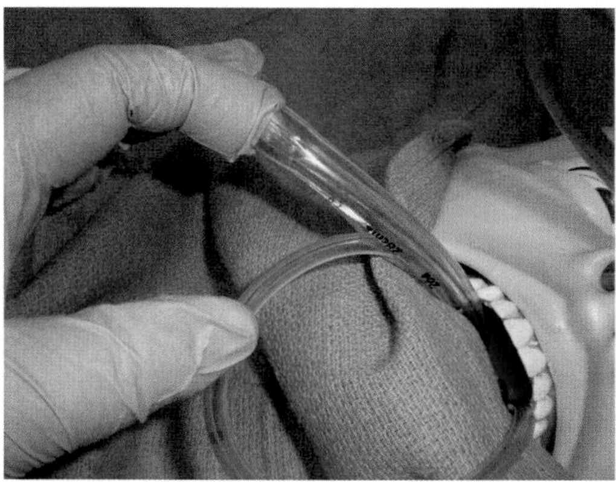

Fig. 28.16 Passing the NGT through the ET tube and into the stomach. Photo by Tracy R. Land ACNP-BC, CVNP-BC

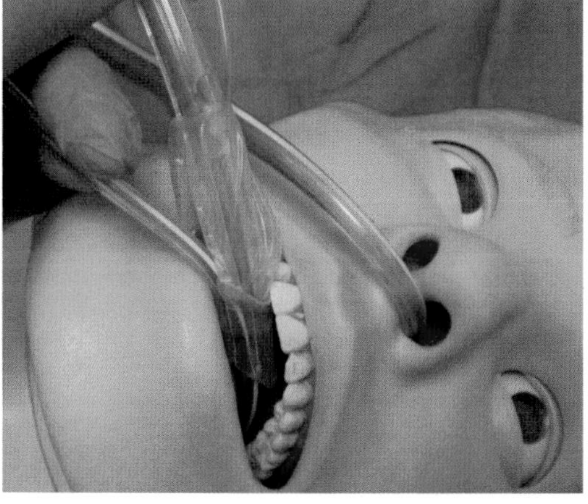

Fig. 28.17 Removal of the ET tube from the NG and patients mouth. Photo by Tracy R. Land ACNP-BC, CVNP-BC

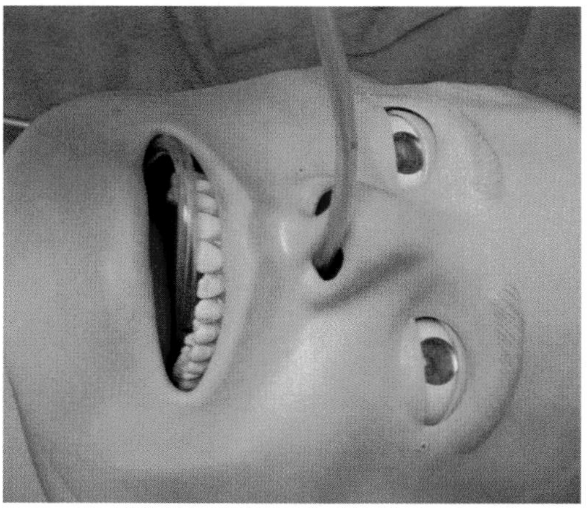

Fig. 28.18 Backing the NG tube out. Photo by Tracy R. Land, ACNP-BC, CVNP-BC

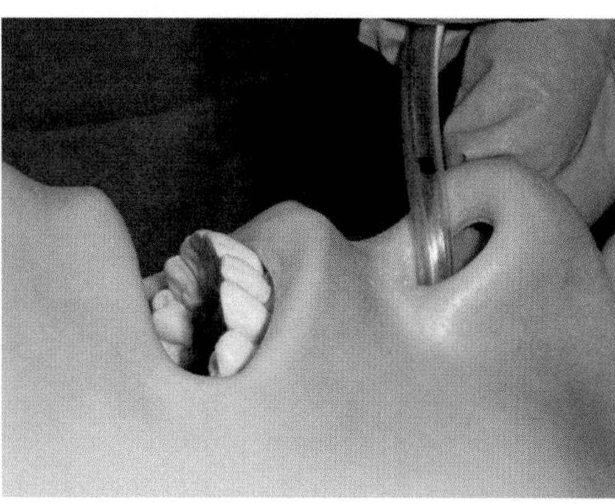

Fig. 28.19 NG tube at proper mark. Photo by Tracy R. Land ACNP-BC, CVNP-BC

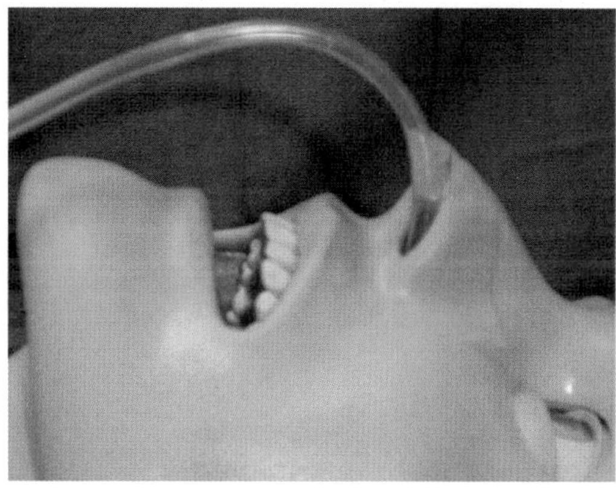

Fig. 28.20 Securing the NG tube. Photo by Tracy R. Land ACNP-BC, CVNP-BC

28.6 Confirmation

X-ray is the gold standard for confirmation of placement of the NG, OG, or nasoenteric tube [15]. A chest X-ray will often be sufficient to confirm placement of the NG or OG tube and will identify any thoracic complications. Visualization of the distal and proximal ports of the gastric tube can be challenging at times, especially in patients with a high body mass index (BMI). Some simple things that can be done to aid in visualizing these tubes are:

- A feeding tube guidewire can be inserted or left in place to aid in the visualization of the tube to be verified.

- Have an assistant, wearing protective lead, inject a bolus of air into the tube to be verified as the X-ray is being obtained. The bolus of air provides a dark background facilitating visualization of the tube.

An abdominal film is required to confirm placement of a nasoenteric tube.

References

1. Lamont T, Beaumont C, Fayaz A, Healey F, Heuhns T, Law R, et al. Checking placement of nasogastric feeding tubes in adults. BMJ. 2011;342:d2586. doi:10.1136/bmj.d2586.
2. Moharari R, Fallah A, Khajavi M, Kashayar P, Lakeh M, Najafi A. The glidescope facilitates nasogastric tube insertion: a randomized clinical trial. Anesth Analg. 2010;110:115–8. doi:10.1213/ANE.0b013e3181be0e43.
3. Chun D-H, Kim N-Y, Shin Y-S, Kim S-H. A randomized, clinical trial of frozen versus standard nasogastric tube placement. World J Surg. 2009;33:1789–92. doi:10.1007/s00268-009-0144-x.
4. Thomas J. Passing a nasogastric tube. Br Med J (Clin Res Ed). 1981;282:1480.
5. Appukutty J, Shroff P. Nasogastric tube insertion using different techniques in anesthetized patients: a prospective, randomized study. Anesth Analg. 2009;109:832–5. doi:10.1213/ane.0b013e3181af5e1f.
6. Ghatak T, Samanta S, Baronia A. A new technique to insert nasogastric tube in an unconscious intubated patient. N Am J Med Sci. 2013;5(1):68–70. doi:10.4103/1947-2714.106215.
7. Kirtania J, Ghose T, Garai D, Ray S. Esophageal guidewire-assisted nasogastric tube insertion in anesthetized and intubated patients: a prospective randomized control study. Anesth Analg. 2012;114:343–8. doi:10.1213/ANE.0b013e31823be0a4.
8. Tsai Y-F, Luo C-F, Illias A, Lin C-C, Yu H-P. Nasogastric tube insertion in anesthetized and intubated patients: a new and reliable method. BMC Gastroenterol. 2012;12:99.
9. Doshi J, Anari S. Seldinger technique for insertion of a nasogastric tube. Laryngoscope. 2006;116:672–3. doi:10.1097/01.MLG.0000201905.19123.99.
10. Ozer S, Benumof L. Oro- and nasogastric tube passage in intubated patients. Anesthesiology. 1999; 91:137–43.
11. Covidien. 2014. http://www.covidien.com/kangaroo-iris/pages.aspx?page=technology. Accessed 13 Nov 2014.
12. Bong C-L, Macachor J, Hwang N-C. Insertion of the nasogastric tube made easy. Anesthesiology. 2004;101:266.
13. Chen Y-C, Wang L-Y, Chang Y-J, Yang C-P, Wu T-J, Lin F-R, et al. Potential risk of malposition nasogastric tube using nose–ear–xiphoid measurement. PLoS One. 2014;9(2):e88046. doi:10.1371/journal.pone.0088046.
14. Taylor DJ, Allan K, McWilliam H, Toher D. Nasogastric tube depth: the 'NEX' guideline is incorrect. Br J Nurs. 2014;23(12):641–4. doi:10.12968/bjon.2014.23.12.641.
15. Pillai J, Vegas A, Brister S. Thoracic complications of nasogastric tube: review of safe practice. Interact Cardiovasc Thorac Surg. 2005;4:429–33. doi:10.1510/icvts.2005.109488.

Percutaneous Endoscopic Gastrostomy

29

Peter S. Sandor, Brennan Bowker, and James E. Lunn

Abbreviations

PEG	Percutaneous endoscopic gastrostomy
GI	Gastrointestinal
ACP	Advance care provider
ICU	Intensive care unit
NGT	Nasogastric tube
OG	Orogastric tube
INR	International normalized ratio
mm^3	Millimeters cubed
BMI	Body mass index
Kg	Kilogram
m^2	Meter squared
CT	Computerized tomography
BBS	Buried bumper syndrome
RCP	Respiratory care practitioner
cm	Centimeter
mL	Milliliter
NPO	Nil per os
ASGE	American Society for Gastrointestinal Endoscopy
EGD	Esophagogastroduodenoscopy
mcg	Microgram
mg	Milligram
IV	Intravenous

P.S. Sandor, RRT, MHSPA-C (✉) • J.E. Lunn, RRT, MHS, PA-C
Department of Surgery, Saint Francis Hospital and Medical Center,
114 Woodland Street, Hartford, CT 06105, USA
e-mail: psandor@stfranciscare.org; Jlunn@Stfranciscare.org

B. Bowker, MHS, PA-C
Yale-New Haven Hospital – St Raphael Campus,
1450 Chapel Street, New Haven, CT 06511, USA
e-mail: Brennan.Bowker@YNHH.org

29.1 Introduction

Nutritional support in the critically ill patient is paramount for optimal recovery. Although some debate the ideal delivery system, most will agree that enteral feeding is the superior route of nutritional support in patients with functional gastrointestinal (GI) tracts. Prior to the advent of the percutaneous endoscopic gastrostomy (PEG) tube, enteral nutrition was delivered via a nasogastric tube (NGT) or a gastrostomy tube that was placed in an open fashion. Open gastrostomy tube placement, although previously felt the procedure of choice when long-term enteral feeding was necessary, is an invasive surgical procedure, which can have significant morbidity in the critically ill patient.

Gauderer and colleagues changed the mindset of clinicians in 1980 when they introduced the PEG tube as a means to deliver enteral feedings, which subsequently bypassed the need to have the patient undergo a more invasive procedure with general anesthetic [1]. Although first described in the pediatric population, PEG placement quickly evolved as a procedure for patients of all ages and can be performed safely and easily at the beside. Several multicenter trials conducted

D.A. Taylor et al. (eds.), *Interventional Critical Care*, DOI 10.1007/978-3-319-25286-5_29

since its inception have determined that PEGs are indeed safe for long-term use [2–5]. Given this data and the ease of placement, PEG placement has become one of the most commonly performed endoscopic procedures. Although data varies, over 200,000 PEGs are placed annually in the United States [6].

29.2 Indication

In the intensive care unit (ICU), PEGs are routinely placed in the setting of trauma or burns, both of which can leave patients unable to take nutrition by mouth for long periods of time despite functioning GI tracts. Prolonged decreased level of consciousness from central nervous system disorders such as tumors, stroke, and motor neuron diseases is also indications for placement of a PEG tube [7]. Additionally, malignancy of the head or neck often precipitates prophylactic placement of a gastrostomy tube as this has been shown to reduce morbidity when placed therapeutically [8]. PEG tubes are also used for gastric decompression especially when the jejunal extension is utilized [9].

29.3 Contraindications

There are a few absolute contraindications to PEG tube placement, and most relative contraindications are a result of a preexisting comorbidity that increases the risk of the procedure. As with any procedure, disorders of coagulation and presence of pharmacologic anticoagulation should draw special attention by the proceduralist. Some argue that elevated international normalized ratio (INR) and thrombocytopenia are relative contraindications, while others favor these deranged lab values as absolute contraindications. Most concur, however, that an INR greater than 1.5, partial thromboplastin time (PTT) greater than 1.5 the normal value, or a platelet count less than 50,000 mm^3 should delay the procedure until corrected. The inability to perform upper endoscopy is the first absolute contraindication to the procedure. These cases would include fully obstructing head or esophageal tumors. Since this is an elective procedure, hemodynamic instability would also require postponement. Other absolute contraindications include severe ascites, peritonitis, infection at the site of PEG tube placement, and history of total gastrectomy [7].

As obesity rates across the United States continue to steadily rise, this condition must be given special consideration to in the placement of PEG tubes. Several studies have shown that, though more technically challenging, no significant increased morbidity is experienced when placing a PEG tube in obese individuals [10–12]. The inability to transilluminate was the most common reason cited for "failure"; one study noted that obese patients with a BMI <35 kg/m^2 had a higher rate of success when compared to those with a BMI>35 kg/m^2 [10]. McGarr and Bochicchio in two separate studies concluded similarly that overall PEGs are safe for placement despite the obese or even morbidly obese body habitus [11, 12].

29.4 Complications

With PEG tube placement, there can be complications related to the endoscopy as well as gastrostomy tube placement, both of which are relatively low [2].

29.4.1 Skin infections

Skin infections at the site of insertion are the most common complication of PEG tube placement. Since the recommendation of prophylactic antibiotics, the incidence of skin infections has decreased significantly although the complication itself has not been eradicated altogether. High-risk individuals typically have other comorbidities including obesity, diabetes mellitus, poor nutritional status, and chronic corticosteroid therapy [13]. Even less common, however, is the presence of necrotizing fasciitis after PEG. Although relatively few case reports exist in the literature, it should still draw the attention of the practitioner and kept in mind, especially in diabetic patients presenting with high fevers, leukocytosis, and erythema at the insertion site [14–17].

29.4.2 Injury to Surrounding Organs

Injuries to the colon, small bowel, and liver during PEG tube placement have all been described in the literature [18–20]. Colonic injury seems more commonplace as the colon can be juxtaposed above the stomach. The incidence in one study revealed the rate of colo-gastrocutaneous fistula to be 6/2384 cases. In these cases, patients typically developed diarrhea and/or were noted to have fecal material draining from or around the tube insertion site [19]. Small bowel injury is less common and might not be recognized as patients may be asymptomatic, however when recognized, requires immediate surgical repair [18].

29.4.3 Pneumoperitoneum

Pneumoperitoneum after PEG tube placement is only of concern when accompanied by other symptoms such as peritonitis. Wojtowycz completed a study in which patients who received PEG tubes underwent computerized tomography (CT) scans 1 h to 9 days after placement. An astounding 56 % of patients were found to have pneumoperitoneum, yet none of the patients required intervention [21]. A more recent study noted that only 20 % of the cohort examined had pneumoperitoneum on post-procedure radiographs. In all of these cases, none were found to have evidence of peritonitis or other life-threatening processes and concluded; pneumoperitoneum was essentially "benign" [22]. Although "benign" in most cases, pneumoperitoneum could indicate a serious complication of the procedure and should be evaluated appropriately in these situations.

29.4.4 Buried Bumper Syndrome

Buried bumper syndrome (BBS) is a rare but serious complication of PEG tube placement that can have fatal outcomes if not recognized expeditiously. This occurs when the internal bumper of the PEG tube erodes through the gastric wall and migrates along the fistulatous tract between the stomach and the skin. It is hypothesized that excess tension placed on the PEG tube, often in an attempt to prevent leakage from around the tube, is the cause of this condition [23]. Treatment in these cases involves removal of the buried bumper and debridement of necrotic tissue as necessary.

29.4.5 Accidental Dislodgement

Accidental removal of PEG tubes is a very common complication and not typically related to procedural technique. Removal of the tube is described as "premature" occurring within 14 days of the initial placement or "late" occurring after the 2-week period. Tube removal within the first 14 days is a serious complication as the fistulatous tract has yet to be formed. These cases should not be taken lightly as attempts at blind replacement of the tube can result in peritonitis and may require surgical exploration [24]. The rate of accidental dislodgement varies from study to study, but Rosenberger and colleagues found that the early accidental dislodgement rate was 4.1 %, which is congruent to other older studies that have been compiled [25]. Late accidental dislodgement of the PEG tube is less of a concern for life-threatening complications, as a tract from the stomach to the skin has usually formed. In the case of tubes that are dislodged well after the fistula has been formed, it is typically safe to perform the replacement without direct visualization although "tube studies" are frequently performed.

29.5 Resources Required

The placement of a percutaneous gastrostomy tube is a two-proceduralist procedure that requires, at minimum, two skilled clinicians working together.

One proceduralist is responsible for the endoscopy and the other proceduralist is responsible for the gastrostomy tube placement. If available, a third clinician is helpful and can assist the endoscopist with the snare/wire and equipment handling.

In addition to the two proceduralists, an experienced ICU nurse plays an integral role in completing the procedure, as they will be responsible for monitoring and documenting the patient's vital signs, administering sedation, and alerting the team of any issues that arise. An experienced respiratory care practitioner (RCP) should be immediately available for airway complications. If the patient is intubated and mechanically ventilated, the RCP is responsible for ventilator management. A bag-valve mask should always be present and utilized when appropriate.

29.6 Monitoring

As in any critical care setting, patients must be maintained on continuous telemetry with a bedside monitor. Vital signs including oxygen saturation, heart rate, and blood pressure should be reassessed frequently during the procedure and documented as required by the individual institution. To avoid undue complications, all equipment must be checked and secured prior to starting the procedure.

29.6.1 Pulse Oximetry

The pulse oximeter is routinely available and should be utilized continuously. Poorly attached probes, dysfunctional devices, and diaphoretic patients will need to be corrected prior to the start of the procedure. Any decrease in the patient's oxygen saturation should be taken seriously and addressed promptly. If there is a decrease in the saturation, stop the procedure immediately and only resume once the oxygen level has stabilized. If the saturation does not return to baseline, consideration should be made to abort the procedure.

29.6.2 Heart Rate

Heart rate is an important indicator when assessing the patient's pain level when chemical paralysis utilized. If tachycardia is present, pain management and sedation should be addressed immediately. Conversely, bradycardia associated with hypoxemia or a pulse oximeter that is "inaccurate" is an ominous sign. In this instance, the procedure should be aborted and the airway reevaluated. Bradycardia can also be a response to vagal stimulation, especially if the patient has a spinal cord injury. If the patient has vagally mediated bradycardia or spinal cord injury, it is prudent to have medication available to resuscitate the patient prior to starting the procedure.

29.6.3 Blood Pressure

Hypertension is most commonly associated with pain and/or agitation and may be seen in conjunction with tachycardia. If hypertension is deemed secondary to pain, the nurse should administer analgesics. Hypotension, while a concerning sign, is also a common response to sedation and chemical paralysis. Fluid bolus will usually improve the patient's hemodynamic status in these cases. If there is hypotension not responsive to a fluid bolus, a myriad of other complications should be considered including bleeding, loss of airway, and vagal stimulation from gastric distention. Aborting the procedure along with performing a thorough head-to-toe examination must be performed to evaluate for any potential life-threatening conditions. At the completion of the procedure, when stimulation is at a minimum, hypotension can still occur. Typically, this resolves after the effects of the sedation have been abated. If chemical paralysis is utilized during the procedure, sedation should be maintained until paralysis has resolved to avoid unnecessary patient discomfort.

29.7 Equipment

Standard upper endoscope with video cart (insufflation, water irrigation, and photo available)

PEG Kit containing the following:

- Silicone feeding tube with or without jejunal extension
- Chlorhexidine preparatory stick or swab stick containing povidone-iodine solution
- Guidewire—0.035 in. diameter, 260 cm length
- Endoscopy snare
- 5 mL syringe with 22 gauge needle
- 1 % lidocaine
- Sterile fenestrated drape
- Trocar needle/catheter assembly
- Surgical blade, No. 11, attached to scalpel
- Sterile water-soluble lubricant
- Scissors
- Surgical marking pen

29.8 Technical Aspects

There are several techniques of PEG tube placement; however, the "pull" technique will be explained. As with any procedure, a formal "time out" should be completed prior to its commencement. The patient's identity will be confirmed with the wristband and medical record number, the procedure will be confirmed as documented on the consent, and all members of the team will verify the procedural consent. A final confirmation of all necessary equipment, medications, and imaging utilized for the procedure should be discussed at this time as well.

29.8.1 Step 1: Preparation and Sedation

In preparation for the PEG procedure, patients are made nil per os (NPO) at least 6 h prior to the procedure. Thirty minutes prior to the procedure, administration of intravenous cefazolin, or its equivalent, should be dosed to reduce the incidence of stomal infection [26].

Once the time out occurs, procedural sedation is initiated, and the patient is positioned supine with the head of the bed slightly elevated to reduce the risk of aspiration. If the patient is mechanically ventilated, the respiratory care practitioner should confirm that the patient is on a controlled ventilator mode and the airway is checked for stability. Although practices are variable, for intubated patients, propofol 0.05 mg/kg IV bolus with a maintenance infusion of 25–50 mcg/kg/min or intermittent midazolam boluses of 1–2 mg IV every 3–5 min can be used to achieve adequate sedation. Propofol is preferred for its short half-life; however, it may cause hypotension, especially when given as a bolus.

Once adequate sedation is achieved, analgesia should be provided with an opiate, such as fentanyl (0.5–2 mcg/kg dosed every 3–5 min). Fentanyl is preferred for its short duration of action and minimal hemodynamic effects. After appropriate sedation and analgesia occurs, a single dose of cisatracurium besilate (0.15–0.2 mg/kg IV) is recommended for temporary chemical paralysis. During the procedure, further doses of analgesia and sedation should be provided every 3–5 min, as needed, based upon perceived pain or agitation.

The bed should be moved to a position that will accommodate the endoscopist either at the head or side of the bed, depending on the endoscopist preference followed by adjustment of the video monitor. If an OG tube is present, it should now be clamped and left in place to be utilized as a guide for the endoscopist to follow into the stomach. Regardless of whether the patient receives chemical paralysis, a bite block should be placed to avoid damage to the endoscope.

29.8.2 Step 2: Esophagogastroduodenoscopy (EGD)

Once the bite block is secured in place and the endoscope is lubricated with a water-soluble lubricant, it is gently placed into the patient's oral pharynx and advanced in a fashion similar to that of placing an oral gastric tube. Insufflation should be utilized to help improve visualization of the anatomic landmarks of the aerodigestive tract. The endoscope should never be advanced without visualization, as this could lead to serious mucosal injury or perforation. The first structure visualized should be the glottis; care should be taken to follow the esophagus and avoid entering the trachea. If an OG tube is in place, it should be followed; the endoscope should be withdrawn if the vocal cords are visualized. Once the esophagus is entered, the endoscope is carefully advanced through the gastroesophageal junction, into the stomach, and continued through the pylorus to evaluate the duodenum for pathology.

29.8.3 Step 3: Landmark

After an adequate EGD has been performed, the endoscope should be retracted into the stomach and insufflation should be carried out until the stomach is completely distended. Now, transillumination should be performed by pressing the "transillumination" feature of the endoscope which will increase the power of the light on the scope. When transilluminating, an orange glow will be visible through the abdominal wall (Fig. 29.1). Finger pressure is then applied at the point of maximum transillumination; this focal indentation should be seen endoscopically as well (Fig. 29.2). The site with the least amount of finger pressure and best indentation is chosen. As a general rule, the area should be at least 1 in. below the costal margin and to the left of the xiphoid process (Fig. 29.3). Once the landmark is identified, a surgical marking pen is used to indicate the location of the PEG tube placement.

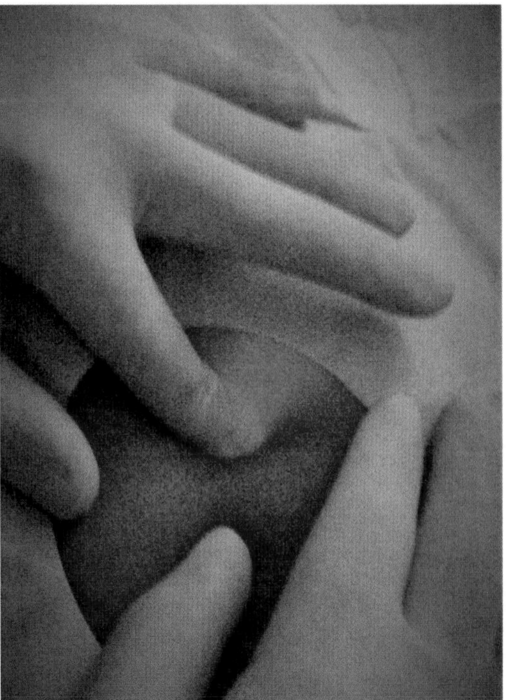

Fig. 29.1 Transillumination

29.8.4 Step 4: Preparation of the Skin

After the landmark has been identified, the site is cleansed with either a chlorhexidine preparatory sticks or a povidone-iodine solution. The abdominal operator performing the skin portion of the procedure will now don a sterile gown and gloves, mask and eye protection, as well as a cap. Next, the sterile drape will be placed over the abdomen with the fenestration over the landmark.

29.8.5 Step 5: Skin Incision and Needle Puncture

Using the 5 mL syringe, the site is anesthetized with lidocaine. Using the scalpel, a horizontal incision 0.5–1 cm wide at the site of the landmark is made. The best technique for this incision is utilizing a gentle stabbing motion creating a 2–3 mm deep incision (Fig. 29.4). Next, place your index finger over the incision and press down on the skin in various directions, paying particular attention to the angle that produces the best indentation on the stomach (which is visualized through the endoscope). Now, place the larger trocar needle with catheter through the incision and advance in the appropriate direction/angle. The maneuver can be described as a "quick poke" which is done in an effort to prevent pushing the stomach away from the anterior abdominal wall. The needle entering the stomach should be visible, through the endoscope, once it is advanced 3–4 cm. If the needle is not visible, it should be removed and the landmark reassessed. If unsure of the direction, depth, or landmark, the decision to abort the procedure should be made.

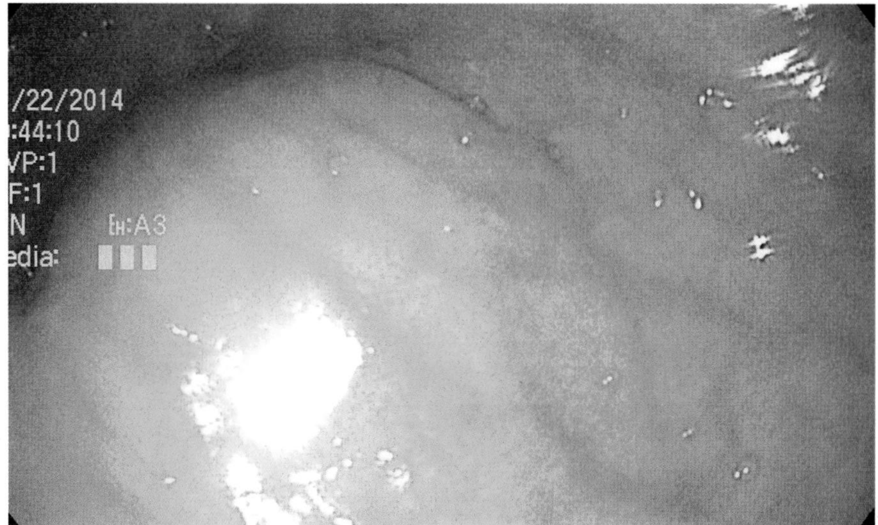

Fig. 29.2 Endoscopic view of finger impression

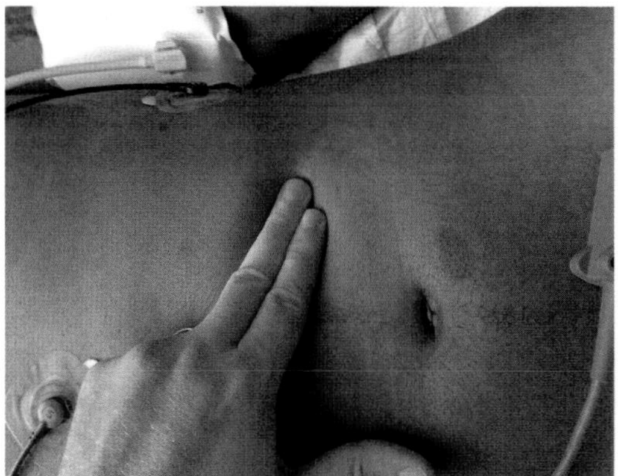

Fig. 29.3 Landmark

29.8.6 Step 7: Snare/Guidewire Coupling

The snare should already be loaded in the endoscope and opened in the general direction of where the trocar needle is to be inserted prior to the gastric puncture (Fig. 29.5). Once the trocar needle is visualized, the snare should be looped around the trocar needle and closed (Fig. 29.6). Next, the abdominal operator will remove the trocar needle making sure to leave the catheter in place. The guidewire is then inserted through the catheter and should be visualized endoscopically. The guidewire tip should always be noted, to prevent accidental gastric puncture or mucosal injury. The snare

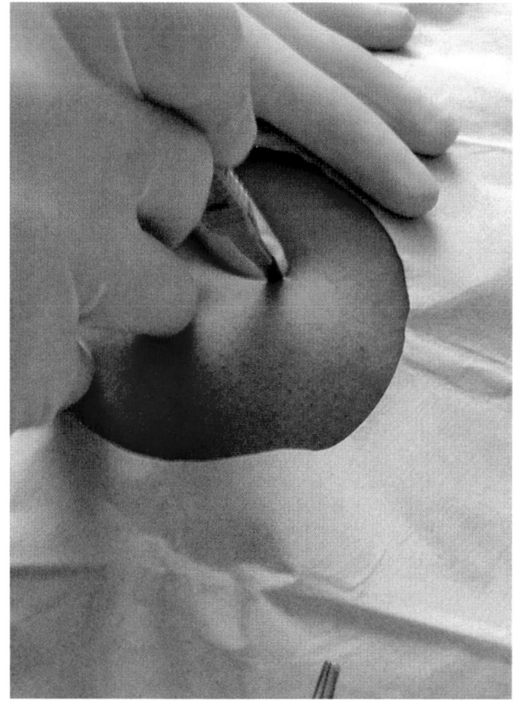

Fig. 29.4 Abdominal incision

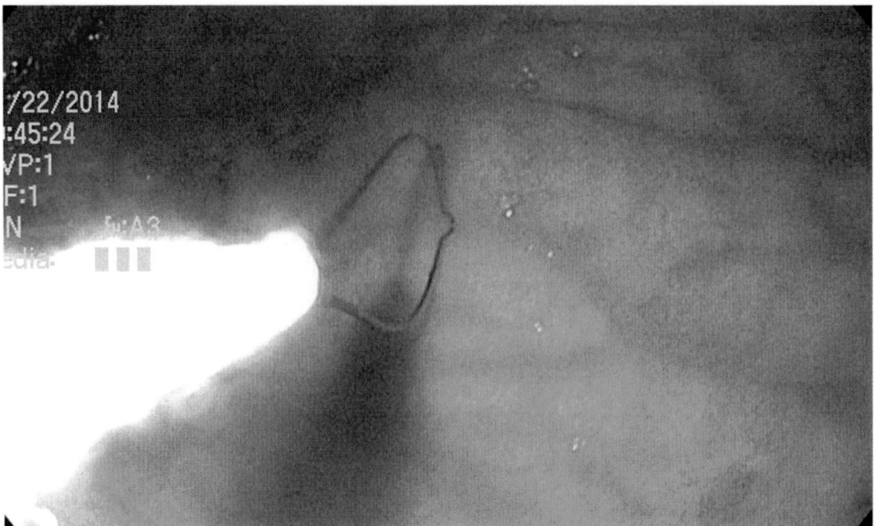

Fig. 29.5 Open snare

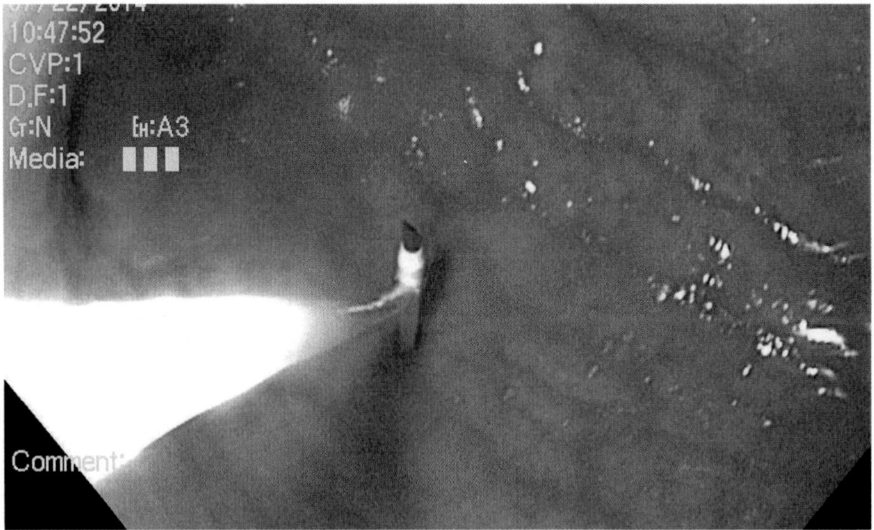

Fig. 29.6 Snare looped on needle

is then loosened slightly to allow the catheter to be removed and then immediately closed to tightly grasp the wire (Fig. 29.7). The endoscopist now begins to slowly remove the endoscope along with the snare and guidewire. The abdominal operator will feed the guidewire through the puncture site (Fig. 29.8) until the endoscope is removed and the wire is visualized exiting the mouth.

29.8.7 Step 8: Insertion of the PEG Tube

While securing the guidewire, the endoscopist lubricates the PEG tube and advances it over the guidewire starting at the tapered end. Once the PEG tube is completely loaded on the guidewire, the distal end of the wire is secured in the endoscopists' hand (Fig. 29.9). The abdominal opera-

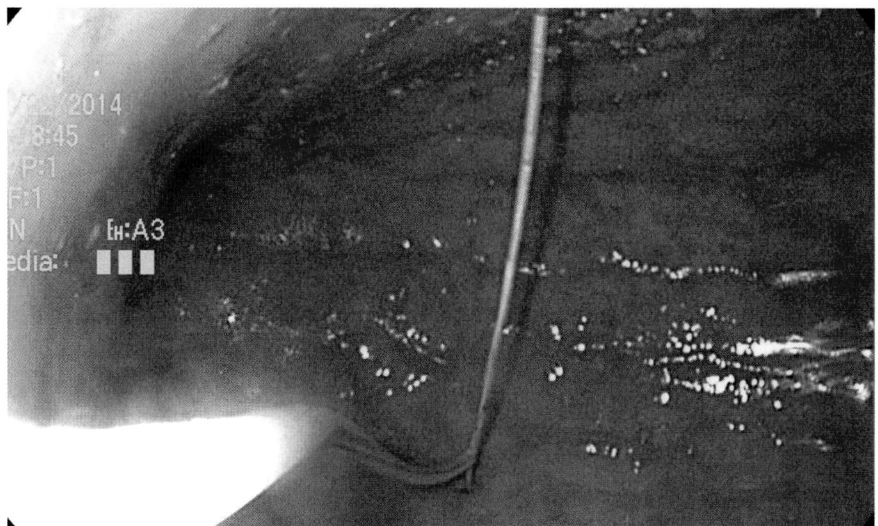

Fig. 29.7 Snare looped on wire

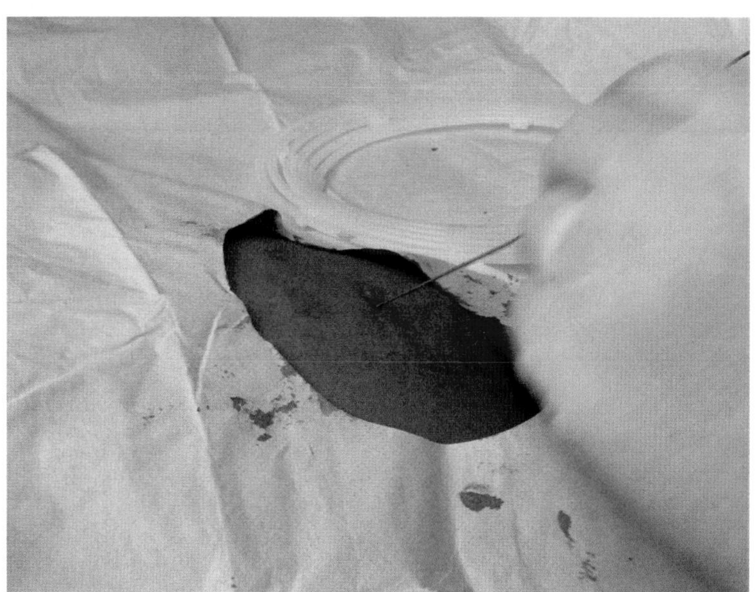

Fig. 29.8 Advancing wire

tor will slowly pull back on the guidewire, while the endoscopist advances the PEG tube into the patient's mouth (always make sure the guidewire exiting the patients' mouth remains secured). This process continues until the abdominal operator visualizes the PEG tube exiting the skin incision (Fig. 29.10). With a short pause, the endoscopist snares the remaining distal end of the guidewire exiting the mouth (Fig. 29.11). The abdominal operator now grasps the PEG tube and resumes traction, while the endoscopist applies gentle pressure on the endoscope/PEG tube assembly to help it advance in to the stomach. It is imperative that the abdominal operator pays strict attention to the PEG tube as care must be taken not to pull the PEG tube completely out of the abdominal incision. Therefore, once the numbers on the PEG tube are visualized exiting the skin, less traction should be applied (Fig. 29.12). The endoscopist can now visualize

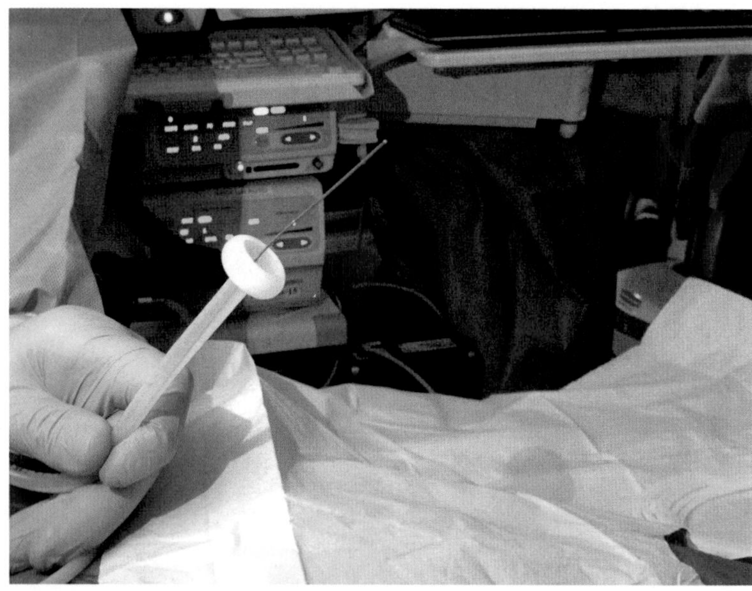

Fig. 29.9 PEG tubeloaded on wire

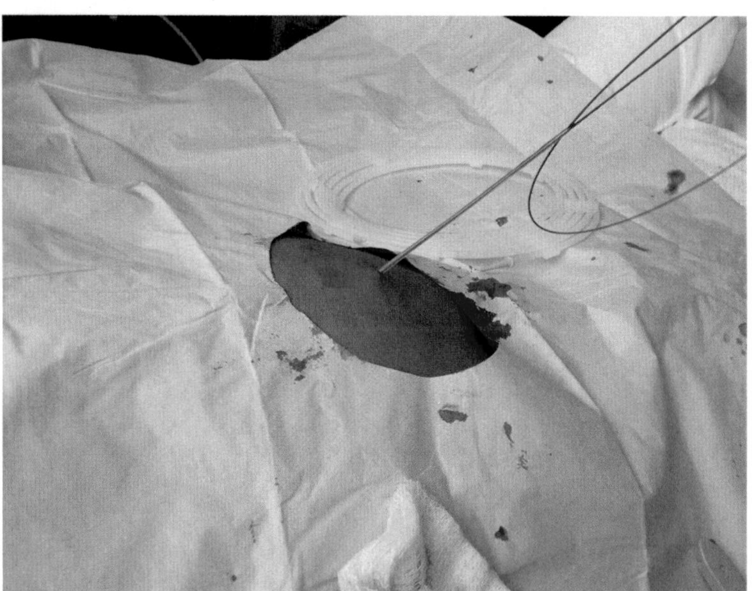

Fig. 29.10 PEG tube exiting abdominal wall

the PEG tube within the stomach, and, while under direct visualization, the abdominal operator pulls the PEG tube until the soft bumper is in contact with the gastric mucosa (Fig. 29.13). The snare is then released and the wire is completely removed, leaving the PEG in place. The number distance, (in centimeters) on the PEG tube, should be noted at the level of the skin (Fig. 29.14).

29.8.8 STEP 9: Crossbar Application and Final Inspection

The abdominal operator now lubricates the external crossbar and slides it over the tapered end of the external portion of the PEG tube advancing it to the skin level. This is done slowly and carefully while the endoscopist continues to visualize the PEG tube bumper. Care must be taken when advancing the crossbar since aggressive advancement can

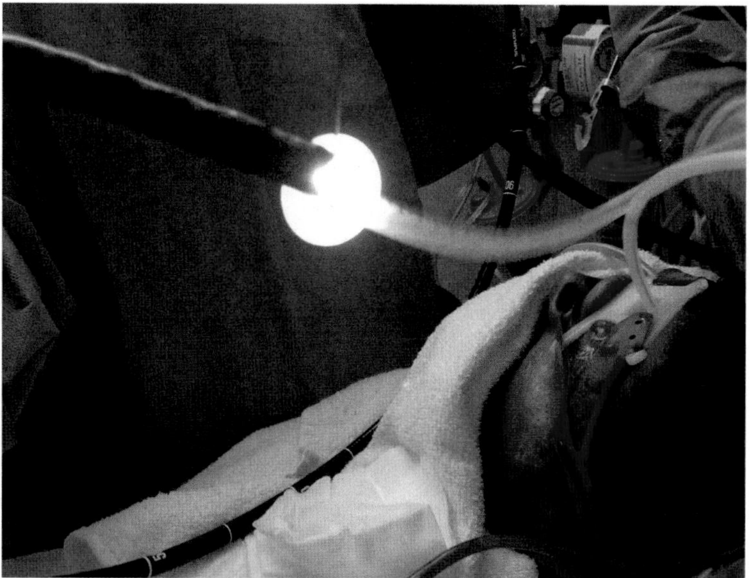

Fig. 29.11 Grasping distal end of wire with PEG tube loaded

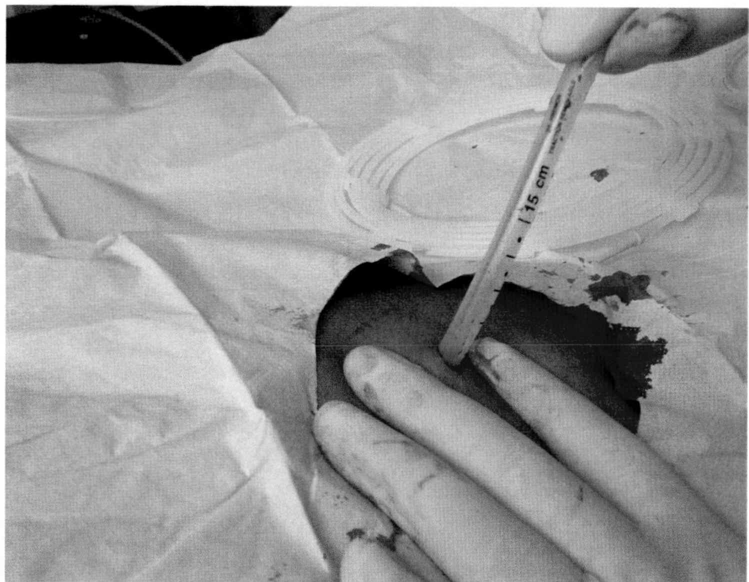

Fig. 29.12 Numbers on PEG tube exiting skin

lead to accidentally dislodgment of the PEG tube, which is a surgical emergency. Depending on abdominal wall thickness, the crossbar typically rests 2–4 cm, at the skin level (Fig. 29.15). The endoscopic portion of the procedure is now complete. However, prior to removal of the endoscope, a picture should be taken for documentation and confirm placement. Then, the stomach is decompressed with continuous suctioning as the endoscope is removed.

29.8.9 Step 10: Procedure Completion

The abdominal operator should now apply the tube clamp supplied with the kit. Next, the PEG tube can be shortened as needed (leaving about 10–12 in. of tubing exiting the skin), and the feeding tube connector can be pressed into the distal end (Fig. 29.16). Initially, the PEG tube should be placed to gravity to allow for

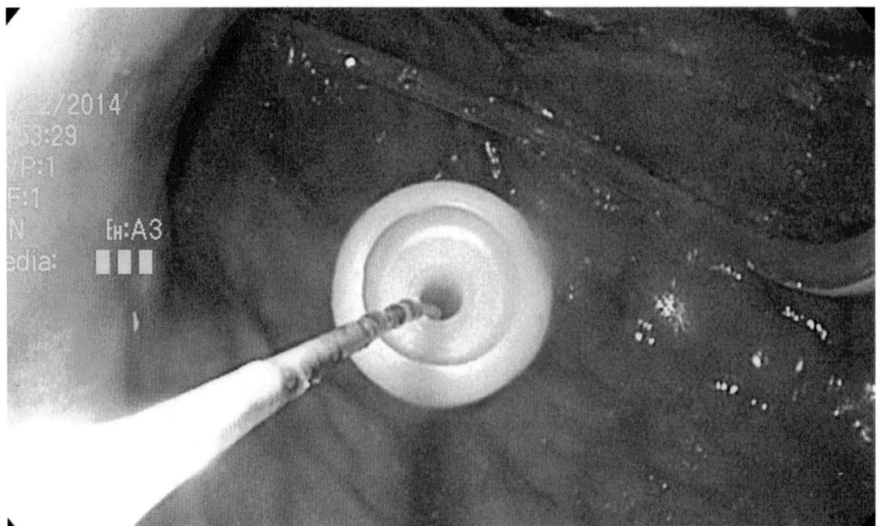

Fig. 29.13 Bumper against gastric mucosa

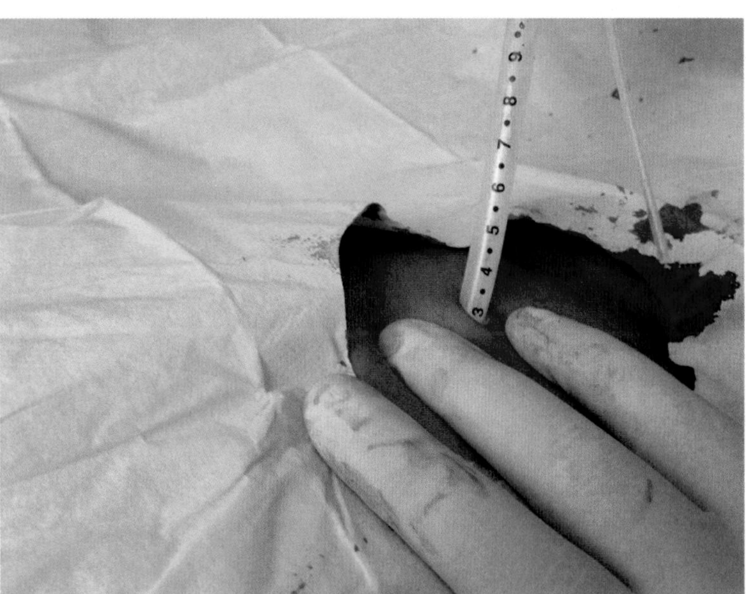

Fig. 29.14 Final location of PEG tube with numbers visualized

complete decompression and a loose dressing applied per hospital policy. If dressings are applied, they should be placed over the crossbar and not between the crossbar and the skin, which will create undue tension on the tube. To prevent dislodgement, care should be taken to avoid tension on the PEG tube; in agitated or active patients, an abdominal binder could be useful in this regard.

29.9 Placement of Percutaneous Endoscopic Gastrojejunostomy

If the decision is made to place a jejunal extension tube, the endoscope should remain in the stomach after the completion of the PEG tube procedure. Once the PEG tube procedure is completed and secured with a crossbar, the abdominal

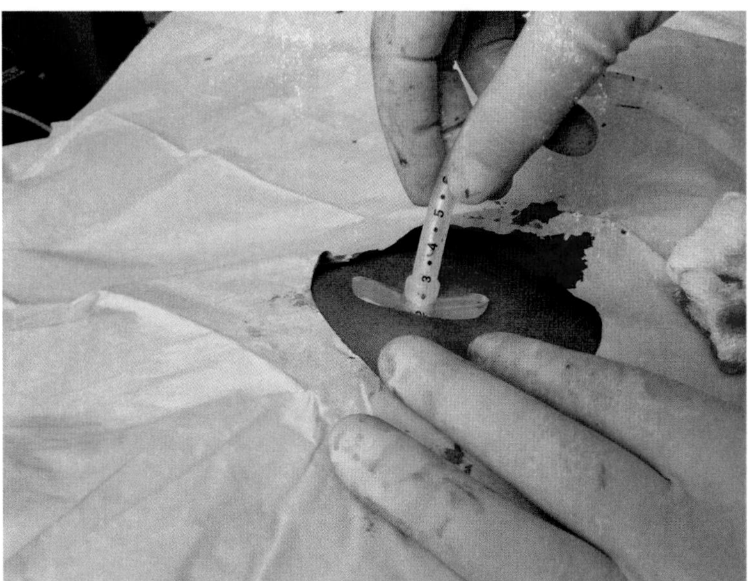

Fig. 29.15 Crossbar in place

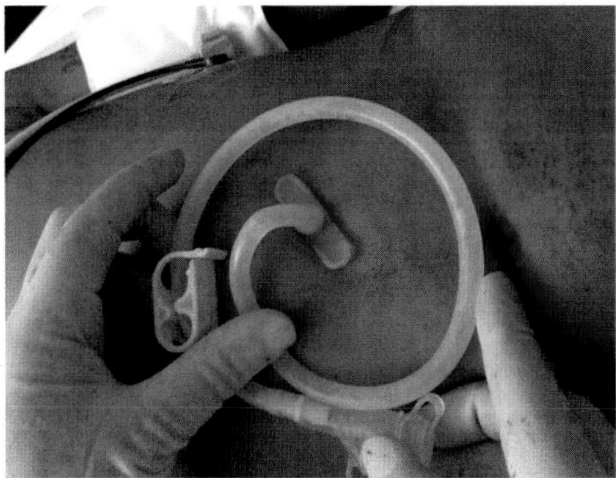

Fig. 29.16 Clamp and distal attachment in place

operator places the jejunal extension guidewire through the lumen of the newly affixed PEG tube. Utilizing a snare or forceps, the endoscopist will grasp this wire as it enters the stomach. Using the endoscope, the endoscopists will drag the wire through the pylorus and advance it as far as possible into the small bowel. At this junction, the goal is to remove the endoscope while maintaining the wire within the small bowel. The forceps/snare will be advanced through the scope as the scope is withdrawn which will help prevent dislodgement of the guidewire. Once the endoscope is in the stomach, the guidewire is released and the snare/forceps is retracted into the scope. The jejunal extension tube is now threaded over the guidewire and advanced into the small bowel. Once in place, the guidewire is removed and the jejunal extension is secured to the gastrostomy tube. The stomach is decompressed and the endoscope is removed. Confirmation of jejunal tube placement can be achieved by injecting 30 mL of water-soluble contrast through the jejunal tube followed by an abdominal radiograph.

References

1. Gauderer MW, Ponsky JL, Izant RJ. Gastrostomy without laparotomy: a percutaneous endoscopic technique. J Pediatr Surg. 1980;15(6):872–5.
2. Grant JP. Percutaneous endoscopic gastrostomy. Initial placement by single endoscopic technique and long-term follow-up. Ann Surg. 1993;217(2):168–74.
3. Amann W, Mischinger HJ, Berger A, Rosanelli G, Schweiger W, Werkgartner G, et al. Percutaneous endoscopic gastrostomy (PEG) 8 years of clinical experience in 232 patients. Surg Endosc. 1997;11(7):741–4.
4. Rabeneck L, Wray N, Petersen N. Long-term outcomes of patients receiving percutaneous endoscopic gastrostomy tubes. J Gen Intern Med. 1996;11(5):287–93.
5. Larson D, Burton D, Schroeder K, DiMagno E. Percutaneous endoscopic gastrostomy: indications, success, complications, and mortality in 314 consecutive patients. Gastroenterology. 1987;93(1):48–52.

6. Gauderer M. Twenty years of percutaneous endoscopic gastrostomy: origin and evolution of a concept and its expanded applications. Gastrointest Endosc. 1999;50(6):879–83.
7. Rahnemai-Azar AA, Rahnemaiazar AA, Naghshizadian R, Kurtz A, Farkas DT. Percutaneous endoscopic gastrostomy: indications, technique, complications, and management. World J Gastroenterol. 2014;20(24):7739–51.
8. Baschnagel AM, Yadav S, Marina O, Parzuchowski A, Lanni TB, Warner JN, et al. Toxicities and costs of placing prophylactic and reactive percutaneous gastrostomy tubes in patients with locally advanced head and neck cancers treated with chemoradiotherapy. Head Neck. 2014;36(8):1155–61.
9. Sakurai Y, Kimura H, Sunagawa R, Furuta S, Inaba K, Isogaki J, et al. Percutaneous endoscopic gastrostomy for gastric decompression after repeated intestinal obstruction after open abdominal surgery. Surg Laparosc Endosc Percutan Tech. 2008;18(6):604–7.
10. Wiggins TF, Garrow DA, DeLegge MH. Evaluation of percutaneous endoscopic feeding tube placement in obese patients. Nutr Clin Pract. 2009;24(6):723–7.
11. McGarr SE, Kirby DF. Percutaneous endoscopic gastrostomy (PEG) placement in the overweight and obese patient. JPEN J Parenter Enteral Nutr. 2007; 31(3):212–6.
12. Bochicchio GV, Guzzo JL, Scalea TM. Percutaneous endoscopic gastrostomy in the super-morbidly obese patient. JSLS. 2006;10(4):409–13.
13. Lee JK, Kim JJ, Kim YH, Jang JK, Son HJ, Peck KR, et al. Increased risk of peristomal wound infection after percutaneous endoscopic gastrostomy in patients with diabetes mellitus. Dig Liver Dis. 2002;34(12):857–61.
14. Greif JM, Ragland JJ, Ochsner MG, Riding R. Fatal necrotizing fasciitis complicating percutaneous endoscopic gastrostomy. Gastrointest Endosc. 1986;32(4):292–4.
15. Cave DR, Robinson WR, Brotschi EA. Necrotising fasciitis complicating percutaneous endoscopic gastrostomy. Gastrointest Endosc. 1986;32(4):294–6.
16. Person JL, Brower RA. Necrotising fasciitis/myositis following percutaneous endoscopic gastrostomy. Gastrointest Endosc. 1986;32(4):309.
17. Korula J, Rice HE. Necrotising fasciitis and percutaneous endoscopic gastrostomy. Gastrointest Endosc. 1987;33(4):335–6.
18. Karhadkar AS, Schwarz HJ, Dutta SK. Jejunocutaneous fistula manifesting as chronic diarrhea after PEG tube replacement. J Clin Gastroenterol. 2006;40(6):560–1.
19. Friedmann R, Feldman H, Sonneblick M. Misplacement of percutaneously inserted gastrostomy tube into the colon: report of 6 cases and review of the literature. JPEN J Parenter Enteral Nutr. 2007;31(6): 469–76.
20. Chaer RA, Rekkas D, Trevino J, Brown R, Espat NJ. Intrahepatic placement of a PEG tube. Gastrointest Endosc. 2003;57(6):763–5.
21. Wojtowycz MW, Arata JA, Micklos TJ, Miller FJ. CT findings after uncomplicated percutaneous gastrostomy. AJR Am J Roentgenol. 1988;151(2):307–9.
22. Wiesen AJ, Sideridis K, Fernandes A, Hines J, Indaram A, Weinstein L. True incidence and clinical significance of pneumoperitoneum after PEG placement: a prospective study. Gastrointest Endosc. 2006; 64(6):886–9.
23. Pop GH. Buried bumper syndrome: can we prevent it? Pract Gastroenterol. 2010;34(5):8–13.
24. Marshall JB, Bodnarchuk G, Barthel J. Early accidental dislodgement of PEG tubes. J Clin Gastroenterol. 1994;18(3):210–2.
25. Rosenberger LH, Newhook T, Schirmer B, Sawyer RG. Late accidental dislodgement of a percutaneous endoscopic gastrostomy tube: an underestimated burden on patients and the health care system. Surg Endosc. 2011;25(10):3307–11.
26. Lipp A, Lusardi G. Systemic antimicrobial prophylaxis for percutaneous endoscopic gastrostomy. Cochrane Database Syst Rev 2013; issue 11. Art. No.: CD005571. doi:10.1002/14651858.CD005571.pub3.

Flexible Intestinal Endoscopy 30

Marialice Gulledge and A. Britton Christmas

Flexible upper gastrointestinal endoscopy is generally a safe and common procedure enabling visualization of the oropharynx, esophagus, stomach, and proximal duodenum [1]. Lower intestinal endoscopy or colonoscopy allows visualization of the entire colon, rectum, and the terminal ileum. Both procedures are undertaken for a variety of diagnostic or therapeutic reasons [2]. Many upper endoscopies are performed for the evaluation of symptoms or abnormal findings on gastrointestinal (GI) radiology [1]. It can also be used for surveillance (as in Barrett's esophagus) or to screen for gastric cancer. In the United States, lower intestinal endoscopy (colonoscopy) is the most commonly used screening test for colorectal cancer in the asymptomatic patient [3]. Evidence suggests that early detection and removal of adenomatous polyps may prevent some cancers and reduce mortality [4].

While flexible intestinal endoscopy is routinely scheduled and performed in the inpatient and outpatient setting, it remains a fairly uncommon procedure in the critical care area. In this setting, the endoscopist is challenged with a unique set of circumstances as opposed to routine surveillance examinations [5]. Additionally, the indications are often somewhat different than for elective procedures and necessitating variability in techniques [5].

Urgent endoscopy may be employed to (1) determine the location and type of bleeding, (2) identify patients with ongoing hemorrhage or those at risk for rebleeding, (3) identify those patients that may be amenable to endoscopic intervention, and (4) guide and direct subsequent treatment [6, 7].

Risks of endoscopy include aspiration, adverse reactions to sedation, perforation, and increased hemorrhage during therapeutic intervention attempts [8]. In patients who have had a recent myocardial infarction (within 30 days), a careful assessment of the risks and benefits must be considered prior to upper endoscopy. While this particular patient population may be vulnerable to complications from continued bleeding without endoscopy, they are also at increased risk for fatal ventricular tachycardia, hypotension, and respiratory arrest during the procedure [9].

30.1 The Role of Endoscopy for Diagnosis

The American College of Gastroenterology 2012 guidelines recommend endoscopy within 24 h of admission following optimization of hemodynamics for patients with upper gastrointestinal bleeding (UGIB) [10, p. 345]. For patients who are hemodynamically stable and without serious comorbidities, endoscopy should be performed in a nonurgent setting as soon as possible to dis-

M. Gulledge, DNP, ANP-BC
A.B. Christmas, MD, FACS (✉)
Department of Surgery, Acute Care Surgery,
Carolinas Medical Center, Charlotte, NC 28203, USA
e-mail: marialice.gulledge@carolinashealthcare.org;
ashley.christmas@carolinashealthcare.org

D.A. Taylor et al. (eds.), *Interventional Critical Care*, DOI 10.1007/978-3-319-25286-5_30

cern low-risk endoscopy findings in patients who may potentially be safely discharged home [10, p. 346]. For those with higher-risk features (tachycardia, hypotension, bloody emesis, or nasogastric aspirate in hospital), endoscopy within 12 h should be considered to potentially improve clinical outcomes [10, p. 346].

30.2 Indications

Acute gastrointestinal (GI) bleeding represents one of the most common GI disorders. It involves any bleeding from the mouth, esophagus, stomach, and small and large intestines to the rectum [11]. Bleeding can range from the occult, notable on laboratory surveillance and guaiac testing, to the overt hemorrhage. The mortality rate increases with patients age>65 years and in presence of comorbid conditions such as renal and/or hepatic dysfunction, heart disease, and malignancy [12].

Acute upper GI bleeding (AUGIB) carries a mortality of 6–10 % and an incidence of 40–150 per 100,000 persons [12]. Common causes of AUGIB include ulcers (peptic, gastric, and duodenal), Dieulafoy's lesions, arterial-venous malformations, varices, and aortoesophageal fistula [7, 12]. Other causes may include infectious diarrhea caused by enteric pathogens such as *Salmonella*, *Shigella*, and *Clostridium difficile* [12].

Acute upper gastrointestinal (UGI) hemorrhage is a common and potentially life-threatening diagnosis which accounts for more than 300,000 hospitalizations at a cost of approximately 2.5 billion dollars annually [13]. UGIB is defined as bleeding from a source proximate to the ligament of Treitz and is categorized at variceal or non-variceal [13]. Bleeding from the UGI tract is four times more common than bleeding from the lower GI tract with a higher incidence in men than woman [13, p. 7].

Initial management of UGI includes obtaining an accurate history and physical examination, laboratory analysis, and appropriate diagnostic studies with ongoing assessment of hemodynamic stability and active resuscitation [8]. The physical examination should focus on clinical signs which indicate the severity of blood loss, help localize the source of bleeding, and suggest potential complications [8]. The presence of abdominal pain associated with rebound tenderness or involuntary guarding suggests peritonitis and raises the concern of perforation [8]. If any of these signs are present, the possibility of perforation must be excluded prior to endoscopy [8].

The management of UGI bleeding in critically ill patients is often confounded by an association of comorbidities, the risk for recurrent GI bleeding, and advanced age. A risk assessment should be performed to help stratify patients into high- and low-risk categories which may assist with clinical decision making regarding the timing of endoscopic evaluation and the appropriate admission level of care [10, p. 347]. A variety of triage and risk assessment scores exist to help differentiate risk and mortality in patients who present with acute upper gastrointestinal hemorrhage (UGIH). The pre-endoscopic Rockall score uses clinical data available at time of presentation which relates the severity of the bleeding episode (systolic blood pressure and pulse) to patient factors (age and comorbidities) [14]. The Blatchford score has a range of 0–23 and uses clinical and laboratory data available soon after admission to predict the risk of intervention and death (systolic blood pressure, pulse, melena, syncope, hepatic disease, heart failure, hemoglobin, and blood urea nitrogen) [15].

Factors that predict bleeding from an upper GI source include a patient reported history of melena, melenic stool on examination, blood or coffee grounds appearing gastric drainage on nasogastric lavage, and a blood urea nitrogen to serum creatinine greater than 30 [16]. However, the presence of blood clots in stool decreased the likelihood of an UGIB. The presence of tachycardia, nasogastric lavage with red blood, or a hemoglobin of less than 8 g/dl increased the likelihood of severe UGIB requiring urgent intervention [16].

The severity of illness should direct resuscitative efforts. Patients with hemodynamic instability must be managed with rapid intervention to secure the airway, breathing, and circulation (ABCs). During the initial resuscitation, it is important to determine if the bleeding is from an upper or lower GI source as this will help guide the diagnostic approach. In the hemodynamically unstable patient with hematochezia and an unclear GI bleeding source, esophagogastroduodenoscopy (EGD) is recommended prior to colonoscopy to rule out upper GI bleeding [17].

30.3 Indications for Lower Intestinal Endoscopy

Acute lower GI bleeding (ALGIB) is typically less dramatic than upper GI bleeding and is often self-limiting in nature [7]. Common causes of ALGIB include diverticulosis, ischemic colitis, vascular ectasias, hemorrhoids, rectal varices, nonsteroidal anti-inflammatory drug (NSAID) use, inflammatory bowel disease, and malignancy [7, 12]. Of note, the use of enteric-coated aspirin does not reduce the risk of GI bleed [12].

Acute colonic pseudo-obstruction (ACPO or Ogilvie syndrome) is characterized by massive colonic dilation in the absence of mechanical obstruction. Ischemia and perforation are potential life-threatening complications from this syndrome. The rate of ischemia and perforation increases significantly with cecal diameters of >10 cm as the tension increases on the colon wall. See Fig. 30.1.

Initial management is typically conservative with orders for nothing by mouth, nasogastric tube placement and decompression, rectal tube decompression, and patient ambulation (as clinically indicated).

Additionally, the advanced care practitioner (ACP) should evaluate and correct electrolyte and metabolic abnormalities. Laboratory testing may include phosphorus, magnesium, calcium, and thyroid function [18, p. 673]. If sepsis is suspected, obtain blood cultures and initiate antibiotics. Management should also include the discontinuation of narcotics and anticholinergic medications. Frequent physical examinations should be performed to assess for abdominal tenderness or any signs of peritonitis [18] with ongoing plans for operative intervention as appropriate.

Colonic volvulus occurs a bowel segment twists upon itself resulting in colonic obstruction, venous congestion, and arterial inflow obstruction to the affected area [18]. See Fig. 30.2. Endoscopic decompression and rectal tube placement may successfully reestablish integrity of the bowel. Following the procedure, the clinician must monitor for ongoing peritonitis from perforation, ischemia, or bowel infarction after detorsion.

Left-sided colonic or rectal ischemia (see Fig. 30.3) is a possible complication following surgical repair of ruptured abdominal aortic aneurysm (AAA). The reported incidence ranges from 10 % to 42 % following open repair of ruptured

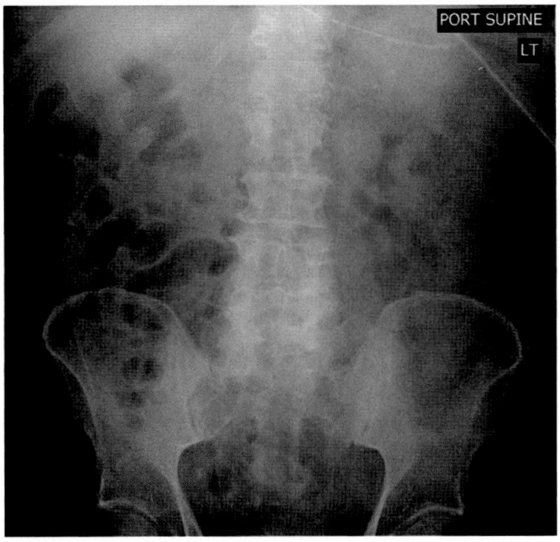

Fig. 30.1 X-ray of ACPO

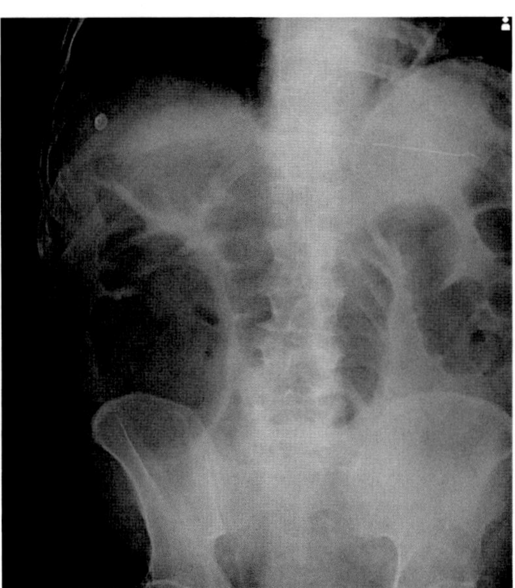

Fig. 30.2 Colonic volvulus

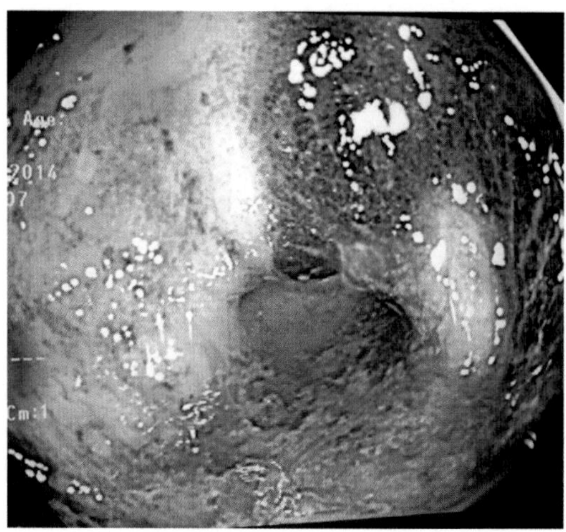

Fig. 30.3 Colonoscopic demonstration of colonic ischemia following open repair of ruptured AAA

AAA [19, 20]. The origin of colonic ischemia (CI) following AAA repair is multifactorial and includes operative repairs lasting longer than 4 h, hypotension and underlying shock, the use of vasopressive medications, inferior mesenteric artery and/or internal iliac artery occlusion, micro-embolization, and underlying renal disease. In some cases, rigid sigmoidoscopy or colonoscopy may be necessary to evaluate the possibility of bowel ischemia at the bedside [19]. However, once the diagnosis of CI is confirmed, colectomy should be considered. The patient should undergo ongoing diligent surveillance until returned to the operating room.

30.4 Preparation Step-Up

If time allows, the ACP can facilitate family notification and obtain consent. During this discussion, the ACP should include the possibility of the need for further diagnostic workup and interventions. This may include the need for angiography/arteriography or operative intervention with the possibility of exploratory laparotomy.

Endoscopic carts and equipment are often retrieved from the surgical or endoscopy suite. See Fig. 30.4. The endoscope is a flexible tube that contains a control section, an insertion tube, and a connector area.

- The control section is held in the physicians' left hand and has two stacked dials or wheels that control direction by deflecting the instrument up/down or left/right. Buttons on the control section are used for insufflation, air, and suction [21]. Additionally, the control section has an entry port to use to introduce or insert accessories through the channel of the device [21]. See Fig. 30.5.
- The insertion tube is a flexible shaft and is attached to the control section. See Fig. 30.6. It varies in length according to primary use. This tube contains an air and water channel and either a fiber-optic source or an electronic video system [21].
- The connector area attaches the endoscope to an image processor, a light and electrical source, air, and water [21]. See Fig. 30. 7.

Ideally for upper endoscopy, the patient should have had nothing by mouth for 4–8 h. The requirements for the patient bowel preparation for lower GI endoscopy may vary from physician to physician; therefore, the ACP should have ongoing dialogue with the attending physician regarding the proposed plan for either procedure and enter physician orders accordingly. Some physicians perform colonoscopy on the un-prepped bowel, as blood acts as a laxative and its presence may provide additional information regarding the location of the bleed [7]. In patients with ACPO, colonoscopy is performed without the administration of oral laxatives or bowel preparation [18]. Additionally, sedation with benzodiazepines alone is preferred because the use of narcotics can further inhibit colonic motility [18, p. 675].

30.5 Procedure

1. Conduct a complete history and physical examination.
2. Obtain informed consent. If emergent, document a detailed note in the medical record of the indications addressing the emergent nature of the procedure.
3. Upper or lower GI preparation orders at the direction of the attending physician (typically four or more liters of polyethylene

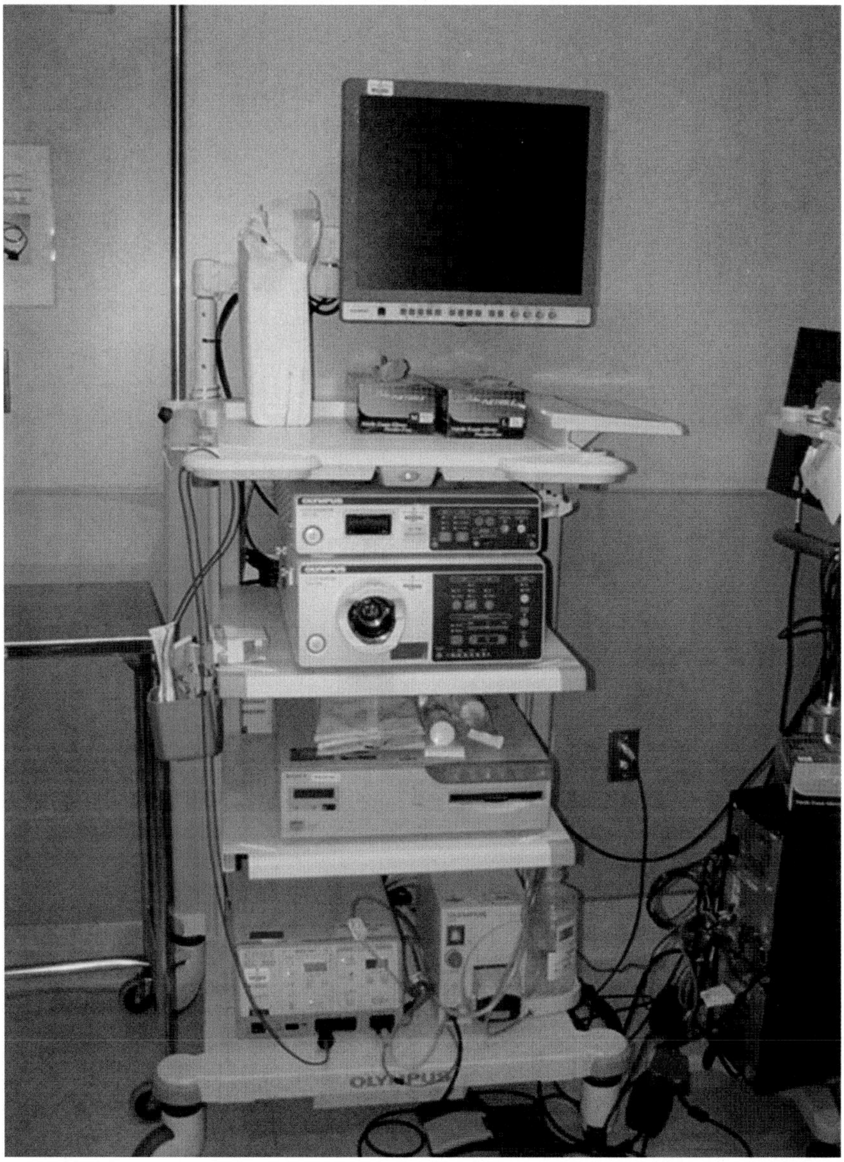

Fig. 30.4 Endoscopy cart

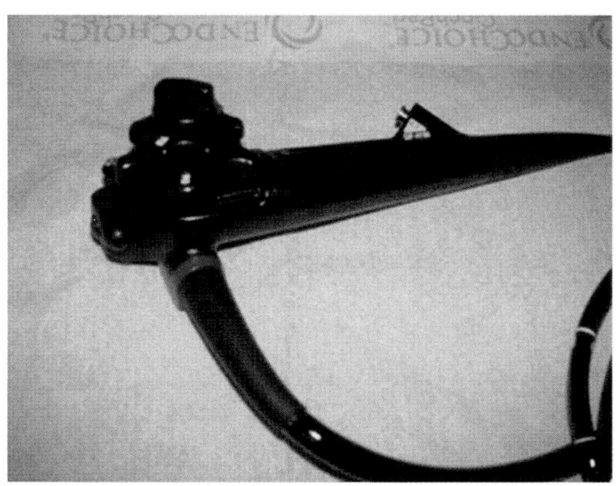

Fig. 30.5 Control buttons for colonoscope

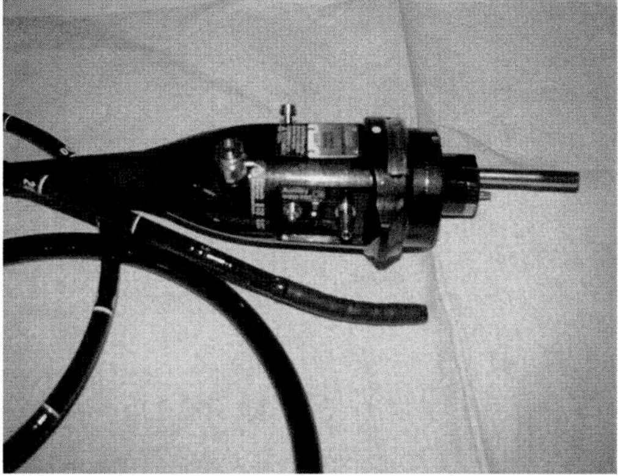

Fig. 30.6 Flexible shaft

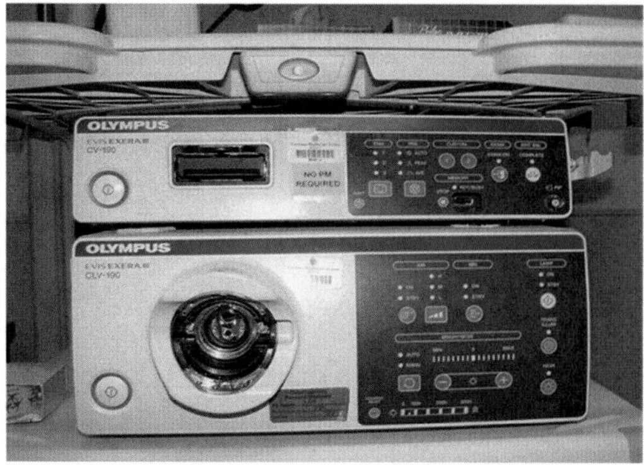

Fig. 30.7 Air/water/light source

glycol-based solutions for lower GI preparation).

4. Perform a "time out" to verify patient and procedure and address any possible concerns that may arise.
5. Ensure appropriate hemodynamic monitoring.
6. Attach the endo-videoscope connector to the endoscopy video system.
7. Attach wall suction to the endo-videoscope.
8. Pretreatment with appropriate sedatives/analgesia as appropriate.
9. Prep, position, and drape the patient in the proper position.
10. During the colonoscopy procedure, the ACP can ensure proper documentation of:
    (a) Vital signs (including pulse oximetry)
    (b) Cardiac rhythm
    (c) Level of sedation/consciousness
    (d) Endoscopy depth of insertion
        - For lower GI:
            - Cecal intubation time
            - Colonoscopy withdrawal time from the cecum
    (e) Presence of any pathology
    (f) Interventions performed
    (g) Any unexpected or untoward outcomes/events

30.6 Complications/Pitfalls in ICU

Patients must have continuous cardiac monitoring, pulse oximetry, and blood pressure monitoring throughout the procedure. Additionally, the ACP should prepare the staff and the patient to prepare for possible invasive hemodynamic monitoring. In the hemodynamically labile or unstable patient undergoing intubation with rapid sequence intubation, one must anticipate the potential side effects of medication administration on the hemodynamics of the patient. It is not uncommon for hypotension to occur following induction. The ACP must anticipate untoward effects and ensure that intravenous crystalloid fluids are available for infusion via pressure bags if needed. Additionally, vasopressors should be premixed and readily available.

Initial laboratory evaluation should include a complete blood count, a coagulation profile, serum chemistry, and type and crossmatch for blood products. Consideration for serum lactate monitoring and arterial blood gas evaluation may be of additional diagnostic value. Fresh frozen plasma (FFP), platelets, and cryoprecipitate may be considered for treatment of coagulopathy. For patients who receive warfarin, vitamin K may also be considered with the use of FFP or prothrombin complex.

Patients should receive appropriate ongoing volume resuscitation, correction of electrolytes, and intermittent nasogastric suction for decompression. Under-recognition of shock is a pitfall that must be avoided. The treatment of shock should occur concomitantly as the differential sources of GI emergency are being evaluated and determined. The ACP must understand that a "normal blood pressure" does not exclude the diagnosis of shock. Ongoing monitoring of end-organ perfusion includes the patients' level of consciousness, serum lactate monitoring, central venous oxygen saturation ($ScvO_2$) or mixed venous oxygen saturation (SvO_2), hourly urine output, as well as other clinical indicators. While intravenous fluids should be ordered and administered, consideration for the use of vasopressors may be needed to further support adequate perfusion of the organs. Additionally, when bleeding cannot be controlled endoscopically, preparation for arteriography or intraoperative intervention must be considered and initiated.

The ACP should possess an understanding of the relative contraindications to endoscopy which include severe coagulopathy, severe thrombocytopenia, and severe neutropenia. Additional relative surgical complications include colonic necrosis, fulminant colitis, toxic megacolon, acute severe diverticulitis, recent colonic surgery, and acute peritonitis [22]. In patients with peritoneal signs or suspicion for perforation, prompt surgical consultation is necessary and recommended [18].

References

1. Greenwald DA, Cohen J. Overview of upper gastrointestinal endoscopy (esophagogastroduodenoscopy) [up to date, cited 2015 Oct 15]. Available from: http://www.uptodate.com/contents/overview-of-upper-gastrointestinal-endoscopy-esophagogastroduodenoscopy?source=search_result&search=role+of+endoscopy&selectedTitle=1%7E150
2. Grassini M, Verna C, Niola P, Navino M, Battaglia E, Bassotti G. Appropriateness of colonoscopy: diagnostic yield and safety in guidelines. World J Gastroenterol. 2007;13(12):1816–9. Available from http://www.ncbi.nlm.nih.gov/pubmed/17465472.
3. Lieberman DA, Rex DK, Winawer SJ, Giardiello FM, Johnson DA, Levin TR. Guidelines for colonoscopy surveillance after screening and polypectomy: a consensus update by the US Multi-Society Task Force on colorectal cancer. Gastroenterology. 2012;143(3):844–57. Available from http://dx.doi.org/10.1053/j.gastro.2012.06.001.
4. Zauber AG, Winawer SJ, O'Brien MJ, Volelaar IL, et al. Colonoscopic polypectomy and long-term prevention of colorectal-cancer deaths. N Engl J Med. 2012;366(8):687–96. Available from https://www.med.upenn.edu/gastro/documents/nejmoa1100370.pdf.
5. Church J, Kao J. Bedside colonoscopy in intensive care units: indications, techniques and outcomes. Surg Endosc. 2014;28(9):2679–82. doi:10.1007/s00464-014-3526-6. Available from http://www.ncbi.nlm.nih.gov/pubmed/24771194. Epub 26 Apr 2014.
6. Albeldawi M, Ha D, Mehta P, Lopez R, Jang S, Vargo JJ, et al. Utility of urgent colonoscopy in acute lower gastrointestinal bleeding: a single center experience. Gastroenterol Rep (Oxf). 2014;2(4):300–5.
7. Barnert J, Messmann H. Management of lower gastrointestinal tract bleeding. Best Pract Res Clin Gastroenterol. 2008;22(2):295–312. Available from http://www.bpgastro.com/article/S1521-6918(07)00131-X/abstract.
8. Saltzman JR, Feldman M (editor), Travis AC (editor). Approach to the acute upper gastrointestinal bleeding in adults [up to date cited 2014 Sep 22). Available from up to date: http://www.uptodate.com/contents/approach-to-acute-upper-gastrointestinal-bleeding-in-adults?source=machineLearning&search=upper+GI+bleed+in+the+ICU&selectedTitle=1%7E150§ionRank=1&anchor=H4#H4
9. Cappell MS, Iacovone FM. Safety and efficacy of esophagogastroduodenoscopy after myocardial infarction. Am J Med. 1999;106(1):29–35. Available from http://www.ncbi.nlm.nih.gov/pubmed/10320114.
10. Laine L, Jensen DM. Management of patients with ulcer bleeding. Am J Gastroenterol. 2012;107:345–60. doi:10.1038/ajg.2011.480.
11. El-Tawil AM. Trends on gastrointestinal bleeding and mortality: where are we standing? World J Gastroenterol. 2012;18(11):1154–8. doi:10.3748/wjg.v18.i11.1154.
12. Manning-Dimmitt LL, Dimmitt SG, Wilson GR. Diagnosis of gastrointestinal bleeding in adults. Am Fam Physician. 2005;71(7):1339–46. Available from http://www.aafp.org/afp/2005/0401/p1339.html.
13. Kim J. Management and prevention of upper GI bleeding. Gastroenterology and Nutrition Series PSAP–VII. 2012:7–26 [cited 2014 Sep 22]. Available from: http://www.accp.com/docs/bookstore/psap/p7b11sample01.pdf
14. Rockall T, Logan RF, Devlin HB, Northfield TC. Risk assessment after acute upper gastrointestinal hemorrhage. Gut. 1996;38(3):316–21. Available from http://www.ncbi.nlm.nih.gov/pmc/articles/PMC1383057/.
15. Blatchford O, Murray WR, Blatchford M. A risk score to predict need for treatment for upper gastrointestinal hemorrhage. Lancet. 2000;356(9238):1318–21.
16. Srygley FD, Gerardo CJ, Tran T, Fisher DA. Does this patient have a severe upper gastrointestinal bleed? JAMA. 2012;307(10):1072–9.
17. Barnert J, Messmann H. Diagnosis and management of lower gastrointestinal bleeding. Gastroenterol Hepatol. 2009;11:637–46. doi:10.1038/nrgastro.2009.167.
18. American Society for Gastrointestinal Endoscopy (ASGE). The role of endoscopy in the management of patients with known and suspected colonic obstruction and pseudo-obstruction. Gastrointest Endosc. 2010;71(4):669–79. doi:10.1016/j.gie.2009.11.027. Available from: http://www.asge.org/uploadedFiles/Publications_and_Products/Practice_Guidelines/The%20role%20of%20endoscopy%20in%20the%20management%20of%20patients%20with%20known%20and%20suspected%20colonic%20obstruction%20and%20pseudo-obstruction.pdf.
19. Becquemin JP, Majewski M, Fermani N, Marzell J, Desgrandes P, Allaire E, et al. Colon ischemia following abdominal aortic aneurysm repair in the era of endovascular abdominal aortic repair. J Vasc Surg. 2008;47(2):258–62. doi:10.1016/j.jvs.2007.10.001.
20. Champagne BJ, Lee C, Valerian B, Mulhotra N, Mehta M. Incidence of colonic ischemia after repair of ruptured abdominal aortic aneurysm with Endograft. J Am Coll Surg. 2007;204(4):597–602.
21. Bosco JJ, Barkun AN, Isenberg GA, Nhuyen CC, Petersen BT, Silverman WB, et al. Gastrointestinal endoscopes. Gastrointest Endosc. 2003;58(6):822–30.
22. Bayat I, Hirst, J, Miller, BJ, Kate V (editor). MEDSCAPE [2014 Aug 13). Introduction to rigid sigmoidoscopy. Available from: http://emedicine.medscape.com/article/81001-overview

31 Common Urologic Procedures

Timothy M. Fain and Chris Teigland

31.1 Proper Technique for the Insertion of Foley Catheters

While most Foley catheters are usually inserted by nurses in the Emergency Department prior to the patient's arrival in the ICU setting, a good percentage of these patients will eventually require a Foley to be placed for various reasons. Therefore, it is a good practice to know proper sterile technique. Since this is taught in detail in most nursing institutions, we will briefly review it here [1]. This chapter will cover general technique and will not address some of the more complicated insertions, such as in the morbidly obese patient with a buried penis.

1. Wearing clean gloves, cleanse the patient's genitals with either a betadine solution or chlorhexidine solution (usually provided in Foley catheter kit). Be sure to check patient's allergies first (particularly to iodine/betadine). When halfway through the prep, don a pair of sterile gloves (also provided in the Foley kit) and finish the prep. This is to prevent the sterile gloves from becoming contaminated early on in the prep.
2. In males, pay attention to prepping the scrotum/inner thighs as the penis is often set back down after prepping, and it may touch these adjacent surfaces, contaminating the cleansed surface.
3. In heavily soiled patients (from bodily fluids such as blood, stool, or purulent material), make sure patient is bathed adequately before attempting any prep.
4. Drape the patient with a sterile drape or field if desired and provided; most simple insertions do not necessitate this step.
5. In females, spread the labia before inserting the Foley. In males, firmly elevate the penis with one hand while inserting the tip of the Foley with the other. Be sure to apply adequate lubrication. In most kits, a syringe of lubricating jelly is provided; with males, apply a small amount of this jelly to the Foley and inject the rest directly into the urethra. This will maximize the amount of lubrication used.
6. In females, insert the Foley well beyond when you begin to see urine emanating from the tip of the Foley; for males, insert every Foley to the hub/balloon port. This will ensure that you get good placement and do not injure the prostatic urethra with the balloon.
7. Finally, once you feel the catheter is in appropriate position in the bladder (the Foley will not be extruding itself from the urethra in males), gently inflate the balloon with 10 ml of sterile water (not saline, which can crystallize

T.M. Fain, MSN, BSN, NP (✉)
C. Teigland, MD, FACS
Department of Urology, Carolinas Medical Center, 1023 Edgehill Rd South, Charlotte, NC 28173, USA
e-mail: tim.fain@carolinashealthcare.org

D.A. Taylor et al. (eds.), *Interventional Critical Care*, DOI 10.1007/978-3-319-25286-5_31

and prevent balloon from deflating), gently pull balloon down to bladder neck, and place catheter to straight drainage. If the patient has obvious discomfort while inflating the balloon, take care that you are not still in the urethra.

31.2 Difficult Foley Catheter Insertions

31.2.1 Benign Prostatic Hypertrophy (BPH)

Most of the consults we see for this issue have usually a significant history of voiding complaints or lower urinary tract symptoms; often the history is not immediately revealed because of the critical nature of the patient's illness, other than as evidenced in the medical record. Often at the point of consultation, there have been at least several attempts by the nursing staff and/or ICU providers to place a Foley catheter, albeit unsuccessfully. Usually, the types of catheters that have been attempted are standard latex Foleys (16 or 18fr) and sometimes a Coude, which is a type of curved tip catheter that is good for advancing beyond the area of the prostate (Fig. 31.2).

Generally speaking, the setup used for placing a Foley in a patient with suspected BPH is the same as other difficult catheter insertions [2]: first obtain the urology cart from medical equipment so that the person inserting the catheter has good access to whatever equipment/supplies that may be needed. Typically in this scenario, without knowing whether the difficulty in placing the Foley is from BPH or another issue (such as urethral stricture), the usual supplies brought into the room include a standard Foley kit, a boat of 4×4s or gauze, a Uro-jet syringe (Fig. 31.1), a 20fr Coude-tip Foley (Fig. 31.2), and a 12fr all-silicone Foley (Fig. 31.3).

1. Using the standard Foley kit, prep the patient using sterile technique.
2. Drape the patient with sterile towels or a sterile field/drape (using the supplies in the Foley kit), and if using a specialty catheter, remove the 16 or 18fr Foley from the tubing in the box, being careful to separate these items from the rest of the contents in the kit in order to maintain a sterile field. Make sure you open any items you intend to use while in sterile gloves first, i.e., the Uro-jet syringe. Then open the outer wrapper of the Foley you intend to use and place the Foley on the sterile field (there should still be a plastic wrapper around it).

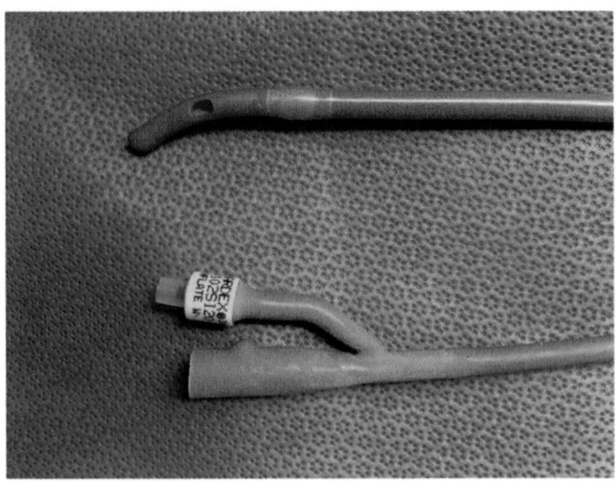

Fig. 31.2 Coude Foley catheter

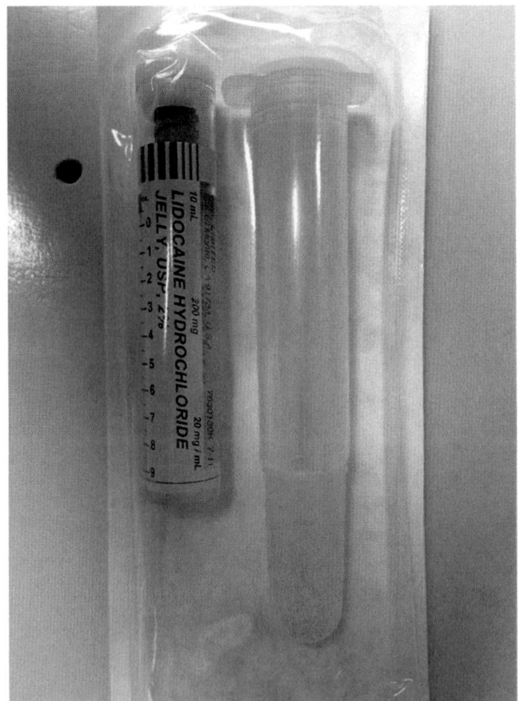

Fig. 31.1 Uro-jet syringe

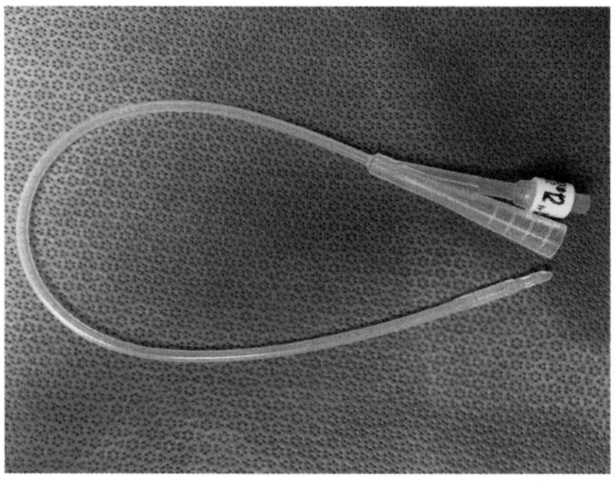

Fig. 31.3 All-silicone Foley catheter

3. Make sure you have sterile gloves on at this point (if not done during the prep).
4. Open the Foley intended for use and place it on the sterile field.
5. Administer a Uro-jet syringe with viscous lidocaine jelly directly into the patient's urethral meatus. This adds the advantage of dilating the urethra, providing local analgesia, and potentially closing any posterior flaps in the urethra that have been unearthed by multiple Foley attempts (these are called false passages). This extra lubrication can actually make the difference when placing a Foley in these type of circumstances, whether the obstruction is due to BPH or another issue.
6. Once the Uro-jet has been administered and adequate time has passed to provide analgesia, usually 20–30 s anecdotally—however some literature suggests up to 10 min may be necessary in some cases [2]—the Foley catheter should then be heavily lubricated on the distal third and then, with the tip of the Coude facing upward, inserted gently until resistance is met. The way to tell if the Coude Foley tip is facing upward while in the urethra is to keep the balloon port of the catheter facing up at all times. This will give you the greatest chance of passing the Foley catheter beyond the prostate or a false urethral passage.
7. If the Foley will not advance, depending on your comfort level, some pressure may be necessary if the prostate hypertrophy is significant. If the Foley still will not advance, make sure a urology provider is the only person performing further attempts.
8. If the Foley advances into the bladder, do not inflate the balloon unless urine is seen effluxing from the Foley port. Make sure to advance the Foley all the way to the hub, and if it is not extruding itself from the urethra, you can be fairly confident you are in the bladder, particularly if confirmed with urine output. Sometimes the gel from the Uro-jet will clog the Foley tip, and to confirm you are in the bladder, you may have to take a syringe and aspirate the main Foley port to bring urine into the Foley or hand irrigate the Foley with a Toomey syringe.
9. Gently inflate the balloon with the 10 ml of sterile water provided with the kit. If resistance is noted to balloon inflation or if you note the patient becoming agitated when you attempt to inflate it, the Foley may still be in the prostate or not in the right place. You may consider using 30 ml if the patient has already pulled another Foley out with the balloon inflated or if you are inserting a three-way hematuria catheter (covered in another section).
10. Gently pull down the catheter balloon until it rests at the bladder neck, then attach the Foley tubing to the patient's leg using a leg strap or securing device (stat-lock; see illustration). Depending on the patient's condition, one application may be more suitable than the other (if there is not much length of Foley protruding from the urethra, a stat-lock will not work).
11. Watch the Foley drain to see if there are any indications of a problem (sudden output of bright red blood, clots in the tubing, no urine output, or blood/urine coming out around the Foley).

31.2.2 Urethral Stricture Disease

Most of the patients with this problem have some degree of voiding complaints, although they may not be able to give you any information in the critical care setting. Most urethral strictures are discovered when a Foley is being attempted, and it will not pass into the bladder. About 99 % of these patients are male; true urethral stricture disease in females is extremely rare. These can seem or feel like BPH, when in reality, a more involved process is indicated. Prompt urologic consultation is indicated in these situations, as nearly all complex strictures require a surgical procedure to bypass with a Foley. For the sake of instruction, we will include the usual techniques utilized to dilate or open strictures. The goal of dilation with urethral strictures should be the minimal amount to allow the smallest effective catheter to pass, usually dilate to two French sizes above planned size of Foley to be placed, e.g., to 16fr to place 12fr catheter. If suspect a larger diameter is needed due to debris or blood in urine, may dilate further [3].

1. In an attempt at brevity, presume that the patient has been prepped using sterile technique. The difference with this procedure is that we will usually drape the patient with sterile towels to form a large sterile field; this necessitates the usual OR pack of blue towels that can be obtained from the urology cart or sterile processing. A large prepacked sterile drape is also available on the cart.
2. Once draped, we will then administer a Urojet per the urethra and await adequate analgesia (at least 20–30 s). A fairly good amount of KY jelly should be available on the field for lubricating dilators/catheters.
3. In an effort to minimize urethral trauma at the bedside, we will sometimes obtain a 12fr all-silicone Foley, which can bypass a stricture without too much difficulty [3]. Make sure adequate lubrication is applied prior to attempting to pass. A significant amount of pressure will generally be required to advance the Foley. Urologic expertise is of course recommended.
4. If the 12fr Foley will not advance and the feel of the urethra indicates a stricture (and not a false passage), we will obtain a set of filiforms and followers, a flexible cystoscope, or a guide wire and angiocath needle. These techniques will be broken down further as noted below.

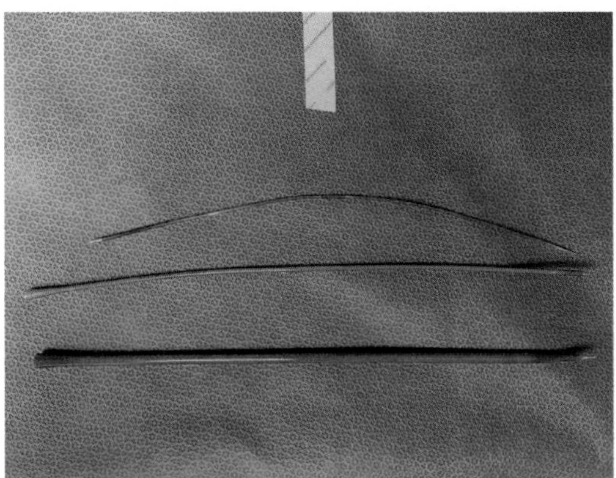

Fig. 31.4 Filiform with followers

(a) Dilation of urethral stricture using filiforms and followers (Fig. 31.4). Filiforms are very small, stiff composite catheters that measure from < 1 mm to 2 mm thick and usually have a curved tip. They come in various lengths and have a small threaded bolt on the tip that a follower (sized from 6fr all the way to 24fr), woven of the same material but sometimes strengthened with braided steel covered in composite, and can be threaded into and be inserted behind the filiform to dilate the stricture. Proper technique heavily relies on a good tactile sense of one's position in the urethra and whether the filiform/follower has exited the urethra. They allow blind navigation of the true urethral lumen and access to the bladder.

- After applying lubrication to the filiform, the filiform is inserted gently, and attempts are made to maneuver the tip through the strictured area and beyond, into the bladder. One can tell if the filiform has successfully passed into the bladder if it does not extrude itself once passed all the way up to the bolt on the end.
- Once the filiform is felt to be secure within the bladder, successive followers are attached beginning often with 8fr then allowing for the density of the stricture; dilation may proceed up to 24fr in size. Usually, dilation of two sizes above the planned size of the Foley to be inserted is required (i.e., dilate to 20fr if an 18fr Foley is planned to be inserted).

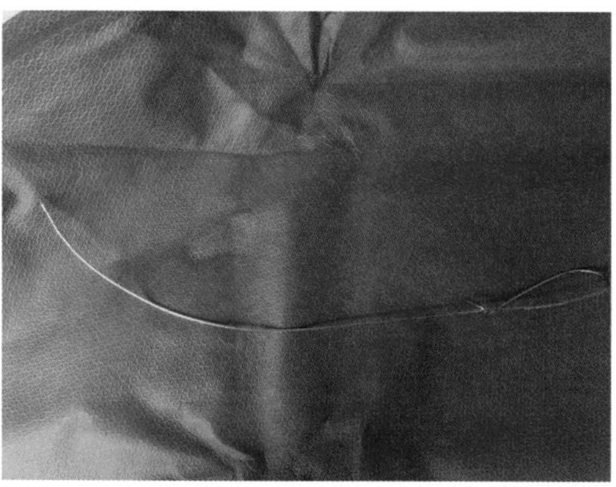

Fig. 31.5 Catheter stylet with threaded tip

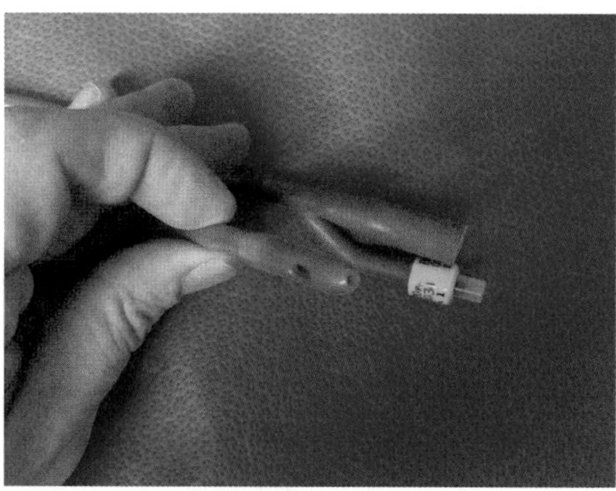

Fig. 31.6 Council-tip Foley catheter

- As successive followers are passed, there are eyelets in the end of each follower that allow in most cases for urine to drain from the end of the follower confirming as one dilates; they are indeed still in the bladder.
- Once adequate dilation has been accomplished, the filiform and follower are both removed. An all-silicone Foley is then utilized because of its stiffness and likelihood of passing; generally 2–3 sizes less than the size of the last follower used are appropriate. If there is concern for a false passage, the follower is removed only, and a Le Forte stylet/Council catheter guide is obtained (Fig. 31.5), which can be threaded onto the filiform. One can place a Council-tip Foley, a special catheter with a hole manufactured in the very tip (Fig. 31.6), over the stylet in a retrograde fashion. Once the catheter is fully loaded on the stylet, the stylet can then in turn be threaded into the indwelling filiform and the Council Foley slid over both devices and into the bladder.

  (b) If the urethral stricture is unable to be bypassed by a filiform, an alternative could be to obtain a flexible guide wire or "glide wire." This is often a flexible, composite/nylon guide wire, which is hydrophilic, 0.89 mm in diameter, and usually 150 cm long that due to its flexibility, in some cases, can be navigated blindly beyond a tight urethral stricture. The technique discussed here is called the "Blitz" technique (Fig. 31.7). It involves blindly passing the glide wire to the bladder then advancing a small diameter Foley (12fr all silicone) over the wire after back-loading it onto the wire [4]. This technique is used generally in male patients with either false passage and/or urethral stricture disease, but other applications may be feasible [5].

- Provided the patient has been prepped and draped appropriately, a 0.89 mm glide wire is moistened and inserted with the flexible tip first. The wire is manipulated until it easily passes beyond the area of stricture. We advocate advancing the wire until most of it is curled in the bladder and only about 30–40 cm remain outside the urethra. This will make certain of placement as the wire will curl back on itself and the tip exit the penis if not in the bladder. It will also make it less likely that the wire will be dislodged while attempting Foley placement.
- Then obtain an 18 gauge angiocath and 12fr all-silicone Foley. After piercing the tip of the Foley with the angiocath, retract the needle and leave the sheath intact. Backload the wire into the Foley and then remove the sheath. Manipulate the wire so that it pulls back into the tube and out of the eyelet. Once the Foley is properly loaded, advance the Foley with ample lubrication over the wire and into the bladder. It can act as a soft dilator due to the stiffness and shape of the Foley. Once the Foley is pushed to the hub and urine is confirmed draining from the tip, the wire can be

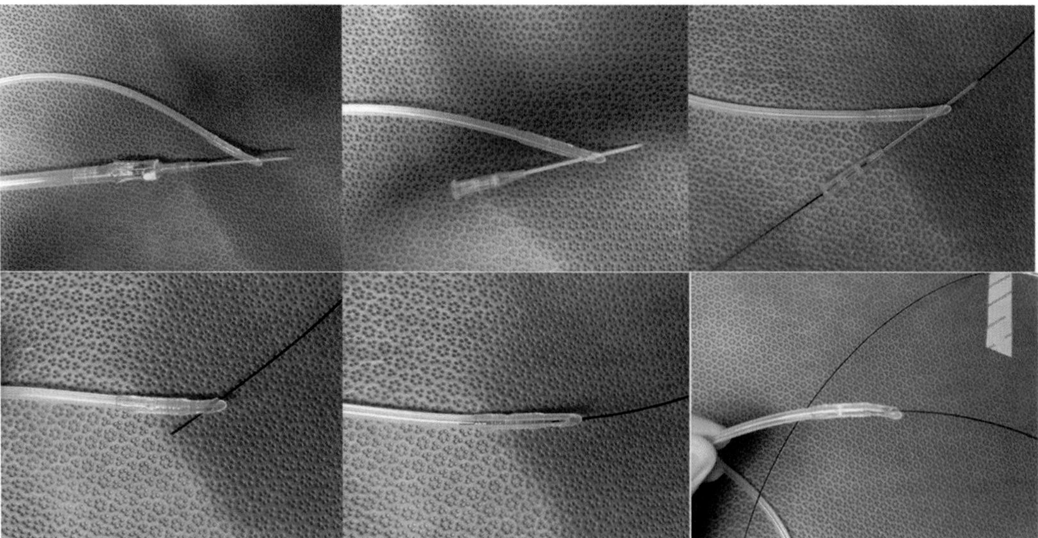

Fig. 31.7 Blitz technique

removed from inside the Foley. Then all that remains is to inflate the balloon and place the Foley to drainage.

(c) Lastly, the standard of care for difficult Foley catheterizations in general, not just for urethral strictures, is flexible cystoscopy (Fig. 31.8). This technique is generally reserved for persons trained in general urology. Cystoscopy provides direct visualization of the problem and, in most cases, quick access to the bladder. However, it is more expensive, and setting up all of the needed equipment can be time consuming. It may be difficult to tell the difference between a bladder neck contracture (BNC) and a urethral stricture, something cystoscopy can readily differentiate between. This is the gold standard when applied to urethral disruptions from trauma, when blind catheterization is not necessarily recommended.

- In general, the same prep applies to patients undergoing cystoscopy as with dilation of urethral strictures; a large sterile field is important as a place to set the cystoscope and assorted equipment is needed.
- The cystoscope tip is amply lubricated, and after the Uro-jet has taken effect, the scope is introduced into the urethra. Care must be taken to elevate the patient's penis firmly while using the cystoscope; otherwise adequate visualization may not be possible.

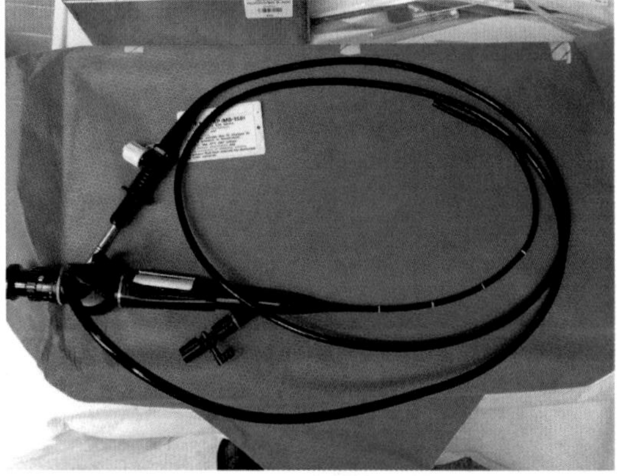

Fig. 31.8 Olympus flexible cystoscope

- Once the area of stricture has been visualized, a flexible guide wire (preferably a stiff guide wire with a flexible tip) can be advanced through the scope beyond the area of stricture, with the flexible tip foremost. If the wire advances without much resistance, continue advancing the wire until most of it is coiled in the bladder and only about 30–40 cm remains outside the urethra. This will make it easier to work with dilators.

Then remove the cystoscope over the wire while preventing the wire from being removed (push-pull or "Seldinger" technique).

- Once the scope has been removed, obtain a set of Cook or similar dilators. These are stiff, plastic/composite, hollow, cone-tip dilators that fit over a wire and are sized from 6fr to 30fr. After ample lubrication, the dilators can be used successively to dilate the stricture. The goal is of course to dilate the minimal amount to allow the smallest catheter to pass. In general, most strictures are dilated to 18 or 20fr to allow regularly sized catheters to pass.
- Once the last dilator has been utilized, a Council-tip Foley is obtained; usually the 16 or 18fr size is selected for its likelihood of passing. After applying ample lubrication, the catheter is inserted over the wire and into the bladder. Often, at the narrowest point in the urethra (where the stricture was dilated) or at the bladder neck, the catheter will meet significant resistance. This is where having a second set of hands to help pull back on the wire to keep it tense while the Foley is advanced comes in handy. The catheter will usually pass. If not, the wire may have to be removed and loaded back into the cystoscope, and the urethra visually inspected. This can determine if a false passage has developed or if the stricture was adequately dilated. In some cases, a BNC is discovered, which can be notoriously difficult to dilate adequately to allow for Foley placement. Another advantage of cystoscopy is that if a BNC is noted, one may dilate this a little more than a typical stricture (up to 24fr) to facilitate passage of the catheter.
- If, despite multiple attempts, a Foley cannot be placed, the next step may be a suprapubic tube [4].

31.2.3 Bladder Neck Contractures

These are usually detected either by careful placement of a Foley with some urine noted draining from the catheter, but the catheter could not be advanced into the bladder or by cystoscopy. This is a male problem, and most if not all patients with this issue have had some type of procedure or treatment of their prostate. The most common treatments associated with this problem are transurethral resection of the prostate (TURP), radical prostatectomy, and brachytherapy (radioactive seed implantation into the prostate). They can be very resilient and difficult to dilate large enough to place a Foley. This is a procedure that should only be attempted by a provider trained in urologic procedures. Presume that filiforms and followers can be used just as effectively as cystoscopy with dilation of the contracture over a wire. Having previously outlined the use of cystoscopy and dilators to open a urethral stricture as discussed above in section (c), we will refer to this section for guidance as the methodology would be essentially no different here in the treatment of BNCs [6].

31.2.4 Meatal Stenosis

This is an often perplexing problem that is nearly as common as urethral stricture disease, although the actual incidence is unknown. The solutions to dilating the stenosis and passing a Foley are relatively simple, but require the services of a trained provider.

1. Standard prep and drape.
2. Small mosquito clamp or pair of hemostats can be inserted into the meatus after local analgesia (Uro-jet) and gently opened to dilate the stenosis.
3. A more subtle approach may be to utilize Van Buren sounds (Fig. 31.9), dilating progressively from the largest size that will fit in the meatus until adequate dilation allows for Foley placement [2].
4. Often, after the Foley has been placed, patient will require an elective procedure called a meatotomy and/or meatoplasty, in order to extract the scar tissue contributing to the stenosis.

31.2.5 Suprapubic Cystostomy

This procedure is not routinely performed in the ICU setting due to the proficiency of catheter placement associated with advanced technology

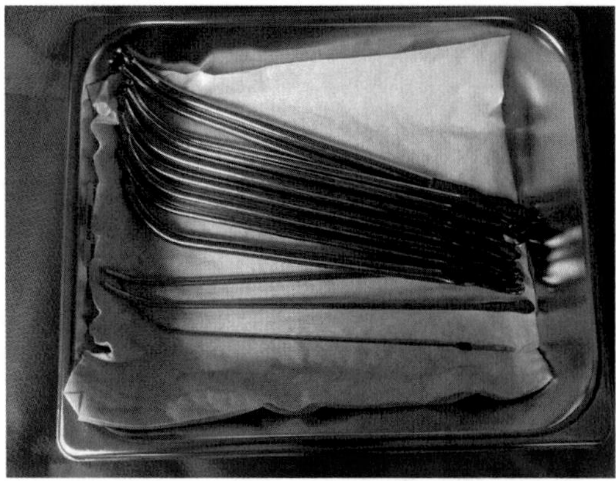

Fig. 31.9 Van Buren sounds

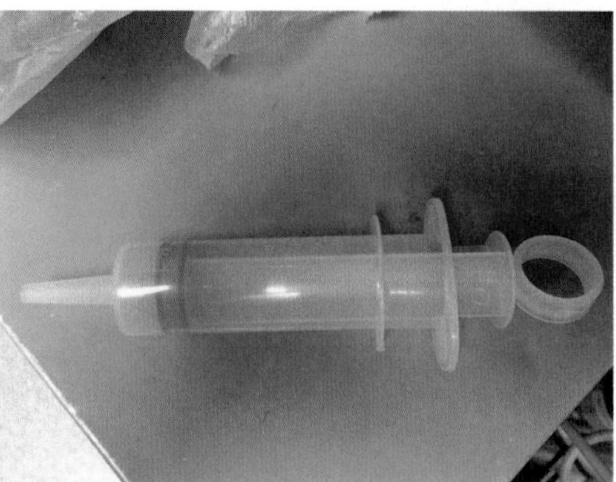

Fig. 31.10 Toomey syringe

and training, as well as the ease by which suprapubic tubes can be placed under US guidance with fluoroscopy by the Interventional Radiology department. Urologists typically perform this procedure in the OR under a more controlled environment with available fluoroscopy.

31.3 Clot Evacuation Due to Hematuria

Gross hematuria with clot retention is a vexing problem that can require a patient to go to the operating room in order to correct. Several measures can be done at the bedside in order to hopefully prevent this, though not always. There are multiple possible underlying reasons for a patient to have gross hematuria, and sometimes until the cause is isolated and addressed, some of the measures we recommend can be merely "putting a Band-Aid" on the problem. However, these can be effective measures that, if introduced early, can help prevent unnecessary trips to the operating room.

31.3.1 Foley Selection

The minimum size to be placed in a patient with hematuria and clots is a 22fr three-way Foley, readily available in most ICU settings, the OR, and urology floor, as well as on the urology cart in medical equipment. Ideally, a 24fr three-way is selected and placed (several types of this Foley exist, but some are more often utilized by trained urology professionals), which, although uncomfortable, allows for the greatest chance of adequately draining the bladder while evacuating clots. Three-way Foleys less than 22fr in size have no useful application in the setting of hematuria with clots; if one is encountered having been placed by the ER or another facility, promptly remove this Foley and replace with a 22 or 24fr three-way (if ongoing hematuria/clots noted).

31.3.2 Clot Evacuation

Three ports are included on three-way Foleys, one for the balloon (which should be inflated to 30 ml with sterile water), one for continuous bladder irrigation (CBI), and the main port for drainage of urine. To evacuate clots from the bladder effectively (presuming a 22 or 24fr Foley in place), one must plug the irrigation/CBI port with a Foley hole plug or clamp the tubing connected to the CBI. A Toomey syringe (Fig. 31.10) is most effective in irrigating/evacuating clots at the bedside. It is helpful to test the bladder for clot retention by first attempting to withdraw from the main port to evacuate clots/excess urine. Then, one must introduce a minimum of 60 ml sterile saline/water and up to 180 ml to successfully hand irrigate the bladder of clots. This can be continued until the urine is clear or at least until no further clots are evacuated.

31.3.3 Continuous Bladder Irrigation

Initiated when as many clots have been evacuated from the bladder as possible and when gross hematuria is persistent. This can help with hemorrhagic cystitis, prostatic bleeding, or when there has been an injury from a Foley catheter. To reiterate, *CBI should not be attempted when there are a large amount of known persistent clots within the bladder or when the catheter is less than 22fr in size*. This can lead to bladder rupture.

31.4 Reduction of Paraphimosis

This is a common problem experienced in the ICU when for whatever reason, the foreskin is retracted (pulled back toward the body) to facilitate hygiene or place a Foley catheter and then left in a retracted position. The glans may begin to swell and the foreskin contract, forming a stenotic ring of tissue that can become necrotic and constrict the glans, causing further swelling and ischemia. This can only happen in uncircumcised males and is often mistaken for penile edema. Exacerbating factors can be anasarca/third spacing of fluid or pelvic fractures/injury resulting in pelvic hematoma/bleeding into genitals.

31.4.1 Technique

Firm pressure is exerted on the foreskin and glans penis, with an effort to massage the edema/fluid back from the distal shaft and into the pelvis. This may take quite a while, and you may need to apply pressure in multiple areas of the foreskin/glans to effectively reduce the edema. Then you may observe where the constrictive ring of tissue is in regard to where the glans penis is and begin to apply pressure to the glans directly inward while stretching out the penis and holding the foreskin by at least two opposite sides. This may take a trained professional to perform, but can easily be learned by performing several difficult reductions.

31.4.2 Follow-Up

Once the glans is seen to "pop" back down below the constricted ring of foreskin, the foreskin should be left reduced or pulled away from the body to allow for healing/swelling to resolve. In most cases there is minor bleeding from the trauma of the procedure. Consider pre-procedural narcotics or sedation if the patient is very uncomfortable.

Herein, this concludes our discussion covering common urologic procedures performed in the ICU setting. References are cited below.

References

1. Gould CV, Umscheid CA, Agarwal RK, Kuntz G, Pegues DA, the Healthcare Infection Control Practices Advisory Committee. Guideline for prevention of catheter-associated urinary tract infections. Atlanta, GA: DHHS/CDC; 2009.
2. Ghaffary C, Yohannes A, Villanueva C, Leslie SW. A practical approach to difficult urinary catheterizations. Curr Urol Rep. 2013;14:565–79.
3. Villanueva C, Hemstreet III GP. Difficult male urethral catheterization: a review of different approaches. Int Braz J Urol. 2008;34:401–12.
4. Villanueva C, Hemstreet III, GP. AUA Update Series. 2011; 30(5):42–47. Difficult catheterizations: tricks of the trade.
5. Blitz B. A simple method using hydrophilic guide wires for the difficult urethral catheterization. Urology. 1995;46:99–100.
6. Lachat ML, Moehrlen U, Bruetsch HP, et al. The Seldinger technique for difficult transurethral catheterization: a gentle alternative to suprapubic puncture. Br J Surg. 2000;87:1729.

Part VIII

Abdominal Procedures

Paracentesis

32

David Carpenter, Michael Bowen, and Ram Subramanian

32.1 Introduction

Paracentesis is a relatively simple procedure where a needle is inserted into the peritoneal cavity to obtain ascitic fluid [1]. Traditionally paracentesis are divided into diagnostic and therapeutic procedures. Diagnostic paracentesis refers to removal of a small amount of fluid for testing purposes. Therapeutic paracentesis refers to the removal of large volumes of fluid for relief of symptoms [2].

32.2 Indications

Paracentesis should be performed on all patients with new onset ascites [2]. This includes differentiating between exudative and transudative ascites. Any patient with suspected spontaneous bacterial peritonitis (SBP) should also undergo paracentesis. Finally any patient with end-stage liver disease and ascites who is hospitalized should undergo diagnostic paracentesis to rule out occult SBP [3] (Table 32.1).

Therapeutic paracentesis is indicated for symptomatic tense ascites and to relieve associated dyspnea or abdominal pain.

32.3 Contraindications

The only absolute contraindication is an acute abdomen requiring surgery. Paracentesis should also be avoided in patients with active disseminated intravascular coagulation. Care should be taken in pregnant patients and patients with bowel distension, intra-abdominal adhesions, and distended bladder. The provider should avoid sites with skin infection, enlarged surface vessels, surgical scars, or hematomas. Recannulated umbilical veins and varices should also be avoided.

Many of the patients undergoing paracentesis will have significant abnormalities of coagulation or thrombocytopenia due to their underlying liver disease. However, despite the seeming risks of coagulopathy or thrombocytopenia, routine administration of fresh frozen plasma or platelets is not needed [4, 5]. This delays the procedure and exposes the patient to transfusion risk.

D. Carpenter, MPAS, PA-C (✉)
Emory Critical Care Center, Atlanta, GA, USA
e-mail: david.carpenter@emoryhealthcare.org

M. Bowen, MN, ACNP
Department of Radiology, Emory School of Medicine, 1365 Clifton Road, Atlanta, GA 30322, USA
e-mail: mbowen@emory.edu

R. Subramanian, MD, FCCM, FCCP
Departments of Surgery and Medicine, Emory School of Medicine, Atlanta, GA, USA
e-mail: RMSUBRA@emory.edu

D.A. Taylor et al. (eds.), *Interventional Critical Care*, DOI 10.1007/978-3-319-25286-5_32

Table 32.1 Indications of SBP

Fever
Abdominal pain
Worsening encephalopathy
Leukocytosis
Shock

32.4 Preparation

Prior to the procedure, explain the procedure to the patient and obtained informed consent. Risks for paracentesis are listed below:

In addition the provider should gather necessary equipment and prepare any laboratory paperwork. The supplies will depend on whether the paracentesis is a diagnostic or therapeutic paracentesis (Tables 32.2, 32.3 and 32.4).

For a therapeutic paracentesis, there are a number or prepackaged kits containing the majority of supplies. In addition for those who desire a needle over catheter approach, a thoracentesis kit can be used (see Fig. 32.1).

32.4.1 Needle Selection

In general for a therapeutic paracentesis, there are two choices of needles. Traditionally, a Caldwell needle (see Fig. 32.2) with metal cannula has been used. Other providers prefer a large-bore catheter over needle device (see Fig. 32.3). While catheter shear has been mentioned as a possible complication of the catheter over needle device, in the author's experience, this is not the case with experienced operators.

32.4.2 Patient Position

The patient is usually supine or with the head slightly elevated. The patient is usually positioned with the needle site slightly dependent to help with fluid accumulation.

32.4.3 Selecting Needle Entry Site

Traditionally the left or right lower quadrant is the preferred site for paracentesis. The site used is 2 finger widths medial and cephalad to the anterior iliac spine. In addition a midline approach 2 cm below the umbilicus is generally devoid of vessels. However, with increasingly obese patients, this site has become more difficult to use.

Typically shifting dullness (percussing for resonance and moving laterally until dullness is percussed) has been used to identify areas of fluid for paracentesis [6]. However, with the ubiquity of ultrasound, there is little reason not

Table 32.2 Risk for paracentesis

Bleeding
Infection
Injury to intra-abdominal organs
Post-procedural hypotension

Table 32.3 Supplies for a diagnostic paracentesis

20 cc syringe
10 cc syringe
Chlorhexidine prep
1.5 inch 22 gauge needle x 2
1 % lidocaine
Sterile gloves
Surgical cap
Surgical mask
Alcohol prep
Sterile towel or small drape
Specimen bottle

Table 32.4 Supplies for therapeutic paracentesis

60 cc syringe
10 cc syringe x 2
TB syringe or 27 gauge 1 inch needle
1.5 inch 22 gauge needle x 2
1 % lidocaine
Sterile gloves
Surgical cap
Surgical mask
Alcohol prep
Sterile towel or small drape
Specimen bottle
1 L vacuum bottle or suction drainage bottle
#11 disposable scalpel
Chlorhexidine prep
Paracentesis needle
Sterile 4 × 4 gauze sponge
Suction tubing
Luer lock adapter

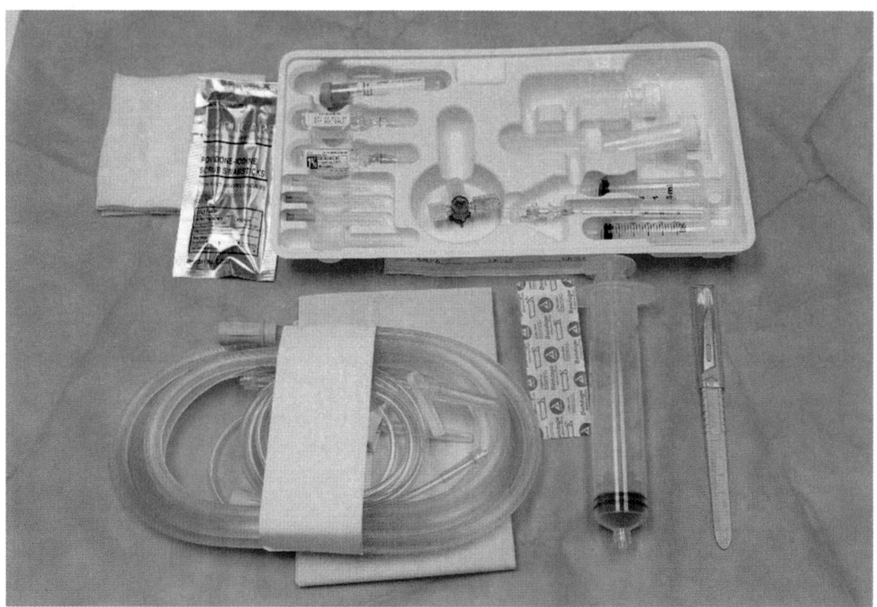

Fig. 32.1 Example of paracentesis kit

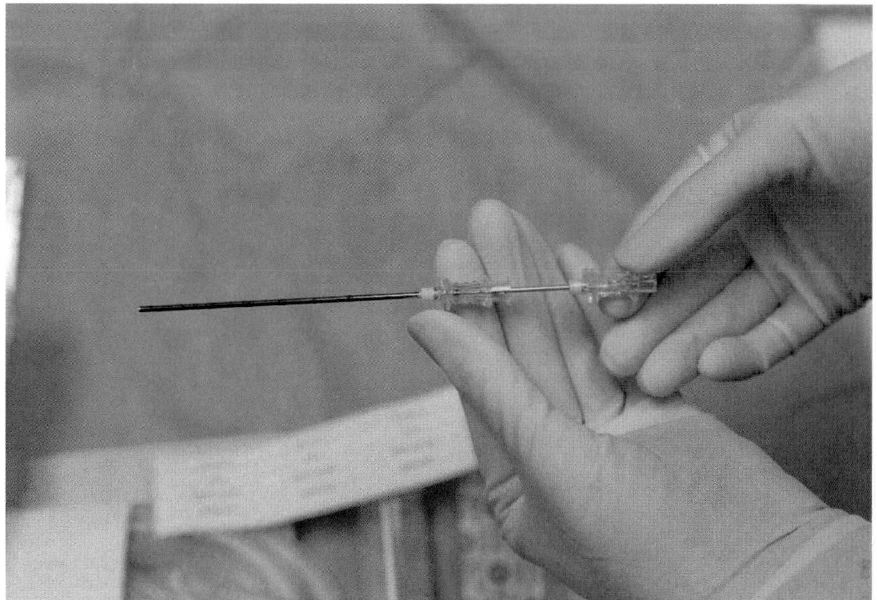

Fig 32.2 Caldwell needle

to use this modality when selecting the site. Generally a phased array probe is used to find an area of adequate fluid at a sufficient distance from the bowel. The use of ultrasound also helps avoid other anatomic structures such as the urinary bladder. In addition measurements can be taken to show depth needed to obtain ascetic fluid. Finally, a linear probe can be used to examine the surface anatomy to avoid unanticipated vasculature. As mentioned above, avoid sites with hematomas, skin infections, obvious vasculature, or surgical scars. Once an appropriate site is found, the site is marked with surgical marker (see Figs. 32.4 and 32.5).

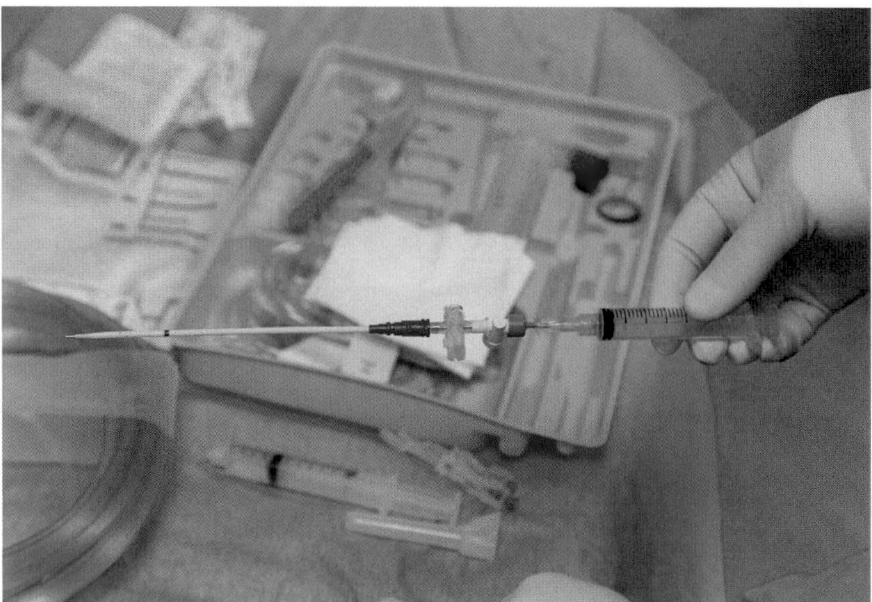

Fig. 32.3 Gauge needle with 8 French catheter

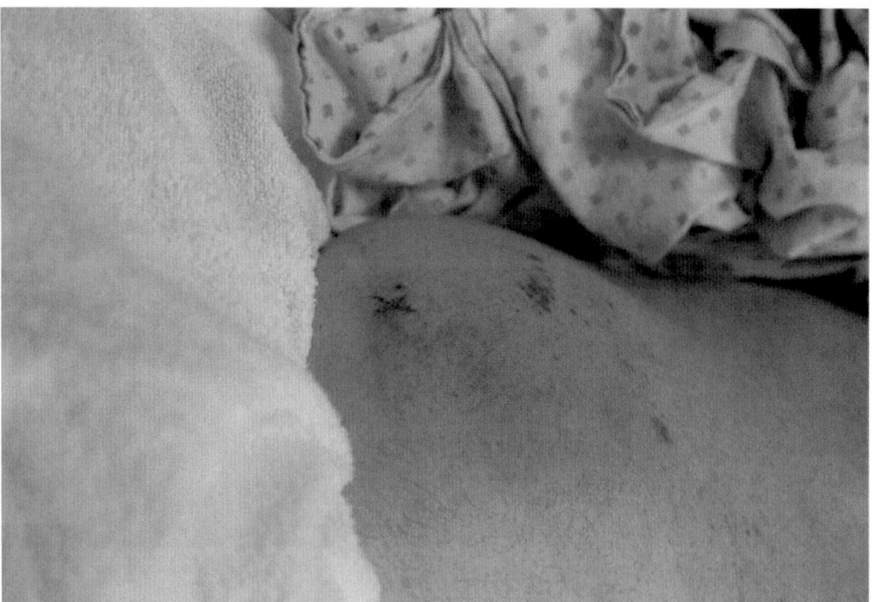

Fig. 32.4 Site marked with surgical marker

32.4.4 Preparing the Site

Using non-sterile gloves, the area is prepared with chlorhexidine. The prep is administered in a circular manner starting at the site and proceeding outward (see Fig. 32.6).

After preparing the site, place the sterile drape over the area with the site exposed (see Fig. 32.7). As an alternative to a sterile drape, sterile towels can be used.

32.4.5 Anesthetizing the Site

Using 1 % lidocaine, local anesthesia is injected into the site. Using a small gauge

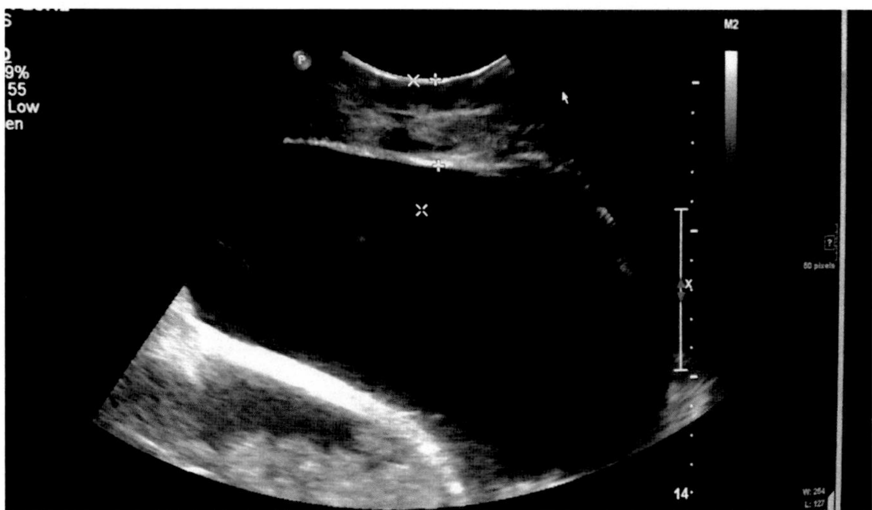

Fig. 32.5 Ultrasound showing abdominal wall, ascetic fluid, and bowel

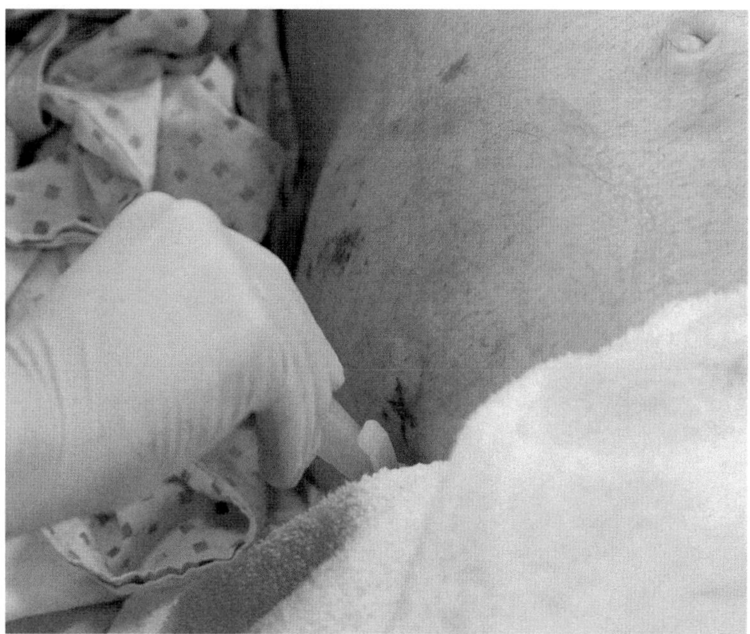

Fig. 32.6 Using chlorhexidine prep on the site in a circular motion

(TB or 25 gauge) needle, a small skin weal is created (see Fig 32.8).

Alternatively a 22 gauge needle can be used for both the skin wheal and deeper injection. After forming the skin wheal, the needle is advanced 1/2 cm at a time aspirating and injecting 1 cc of lidocaine each time until ascites is aspirated (see Fig. 32.9). The remaining lidocaine should then be injected to anesthetize the peritoneum.

32.5 Diagnostic Paracentesis

For a diagnostic paracentesis, a fresh 20 cc syringe is advanced along the same track as the anesthetic needle until ascites is aspirated. Generally 20 ccs of ascites is sufficient for tests needed for a diagnostic paracentesis. In obese patients, a 1.5 cm needle may not be sufficient to reach the ascites. In this case, a 2.5 inch 22 gauge

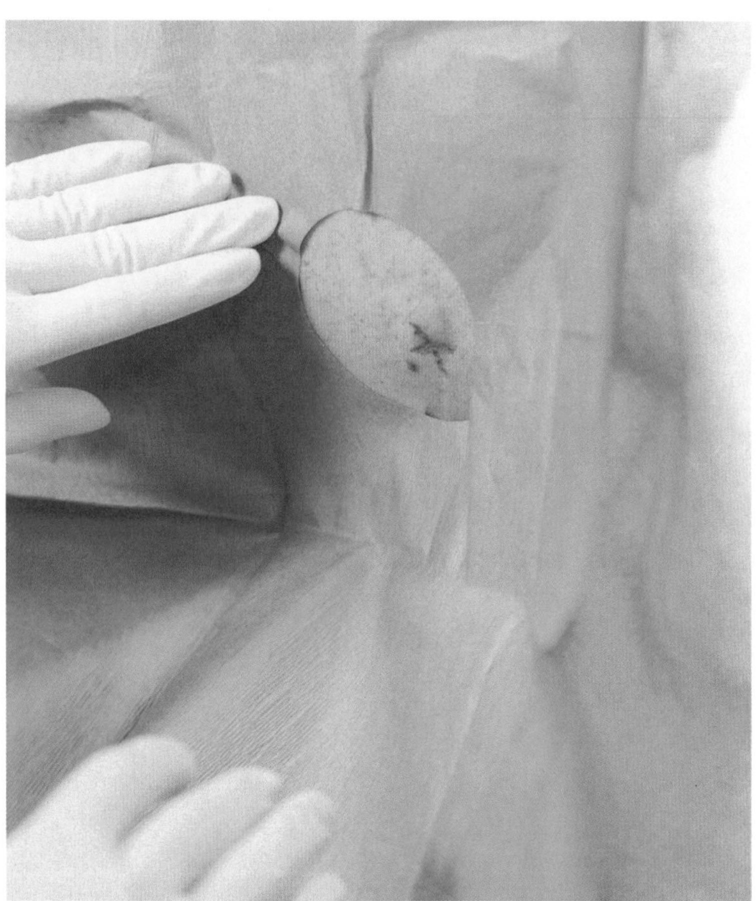

Fig. 32.7 Applying the drape with site exposed

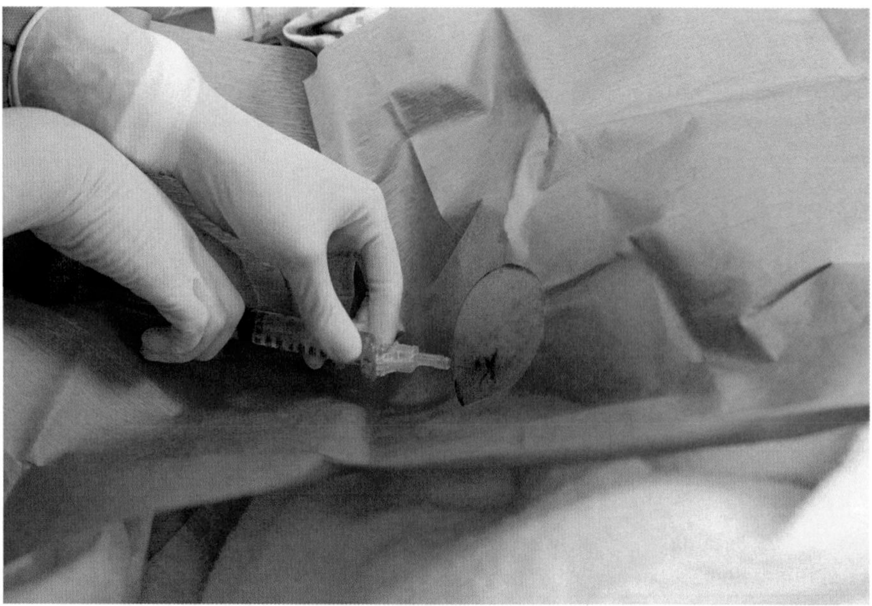

Fig. 32.8 Using a small gauge needle, a skin wheal is created at the site

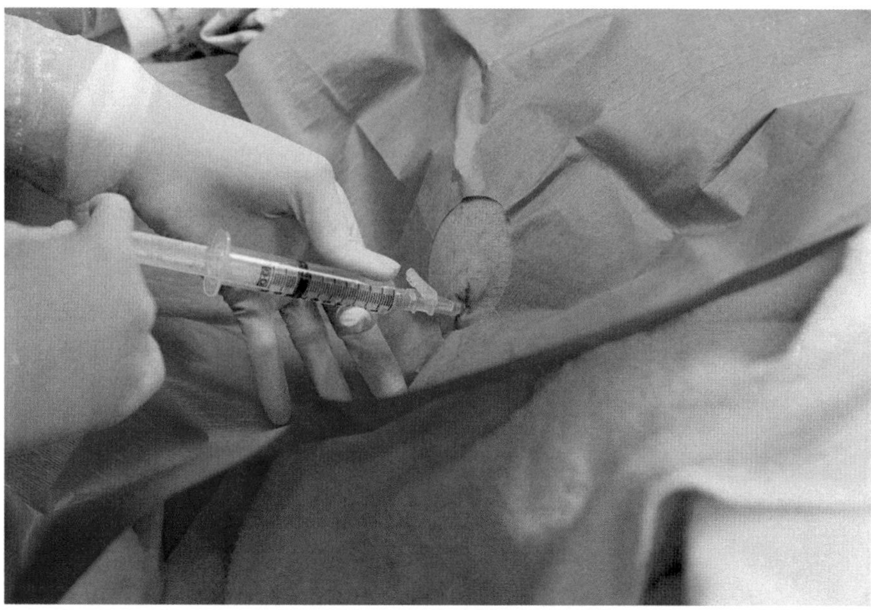

Fig. 32.9 A 22 gauge needle is then advanced aspirating and injecting lidocaine at ½ cm intervals

needle such as those used for lumbar puncture may be needed. For small fluid collections, direct visualization of the needle with ultrasound may add an extra measure of safety. Our center generally sends fluid for cytology on an initial diagnostic paracentesis. If cytology is done, most laboratories require at least 100 ccs of ascites for a total of 120 ccs of ascites on an initial diagnostic paracentesis.

32.6 Therapeutic Paracentesis

For a therapeutic paracentesis, once the area has been anesthetized, a small skin nick is made with a #11 blade to facilitate catheter entry (see Fig. 32.10).

The catheter is then advanced into the tissue at 90° to the skin until ascitic fluid is obtained (see Fig. 32.11).

Once ascites is aspirated, holding the needle in place, the catheter is advanced into the peritoneum (see Fig. 32.12).

Once the catheter is advanced, a 20 cc or 60 cc syringe is attached to the catheter, and ascites is obtained for testing (see Fig. 32.13). Using a Caldwell needle, a separate three-way valve is attached to the needle.

Suction tubing is then connected to the catheter running either to a vacuum bottle or suction catheter (see Fig. 32.14).

For a large-volume paracentesis, removal should continue until 5 L is reached or flow stops (see Fig. 32.15). Larger-volume paracentesis can be done to decrease frequency of paracentesis but increase the risk of periprocedural hypertension. As the pocket collapses, bowel or omentum may occlude the catheter. Resumption of flow can be achieved by shifting the position of the patient or having an assistant gently press on the contralateral side. The catheter can be redirected by stopping suction with the three-way valve attached to the catheter. The catheter can be pulled back slightly and redirected to obtain more fluid.

Once the desired fluid had been removed, the catheter is withdrawn and pressure applied to the site. For diagnostic paracentesis, a bandage will usually suffice as a dressing. For therapeutic paracentesis, a pressure dressing is sometimes required. The patient should lie flat for 2 h. Having the patient lie with the paracentesis site up may reduce leakage from the site. Persistent leakage may be treated with a purse string suture. Dermabond can also be used on paracentesis sites with good effect.

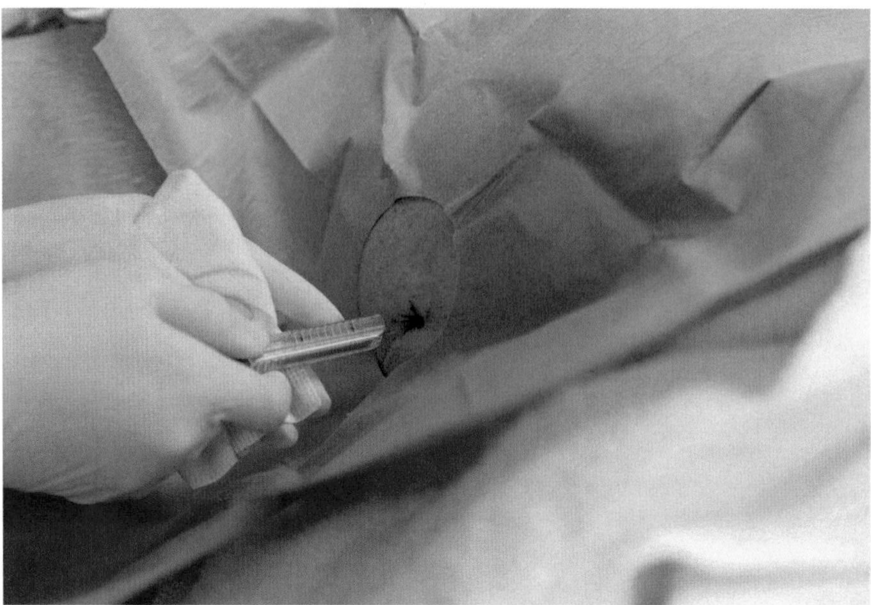

Fig. 32.10 Using a #11 blade to make a small skin nick

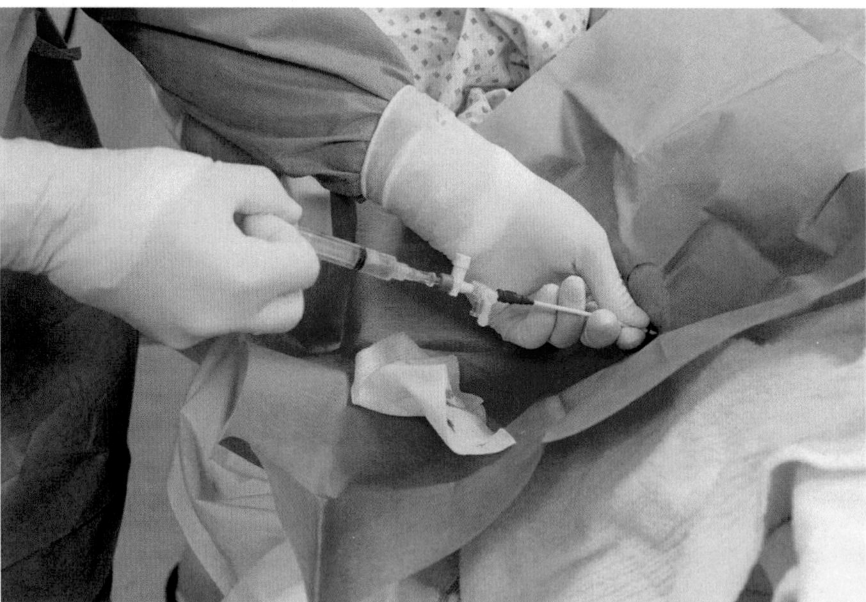

Fig. 32.11 Catheter is advanced until ascites is aspirated

32.6.1 Administration of Albumin After Large-Volume Paracentesis

For paracentesis less than 5 L, albumin is generally not required. When more fluid is removed, 8–10 g/L of 25 % albumin is recommended to prevent hepatorenal syndrome [7–9].

32.7 Analysis of Peritoneal Fluid

Handling of peritoneal fluid is institution dependent. Generally a tube without additive should be sent for albumin measurement. Some institutions may use an EDTA-treated tube for cell count and differential. Institutions may also use aerobic and anaerobic bottles for culture, while

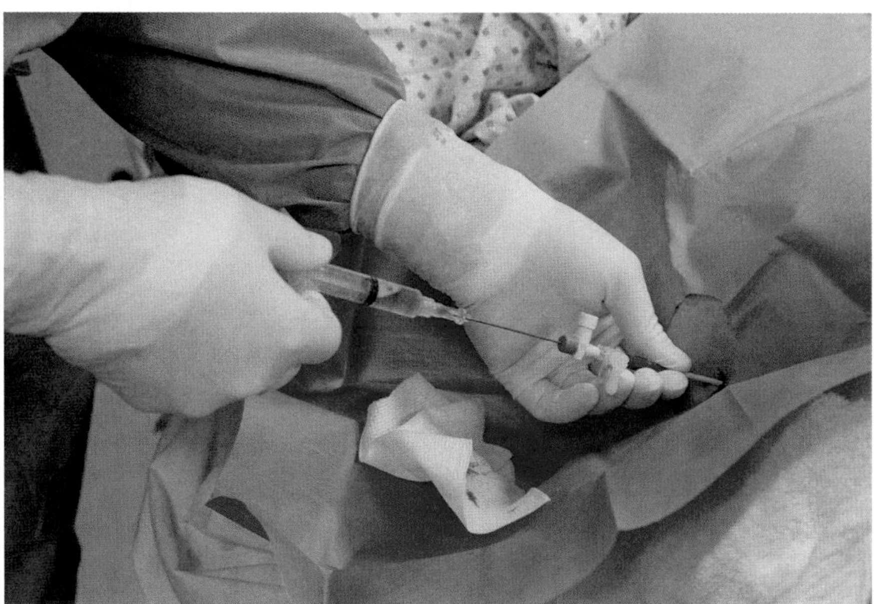

Fig. 32.12 With needle held in place, catheter is advanced into the peritoneum

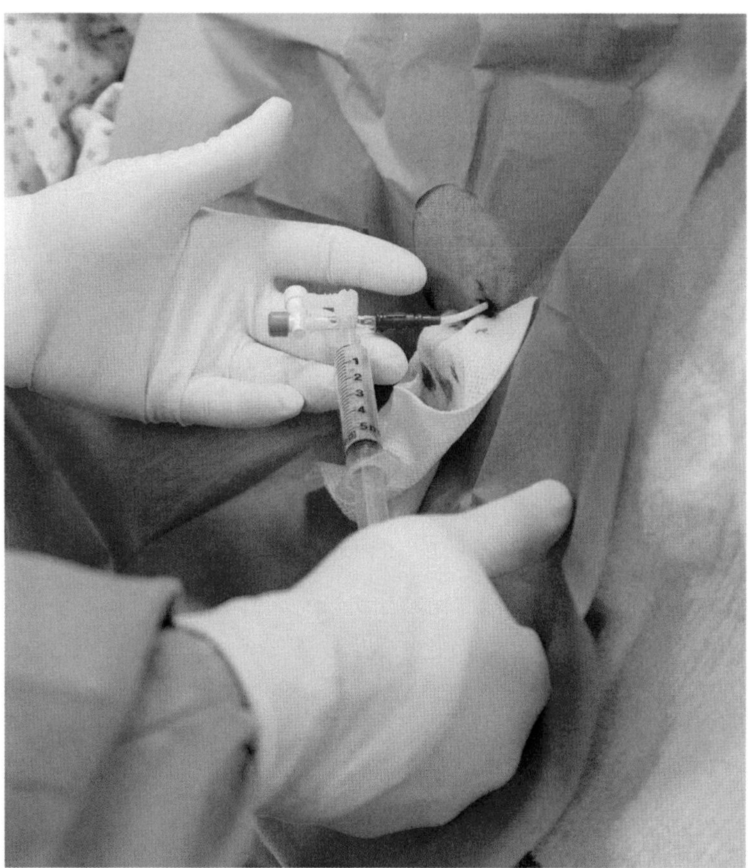

Fig. 32.13 Ascites is obtained for testing

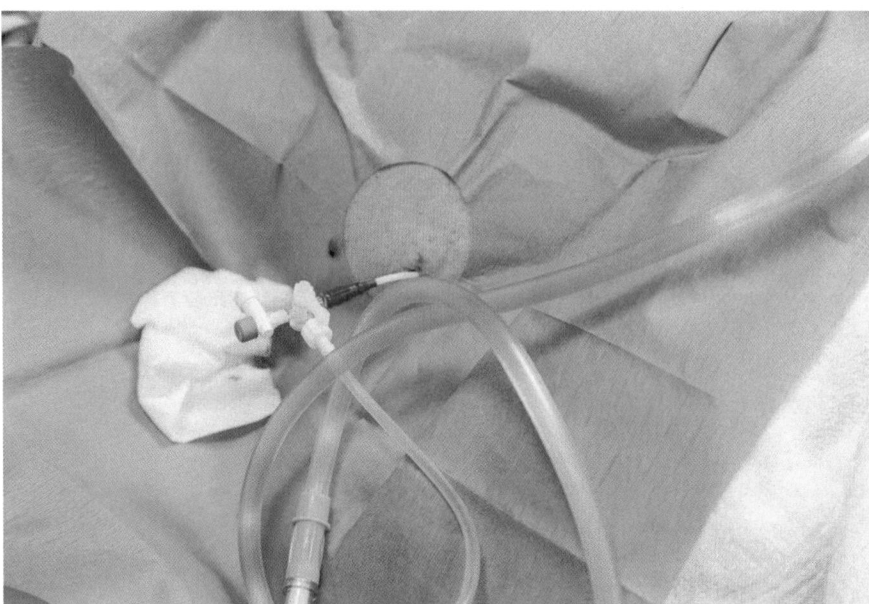

Fig. 32.14 Catheter is attached to suction tubing

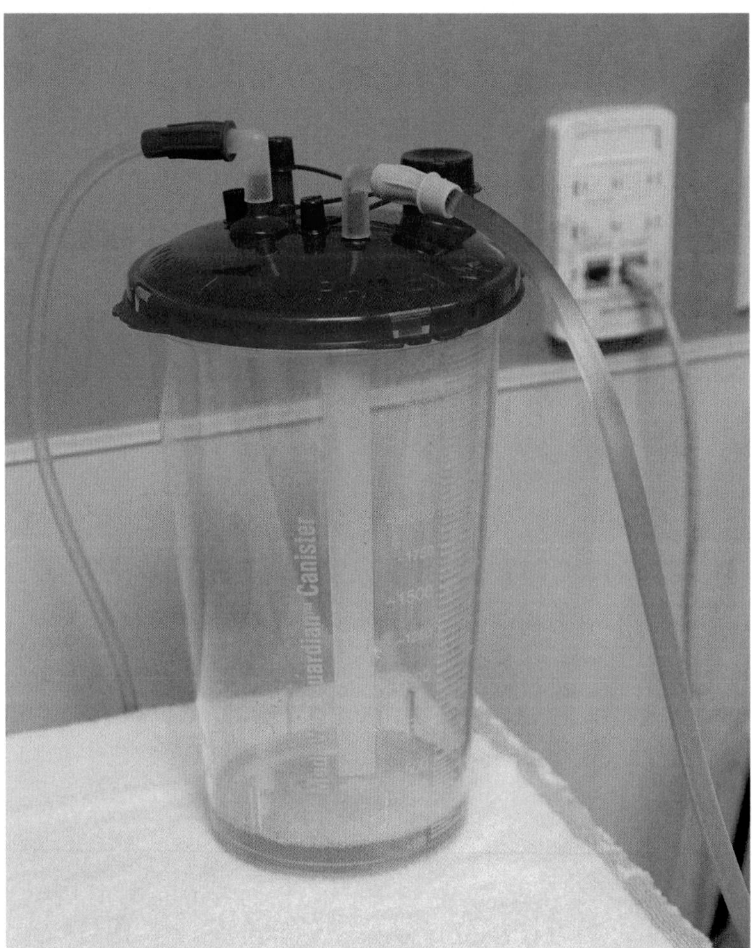

Fig. 32.15 Ascites flowing into a suction canister

Table 32.5 Differential diagnosis of ascites based on serum-ascites albumin gradient

Gradient ≥ 1.1 g/dL (portal hypertension)	Gradient < 1.1 g/dL
Cirrhosis	Peritoneal carcinomatosis
Alcoholic hepatitis	Peritoneal tuberculosis
Right heart failure	Pancreatic ascites
Portal vein thrombosis	Nephrotic syndrome
Budd-Chiari syndrome	Biliary ascites

others may reserve these for blood cultures due to automated testing. Close coordination with the clinical laboratory will help ensure ascites testing is in the proper medium.

When checking for spontaneous bacterial peritonitis, an absolute neutrophil count of 250 cells/μL is considered diagnostic [10]. Whether a cell count should be sent on all repeat outpatient paracentesis is debateable, but the authors generally believe that its use for the detection of occult SBP is helpful. At the very least, cell count should be sent on any hospitalized patient [2].

Other common tests include albumin, total protein, culture, glucose, lactase dehydrogenase, and amylase. Uncommon tests include acid fast bacteria, cytology, triglyceride, and bilirubin.

32.7.1 Serum-Ascites Albumin Gradient

Subtracting the ascites albumin level from a concurrent serum albumin level will give a serum-ascites albumin gradient. A gradient ≥ 1.1 g/dL is indicative of portal hypertension. A value of less than 1.1 g/dL indicates other causes [11] (Table 32.5).

32.8 Complications

Complications are rare and generally self-limiting. However, given the decompensated nature of the patient population, some complications can be devastating [12]. The most common complication is persistent leak from the puncture site. As mentioned above, having the patient lay on the contralateral side may help. If the leak is persistent, placement of an ostomy bag will help determine the amount of the leak. Gauze dressings generally soak through and may lead to skin breakdown. For large persistent leaks, a purse string or figure of eight suture may help halt the leak. A repeat large-volume paracentesis may help relieve the pressure and resolve the leak.

Another relatively rare complication of large-volume paracentesis is post-procedural hypotension. This usually responds to fluid bolus of either albumin or crystalloid. Hepatorenal syndrome is another complication of large-volume paracentesis [7, 9]. While administration of 25 % albumin may help alleviate the risk, it does not completely reduce it.

Other rare complications include abdominal wall or retroperitoneal hematoma, perforation of the bowel or bladder, or laceration of a major blood vessel. While the overall rate of these is unknown, studies suggest the rate is under 1 %.

32.9 Conclusion

Paracentesis is a common ICU procedure, especially with those dealing with advanced liver disease. The procedure is generally safe and effective in both relieving symptoms and diagnosing infection. Knowledge of the anatomy, adherence to procedures, and understanding contraindications will help avoid complications.

References

1. Runyon BA. Paracentesis of ascitic fluid: a safe procedure. Arch Intern Med. 1986;146(11):2259–61.
2. Runyon BA. Introduction to the revised American Association for the study of liver diseases practice guideline management of adult patients with ascites due to cirrhosis 2012. Hepatology. 2013;57(4):1651–3.
3. Wong CL, Holroyd-Leduc J, Thorpe KE, Straus SE. Does this patient have bacterial peritonitis or portal hypertension? How do I perform a paracentesis and analyze the results? JAMA. 2008;299(10):1166–78.
4. Mannucci P. Abnormal hemostasis tests and bleeding in chronic liver disease: are they related? No. J Thromb Haemost. 2006;4(4):721–3.

5. McVay P, Toy P. Lack of increased bleeding after paracentesis and thoracentesis in patients with mild coagulation abnormalities. Transfusion. 1991;31(2):164–71.
6. Sakai H, Sheer TA, Mendler MH, Runyon BA. Choosing the location for non-image guided abdominal paracentesis. Liver Int. 2005;25(5):984–6.
7. Bernardi M, Caraceni P, Navickis RJ, Wilkes MM. Albumin infusion in patients undergoing large-volume paracentesis: a meta-analysis of randomized trials. Hepatology. 2012;55(4):1172–81.
8. GINES P, Tito L, Arroyo V. Randomized comparative study of therapeutic paracentesis with and without intravenous albumin in cirrhosis. Gastroenterology. 1988;94:1493–502.
9. Planas JP, Rimola A, Llach J, Humbert P, Badalamenti S, Jimenez W, et al. Total paracentesis associated with intravenous albumin management patients with cirrhosis and ascites. Gastroenterology. 1990;98:146–51.
10. Such J, Runyon BA. Spontaneous bacterial peritonitis. Clin Infect Dis. 1998;27:669–74.
11. Runyon BA, Montano AA, Akriviadis EA, Antillon MR, Irving MA, McHutchison JG. The serum-ascites albumin gradient is superior to the exudate-transudate concept in the differential diagnosis of ascites. Ann Intern Med. 1992;117(3):215–20.
12. Sandhu BS, Sanyal AJ. Management of ascites in cirrhosis. Clin Liver Dis. 2005;9(4):715–32.

Diagnostic Peritoneal Lavage 33

Heather Meissen and Kevin McConnell

33.1 History/Introduction

Diagnostic peritoneal lavage (DPL) was first described in 1965 by Root et al., as a diagnostic evaluation method for hemoperitoneum or bowel injury in patients who have experienced blunt or penetrating abdominal trauma [1]. Prior to this, physical examination was the only tool trauma surgeons had to evaluate for intra-abdominal injuries, subsequently determining the need for exploratory laparotomy. Since then other methods of evaluation have served as an adjunct to the primary survey including computed tomography (CT) and focused assessment with sonography for trauma (FAST). Over the last two decades, the FAST exam has become first line in diagnosing hemoperitoneum in the hemodynamically unstable patient with blunt or penetrating trauma because it is noninvasive and quick and can be done while resuscitation continues [2]. Due to the rapidly progressing use of FAST and CT, DPL is no longer considered the primary modality for diagnosing blood in the abdominal cavity. DPL is now limited to patients who are hemodynamically unstable where the FAST exam was negative or indeterminate [3].

H. Meissen, ACNP, CCRN, FCCM (✉) •
K. McConnell, MD
Emory Healthcare, Emory Critical Care Center,
550 Peachtree Street, NE, 3rd Floor Room 3250-DF,
Atlanta, GA 30308, USA

1394 Noel Drive, Atlanta, GA 30319, USA
e-mail: heather.meissen@emoryhealthcare.org

Most recently, the American College of Surgeons has adopted FAST into the Advanced Trauma Life Support (ATLS) protocol. DPL has been removed as the first-line diagnostic tool for intra-abdominal hemorrhage, and it has been listed as an optional skill set [4]. Even in the light of that change, DPL still remains valuable for patients who are hemodynamically stable where the FAST exam is negative or indeterminate [3]. FAST has a sensitivity and specificity of 80–85 % and 97–99 %, respectively [2]. DPL carries a similar sensitivity of 82–96 % and specificity of 87–99 % [3]. Furthermore, some studies suggest that the FAST exam has led to fewer nontherapeutic exploratory laparotomies as compared to DPL, 13 % and 36 %, respectively [3, 5].

Consistent with its acronym, FAST can be performed more quickly than DPL. One study found mean performance time for FAST to be 2.53 ± 0.52 min, whereas the mean time taken to perform DPL was 12.19 ± 2.49 min [2]. It must be noted that the DPL procedure in this study was performed as open technique which is considered a slower procedure as compared to the closed technique [6]. However, a separate meta-analysis study compared procedure times of open versus closed techniques and documented the mean procedure time for the closed technique to be 17.8 min and open technique 26.8 min. This same study showed no significant difference in major complications between open and closed technique but suggested a significant difference in minor complications with open technique having more

D.A. Taylor et al. (eds.), *Interventional Critical Care*, DOI 10.1007/978-3-319-25286-5_33

minor complications. Furthermore, this study found a fourfold higher risk of technical difficulties and failures with the closed procedure [7].

In patients who are hemodynamically stable, CT should be the first-line diagnostic tool [6]. Where CT is not available, FAST or DPL should be considered [4]. Some trauma centers do not have CT scanning capabilities within their units; therefore, patients must be transported to the scanner which can delay treatment. However, since CT scans have become helical, the time needed for an adequate study has been greatly reduced. CT has a sensitivity of 92–97 % and a specificity of 98 % [6] when evaluating for hemoperitoneum. Comparing DPL to CT, DPL is invasive, quick, cheap, and accurate for diagnosing intra-abdominal bleeding or enteric injury [8]. DPL fails to diagnose injuries to the diaphragm and cannot rule out retroperitoneal injury. CT is noninvasive, time consuming, expensive, and accurate. CT can accurately diagnose injuries to solid organs and can identify intra-abdominal or retroperitoneal bleeding. However, its sensitivity and specificity for diagnosing enteric injury are inferior to DPL [9].

In summary, both FAST and CT have two key advantages: they are noninvasive and they provide additional anatomic information. DPL will identify blood in the abdomen, but cannot identify the location; thus, injuries such as splenic laceration, liver laceration, and pelvic bleeding that are often treated nonoperatively with embolization or observation will lead to laparotomy under most DPL algorithms.

33.2 Indications

DPL is primarily indicated for hemodynamically unstable patients following blunt or penetrating trauma [10], when ultrasound is not readily available. Blunt trauma refers to physical injury to a particular anatomical region by way of impact, injury, or physical attack. Common mechanisms of injury include motor vehicle accidents, pedestrian hit by car, interpersonal violence or abuse, and contusions from fall. Penetrating trauma refers to an injury where an object penetrates the skin and enters the body. Common mechanisms of injury include gunshot and stab wounds [11, 12].

Indications for a supraumbilical approach include patients with pelvic fractures, patients with previous lower midline surgeries as evidenced by scarring, and patients who are pregnant. All other patients should receive an infraumbilical approach [4, 6]. Indications for open technique include pregnancy, midline scarring, and pelvic fracture. The standard pediatric and adult patient can undergo the closed technique.

33.3 Contraindications

The only absolute contraindication to DPL is an obvious need for laparotomy [4]. Otherwise, relative contraindications can include coagulopathy, prior abdominal surgeries, abdominal wall infections, pregnancy, and morbid obesity. Other relative contraindications can include hemodynamically stable patients, access to ultrasound equipment, and lack of training of the medical provider (Table 33.1).

33.4 Procedure

DPL can be done in two different ways: open or closed. The most common technique is closed with modified Seldinger technique. The standard pediatric and adult patient can undergo the closed technique. Some indications for the open technique include pregnancy, midline scarring, and pelvic fracture. The anatomical location is determined based on the presentation and comorbidities of the patient. The two anatomical locations are infraumbilical and supraumbilical. The infraumbilical location is preferred in the majority of patients. If the patient has a suspected pelvic fracture, is pregnant, or has a history of lower abdominal surgeries as evidenced by scaring, the procedure should be conducted in the supraumbilical location.

Customarily, DPL is performed in two phases [4]. The first phase involves inserting a catheter into the peritoneum through a small incision either above the umbilicus or below depending

Table 33.1 Comparing DPL, FAST, and CT when looking at indications, contraindications, advantages, and disadvantages

	DPL	FAST	CT
Indications	• Hemodynamically unstable • Blunt or penetrating trauma • No access to US or CT scan	• Hemodynamically unstable • Blunt or penetrating trauma	• Hemodynamically stable • Blunt or penetrating trauma
Contraindications	• Obvious need for laparotomy	• None	• Hemodynamically unstable patient
Advantages	• Inexpensive • Detects hollow visceral or bowel injury • Accurate • Quick • High sensitivity • High specificity	• Noninvasive • Easily performed • Can be performed concurrently with resuscitation • Quickest • Accurate • High sensitivity • High specificity • Some anatomic information	• Highly sensitive for determining presence of blood • Accurate • High sensitivity • High specificity • Can detect clinically unsuspected injuries • Can evaluate the retroperitoneal space • Excellent anatomic information
Disadvantages	• Invasive • Cannot identify retroperitoneal injury • Small risk of injury to bowel/other abdominal structures	• Relies on free fluid for diagnosis • Limited detection of injuries not associated with hemoperitoneum, e.g., bowel injury • Results may be variable with morbidly obese patients	• Expensive • Requires transport • Slower • Can miss mesenteric or hollow visceral injury

on the comorbidities of the patient. The catheter is then connected to a syringe. Recovery of 10 cc of blood or enteric contents constitutes a positive finding and the procedure is terminated [4, 10]. If blood or enteric contents cannot be aspirated, the second phase of the procedure begins. The catheter remains in the peritoneal space and intravenous tubing is connected. Next 1 L of warmed balanced salt solution is introduced into the peritoneum [10]. The bag is lowered and gravity removes the fluid from the abdomen. The fluid is then sent for analysis to determine a positive or negative finding.

33.4.1 Closed Technique

1. Place patient in supine position.
2. Place NG tube to decompress stomach and to prevent injury to the stomach.
3. Place Foley catheter to decompress bladder and to prevent injury to the bladder.
4. If the provider is right handed, stand on patient's left side so that your dominant hand faces the patients head.
5. Prep and drape your patient based on the institution protocol which could include full body drape.
6. Draw up and inject local anesthetic 1 % lidocaine with epinephrine to minimize bleeding at the skin which could cause a false-positive.
7. Next, insert the DPL needle and angiocatheter at a 45° angle toward the pelvis.
   a. Infraumbilical: Insert the needle just below the umbilicus.
   b. Supraumbilical: Insert the needle just above the umbilicus.
   c. Note: The bifurcation of the aorta lies directly below the umbilicus; to ensure you do not damage the aorta, please angle your needle at a 45° angle toward the pelvis.
8. Resistance will be encountered as the needle traverses the fascia and once again as it penetrates the peritoneum.

9. Aspirate continuously as the needle enters the peritoneal cavity. If more than 10 cc of frank blood or bowel contents is aspirated, the procedure will end.
   a. At this point, this is a positive DPL, and the patient must go to the operating room immediately for exploratory laparotomy.
10. If 10 cc of frank blood or bowel contents is not aspirated, then remove the syringe and needle leaving the angiocatheter.
11. Next, insert the guide wire through the angiocatheter.
12. Remove angiocatheter.
13. Use an 11 blade to make a small 2–3 mm vertical incision just along the guidewire toward the umbilicus. The incision should be through the skin and subcutaneous tissues.
14. Place DPL catheter over guidewire and insert catheter into the abdomen.
15. Remove guidewire.
16. Connect IV tubing to catheter and instill 900 cc of warm isotonic fluid into abdominal cavity. If the patient is a pediatric patient, only instill 10 cc/kg of fluid into the abdomen.
    a. Note: Do not instill the total volume of the fluid from the bag.
    b. Fluids should be isotonic crystalloid and should be warmed to prevent hypothermia.
    c. Do not introduce air into the system.
17. Once 900 cc of fluid has been instilled into the abdomen, take the fluid bag and place it on the floor or below the level of the patient's abdomen. Gravity allows for fluid to drain back into the bag.
    a. Note: Ideally, the entirety of the fluid should return to the bag. At a minimum, 75 % of the fluid should come back.
    b. You must retrieve a minimum of 600 cc of fluid to make findings valid.

33.4.2 Open Technique (Considered Surgical Procedure)

1. Place patient in supine position.
2. Place NG tube to decompress stomach and to prevent injury to the stomach.
3. Place Foley catheter to decompress bladder and to prevent injury to the bladder.
4. If the provider is right handed, stand on patient's left side so that your dominant hand faces the patients head.
5. Prep and drape your patient based on the institution protocol which could include full body drape.
6. Draw up and inject local anesthetic 1 % lidocaine with epinephrine to minimize bleeding at the skin which could cause a false-positive.
7. Use 11 blade to make a small 2–3 cm vertical incision. The incision should be through the skin and subcutaneous tissues.
   a. Infraumbilical: Incision should be made just below the umbilicus.
   b. Supraumbilical: Incision should be made just above the umbilicus.
8. Spread subcutaneous fat bluntly with a hemostat or retractors until anterior abdominal fascia is visualized.
9. When the abdominal fascia is visualized, place two stay 2.0 vicryl sutures on both sides of incision. Do not tie off. Drape the four ends of the sutures to the side.
10. Next, make a 1–2 cm vertical incision into the fascia between the sutures.
11. The pre-peritoneal fat is then spread open with hemostats and the peritoneum is grasped with the hemostats.
12. The peritoneum is then grasped a second time and tented up.
13. Next, make a 2–3 mm vertical incision in the peritoneum.
14. Then insert the catheter inferiorly toward the pelvis.
15. Attach the syringe and aspirate contents.
16. If more than 10 cc of frank blood or bowel contents is aspirated, the procedure will end.
    a. At this point, this is a positive DPL, and the patient must go to the operating room immediately for exploratory laparotomy.
17. Next, if the aspirate is not positive, connect IV tubing to catheter and instill 900 cc of warm isotonic fluid into abdominal cavity. If the patient is a pediatric patient, only instill 10 cc/kg of fluid into the abdomen.

   a. Note: Do not instill the total volume of the fluid from the bag.
   b. Fluids should be isotonic crystalloid and should be warmed to prevent hypothermia.
   c. Do not introduce air into the system.
18. Once 900 cc of fluid has been instilled into the abdomen, take the fluid bag and place it on the floor or below the level of the patient's abdomen. Gravity allows for fluid to drain back into the bag.
   a. Note: Ideally, the entirety of the fluid should return to the bag. At a minimum, 75 % of the fluid should come back.
   b. You must retrieve a minimum of 600 cc of fluid to make findings valid.
19. Finally, if the initial findings are inconclusive, then tie together the fascia with your two stay sutures while awaiting analysis.

33.5 Diagnostic Criteria

Positive findings during a DPL will indicate and necessitate emergent exploratory laparotomy for the hemodynamically unstable patient. It is important to understand what criteria constitute a positive finding. Traditionally, DPL is done in two phases. Therefore, positive findings can be separated into two phases. During phase 1, if >10 cc of frank blood or enteric contents is aspirated, the procedure is terminated as the findings are positive and the patient will need to go to the operating room [4]. One study suggested aspiration of at least 10 cc of blood had a positive predictive value of greater than 90 % for intraperitoneal injury due to blunt trauma [13] (Table 33.2).

During phase 2, fluid instilled into the abdomen, and then drained, is sent to the lab for biochemical analysis. Much controversy has surrounded the interpretation of the findings during this phase. Many have agreed on the positive criteria for blunt trauma but some have argued for the criteria in penetrating trauma. One retrospective study determined that decreasing the red blood cell count (RBC) criteria for operation from >100,000 RBC/mm^3 to >10,000 RBC/mm^3 significantly increased the number of nontherapeutic procedures and did not decrease the number of missed injuries [14].

A white blood cell count (WBC) of >500 WBC/mm^3 can be determinate of a hollow viscus injury otherwise known as bowel injury. Let it be noted, the WBC can tend to lag by 3–6 h [13]. Some studies have also evaluated the efficacy of measuring amylase and alkaline phosphatase levels. One study determined these parameters to be useful when combined with a positive WBC count [14].

Finally, the volume of lavage returned was directly proportional to the number of RBCs seen. Meaning, the RBC count increased with more fluid recovery. To avoid a false negative, the provider should remove a minimum of 600 cc [13].

33.6 Complications

DPL is an invasive procedure that carries some risk of complication and subsequent injury to the patient. Many studies show a low risk when the provider is a seasoned proceduralist and is familiar with the technique. One study suggested the risk of complication as low as 0.8–2.3 % [3]. However, significant

Table 33.2 Biochemical analysis: positive findings

Procedure phase		Blunt trauma	Penetrating trauma
Phase 1	Frank blood	10 cc	10 cc
	Frank enteric contents	10 cc	10 cc
Phase 2	RBC count	>100,000 RBC/mm^3	>100,000 RBC/mm^3
	WBC count	>500 WBC/mm^3	>500 WBC/mm^3
	Amylase	>20 IU/L	>20 IU/L
	Alkaline phosphate	>3 IU/L	>3 IU/L
	Enteric contents	+	+

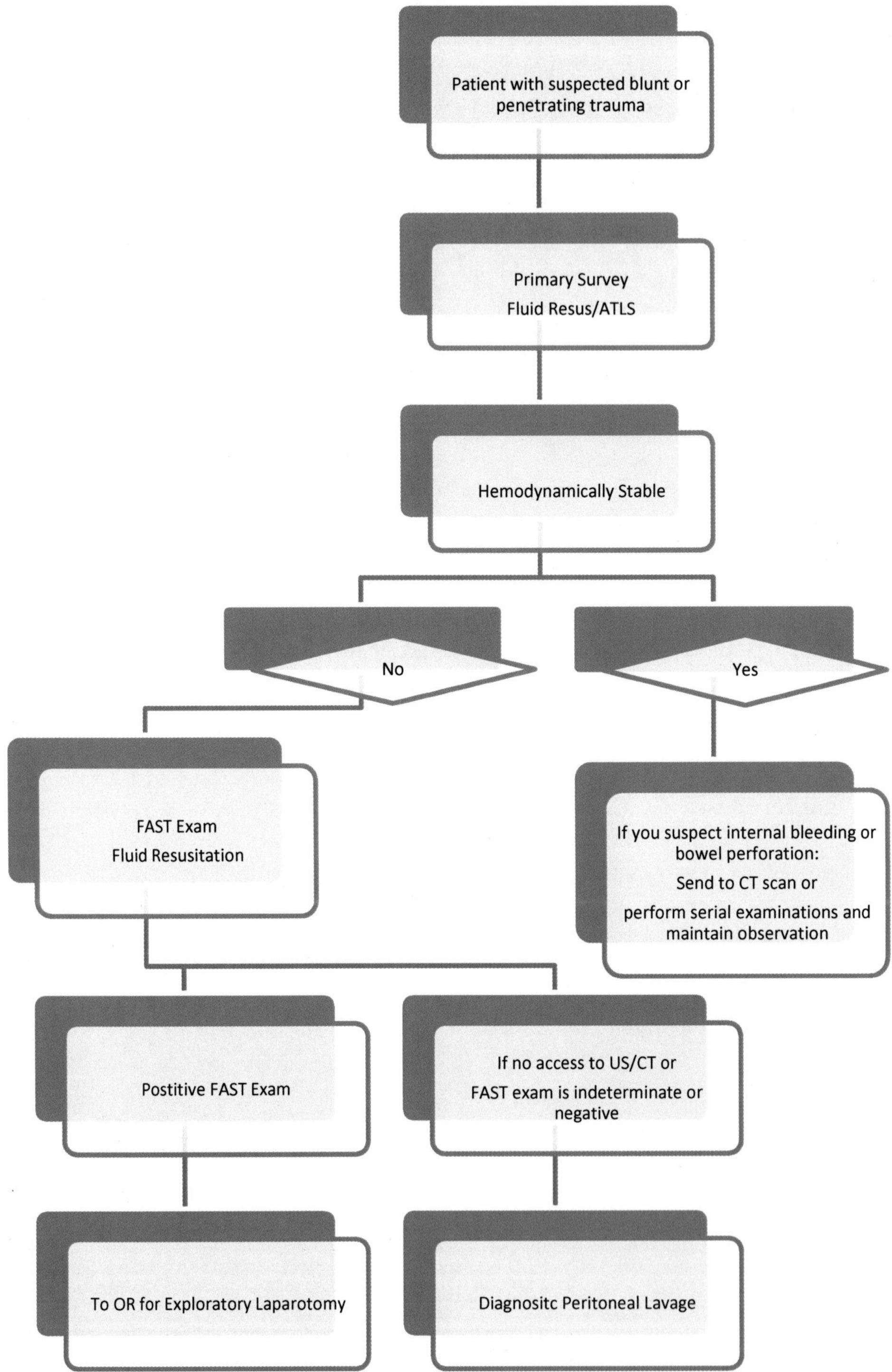

Fig. 33.1 Blunt and penetrating abdominal trauma decision tree

expertise and judgment is required in patients with prior abdominal surgery, pregnancy, or obesity, where the anatomy makes DPL more technically difficult and there is increased risk of damage to structures underlying the abdominal wall.

Some common complications include:

1. Catheter misplacement
2. Local or systemic infection—wound infection
3. Site hematoma
4. Hemorrhage
   a. Note: The bifurcation of the aorta is anatomically posterior or below the umbilicus. To avoid hitting the aorta, make sure the needle enters at a 45° angle toward the pelvis.
5. Bowel perforation
6. Intra-abdominal organ or retroperitoneal injury
7. Damage to surrounding structures
8. Failure to recover warm fluids instilled
   a. Could create false-positive on CT scan if CT is performed after DPL
9. False-positive leading to unnecessary laparotomy
10. Long-term scar tissue

33.7 Troubleshooting

1. Fluids remain in the peritoneal space.
   a. Make sure the bag is on the floor or at the lowest level below the patient.
   b. The patient may need to be repositioned.
      i. Reverse Trendelenburg
   c. Slosh the abdomen to move and shift bowel and fluids.
   d. Keep some fluid in the bag to allow for a vacuum. If no fluid is left in the bag, fluid will not drain back out.
2. If a DPL is performed prior to CT scan, the CT results may be inconclusive due to remaining fluid from the lavage.
3. DPL cannot be performed more than once.

33.8 Conclusion

For many years, physical exam and DPL were the gold standard in identifying patients who needed emergent exploratory laparotomy. However, as technology and medicine evolve, so do the procedures medical providers perform to evaluate intra-abdominal injury. Understanding that every invasive procedure carries a risk, medical providers have now transitioned to primarily using noninvasive alternatives such as CT scan and FAST. The ATLS guidelines for managing blunt or penetrating trauma to the abdomen have been changed to echo these sentiments. Most patients who are hemodynamically stable are evaluated with physical examination and CT scans to assess for intra-abdominal injury. Hemodynamically unstable patients after blunt or penetrating abdominal trauma should be evaluated by ultrasound, as it is noninvasive and FAST and can be done while resuscitation continues. Both ultrasound and CT scan provide additional anatomical information not available from DPL. If the medical provider does not have access to or experience with ultrasound, and the patient is not safe for transport to CT scan, a DPL can be a useful tool to assess for intra-abdominal injury. DPL is fast and accurate in diagnosing hemoperitoneum or hollow viscus injury (Fig. 33.1).

References

1. Root HD, Hauser CW, McKinley CR, et al. Diagnostic peritoneal lavage. Surgery. 1965;57:633–7.
2. Kumar S, Kumar A, Joshi MK, Rathi V. Comparison of diagnostic peritoneal lavage and focused assessment by sonography in trauma as an adjunct to primary survey in torso trauma: a prospective randomized clinical trial. Ulus Travma Acil Cerrahi Derg. 2014;20(2):101–6.
3. Jansen JO, Logie JR. Diagnostic peritoneal lavage-an obituary. Br J Surg. 2005;92:517–8.
4. Jagminas L, Kulkarni, R, et al. Diagnostic peritoneal lavage. Medscape [updated 2014 Mar 21]. Available from: http://emedicine.medscape.com/article/82888-overview. Accessed 18 Sep 2014.
5. Falcone RE, Thomas B, Hrutkay L. Safety and efficacy of diagnostic peritoneal lavage performed by supervised surgical and emergency medicine residents. Eur J Emerg Med. 1997;4:150–5.
6. Hoff WS, Holevar M, Nagy KK, Patterson L, Young JS, Arrillaga A, Najarian MP, Valenziano CP. Practice management guidelines for the evaluation of blunt abdominal trauma: the EAST practice management guidelines work group. J Trauma. 2002;53:602–15.
7. Hodgson NF, Stewart TC, Girotti MJ. Open or closed diagnostic peritoneal lavage for abdominal trauma? A meta-analysis. J Trauma. 2000;48(6):1091–5.
8. Feliciano DV. Diagnostic modalities in abdominal trauma. Peritoneal lavage, ultrasonography, computed tomography scanning, and arteriography. Surg Clin North Am. 1991;71:241–56.

9. Ekeh AP, Saxe J, Walusimbi M, et al. Diagnosis of blunt intestinal and mesenteric injury in the era of multidetector CT technology—are results better? J Trauma. 2008;65(2):354–9.
10. Jahadi MR. Diagnostic peritoneal lavage. J Trauma. 1972;12(11):936–8.
11. McKenny M, Lentz K, Nunez D, et al. Can ultrasound replace diagnostic peritoneal lavage in the assessment of blunt trauma? J Trauma. 1994;37(3):439–41.
12. Monzon-Torres BI, Ortega-Gonzalez M. Penetrating abdominal trauma. S Afr J Sci. 2004;42(1):11–3.
13. Marx JA. Blunt abdominal trauma: priorities, procedures and pragmatic thinking. Emerg Med Pract. 2001;3(5):1–28.
14. Thacker LK, Parks J, Thal E. Diagnostic peritoneal lavage: is 100,000 RBCs a valid figure for penetrating abdominal trauma? J Trauma. 2007;62(4):853–7.

34 Bedside Laparoscopy in the ICU

Jennifer J. Marrero and A. Britton Christmas

Despite the tremendous advances in the treatment of sepsis, it is clear that source control is paramount to success. Equally important is the rapid identification of that source. Critically ill patients in the intensive care unit (ICU) can often pose many significant diagnostic challenges. While many patients initially present with acute intra-abdominal processes such as intestinal ischemia or sepsis, others can develop a number of acute processes unrelated to their admission diagnosis. These include pseudomembranous colitis, acalculous cholecystitis, intestinal or gastric perforation, or pancreatitis. Subsequently, these complications yield dramatic increases in morbidity and mortality, with mortality rates of 50–100 % [1].

J.J. Marrero, MSN, ACNP-BC (✉)
Department of Surgery, Carolinas Medical Center, 1000 Blythe Blvd., MEB 6th Floor, Charlotte, NC 28203, USA

Department of Trauma and Surgical Critical Care, Carolinas Medical Center, 1000 Blythe Blvd., Charlotte, NC 28203, USA
e-mail: jennifer.marrero@carolinashealthcare.org

A.B. Christmas, MD, FACS
Department of Surgery, Carolinas Medical Center, 1000 Blythe Blvd., MEB 6th Floor, Charlotte, NC 28203, USA
e-mail: ashley.christmas@carolinashealthcare.org

The physical examination is typically impaired in the ICU setting from a variety of factors. Critically ill ICU patients commonly have impaired mental status due to metabolic encephalopathy, brain injury, or pharmacologic sedation. As such, the abdominal exam is also much less reliable mandating a high degree of clinical suspicion. Furthermore, most of these patients are hemodynamically labile requiring multiple vasopressors and escalating ventilatory support thereby imposing significant risks during patient transport for imaging or even to the operating room. Life-threatening complications incurred during patient transport, including hypotension, respiratory distress, central line disconnections, and dysrhythmias, are not uncommon and have been reported to occur in up to 45 % of ICU patient transports [1].

Historically, the association between occult intra-abdominal infection and organ dysfunction was deemed sufficiently strong enough to justify empiric laparotomy for the patient with progressive organ dysfunction but no defined focus of infection [1]. However, exploratory laparotomy has not demonstrated an overall decrease in mortality given the large percentage of negative or nontherapeutic results. Of note, laparotomies under these circumstances are associated with reported morbidity rates ranging from 5 to 22 % [2]. Given the high rates of negative or nontherapeutic laparotomies, diagnostic laparoscopy offers a viable alternative to laparotomy in 25–50 % of these patients, particularly in the setting of acalculous choleycystitis [3].

D.A. Taylor et al. (eds.), *Interventional Critical Care*, DOI 10.1007/978-3-319-25286-5_34

The Society of American Gastrointestinal and Endoscopic Surgeons (SAGES) recommends that diagnostic laparoscopy is technically feasible and can be applied safely in appropriately selected ICU patients (grade B). Diagnostic laparoscopy is generally well tolerated in the ICU population with overall morbidity rates reported from 0 to 8 % with no mortality directly associated with the procedure being described [4]. Level II and III data demonstrate diagnostic accuracy ranging between 90 and 100 % with the main limitation being the evaluation of retroperitoneal structures [4]. Therefore, despite the technical challenges associated with bedside laparoscopy, it offers a viable alternative to exploratory laparotomy which has traditionally yielded higher mortality rates, particularly in ICU patients with multisystem organ failure [5–7].

34.1 Indications

The most common indication for diagnostic laparoscopy occurs in the setting of unexplained sepsis with clinical suspicion for an intra-abdominal process or secondary process. Frequently suspicion is heightened by progressive metabolic acidosis and other physiologic derangements such as tachycardia and hypotension unexplained by other causes or abdominal pain or tenderness in an obtunded or sedated patient [8]. In most cases, diagnostic workup to identify other causes of sepsis including bacteremia, urinary tract infections, and pneumonia has been negative. Bedside laparoscopy can facilitate clinical decisions, avoid unnecessary transport to CT, and also provide the potential for therapeutic intervention.

34.2 Preparation and Setup

A detailed history and physical examination help to identify potential pitfalls. Specifically, prior abdominal surgeries can complicate or even preclude laparoscopic evaluation of the abdominal cavity. Physical examination is extremely important to identify any abdominal scarring. It is imperative to ascertain any information related to previous or recent abdominal surgeries and any possibility for the presence of intraperitoneal mesh, such as from a prior ventral hernia repair. Laboratory studies including coagulation survey, complete blood count (CBC) and basic metabolic panel (BMP), electrocardiogram (ECG) and chest radiographic imaging, and arterial blood gas should be performed prior to the planned procedure if feasible. Obtain consent from the family and ensure the risks (including death), potential benefits, and procedure are explained in detail.

Proper equipment and personnel are gathered to the bedside for the procedure. Equipment should include a laparoscopic mobile tower, operative materials, and backup equipment (Table 34.1). The mobile tower includes a large screen video monitor, insufflator with CO_2, light source, and camera (Fig. 34.1). Sterile equipment includes the laparoscope, access trocars, and their associated insufflation tubing and video and light source cables. Instruments include laparoscopic graspers. The operative team includes the surgeon, operating room nurse, first assistant (ACP), and circulating nurse for equipment needs. The bedside nurse should be present for additional medication and supply needs. Anesthesia and monitoring can be managed by either an anesthesiologist or critical care ACP. Physiologic monitoring should include: blood pressure, electrocardiogram, pulse oximetry, and end-tidal carbon dioxide (CO_2) monitoring during and after the procedure (Figs. 34.2, 34.3, 34.4, and 34.5).

Table 34.1 Equipment

Laparoscopic mobile tower	Operative materials	Backup equipment
Insufflator	Laparoscopic instruments	Open set
Image processor	Needle drivers	Lap sponges
Light source	Clip appliers	Suture
Cautery	Various sutures	Open suction
Monitor	Ports	Retraction instruments
Second monitor	Coagulating substrates	Lighting (overhead and headlamp)
–	Bipolar vessel sealing system or harmonic scalpel of choice	–

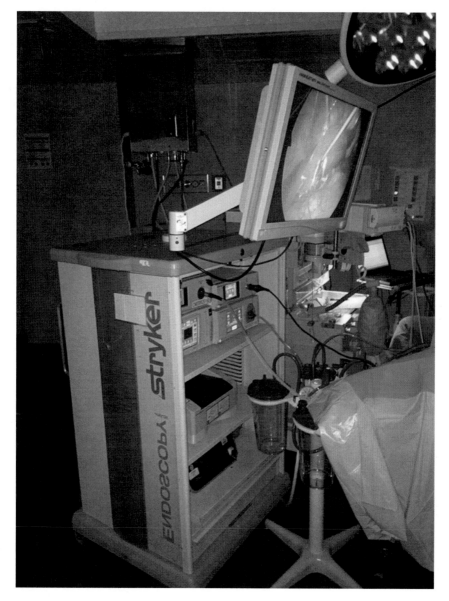

Fig. 34.1 Laparoscopic mobile tower

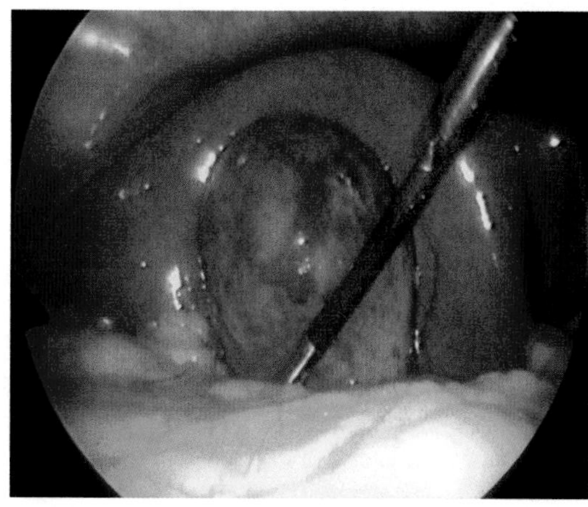

Fig. 34.2 Acalculous cholecystitis

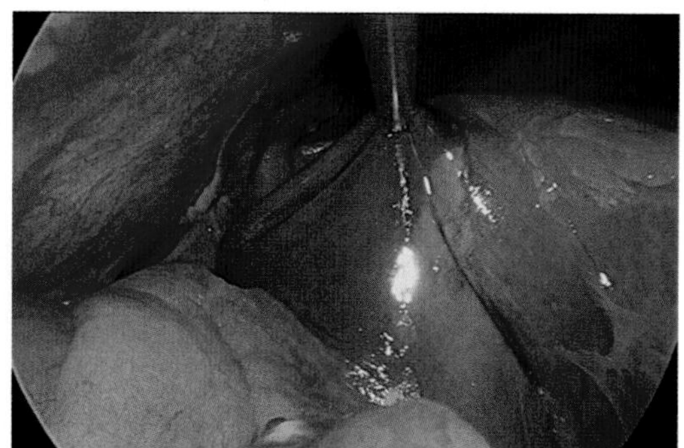

Fig. 34.3 Gangrenous cholecystitis

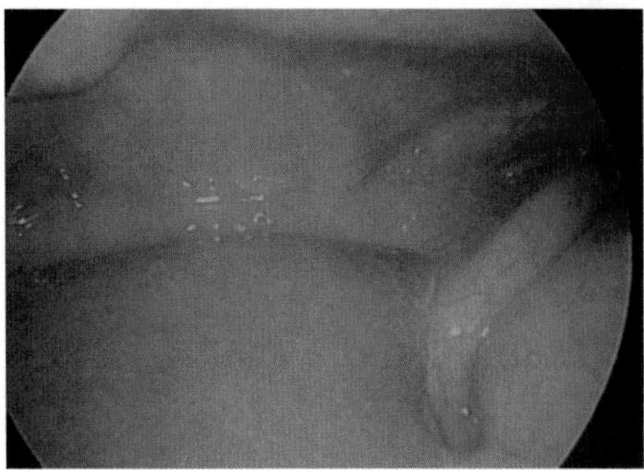

Fig. 34.4 Peritonitis

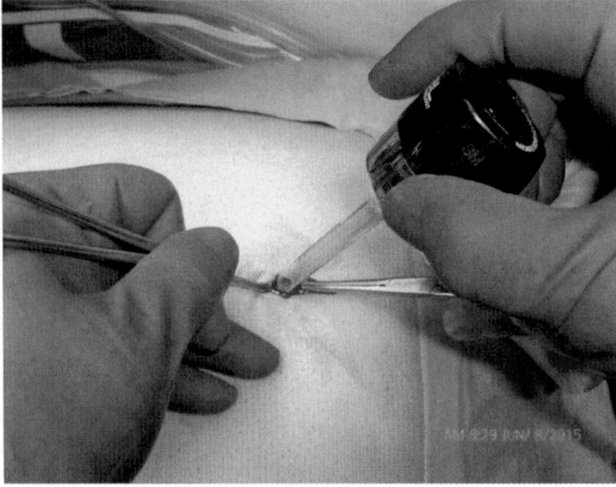

Fig. 34.5 Insertion of trocar

The patient is prepped and draped in the typical sterile fashion. All team members present in the room should wear caps and masks, with the operative team wearing sterile gowns, gloves, and masks. Our typical abdominal access is with an open technique rather than using a Veress needle [9]. In patients with previous abdominal operations, we access laterally [10]. Once access is obtained, we insufflate to the minimal pressure that allows visual exploration. Hemodynamics are constantly monitored and communicated to the operating team. Exploration should examine the liver, gallbladder, both diaphragmatic spaces, the pelvis, and entire gut. Dependent areas such as Morrison's pouch and the pelvis are common areas for purulence and enteric contents to accumulate (Figs. 34.6, 34.7, and 34.8).

34.3 Pitfalls

The ACP should be aware of patient selection and understand the absolute and relative contraindications for diagnostic laparoscopy. Prior abdominal surgeries can make laparoscopy difficult and increase potential risk due to intra-abdominal adhesions, i.e., enterotomy. Uncorrected coagulopathy, known or obvious indication for therapeutic intervention such as perforation or peritonitis, suspected intra-abdominal compartment syndrome, intestinal obstruction with associated massive bowel dilation, wound dehiscence, or clear indications of bowel injuries such as the presence of bile or evisceration are absolute contraindications for diagnostic laparoscopy [11]. Should any of these circumstances be present, an exploratory laparotomy is mandated. Morbid obesity, pregnancy, presence of anterior abdominal wall infection, recent laparotomy (4–6 weeks), or extensive adhesions from previous surgery or aortoiliac aneurysmal disease represent relative contraindications and should be weighed very carefully when considering diagnostic laparoscopy [11].

The potential physiological complications of laparoscopic surgery are increased in the critically ill patient, including the chemical effect of carbon dioxide and the inherent increased intraperitoneal pressure associated with pneumoperitoneum and adequate insufflation. The increased intra-abdominal pressure elevates the diaphragm and subsequently results in the collapse of basal lung tissue. Potential deleterious physiologic effects include decreased functional residual capacity, ventilation perfusion mismatch, and increased intrapulmonary shunting of blood leading to hypoxemia and increased alveolar arterial oxygen gradient [12]. Increasing the frequency of mechanical ventilation with positive end expiatory pressure (PEEP) and increasing the fraction of inspired oxygen during the procedure will decrease the intraoperative atelectasis and improve the gas exchange and oxygenation [12].

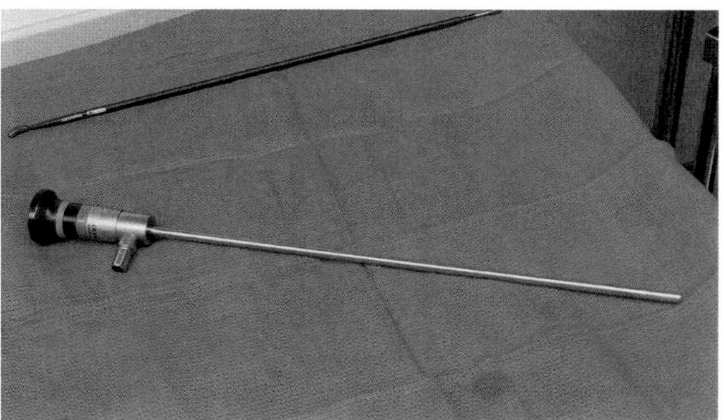

Fig. 34.6 Laparoscopic camera and electrocautery

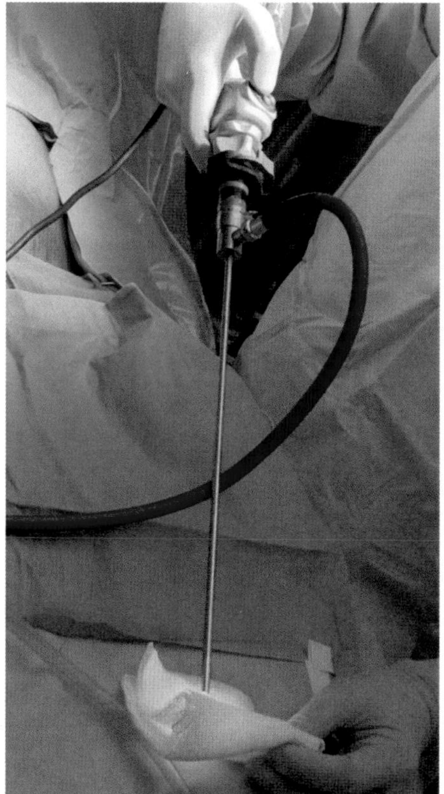

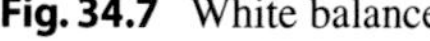

Fig. 34.7 White balance

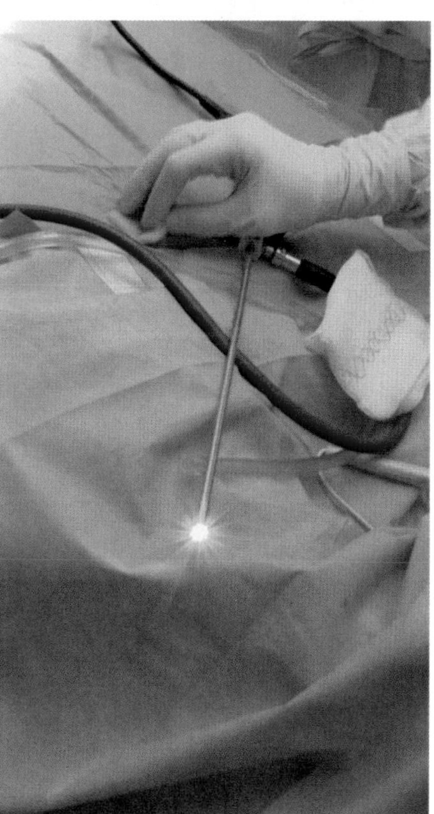

Fig. 34.8 Light activation

Compression of the vena cava may occur during insufflation yielding decreased preload (thus cardiac output) and increased vascular resistance in the arterial circulation [12]. This effect can be minimized with adequate fluid resuscitation. Furthermore, limiting insufflation pressures (<10 mmHg) leads to less hemodynamic compromise. Cardiac arrhythmias including bradycardia from vagal stimulation, premature ventricular contractions, or ventricular tachycardia can also occur and should be closely monitored. Hypercarbia can also result due to the reabsorption of the carbon dioxide into the circulation. This hypercarbia coupled with hypoventilation can yield acidosis and further depression of the cardiopulmonary system [13]. The use of continu-

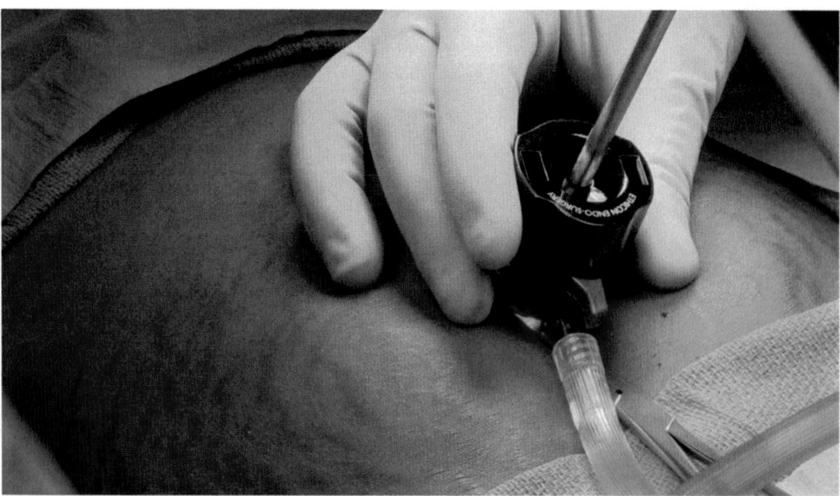

Fig. 34.9 Insertion of laparoscope

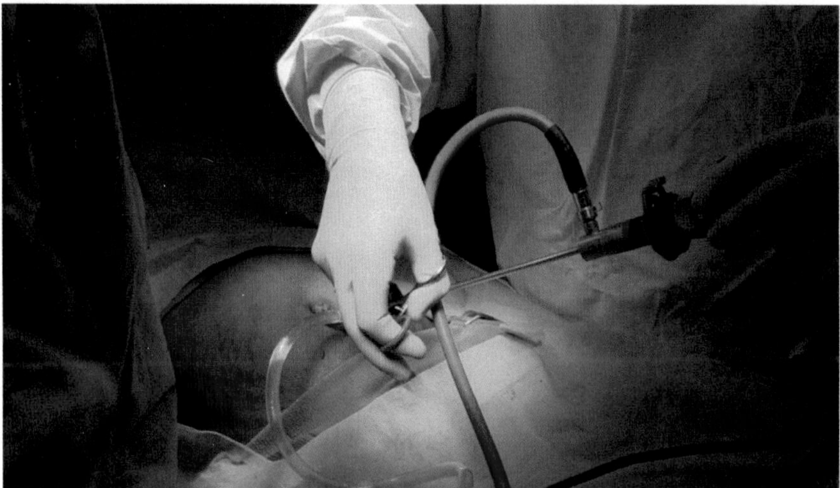

Fig. 34.10 Removal of Kocher clamp

ous end-tidal carbon dioxide monitoring may help to prevent worsening acidosis in these circumstances. If the physiologic effects of the pneumoperitoneum are not adequately tolerated, then laparoscopy is aborted (Figs. 34.9 and 34.10).

34.4 Conclusion

The critically ill ICU population poses difficult diagnostic challenges, and transportation of these patients for further testing can carry significant mortality and morbidity risks [1]. Diagnostic laparoscopy provides a sensitive modality for diagnosis of intra-abdominal pathology for patients exhibiting sepsis or systemic inflammatory response (SIRS) in the ICU [4, 5, 14].

References

1. Jaramillo EJ, Trevino JM, Berghoff KR, Franklin Jr ME. Bedside diagnostic laparoscopy in the intensive care unit: a 13-year experience. J Soc Laparoendosc Surg. 2006;10:155–9.
2. Gagne DJ, Malay M, Hogle N, Fowler D. Bedside diagnostic minilaparoscopy in the intensive care patient. Surgery. 2002;131:491–6.
3. Ceribeli C, Adami EA, Mattia S, Benini B. Bedside diagnostic laparoscopy for critically ill patients: a

retrospective study of 62 patients. Surg Endosc. 2012;26(12):3612–5.
4. Society of American Gastrointestinal Endoscopic Surgeons. Diagnostic laparoscopy in the ICU. In: Guidelines for diagnostic laparoscopy. 2010. Retrieved from http://www.sages.org/publications/guidelines/guidelines-for-diagnostic-laparoscopy/
5. Zemlyak A, Heniford T, Sing RF. Diagnostic laparoscopy in the intensive care unit. J Intensive Care Med. 2015;30(5):297–302.
6. Crandall M, West MA. Evaluation of the abdomen in the critically ill patient: opening the black box. Curr Opin Crit Care. 2006;12(4):333–9.
7. Hutchins RR, Gunning, Lucas DN, Allen-Mersh TG, Soni NC. Relaparotomy for suspected intraperitoneal sepsis after abdominal surgery. World J Surg. 2004;28(2):137–41.
8. Peris A, Matano S, Manca G, Zagli G, Bonizzoli M, Cianchi G, Pasquini A, Batacchi S, DiFilippo A, Anichini V, Nicoletti P, Benemei S, Geppetti P. Bedside diagnostic laparoscopy to diagnose intraabdominal pathology in the intensive care unit. Crit Care. 2009;13(1):R25.
9. Carbonell AM, Harold KL, Smith TI, Matthews BD, Sing RF, Kercher KW, Heniford BT. Umbilical stalk technique for establishing pneumoperitoneum. J Laparoendosc Adv Surg Tech. 2002;12(3):203–6.
10. Goldstein SL, Matthews BD, Sing RF, Kercher KW, Heniford BT. Lateral approach to laparoscopic cholecystectomy in the previously operated abdomen. J Laparoendosc Adv Surg Tech. 2001;11(4):183–6.
11. Ballehaninna U, Chamberlain R. Exploratory laparoscopy. 2014. Retrieved from http://emedicine.medscape.com/article/1829816-overview#aw2aab6b2b2
12. Srivastava A, Niranjan A. Secrets of safe laparoscopic surgery: anaesthetic and surgical considerations. J Minim Access Surg. 2012;6(4):91–4.
13. Henny CP, Hoflank J. Laparoscopic surgery: pitfalls due to anesthesia, positioning and pneumoperitoneum. Surg Endosc. 2005;19(9):1163–71.
14. Pecaro AP, Cacchoinoe RN, Sayad P, Williams ME, Ferzli GS. The routine use of diagnostic laparoscopy in the intensive care unit. Surg Endosc. 2001;15(7):638–41.

35 Decompressive Laparotomy

Michael Pisa, Jason Saucier, and Niels D. Martin

35.1 Introduction

Bedside exploratory laparotomy in the intensive care unit (ICU) is a diagnostic and therapeutic procedure that warrants significant consideration with regard to patient selection, indication, provider skill set, and resource availability. In general, patients selected for bedside surgery are most often those with a high potential for morbidity and mortality, especially as related to transiting through the hospital to the operating room [1]. Objectively, these patients are frequently those on high doses of vasoactive medications and on advanced modes of ventilation unable to be easily replicated during transport or in the operating room, those reliant on invasive therapies such as continuous renal replacement therapy or extracorporeal membrane oxygenation, or those with profound hemodynamic instability requiring immediate surgical intervention.

There are two main types of bedside exploratory laparotomy: those performed as an index or primary opening of the abdomen or reopening of a previous laparotomy. Common indications for either type include intra-abdominal hemorrhage, intra-abdominal contamination or ischemia, abdominal compartment syndrome, or washout of the abdominal compartment with or without closure (Fig. 35.1). Specific considerations in the patient preparation and surgical technique unique to each of these indications will be discussed in the following sections of this chapter.

Bedside laparotomy is resource intensive, both on the part of human capital and instrumentation. For most ICUs, these resources are not typically available, and preplanning and infrastructure placement are essential. Understanding the constraints and technical limitations of the ICU's "operative" environment is essential in patient and procedure selection. Having a complete understanding of the equipment and supplies necessary for the intended operation is critical. All of these concepts and steps will be elaborated in the following sections.

This chapter will not specify the needs for every ICU. Every ICU is different, with different limitations and protocols. Thus, this chapter should be used more for the concepts rather than a "cookie-cutter" approach. For these reasons, there is a paucity of readily applicable literature available on bedside surgery in the ICU. Further, due to the critically ill nature of this patient population, randomized and blinded trials are not easily accomplished, and thus there is a relative paucity of randomized, controlled data surrounding

M. Pisa, CRNP • J. Saucier, CRNP
N.D. Martin, MD, FACS (✉)
Division of Traumatology, Surgical Critical Care, and Emergency Surgery, Perelman School of Medicine at the University of Pennsylvania, 3400 Spruce Street, 5 Maloney Building, Philadelphia, PA 19104, USA
e-mail: Michael.pisa@uphs.upenn.edu; Jason.saucier@uphs.upenn.edu niels.martin@uphs.upenn.edu

D.A. Taylor et al. (eds.), *Interventional Critical Care*, DOI 10.1007/978-3-319-25286-5_35

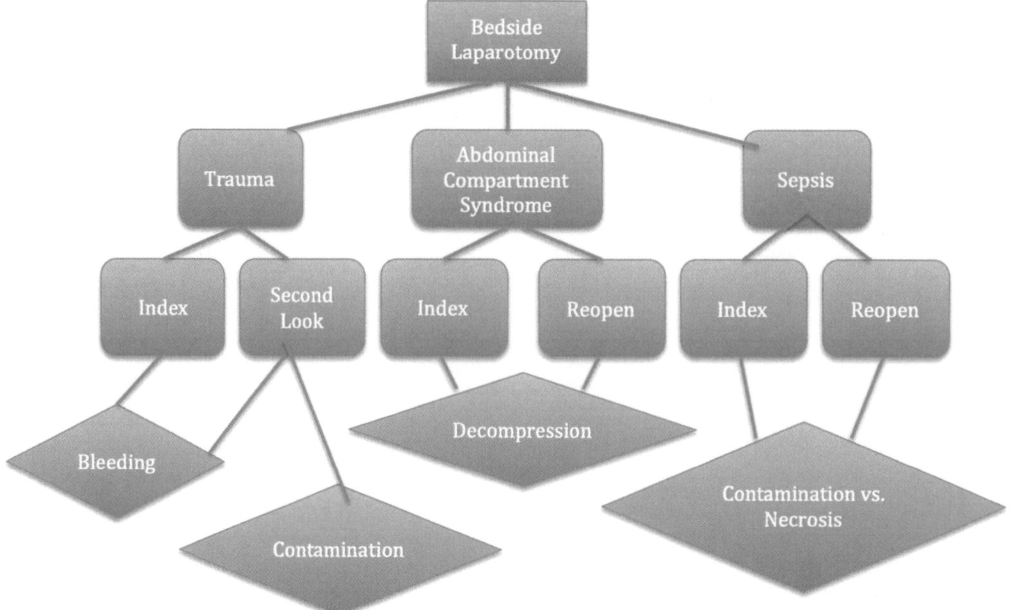

Fig. 35.1 Conceptual algorithm for bedside laparotomy etiology

bedside laparotomy. Therefore, for this population, the best overlap with clinical evidence is the broadly accepted conceptual framework of damage control surgery [2].

Damage control surgery is a strategy that aims to expediently address immediate life-threatening injuries such as bleeding, abdominal hypertension, and contamination while deferring definitive management of less mortal insults for a later time when shock, coagulopathy, and hypothermia have been corrected. By definition, as part of damage control, the abdominal wall is left open for later re-exploration and closure [3, 4]. This approach was initially implemented in the care of critically injured trauma patients, but its use has since been applied with mortality benefit to non-trauma patients requiring acute surgery for other abdominal insults [5].

Of note, the term "damage control" is a naval term referring to a ship's ability to sustain damage and maintain mission integrity [4]. In its current form, damage control surgery is a staged process in the following paradigm: (1) hemorrhage control and prevention of contamination, (2) physiologic restoration in the ICU, (3) second look for missed injury and definitive repair, and (4) abdominal wall closure/reconstruction [4]. Because of the acuity of bedside laparotomy, they almost universally follow damage control methodologies.

35.2 Indications

Bedside laparotomy denotes urgency, acuity, and critical illness. The contributing underlying processes commonly include intra-abdominal hemorrhage, contamination or ischemia, abdominal compartment syndrome, or re-exploration of a previously open abdomen for washout or closure [3, 4, 6]. In most cases, a bedside laparotomy is utilized when operative focus can be directed at just one of the above indications with high probability of a single, addressable insult. This focus will give rise to general, indication-specific considerations.

- Intra-abdominal Hemorrhage
- The focus of this bedside exploration is control of bleeding. These patients have generally

already undergone their primary operation and this is a reopening. The comfort of knowing what intra-abdominal processes are present from the previous operation allows for confident bedside exploration. Primary laparotomy for bleeding has a much higher potential for morbidity as the etiology and thus the required resources are unknown. Additional resources for ICU hemorrhage resuscitation during bedside surgery should be considered and will be discussed later in this chapter [4].

- Sepsis from Contamination/Ischemia
- Operations for this indication may be undertaken at the bedside as either an index case or reopening of a previous laparotomy. The focus of this exploration is source control in the setting of abdominal sepsis. Common etiologies include perforated viscous from diverticulitis, peptic ulcer disease, ischemia, infection, or surgical misadventure. Important operative tenants include removal of the septic source and washout of abscess cavities. The necessary adjuncts to surgery will be discussed shortly.
- Abdominal Compartment Syndrome
- Abdominal compartment syndrome encompasses the clinical manifestations associated with intra-abdominal hypertension. Decompression is preferable prior to the development of formal abdominal compartment syndrome. This etiology is the most common bedside indication for primary laparotomy although it can also be seen with reopenings of recent laparotomies. This etiology is also commonly seen in both medical and surgical intensive care environments. Immediate surgical decompression is the gold standard of treatment for abdominal compartment syndrome [7]. Although most bedside surgery results in an open abdomen, by definition, abdominal compartment syndrome requires temporary abdominal closure that expands the peritoneal volume, unless a space occupying substance (ascites) is removed. This temporary closure is most commonly a negative pressure wound therapy system or "vacuum dressings" [8, 9].
- It should be noted that even with a vacuum dressing, a patient can develop or redevelop abdominal compartment syndrome [10]. The high-risk patient should therefore be monitored closely for the development of intra-abdominal hypertension and abdominal compartment syndrome [7]. This ongoing assessment generally includes hemodynamic and bladder pressure monitoring.
- Re-exploration of an Open Abdomen for Washout or Closure
- This re-exploration functions twofold: as a washout of any purulent fluid for additional source control and as a second look to rule out new or previously unrecognized intra-abdominal pathology. In a clinically deteriorating patient, missed hollow viscus injury should be high on the differential, especially if there is a known solid organ injury [11]. Formal closure at the bedside is less common, as this is generally performed after clinical improvement, when transit to an operating room is safe for the patient.

35.3 Patient Selection

Published clinical studies have reported similar complication and mortality rates for bedside versus operating room laparotomy [6]. However, the operating room environment clearly has additional resources not available in an ICU. Therefore, patient selection based on physiology and suspected operative needs should be considered. Bedside laparotomy should be reserved for those patients in whom a trip to the operating room is deemed overly risky. Necessitating features may include profound hemodynamic instability or the requirement for ventilator strategies not sustainable during travel to or in the operating room [1].

35.4 The Intensive Care Unit as an Operative Suite

The operating room is pre-equipped with all of the necessary equipment required for an exploratory laparotomy and all of its potential avenues. It generally has an efficient layout, both in the actual operating space and also in adjacent equipment storage areas with easy access. Also available in the operative suite is a full complement of specialized machinery such as cell saver, cardiopulmonary bypass, etc. The ICU generally does not have these resources; however, with preplanning, some infrastructure can be owned by the ICU and other resources can be brought in by the operating room staff. Elements of the ICU preplanning and preparation will be discussed in an upcoming section.

Beyond physical equipment, effectively utilizing the ICU can maximize operative effectiveness. Patient and operative provider positioning is one component. Bed height, use of footstools, and patient positioning on the ICU bed can improve performance. Temperature control is another important factor as hypothermia can lead to coagulopathy. The decision to perform surgery can sometimes be based on minimizing heat loss by not moving to an operative suite. If a thermostat is present in the ICU room, considerations toward raising the temperature should be employed.

35.5 ICU Logistics

Most ICUs are not designed to function as an operating room. Whereas operative suites are generally restricted access areas with personnel familiar with operative choreography, sterile fields, and patient flow, the ICU is not. Most ICUs have open corridors with transiting visitors and unfamiliar staff. In order to best preserve a sterile operative environment and protect the privacy of the patient, every effort should be made to limit access to the area immediately around the "ICU room turned operative suite."

All those in the ICU room turned operative suite should be outfitted with personal protective gear including surgical caps, surgical masks, and eye protection. Those at the bedside should be outfitted with sterile gowns and gloves. When possible, the door to the room should be shut. If lack of space dictates overflow to the hall, portable privacy screens should be used.

While many ICUs are equipped with small boom mounted procedure lights, the amount of focused light they provide is often considerably less than that provided by operating room lighting. Portable lighting is available and should be considered for capital purchase if bedside procedures become routine in an ICU. Additional lighting may be provided by surgical headlamps. These headlamps come with light sources that can be mounted on a procedure cart or can be completely housed on the user.

35.6 Durable Equipment

Most ICU rooms are pre-equipped with cardiovascular monitoring devices, ventilators, suction, and oxygen sources that can facilitate bedside laparotomy. Additional equipment, with preplanning, can be easily acquired or improvised. ICU tray tables can be used as a surgical table once draped with a sterile sheet. Practitioners should avoid placing instruments on the patient or the bed as they may shift and/or fall off the bed; further, they may injure the underlying patient if not properly placed down. As the ICU bed was not intended for surgery, bed parts and surrounding ICU equipment are vulnerable to breeching the surgical field. Appropriate and additional draping may be necessary.

Standard ICU equipment and clean supply are dwarfed by the quantity and variety of surgical implements available in most operative suites. Adequate preplanning is needed to stock essential elements for bedside laparotomy. Table 35.1 and Fig. 35.2, respectively, list and display specialized equipment that should be available for bedside laparotomy. The durable equipment should dwell in the ICU and be ever present. If components need to be acquired from other locations, that will likely impede the decision to do bedside surgery. Notable elements here include an electrocautery with corresponding pencils and grounding pads that are kept on an operative procedure cart. This procedure cart is an essential component of ICU readiness. Its contents, however, must be kept stocked and frequently reviewed for not only used resources but expired equipment as well.

Table 35.1 Bedside laparotomy procedure cart contents

Instrument trays and kits	Adjuncts
Thoracotomy tray	Bovie pencils and grounding pads
Open tracheostomy tray	Scalpels
Minor procedure tray	GIA staplers with reloads
Internal defibrillation paddles	Vessel loops
Laceration kit	Umbilical tape
Percutaneous tracheostomy kit	Skin staplers
Pigtail catheter kit	Surgicel
	QuickClot
	Gelfoam
Additional equipment	
Drawer full of sterile gloves	
Freestanding suture tree (broad selection)	

Non-disposable instruments, as prepared by central sterile supply, should also be present in the ICU. Trays such as a thoracotomy tray must be available, even if just singularly, with the understanding that it will be replaced when used. A thoracotomy tray is a good universal tray, even for laparotomies as most major general instruments are present. Depending on the contents of a thoracotomy tray, the only additions possibly needed are handheld retractors. In rare circumstances, the operating room itself can bring specialized equipment and staff if needed, but this adds to complexity and can be an impediment.

35.7 Disposables

Disposables can be divided into two main groups: those used during every bedside laparotomy and those that just need to be available but not opened. For those elements used in every bedside laparotomy, central supply can assemble a kit ready for use that does not overload your procedure cart. This kit can be housed in a large tote box. Several tote boxes are recommended as tote turnover may take several days. Totes should have expiration dates and be sealed to ensure their contents have not been tampered with. Table 35.2 displays the recommended contents of a tote box. These contents can be adjusted based on local practice patterns, especially in reference to the technique used to ultimately but temporarily close the abdomen. The tote box also contains saline irrigation. This will be at room temperature. If copious irrigation is used, irrigation from a warmer is recommended so as not to induce or worsen hypothermia.

Additional disposable equipment frequently utilized can also be stocked in the bedside

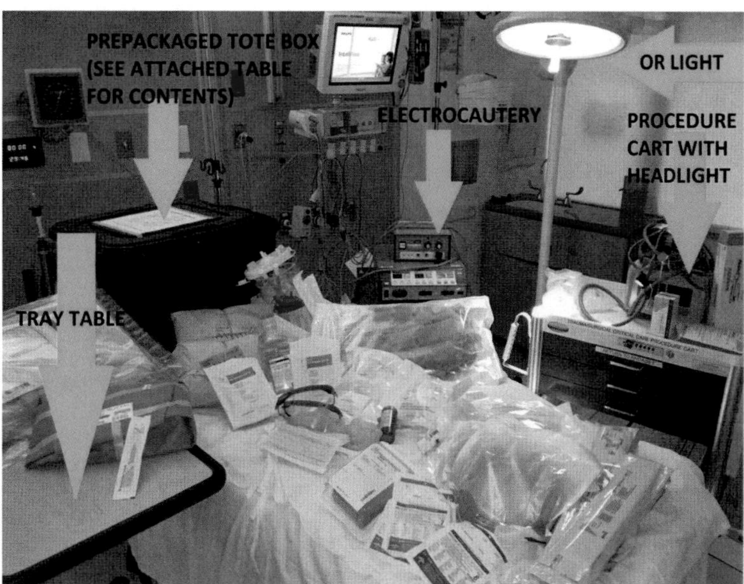

Fig. 35.2 Pre-stocked and pre-arranged equipement needed for bedside laparotomy

Table 35.2 Bedside laparotomy prepackaged tote box contents

Item	Par
ABThera VAC dressing	1 each
Ioban small	1 each
Ioban large 60 × 85	1 each
Jackson-Pratt drain	2 each
Canister suction Lg	2 each
Suction tubing 25 ft	2 each
Suction, Yankauer	2 each
Suction, Poole	1 each
Betadine 4 oz	1 each
Benzoin 2 oz	1 each
Irrigation solution 1500 mL	2 each
Wound closure kit	1 each
Scalpel#10	1 each
Gown pack (sterile)	1 each
Linen pack (sterile)	1 each
Gloves, Neolon sz 7	2 each
Gloves, Neolon sz 8	2 each
Lap sponges 18 × 18	4 each

laparotomy procedure cart. Examples of this are laparotomy pads: the tote contains a starting amount, but if additional are needed, they can be quickly obtained from the cart and placed on the operative field. Some disposables that are important to have on hand, like hemostatic agents, can be placed solely on the cart for ready availability.

35.8 Personnel

Operative procedures, regardless of location, are a human resource-intensive endeavor. The operating room is staffed by a full complement of highly trained specialized providers free to assist in all aspects of the procedure. At the bedside in the ICU, staffing may be very different. The bedside nurse may be responsible for more than one patient. There may not always be nursing assistants or techs free to run and obtain missing equipment. The bedside surgical team must be aware of their ICU personnel resources and work within the confines of their limitations. Operating room personnel can be called to the bedside in an ICU, but depending on the logistics of the institution, this may be met with resistance and increase the threshold for future bedside surgery.

35.9 Imminent Preparations

Patient preparation and anticipating components of patient care during this invasive procedure is a key role. Considerations such as patient positioning, analgesia and sedation, mechanical ventilator management, fluid volume management, supporting hemorrhage control, and understanding all of the equipment and devices that are to be utilized during the procedure should all be anticipated.

Consideration should be given to analgesia and sedation. Whereas in the operating room, anesthesiology clearly performs this role, when at the bedside, the ICU team is generally responsible for providing analgesia and sedation. Paralytic medications are frequently required during exploratory laparotomies; thus, anticipating this medication is important.

Airway and ventilator management must also be actively monitored and optimized during any bedside laparotomy. The ICU team, in conjunction to the surgical team, should discuss the ventilatory needs and potential issues prior to the surgery start time.

Adequate peripheral or central intravenous access should also be established prior to starting an abdominal exploration. Changes in hemodynamics should be expected with sedation, analgesia, and volume losses due to bleeding or insensible operative losses. Laboratory values should be evaluated for the presence of correctible electrolyte abnormalities, anemia, and coagulopathies. When possible, type and crossed blood should be available. The blood bank should be notified of a potential need for cross-matched or uncross-matched blood if applicable.

35.10 Intraoperative Considerations

The operative focus and technique may vary depending on indication and the nature of the procedure. Exploratory laparotomies can either be an index abdominal operation where the abdomen is incised primarily or a reopening of a recent laparotomy where recent sutures are cut or a temporary dressing is removed and the peritoneal cavity is entered directly. For an urgent index bedside exploratory laparotomy, a midline incision is typically chosen. Re-exploration surgeries should reenter through the previous open abdomen or through the previously developed healing wound.

Exploratory laparotomies associated with trauma are often correlated with organ injury and hemorrhage; therefore, blood in the peritoneum should be expected. Significant abdominal organ mobilization may be required to find the focus of injury and should be planned for during incision. Following explorations for trauma, the abdomen is frequently left open in a damage control fashion to facilitate future washouts. This will also expedite the bedside surgery.

Intra-abdominal hypertension and abdominal compartment syndrome (ACS) are caused by increasing pressure within the abdominal cavity. This occurs by volume expansion of either free fluid (or blood) or tissue edema in the mesentery and retroperitoneum. Ultimately, if this pressure becomes too high, it can result in end-organ dysfunction [12]. The aim of the index operation is to decompress the underlying organs and restore function. Examining the bowel and other structures for ischemia during the decompression and looking for evidence of reperfusion is an essential component of the procedure. At the end of this exploration, the abdominal wall is left open to allow contents to partially eviscerate in a controlled fashion (with a dressing), thus any further pressure buildup. It should be noted that, depending on the dressing selected, new, additional pressure can be created and the dressing may need revision at a later date. Various temporary closing techniques will be described in the next section.

Abdominal sepsis generally evolves from a perforated viscous stemming from ischemic necrosis or an anastomotic leak. Occasionally, bacterial organisms primarily invading the peritoneum can also cause abdominal sepsis. When indicated, treatment involves the washout of the abdominal cavity and control of further contamination. The bedside laparotomy technique therefore involves source identification. These patients are often septic from the distributive shock state and require significant fluid administration [13]. Development of abdominal compartment syndrome should be considered as the infectious inflammatory response commonly draws fluid into the abdominal tissues.

A unique indication for bedside laparotomy is intracranial hypertension where decompression of the abdominal wall augments cerebral venous outflow and thus secondarily decreases intracranial pressure [14]. Under this indication, a generous midline incision is created and the viscera are allowed to protrude. A temporary dressing is placed to protect the abdominal contents.

After meeting goals of the bedside exploratory laparotomy, a decision regarding abdominal closure must be made. This decision will hinge on an evaluation of the abdomen, the anticipation of re-exploration, and any need for continued decompressive therapy. Definitive closure is beyond the scope of this chapter and is generally not performed at the bedside.

35.11 Temporary Abdominal Closure Theory and Techniques

Temporary abdominal closure methods include skin closure techniques, mesh products, and negative pressure wound therapy (NPWT) systems [15]. The overall goal of temporary closure is to protect the abdomen from uncontrolled evisceration, to prevent adherence to the abdominal wall prior to definitive closure, and to reduce edema and promote abdominal drainage [15]. The following are several common techniques that facilitate temporary abdominal closure.

In a silo technique, a sterile bag, also known as a "Bogota bag," is sewn into the skin or fascia of the anterior abdominal wall that protects the abdominal contents and reduces fluid losses while the abdomen is open [16]. Direct visualization of the underlying viscera is an advantage of this therapy, although the benefits of fluid reduction and negative pressure are not possible with this technique. This technique is time-consuming and relatively static in size and requires full removal and replacement for size changes.

Dynamic-retention sutures provide a useful technique in facilitating eventual abdominal closure where several elastic retention sutures are placed at the skin or fascia level and allow for constant and adjustable tension toward the midline [17]. When this method is utilized, a protective layer must be placed between the retention sutures and the bowels; this can range from a thick silastic sheet to a commercial dressing.

Towel-based negative pressure systems, also known as a "Barker VAC," utilize a surgical towel and a polyethylene sheet as a base to protect the viscera. The sheet has a few small holes to allow fluid removal, and drain tubing is placed above the towel in the subcutaneous space and is often connected to Jackson-Pratt bulbs or wall suction. An outer plastic adherent dressing is placed. This system is simple and inexpensive, but has limited ability to remove fluid.

Commercial NPWT can be used alone or paired with a dynamic closure strategy as well. It has been shown to increase closure rates without inciting a higher rate of enterocutaneous fistulas [8]. There are several systems on the market but their underlying principles are the same. There is a protective, non-adherent inner layer that is placed directly overlying the bowel. Its function is to prevent the abdominal wall from adhering to the underlying viscera and thus allowing for movement back to the midline for eventual closure. Next is a layer of foam that is tailored to the dimensions of the subcutaneous defect. Finally, an outer adherent, watertight plastic drape is placed. The subcutaneous sponge is placed on suction. This type of dressing allows for a controlled and measurable fluid removal and the ability to slowly tighten the dynamic retention sutures as the inflammation and edema improve.

Each of these techniques can be adapted based on available resources and patient specific needs. Many other techniques exist such as various fascial closures, skin-only closures, and definitive closure. However, their scope is larger than the immediate urgency required in the bedside laparotomy.

In the event that the abdomen is closed formally at the bedside, the usual operating room procedures that involve counting instruments should be performed in the ICU as well. Additionally, routine use of x-rays to document the absence of retained instruments or sponges should be done.

35.12 Management Considerations

The tenants of damage control surgery are to reduce operative time by only completing life-saving surgical interventions [3, 4]. This approach has led to decreased mortality, less hypothermia, and less coagulopathy [18]. However, these same physiologic improvements still require active prevention because even bedside surgery can lead to these untoward consequences [19]. Owing to the limitations of the intensive care unit as an operating room, special consideration should be given to guarding against these potential pitfalls.

Hypothermia Simply opening the abdominal compartment and exposing the abdominal mucosa to the atmosphere drastically increases the surface area available for temperature exchange. Additionally, the instillation of room temperature of irrigation fluid, intravenous fluids, and blood products can hasten hypothermia. Where possible, the ICU room should be warmed. Warm irrigation fluid should be used and stocked on the unit where bedside exploratory laparotomies may take place. Additionally, intravenous fluids and blood products should be warmed prior to administration.

Hypovolemia In elective cases, a restrictive approach to crystalloid fluid administration targeted to specific physiologic endpoints is often utilized and has shown to have improved outcomes [20]. A low-volume resuscitative approach has also shown survival benefit and decreased intensive care length of stay in the patient with acute intra-abdominal bleeding prior to hemorrhage control [21]. While this restrictive approach may serve well acutely, in the patient with ongoing bleeding, a balanced "damage control" approach favoring the administration of blood products in an equal packed red blood cell to fresh frozen plasma ratio has shown mortality benefit [22, 23].

Anemia Bleeding accounts for a large percentage of the preventable deaths associated with trauma [24]. In the bleeding patient with hemodynamic instability, a resuscitation strategy repleting losses with PRBC and FFP in a ratio of 1:1 should be employed targeting restoration of hemodynamic stability [25]. Additional platelet transfusions have also been found to be beneficial. In the patient who is not actively bleeding and is without signs of sepsis or cardiac ischemia, a hemoglobin of 7 as a transfusion trigger is generally supported in the literature [26].

Coagulopathy Trauma-induced coagulopathy is associated with the early phase of injury resulting in diffuse nonsurgical bleeding exacerbating blood loss [27]. This coagulopathy is propagated by hypothermia and the hemodilution associated with large-volume crystalloid resuscitation [24]. A balanced resuscitation favoring early blood product replacement over crystalloid utilizing a ratio of FFP to pRBC of 1:1 has shown a mortality and intensive care unit length of stay benefit over resuscitation strategies relying more heavily on pRBC alone [25].

Abdominal Compartment Syndrome Abdominal compartment syndrome is a state that occurs when abdominal perfusion pressure is insufficient to support end-organ perfusion. The parameter used to establish vulnerability to this state is an intra-abdominal pressure. A measurement by bladder pressure transduction greater than 20 mmHg indicates intra-abdominal hypertension (AIH) [7]. As the pressure rises, evidence of end-organ failure will become evident as AIH becomes ACS. ACS is not only an indication for exploratory laparotomy but is also a complication of the procedure. Care of the devices placed during the ex-lap and continued pressure monitoring is prudent even when the abdominal compartment is left open with a negative pressure wound closure system [10].

35.13 Postoperative Care

Post-exploratory laparotomy patients should receive the same care as any postsurgical ICU patient. Typical routine postoperative laboratory studies should be attained with special attention toward identifying hypoperfusion (lactate), acidosis, coagulopathies, anemia, and correctible electrolyte abnormalities. Many of the patients who are identified as candidates for bedside laparotomies are very ill at baseline; therefore, their postoperative management will need to account for their competing physiologies.

Bleeding All postsurgical patients should be viewed as potentially bleeding until otherwise proven. Post-procedure CBC, hemodynamics, and abdominal dressing output should be scrutinized. Any evidence of hypoperfusion merits bleeding consideration.

Infection Preoperative antibiotics should be given similar to any case in the operating room. If there are concerns for ongoing infection, such as a septic abdomen, appropriate antibiotics should be continued. Cultures should have been taken of any purulent fluids intraoperatively, and these results should be followed closely. In the face of sepsis, antibiotic coverage should be broad spectrum, covering gram positives, gram negatives, anaerobes, and potentially yeast. It is important to note, even in the face of sepsis, in the first few postoperative hours that hypotension should be considered as bleeding until proven otherwise [28].

Pain Control Pain control is important in the postoperative patient. This population has significant cause for pain and should not be underdosed, particularly if still paralyzed. The overall pain management plan should include multimodal therapy in combination with opioid management [29].

Mechanical Ventilation Management Protective lung ventilation may be helpful after abdominal surgery [30] particularly in patients with sepsis or having received a high volume of blood products. Otherwise, minimal ventilator settings paired with spontaneous breathing trials to facilitate fewer ventilator days are important. Patients with an open abdomen do not need to stay mechanically ventilated for the entire time they are open if they can remain un-agitated. All the usual considerations regarding extubation should be employed, and it should be noted that when the abdominal wall is open, the abdominal musculature is not intact and patient's ability to give a forceful cough may be reduced.

Enteral Nutrition Nutritional optimization plays an important role in recovery from critical illness, both from the standpoint of wound healing and immunologically. Following bedside laparotomy and a subsequent open abdomen, enteral nutrition is not contraindicated [31]. Moreover, evidence supports that early enteral nutrition in the open abdomen helps to promote earlier closure, reduce fistula rates, and decrease hospital costs [31]. However, careful detail to the underlying etiology of the ex-lap and any other contraindication that may preclude feeding, such as new small bowel anastomosis, continued profound septic shock, and ACS with high residuals, should be considered.

35.14 Summary

There are significant challenges posed when performing laparotomy at the bedside in the ICU. This approach should be employed only when the risks of transferring a patient to an operating room outweigh the risks of undertaking an operative effort at the bedside. With adequate preparations and preplanning, bedside laparotomy can be safely and successfully performed in an ICU setting.

Conflict of Interest No author has a conflict of interest or financial disclosure necessary.

References

1. Schreiber J, Nierhaus A, Vettorazzi E, Braune SA, Frings DP, Vashist Y, et al. Rescue bedside laparotomy in the intensive care unit in patients too unstable for transport to the operating room. Crit Care. 2014; 18(3):R123.
2. Edelmuth RC, Buscariolli Ydos S, Ribeiro Jr MA. Damage control surgery: an update. Rev Col Bras Cir. 2013;40(2):142–51.
3. Rotondo MF, Schwab CW, McGonigal MD, Phillips III GR, Fruchterman TM, Kauder DR, et al. 'Damage control': an approach for improved survival in exsanguinating penetrating abdominal injury. J Trauma. 1993;35(3):375–82. discussion 382–3.
4. Germanos S, Gourgiotis S, Villias C, Bertucci M, Dimopoulos N, Salemis N. Damage control surgery in the abdomen: an approach for the management of severe injured patients. Int J Surg. 2008;6(3):246–52.
5. Stawicki SP, Brooks A, Bilski T, Scaff D, Gupta R, Schwab CW, et al. The concept of damage control: extending the paradigm to emergency general surgery. Injury. 2008;39(1):93–101.
6. Diaz Jr JJ, Mejia V, Subhawong AP, Subhawong T, Miller RS, O'Neill PJ, et al. Protocol for bedside laparotomy in trauma and emergency general surgery: a low return to the operating room. Am Surg. 2005; 71(11):986–91.
7. An G, West MA. Abdominal compartment syndrome: a concise clinical review. Crit Care Med. 2008;36(4): 1304–10.
8. Bruhin A, Ferreira F, Chariker M, Smith J, Runkel N. Systematic review and evidence based recommendations for the use of negative pressure wound therapy in the open abdomen. Int J Surg. 2014;12(10): 1105–14.
9. Quyn AJ, Johnston C, Hall D, Chambers A, Arapova N, Ogston S, et al. The open abdomen and temporary abdominal closure systems—historical evolution and systematic review. Colorectal Dis. 2012;14(8): e429–38.
10. Gracias VH, Braslow B, Johnson J, Pryor J, Gupta R, Reilly P, et al. Abdominal compartment syndrome in the open abdomen. Arch Surg. 2002;137(11):1298–300.
11. Nance ML, Peden GW, Shapiro MB, Kauder DR, Rotondo MF, Schwab CW. Solid viscus injury predicts major hollow viscus injury in blunt abdominal trauma. J Trauma. 1997;43(4):618–22. discussion 622–3.
12. Cheatham ML. Abdominal compartment syndrome. Curr Opin Crit Care. 2009;15(2):154–62.
13. Holzheimer RG, Gathof B. Re-operation for complicated secondary peritonitis—how to identify patients at risk for persistent sepsis. Eur J Med Res. 2003;8(3):125–34.
14. Joseph DK, Dutton RP, Aarabi B, Scalea TM. Decompressive laparotomy to treat intractable intracranial hypertension after traumatic brain injury. J Trauma. 2004;57(4):687–93. discussion 693–5.
15. Hougaard HT, Ellebaek M, Holst UT, Qvist N. The open abdomen: temporary closure with a modified negative pressure therapy technique. Int Wound J. 2014;11 Suppl 1:13–6.
16. Rutherford EJ, Skeete DA, Brasel KJ. Management of the patient with an open abdomen: techniques in temporary and definitive closure. Curr Probl Surg. 2004;41(10):815–76.

17. Koniaris LG, Hendrickson RJ, Drugas G, Abt P, Schoeniger LO. Dynamic retention: a technique for closure of the complex abdomen in critically ill patients. Arch Surg. 2001;136(12):1359–62. discussion 1363.
18. Johnson JW, Gracias VH, Schwab CW, Reilly PM, Kauder DR, Shapiro MB, et al. Evolution in damage control for exsanguinating penetrating abdominal injury. J Trauma. 2001;51(2):261–9. discussion 269–71.
19. Sagraves SG, Toschlog EA, Rotondo MF. Damage control surgery—the intensivist's role. J Intensive Care Med. 2006;21(1):5–16.
20. Joshi GP. Intraoperative fluid restriction improves outcome after major elective gastrointestinal surgery. Anesth Analg. 2005;101(2):601–5.
21. Duchesne JC, Guidry C, Hoffman JR, Park TS, Bock J, Lawson S, et al. Low-volume resuscitation for severe intraoperative hemorrhage: a step in the right direction. Am Surg. 2012;78(9):936–41.
22. Duchesne JC, Kimonis K, Marr AB, Rennie KV, Wahl G, Wells JE, et al. Damage control resuscitation in combination with damage control laparotomy: a survival advantage. J Trauma. 2010;69(1):46–52.
23. Holcomb JB, Jenkins D, Rhee P, Johannigman J, Mahoney P, Mehta S, et al. Damage control resuscitation: directly addressing the early coagulopathy of trauma. J Trauma. 2007;62(2):307–10.
24. Wafaisade A, Wutzler S, Lefering R, Tjardes T, Banerjee M, Paffrath T, et al. Drivers of acute coagulopathy after severe trauma: a multivariate analysis of 1987 patients. Emerg Med J. 2010;27(12):934–9.
25. Duchesne JC, Islam TM, Stuke L, Timmer JR, Barbeau JM, Marr AB, et al. Hemostatic resuscitation during surgery improves survival in patients with traumatic-induced coagulopathy. J Trauma. 2009; 67(1):33–7. discussion 37–9.
26. Hebert PC, Wells G, Blajchman MA, Marshall J, Martin C, Pagliarello G, et al. A multicenter, randomized, controlled clinical trial of transfusion requirements in critical care. Transfusion requirements in critical care investigators, Canadian Critical Care Trials Group. N Engl J Med. 1999;340(6):409–17.
27. Brohi K, Cohen MJ, Davenport RA. Acute coagulopathy of trauma: mechanism, identification and effect. Curr Opin Crit Care. 2007;13(6):680–5.
28. Weigelt JA. Empiric treatment options in the management of complicated intra-abdominal infections. Cleve Clin J Med. 2007;74 Suppl 4:S29–37.
29. American Society of Anesthesiologists Task Force on Acute Pain Management. Practice guidelines for acute pain management in the perioperative setting: an updated report by the American Society of Anesthesiologists Task Force on Acute Pain Management. Anesthesiology. 2012;116(2):248–73.
30. Futier E, Constantin JM, Paugam-Burtz C, Pascal J, Eurin M, Neuschwander A, et al. A trial of intraoperative low-tidal-volume ventilation in abdominal surgery. N Engl J Med. 2013;369(5):428–37.
31. Collier B, Guillamondegui O, Cotton B, Donahue R, Conrad A, Groh K, et al. Feeding the open abdomen. JPEN J Parenter Enteral Nutr. 2007;31(5):410–5.

The Open Abdomen and Temporary Abdominal Closure Techniques

36

Scott P. Sherry and Martin A. Schreiber

36.1 Introduction

The opening of the abdominal cavity is done for a number of surgical and for some medical reasons. Surgical reasons for opening the abdomen include trauma with inability to close the fascia due to concern for abdominal compartment syndrome, increased airway pressures and intra-abdominal edema or retroperitoneal hemorrhage, need for or desire for second-look operations or repeat procedures to achieve definitive repair, bowel left in discontinuity from damage control surgery, and need for abbreviated operations in order to adequately resuscitate the patient [1–4].

Medical reasons for opening the abdomen include fluid resuscitation leading to intra-abdominal hypertension and abdominal compartment syndrome (e.g., septic shock, hypothermic resuscitation, retroperitoneal hemorrhage, hemorrhagic shock, or ascites) [1–4]. There is also literature that supports the opening of the abdomen for refractory intracranial hypertension [5].

S.P. Sherry, MS, PA-C, FCCM (✉) • M.A. Schreiber, MD, FACS
Department of Surgery, Division of Trauma, Critical Care and Acute Care Surgery, Oregon Health & Science University, 3181 SW Sam Jackson Park Rd., Mailcode L611, Portland, OR 97239, USA
e-mail: sherrys@ohsu.edu; schreibm@ohsu.edu

Conceptually the abdomen cannot be left in a true open state. Once surgery or decompression has been achieved, the abdominal contents must be sealed and protected from the air and the environment. Without a proper seal or closure, there will be massive fluid losses, hypothermia, and high potential for injury of the bowel from exposure to the air. The abdomen is therefore closed with a temporary closure device, and the appropriate term is referred to as temporary abdominal closure (TAC) reflecting the fact the patient's fascial layer is not closed or re-approximated surgically.

Temporary abdominal closure can be achieved with improvised or commercial devices. The benefits and issues surrounding the devices are described below. It is beyond the scope of this chapter to describe each technique in detail.

36.1.1 Improvised Devices

It generally consists of a plastic barrier between the bowel and the atmosphere. A variety of strategies have been adapted through the years. Some are simple devices consisting of a single plastic barrier to more complex devices consisting of a surgical towel or Kerlix between a permeable inner lining and a plastic external seal.

Benefits of improvised devices include their relative simplicity and relative ease of deployment. Most hospitals with operative suites can assemble the necessary materials in order to provide TAC. Overall supply costs are significantly

D.A. Taylor et al. (eds.), *Interventional Critical Care*, DOI 10.1007/978-3-319-25286-5_36

less with improvised devices than commercial ones [1, 6]. There are some challenges associated with the improvised devices including achieving adequate drainage and measurement of effluent losses.

36.1.2 Types of Improvised Devices

Bogota bag: a large sterile irrigation bag that is fashioned to cover the exposed abdominal contents and is sutured to the fascial edges. It provides closure and covering of abdominal contents. This device is not very effective in collecting effluent or measurement of losses.

Towel clip method: the abdomen is closed in a temporary fashion using multiple towel clips to approximate the skin edges. This method is generally not used in the era of modern commercial devices, and there is a high concern for abdominal compartment syndrome from its use.

Barker vacuum pack: a large piece of sterile polyethylene drape is punctured with several small holes in the middle to permit effluent drainage. The drape is then placed over the abdomen down to the abdominal gutters to protect the bowel. Several sterile operating room towels are then placed over the drape with a suction device such as abdominal drains placed in between towels. The drains can be surgically placed through the abdomen through a stab incision or left to exit the open abdomen. The abdomen is then covered with a sterile adhesive drape to provide the seal. Suction is then attached to the drains continuously from the wall-mounted suction device [6, 7]. There are a number of variations to the Barker vacuum pack. Some use Kerlix as a substitute for the towels and utilize different types of drainage tubes, such as chest tubes, nasogastric tubes, JP drains, or track pads from wound vacs. See Fig. 36.1.

36.1.3 Commercial Devices

Commercially manufactured for the purpose of being used for temporary abdominal closures, they generally mimic the standard principle of a permeable inner lining that protects the bowel and an external seal. The commercial device uses the concept of negative pressure wound therapy (NPWT) and a foam dressing covered with an adhesive drape. The dressing is connected to a vacuum device that creates and maintains continuous negative pressure. NPWT has shown some positive effects on wound healing in some studies and may improve fascial closure rates [1, 8]. Other benefits of the commercial devices come with less nursing wound care and dressing needs. With more hospitals using commercial NPWT devices for wounds, they are becoming more accessible and a standard in most major hospitals. Criticisms of the NPWT are the cost associated with the devices and materials as well as the risk of bleeding or

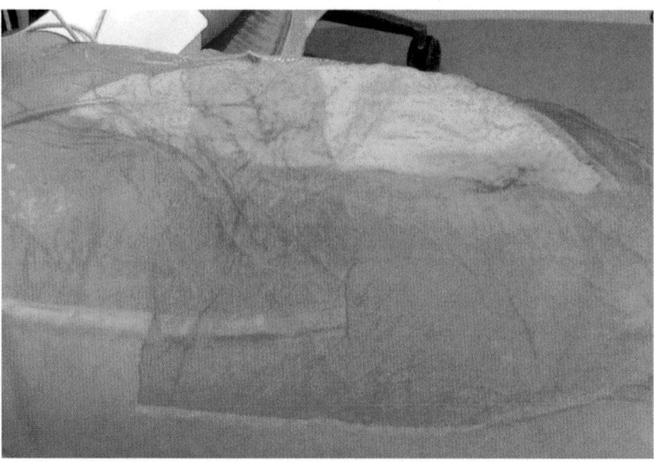

Fig. 36.1 Improvised Barker vacuum pack variant using Kerlix and nasogastric tubing. Photo curtsey of Dr. R. J. Mullins

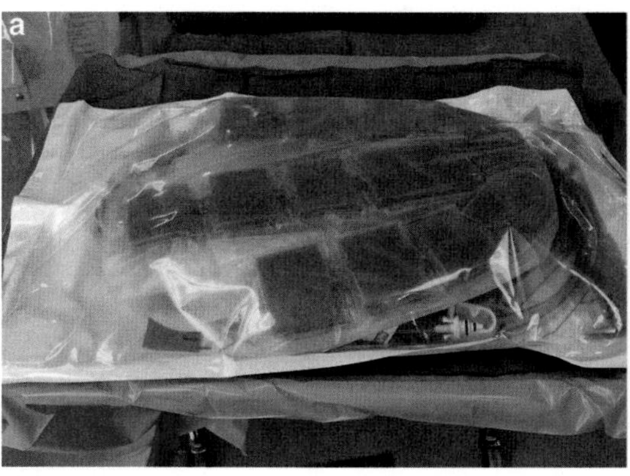
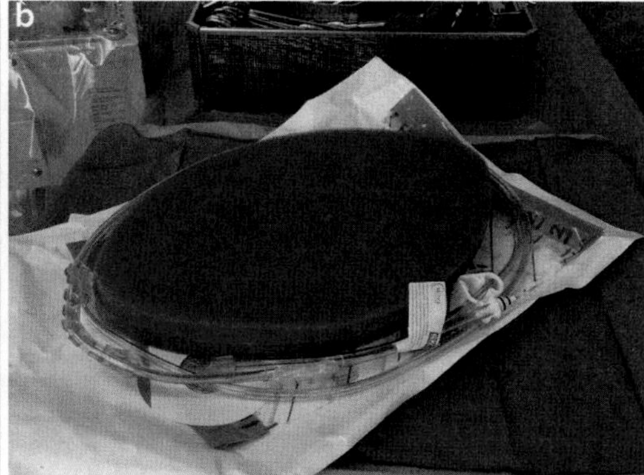

Fig. 36.2 (**a**, **b**) The ABThera device, a commercial NPWT device

enterocutaneous fistulae from continuous suction application to the abdomen and skin edges. To date, there have been no studies to demonstrate clear superiority between the improvised and commercial devices [1].

The ABThera is a recent commercial addition to the management of the open abdomen. Its differences include the use of multiple sponges that are placed into the recesses of the abdomen that provides suction throughout the abdomen. There is some prospective evidence that there may be a survival benefit from the use of this type of commercial device to other improvised devices [8]. See Fig. 36.2a, b.

36.2 Indications

The indications for placement of a TAC device are essentially the inability to close the abdomen primarily at the end of the operative case. The reasoning for this inability to close the abdomen may include:

- Desire to leave abdomen open for concern for or presence of intra-abdominal hypertension or compartment syndrome or high airway pressures.
- The need for further reoperation or exploration of the abdomen including bowel discontinuity second-look operations, edema, or retroperitoneal hemorrhage.

36.3 Contraindications

Absolute: hemodynamic instability where opening the abdomen would not be beneficial and most likely harmful.

Relative: the need to evaluate the abdominal contents in a patient with hemodynamic instability where evaluation and possible therapeutic treatment would be beneficial.

36.4 Preparation

As for any procedure done in the ICU, determine the need for anesthesia, appropriate sedation, analgesia, and chemical paralysis, as well as additional operative support personnel including extra nursing staff and respiratory care. Appropriate equipment should be readily available at the bedside including electrocautery and warm irrigation fluid. If bowel resection or other interventions may be done, have the appropriate instruments, sutures, and devices readily available.

Prepare for blood loss and the need for resuscitation during the procedure with available blood products and appropriate resuscitation fluid. Determine the appropriate dressing device in order to have all the equipment at the bedside. Suction devices should be readied and commercial devices available in the room if used.

If this is a re-exploration or TAC dressing change, it is highly recommended to review the

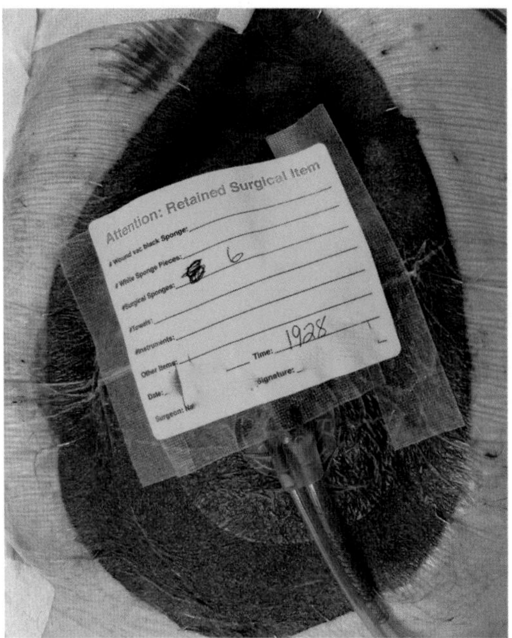

Fig. 36.3 Retained surgical item sticker

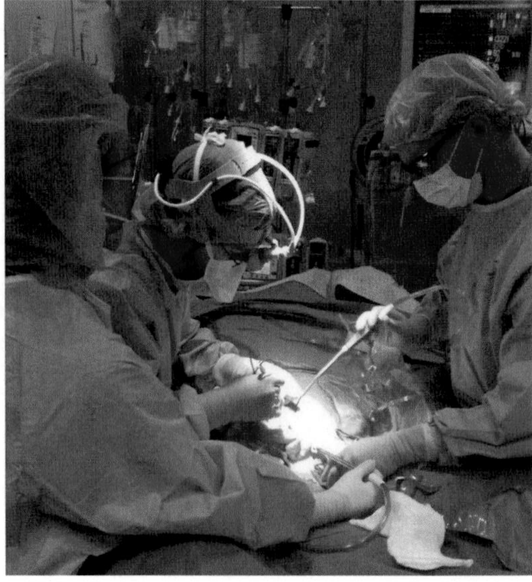

Fig. 36.4 Combined chest and abdominal procedure done in the intensive care unit

previous operative notes to determine if there are any packs or other retained material or devices in the abdomen. Our institution requires a sticker to be placed on the external TAC abdominal dressing that lists retained contents as well as documentation in the chart. This additional layer of safety is intended to prevent retained foreign objects in conjunction with an abdominal X-ray at time of closure of the fascia (Fig. 36.3).

Perform appropriate time-out according to institution practice. This assures correct personnel, equipment, and operative plan including review of consent if not an emergent procedure.

36.5 Procedure

While this procedure is generally done in an operating room setting, it can be done safely and efficiently in the ICU setting both in stable patients and the severely critically ill (Fig. 36.4).

We will describe the steps for placing the ABThera device, a commercial NPWT device. This is our institutions' preferred commercial NPWT device. In general the steps are similar in nature between both improvised and commercial devices.

1. Remove the current TAC device by first removing the adhesive dressing and then the abdominal dressings. Take care in the removal of the abdominal dressing to assure there are no adhesions of the TAC to the bowel. Normal saline or other irrigation fluid may be used to help loosen any adhesions. If staples were used to hold the sponge or towel to the skin, a staple remover or mosquito forceps may be used to remove them from the field. Assure proper disposal of the staples (Figs. 36.5 and 36.6).
2. Prep and drape the abdomen in the standard fashion.
3. Explore the abdomen and perform necessary evaluations and interventions. If applicable, count retained lap pads or devices removed and note additional inserted packs (Fig. 36.7).
4. Once the operative stage is completed, the patient is readied for the TAC. The wound and surrounding skin is cleaned and dried. The TAC device selected is made available.
5. The ABThera device is then sized. The device may be folded or trimmed to fit into the pericolic gutters. If there are drains that need to be laid in the area, cut only between the sponge arm extensions to accommodate

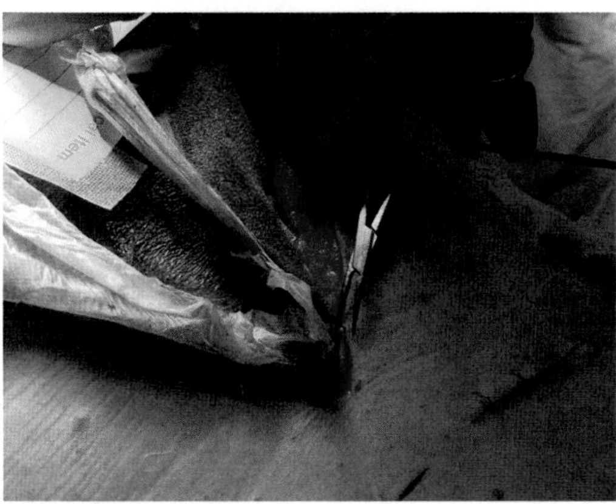

Fig. 36.5 Removal of staples using mosquito clamps

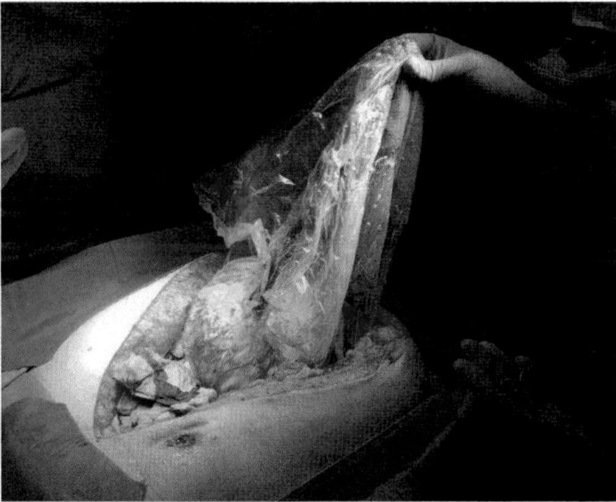

Fig. 36.6 Removal of internal drape

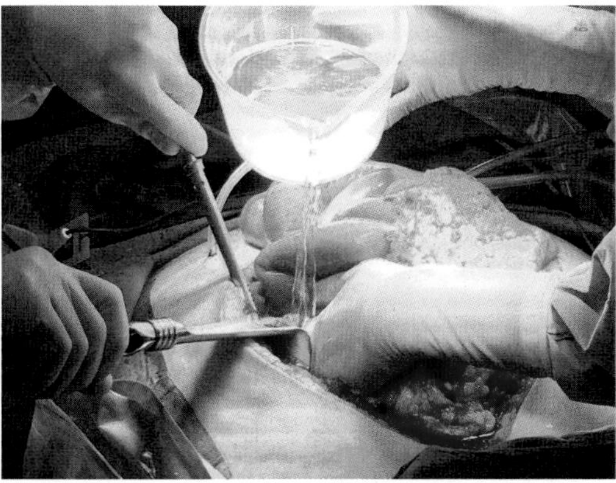

Fig. 36.7 Operative irrigation of the open abdomen

the drains. If the device needs to be smaller in size, cut between the foam square extension and pull the tab portion to assure that there is no exposed foam. Exposed foam may injure bowel and abdominal contents. It is our preference not to cut the device given the risks.

6. Place the device onto the abdominal cavity and with the dressing held up by the edge lower and place the dressings into the pericolic gutter. Retractors may be needed to help achieve proper placement. Use the other hand to bring the dressing down into the gutter. Fold any excess layer up (Fig. 36.8).
7. The sponge is then placed on the abdomen and the sponge is sized and trimmed accordingly if needed (Figs. 36.9 and 36.10).
8. The sponge is then secured to the skin. The device can either be stapled in place or secured along the edges with the adhesive dressing. We prefer to secure with the adhesive dressing (Fig. 36.11).
9. Once the sponge edges are fixed in place, the center portion is secured with the remaining dressing. The suction pad is then obtained and the suction site determined. It is critical to place the suction pad in a convenient spot, usually in the lower midline abdomen, and point the suction drains in an inferior direction. Small superficial lacerations (approximately a 2 cm area) are then made into the plastic covering and into the sponge (less than a 0.25 cm depth) in order to allow the effluent to be removed from the sponge (Fig. 36.12).
10. The suction pad is secured in place over this hole and then attached to suction. With the suction applied, there should be a noticeable change of appearance in the dressing to that of a shriveled raisin. It should be firm. The amount of negative pressure applied to the device should be between 75 and 125 mmHg. If there is concern for fistulae or bowel injury, the lower pressures should be selected. If there is no concern, then the higher suction can be selected to remove effluent from the abdomen (Fig. 36.13).

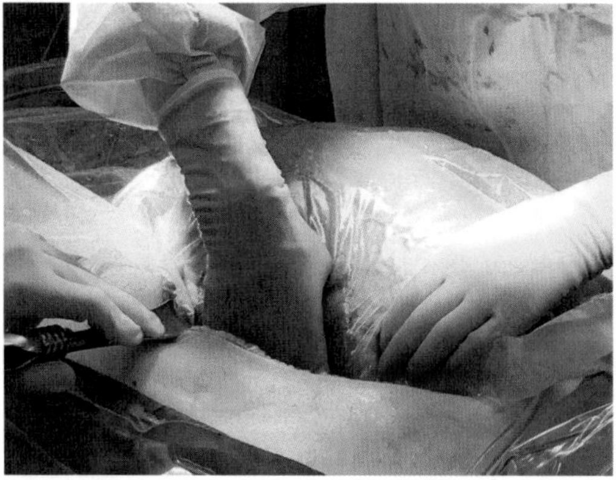

Fig. 36.8 Tucking the ABThera into the abdomen

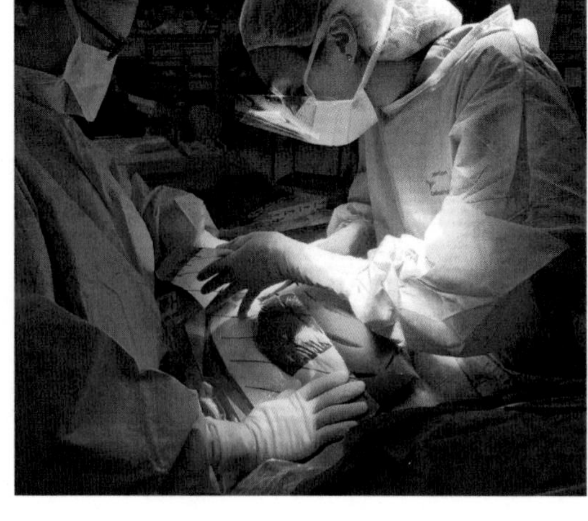

Fig. 36.11 Securing the sponge

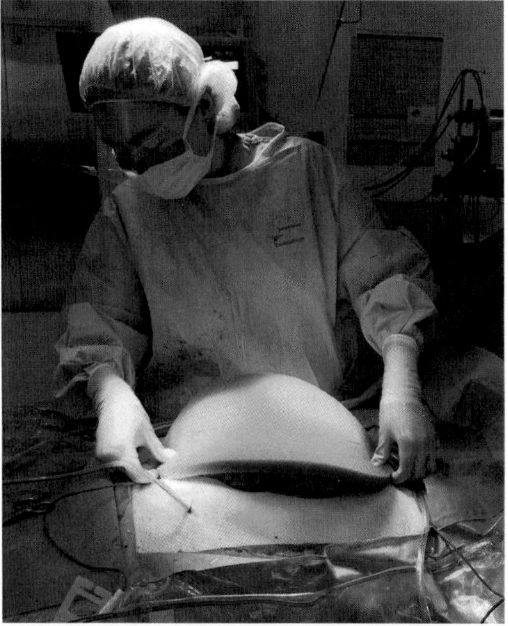

Fig. 36.9 Sizing of the sponge

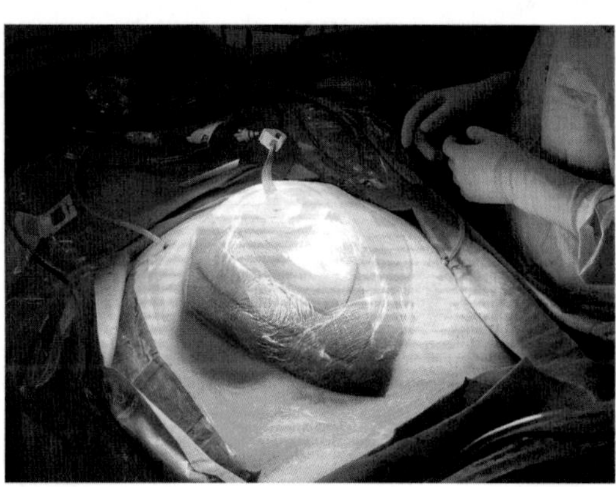

Fig. 36.12 Suction pad in place

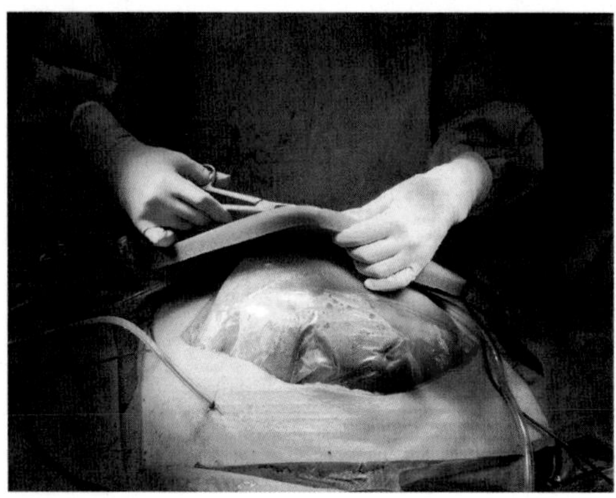

Fig. 36.10 Trimming the sponge

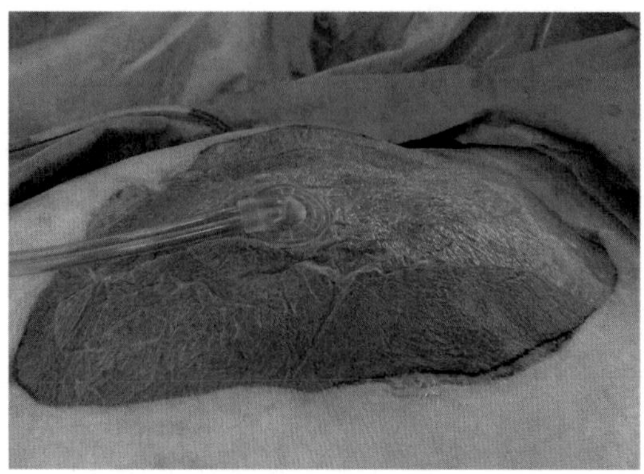

Fig. 36.13 TAC device holding suction

11. Once the device is holding pressure, the remaining dressings and barriers may be removed and the area cleaned. The procedure is then terminated.

36.6 Complications

The following is a list of potential complications from application of a TAC:

- Loss of effluent removal and loss of accurate volume measurement from suction failure.
- Potential contamination of the peritoneal space.
- Direct injury to bowel leading to enterocutaneous fistulae. Prevent this by covering any anastomosis with omentum or other viscera to avoid direct suction from the TAC.
- Abdominal muscle contraction and loss of domain.
- Direct injury to wound edges or other vessels causing bleeding.
- Hypovolemia and shock from volume loss of the effluent. This may progress to or be manifested as acute kidney injury or failure.
- Evisceration or complete failure of the TAC.
- Abdominal compartment syndrome and intra-abdominal hypertension.

36.7 Pearls/Pitfalls

A patient with a TAC device in place can still develop abdominal hypertension and compartment syndrome. The provider must be vigilant and alert to this phenomenon and be prepared to remove the TAC and fully open the abdomen if the patient has clinical symptoms [9].

If the TAC device is not holding appropriate suction or there is a leak in the system, the patient and the device should be evaluated by the provider in a timely fashion. Assessment for leaks begins with holding down around the adhesive draping to determine if that is the source of the leak. If one is found, then additional drape strips or adhesive dressings may be applied to seal. In commercial devices, the suction port is a potential site of clogging or failure and may be in need of replacement. The sponge is sometimes occluded with blood or the suction hole is not large enough and requires revision and replacement. Leaks in the tubing or canister also need investigation. Finally, the vacuum device may be faulty requiring replacement.

36.8 Conclusion

Knowledge of and comfort with removal and replacement of a TAC device are important for the providers taking care of the critically ill or injured patient. Knowledge of the procedure and troubleshooting failures in the system can alert the provider to problems and the need for early interventions such as hemorrhage control and abdominal compartment syndrome.

References

1. Roberts DJ, Zygun DA, Grendar J, et al. Negative-pressure wound therapy for critically ill adults with open abdominal wounds: a systematic review. J Trauma Acute Care Surg. 2012;73:629.
2. Cheatham ML. Abdominal compartment syndrome. Curr Opin Crit Care. 2009;15:154.
3. Diaz JJ, Cullinane DC, Dutton WD, et al. Eastern Association for the Surgery of Trauma: a review of the management of the open abdomen—part 1 "Damage control". J Trauma. 2010;68:1425.
4. Diaz Jr JJ, Dutton WD, Ott MM, et al. Eastern Association for the Surgery of Trauma: a review of the management of the open abdomen—part 2 "Management of the open abdomen". J Trauma. 2011;71:502.
5. Joseph DK, Dutton RP, Aarabi B, Scalea TM. Decompressive laparotomy to treat intractable intracranial hypertension after traumatic brain injury. J Trauma. 2004;57:687.
6. Barker DE, Green JM, Maxwell RA, et al. Experience with vacuum-pack temporary abdominal wound closure in 258 trauma and general and vascular surgical patients. J Am Coll Surg. 2007;204:784.
7. Barker DE, Kaufman HJ, Smith LA, et al. Vacuum pack technique of temporary abdominal closure: a 7-year experience with 112 patients. J Trauma. 2000;48:201.
8. Cheatham ML, Demetriades D, Fabian TC, et al. Prospective study examining clinical outcomes associated with a negative pressure wound therapy system and Barker's vacuum packing technique. World J Surg. 2013;37:2018.
9. Gracias VH, Braslow B, Johnson J, et al. Abdominal compartment syndrome in the open abdomen. Arch Surg. 2002;137:1298.

Part IX

Musculoskeletal Procedures

37 Fracture Immobilization and Splinting

Beth O'Connell and Michael Bosse

37.1 Principles of Splinting

The basic principles for splinting are universally accepted:

1. Immobilize fracture site or reduced dislocation to provide pain relief and assist with inflammatory process/edema resolution.
2. Protect against further soft tissue damage.
3. Correct and prevent deformity.

A thorough and complete physical examination, including appropriate review of necessary radiographs, is fundamental in diagnosis and determination of splinting needs. Once the fracture pattern is recognized, the skin and soft tissue have been evaluated, and appropriate analgesia is provided, the patient is ready for fracture or dislocation reduction and splinting.

Extremity immobilization can be achieved via an off-the-shelf device or with bedside fabricated plaster or fiberglass splints. Prefabricated knee immobilizers, walker boots, Velcro wrist splints, slings, etc. are convenient and universally stocked in medical institutions for sprains and nondisplaced fracture care. These are easily placed by any healthcare provider and allow removal for daily needs and evaluation of soft tissues.

However, for displaced fractures, injuries with soft tissue compromise, or in the setting of significant edema, fiberglass or plaster splinting is usually preferred. Although both mediums are commonly employed for immobilization, there is no data to suggest superiority of either material. An understanding of and respect for the principles and techniques of splint placement is paramount. Achieving and maintaining fracture reduction is vital for skin integrity and pain control. Immobilization of the joint above and below is necessary when addressing diaphyseal fractures.

37.2 Materials

If the fracture is not of a pattern that can be treated with a prefabricated splint, knowledge and skill in the techniques of making and applying a splint made from plaster or fiberglass are required. Basic splinting materials include:

B. O'Connell, MSN, ANP-BC (✉)
Carolinas HealthCare System, Charlotte, NC, USA
e-mail: beth.oconnell@carolinashealthcare.org

M. Bosse, MD, FAAOS
Department of Orthopaedics, Carolinas Medical Center, 1025 Morehead Medical Drive, Suite 300, Charlotte, NC 28204, USA

D.A. Taylor et al. (eds.), *Interventional Critical Care*, DOI 10.1007/978-3-319-25286-5_37

- *Basin or bucket with room temperature water.*
- *Cast padding* is utilized for skin protection and padding of bony prominences under splint material. When placed, it should overlap by 1/2 width to ensure total coverage of underlying skin. For splints, multiple layers are recommended.
- *Plaster* is available in rolls or splint strips of varying widths. The material is made by impregnating crinoline with Plaster of Paris. Once dipped into room temperature water, the powder forms a solid substance and releases heat (an exothermic reaction) during the setting process. Drying time varies by the number of layers used, water temperature, and room temperature [5]. The provider must be thorough in process yet quick with the placement in order to assure desired position before the plaster hardens.
- *Fiberglass* is a lighter-weight product available in prefabricated rolls already padded. It can then be measured, cut, moistened per manufacture's instruction, and placed appropriately.
- *Bias wrap* is a stretchable cloth material used as the final layer of the splint. Because of the possible circumferential compression, ACE wrap and like bandages are not recommended.
- *Tape.*

If a formal orthopedic consult is unavailable for a prolonged time, displaced and angulated fractures must be reduced to restore proper alignment of extremity, relieve pain, and decompress the related soft tissues. Sedation and/or a hematoma block might be required. Once patient comfort is achieved, the extremity is ready for splinting. The non-circumferential placement of plaster or fiberglass allows for continued swelling to occur without fear of vascular or skin compromise and complication, as opposed to immediate casting. Soft tissue concerns can be easily monitored to ensure constant evaluation while continuing to maintain reduced position. With an upper extremity fracture, ensure that any bracelet or rings are removed. Once swelling to the hand or digits occur, they can risk further vascular compromise and difficulty. Attempt removal with any lubricant. At times, a ring cutter is necessary.

37.3 Application Techniques for Commonly Used Upper and Lower Extremity Splints

The actual order and process of splint placement is the same regardless of location or type. Cast padding is placed around the location of the planned plaster or fiberglass splint. Allow for extra padding over bony prominences (elbow, ankle, heel) to avoid breakdown or pressure. Once ensured, take premeasured plaster strips (usually 10–12 layers) or prefabricated fiberglass and dip into room temperature water, squeezing out the excess. Apply the splint material to injured area over cast padding and wrap with the bias. Avoid wrapping too tightly. Ensure desired position, holding until fully hardened. Tape to secure.

Once the splint has set, inspect to ensure that both the proximal and distal ends are well padded and the associated skin is fully protected. Repeat a full neurovascular exam to ensure no change in status post procedure.

37.4 Common Splinting Techniques [1–4]

37.4.1 Thumb Spica

Indicated injuries for use include fracture or ligamentous injury to thumb, first metacarpal fractures, scaphoid fractures, and radial styloid fractures.

Positioning—extend wrist to 20° and abduct thumb, hand in neutral position.

Technique—place cast padding from the level of the interphalangeal (IP) joint of the thumb to the proximal 1/3 of the forearm. Once full skin protection is ensured, take premeasured wet and stripped plaster and apply to radial border of thumb and forearm leaving IP joint of thumb free. Wrap plaster with bias distally from IP joint, proximally to forearm. Avoid wrapping too tightly. Ensure desired position and allow plaster to set. Tape to secure (Fig. 37.1).

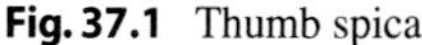

Fig. 37.1 Thumb spica

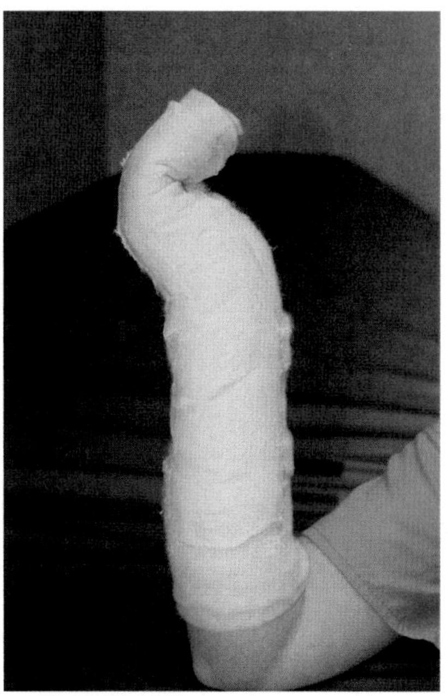

Fig. 37.2 Ulnar gutter splint

37.4.2 Ulnar Gutter Splint

Indicated injuries for use include: fourth/fifth metacarpal fractures, fracture, or ligamentous injuries to ring or small finger.

Positioning—extend wrist 20–30° with flexed metacarpophalangeal (MCP) joint 70–90°.

Technique—place 4×4 gauze between small and ring finger for webspace protection. Use cast padding to wrap the two fingers together and continue proximally up the hand, utilizing the first webspace for hand integration, up to the proximal 1/3 of the forearm. Once full skin protection is ensured, take premeasured wet and stripped plaster and apply to ulnar border of the hand and forearm overlapping the volar and dorsum of the small and ring fingers. Wrap plaster with bias from the distal IP joint proximally up the hand to forearm. Avoid wrapping too tightly. Ensure desired position and allow plaster to set. Tape to secure (Figs. 37.2 and 37.3).

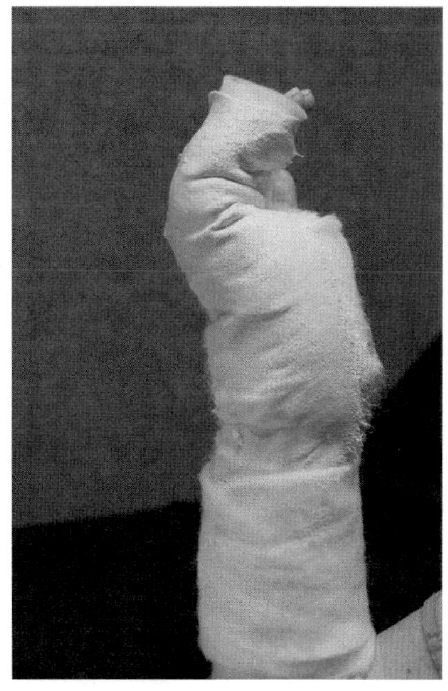

Fig. 37.3 Ulnar gutter splint—example of wrist extension and finger flexion

37.4.3 Radial Gutter Splint

Indicated injuries for use include fractures of index or long finger and second or third metacarpal fractures.

Positioning—extend wrist 20–30° with flexed MCP joints 70–90°.

Technique—place 4×4 gauze between index and long finger for webspace protection.

Use cast padding to wrap the two fingers together and continue proximally up the hand, utilizing the first webspace for hand integration, up to the proximal 1/3 of the forearm. When completed, take the plaster and cut a distal longitudinal slit to allow for the thumb to be excluded from splint. Once full skin protection is ensured, take premeasured wet and stripped plaster and place to the radial aspect of the forearm with the distal portion including the volar and dorsal aspect of the index and long fingers. The remaining digits should be free. Wrap plaster with bias from the distal IP joint proximally up the hand to forearm. Avoid wrapping too tightly. Ensure desired position and allow plaster to set. Tape to secure.

37.4.4 Sugar-Tong Forearm Splint

Indicated injuries for use include distal radius fractures, isolated or both bone fractures of the radius and ulna. It is used to prevent forearm rotation of the wrist or elbow.

Ensure no extreme flexion of the wrist, as this can result in median nerve compression.

Positioning—flexion of elbow at 90°, neutral position of wrist and hand.

Technique—place cast padding beginning distally at the palm of the hand, leaving the MCP joints free, and extend proximally to include the elbow. Ensure extra padding at bony prominence over the olecranon. Once full skin protection is ensured, take premeasured wet and stripped plaster and apply one end to the volar aspect of the hand at the mid-palmar crease. Bring the plaster around the elbow and extend it up to the dorsum of the hand in a U shape, leaving the MCP joints free. This position and elimination of digits should allow for full finger motion. Wrap plaster with bias distally from MCP joints proximally to elbow. Avoid wrapping too tightly. Ensure desired position and allow plaster to set. Tape to secure (Fig. 37.4).

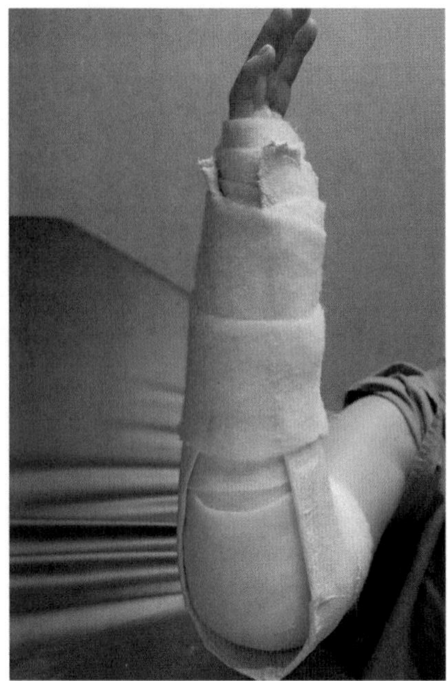

Fig. 37.4 A sugar-tong forearm splint

37.4.5 Posterior Long Arm Splint

Indicated injuries for use include elbow fractures, postreduction of an elbow dislocation, or distal humerus fractures. A posterior component may be utilized in conjunction with a sugar-tong splint for unstable elbow fractures.

Positioning—it may depend on the injury, but typically includes flexion of elbow at 90° with neutral positioning of the forearm and wrist. Ensure no extreme elbow flexion, as this is associated with ulnar nerve compression.

Technique—use cast padding to wrap from wrist crease to the proximal 1/3 of the humerus. Entire hand will be free. Ensure extra padding over bony prominence of olecranon. Once full skin protection is ensured, take premeasured wet and stripped plaster and apply one end to the ulnar aspect of the wrist, proximally up the forearm and over the elbow to the posterior aspect of the humerus. Wrap plaster with bias. Avoid wrapping too tightly. Ensure desired position and allow plaster to set. Tape to secure (Figs. 37.5 and 37.6).

37.4.6 Coaptation Splint for Humerus Fractures

Indicated injury for use includes displaced midshaft humerus fractures.

Positioning—if spine is cleared, elevate head of bed 70–90° to assist with fracture length, elbow in flexion at 90°.

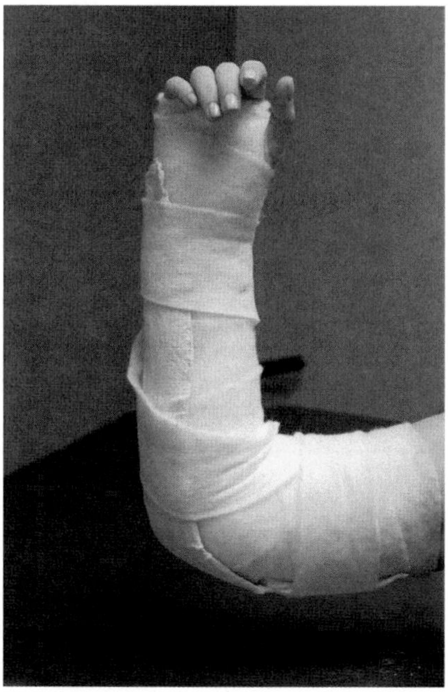

Fig. 37.5 Posterior long arm splint

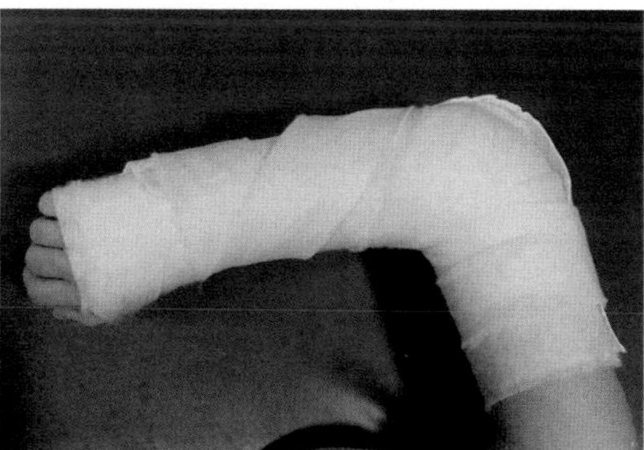

Fig. 37.6 Posterior long arm splint

Technique—coaptation splints are best achieved with two or even three sets of skilled hands. Begin with placing cast padding at proximal forearm and move up the humerus and over the shoulder to include distal clavicle. Ensure that bony prominence over olecranon is well padded. Place one end of premeasured wet and stripped plaster in the axilla and wrap it down under the elbow in a U shape, up and over the shoulder nearing the end of plaster at the base of the neck. Recommend wrapping the ends of the splint both at the axilla and over the shoulder with an abdominal pad or extra cast padding to ensure skin protection. Wrap plaster with bias. Avoid wrapping too tightly. Axial traction would then be held through the elbow and a valgus mold placed on the humerus for fracture reduction. A hand placed firmly on the splint over the shoulder is helpful during the traction and mold placement, in order to keep the splint from slipping. If the plaster is not extended over the distal clavicle, immobilization of the shoulder joint is not achieved. Ensure desired position and allow plaster to set. Tape to secure.

37.4.7 Short Posterior and Sugar-Tong (Stirrup) Leg Splints

Indicated injuries for use include stabilization of severe ankle sprains, metatarsal and midfoot fractures, ankle fractures, and distal tibia fractures. The sugar tong, or stirrup component, increases the stability of splint and prevents inversion, eversion, and plantar flexion of the ankle.

Positioning—for placement of splint, use flexion of knee to allow relaxation of the gastrocnemius, and hold the ankle in neutral position (90°). This is very important with long-term splints in order to prevent an equinus ankle contracture.

Technique—with the leg held in position as described above, use cast padding to wrap from toes proximally to tibial tuberosity. Ensure attention to padding over bony prominences of the medial and lateral ankle and heel. Place premeasured wet and stripped plaster, applying posterior slab from metatarsal heads just distal to popliteal fossa (allows unobstructed motion of knee) (Fig. 37.7). The sugar-tong (stirrup) piece is then added to the medial and lateral aspects of the calf wrapping under the plantar aspect of the foot, terminating just below the fibular head to avoid compression of peroneal nerve (Figs. 37.8 and 37.9). Wrap plaster with bias. Avoid wrapping too tightly. Ensure ankle remains at 90° and allow plaster to set. Tape to secure.

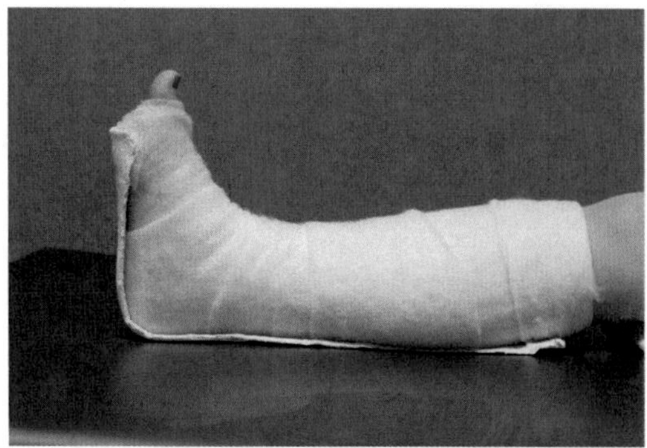

Fig. 37.7 Sugar-tong leg splint—application of posterior slab

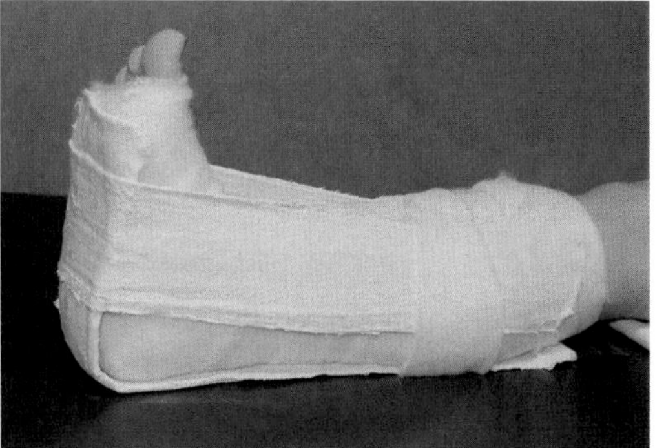

Fig. 37.8 Wrapping the sugar-tong/stirrup portion

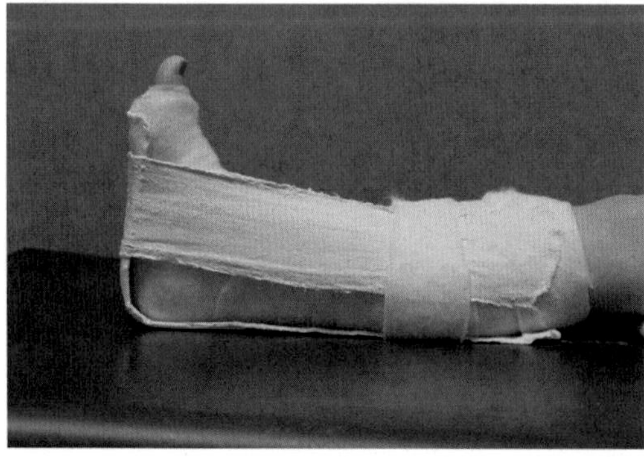

Fig. 37.9 Lateral view of sugar tong/stirrup

37.4.8 Long Leg Splint

Indicated injures for use included proximal or midshaft tibia fractures, knee injuries (postreduction of dislocations, ligamentous injury), distal femur fractures, and patella fractures.

Position—10° of knee flexion and neutral position of ankle at 90°.

Technique—with provider holding gentle axial traction at ankle with leg elevated, and if available, a second assistant supporting leg at the thigh with support under fracture site, place cast padding from toes to proximal thigh just distal to gluteal crease. Ensure that proper bony prominences of ankle and heel are well padded. Place posterior portion of premeasured wet and stripped plaster from metatarsal head to proximal posterior thigh. If ankle immobilization is required for fracture pattern (midshaft tibia fracture), add a long sugar tong (stirrup) as previously described and extend the medial and lateral portion proximally to the distal femur. This ensures immobilization of both ankle and knee joints. With proximal tibia or distal femur fractures, you may opt to place short side slabs of plaster to immobilize knee when ankle is not necessary. Wrap wet plaster with bias. Avoid wrapping too tightly. Ensure desired position and allow to harden. Tape to secure.

37.4.9 Bulky Jones

Indicated injuries for use include calcaneus fractures, ankle injuries, or fractures with significant swelling.

The actual plaster or fiberglass portion is simply a short posterior slab splint. The purpose of bulky cast padding is intended for foot/ankle fractures with notable swelling potential and to ensure appropriate padding to heel with calcaneus fractures.

Position—for placement of splint, use flexion of knee to allow relaxation of gastrocnemius and neutral position (90°) of ankle. With some fracture patterns and those with operative needs, swelling and pain may be such that a fully neutral position may not be attained and slight equinus is accepted.

Technique—with the leg held in position as described above, use cast padding to wrap from metatarsal heads proximally to tibial tuberosity. Ensure attention to padding over bony prominences of medial and lateral ankle and heel

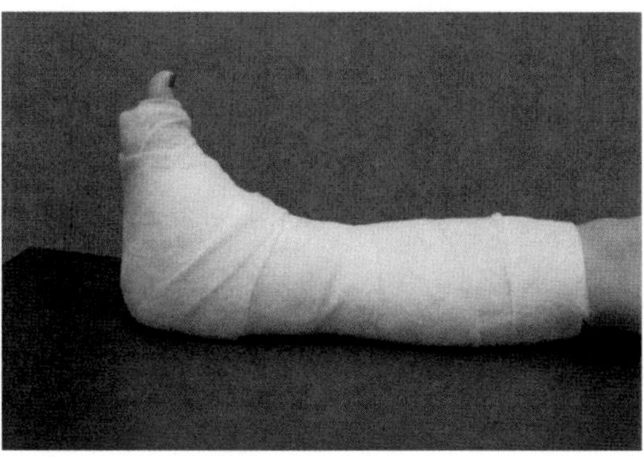

Fig. 37.10 The bulky Jones padding. Note padding to bony prominences and heel

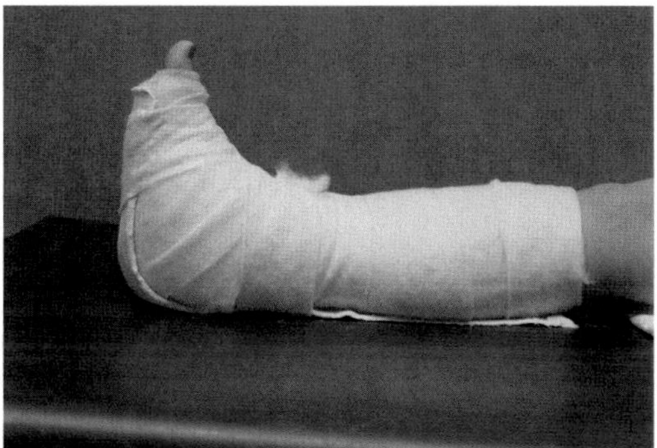

Fig. 37.11 Short posterior splint of the bulky Jones

(Fig. 37.10). The bulky Jones dressing is added by fanning out one complete roll of cast padding and placing this over the heel and both the medial and lateral malleoli. A short posterior splint will then be added as described above terminating at the proximal tibia posteriorly just distal to the popliteal fossa to allow full knee motion (Fig. 37.11). Wrap plaster with bias (Fig. 37.12. Avoid wrapping too tightly. Ensure desired position and allow plaster to set. Tape to secure.

37.5 Splinting Complications

Although splint placement in educated and practiced hands may be seen as a benign procedure, it can cause complications. Attention to detail during placement and careful notation of the finished product is vital to ensure safety.

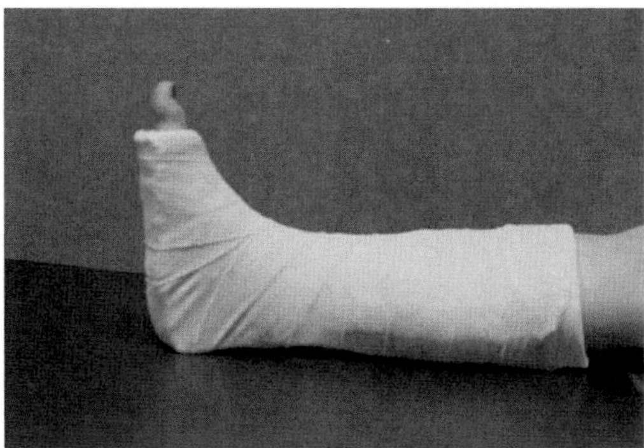

Fig. 37.12 Bias applied to the bulky Jones

Burns [5, 6] Both plaster and fiberglass splint materials harden via a chemical (exothermic) reaction that produces heat. The strength provided by the splint is directly correlated to the layers of material used. Therefore, the more layers used, the more heat is produced at an increased risk of burning a patient's skin. If hot water is used for dipping, more heat is generated leading to an increased risk of burns. Adequate skin protection with cast padding in combination with room temperature water use is imperative in order to avoid thermal burns. Careful attention must be directed to patient concerns and complaints of significant and painful warmth after splint is completed. Have a low threshold for removal and revision if no relief is achieved.

Compartment Syndrome A compartment syndrome is a condition in which increased pressure within a confined space compromises the contents of that space. Although most common in the lower extremities and with circumferential casting, it must be respected that splinting can cause some degree of extremity compression, resulting in further limitation of the available space. In addition to fracture site bleeding, swelling and inflammation are normal responses to trauma. Frequent neurovascular exams must be performed on any patient splinted.

Contractures In the acute setting, most splints are placed with the anticipation of early intervention or fixation. However, if long-term splinting is anticipated, close attention must be placed to the unaffected joints surrounding the fracture site. Any unnecessary joints must be left free to allow unrestricted range of motion. Otherwise, contractures may develop contributing to further immobility and functional deficit.

Skin Compromise A thorough evaluation of the patient's skin condition prior to splint placement is included in the initial exam. Risk of acute skin compromise may occur to areas of pressure whether from fracture pattern or splint material. Adequate protection of bony prominences will decompress and prevent further decline of tenuous soft tissues. Frequent monitoring or scheduled skin checks are encouraged for those deemed at risk. If in doubt of padding sufficiency, add more.

Nerve Compression Final position of the injured extremity when splinted is essential. Specific angles are provided above in application techniques to assist with deterrence of nerve compression secondary to prolonged positioning and/or pressure. For example, if a wrist is hyperflexed and remains splinted for a prolonged course, compression of the median nerve could occur and become a complication not from injury but from splint positioning. Similarly, a hyperflexed elbow with long arm splints could lead to compression and symptoms of the ulnar nerve. Special attention must be given to final positioning of splint in order to avoid splint-related nerve symptoms.

Orthopedic injuries are very common in the trauma population, and they will require appropriate immobilization. A thorough physical examination, review of radiographs, realignment of fracture if displaced, and correct choice of splint based upon injury will be required of the treating orthopedic team. Given the various types of immobilization, practice really does make perfect. Special attention must be given after completion to ensure skin protection and correct position in order to avoid complications.

References

Historical References

1. Swiontkowski M, Stovitz S. Manual of orthopaedics. 6th ed. Philadelphia, PA: Lippincott Williams & Wilkins; 2006. p. 93–118.
2. Sarmiento A, Kinman PB, Galvin ED, Schmitt RH, Phillips JG. Functional bracing of fractures of the shaft of the humerus. J Bone Joint Surg Am. 1977;59(5):596–601.
3. Miller ME, Ada JR. Skeletal trauma. 2nd ed. Philadelphia, PA: WB Saunders; 1992.
4. Connolly J. Fractures and dislocations. Closed management. Philadelphia, PA: WB Saunders; 1995.

Reference List

5. Pope MH, Callahan G, Levarette R. Setting temperatures of synthetic casts. J Bone Joint Surg Am. 1985;67:262–4.
6. Halanski MA, Halanski AD, Oza A, et al. Thermal injury with contemporary cast application techniques and methods to circumvent morbidity. J Bone Joint Surg Am. 2007;89(11):2369–77.

38 Fracture Management: Basic Principles

Jenna Garofalo and Madhav Karunakar

38.1 Fracture Management: Basic Principles

Although no two fractures are identical, the same general principles apply when managing all types of fractures. Once a fracture is identified, it is classified as nondisplaced or displaced. Nondisplaced fractures refer to those types where the bone is anatomically aligned and maintains alignment without undergoing a formal reduction or manipulation. These types of fractures heal well with immobilization in a splint, cast, or brace. Displaced fractures are characterized by fracture patterns where the bone fragments are not in anatomic position and thus require a reduction maneuver to achieve improved alignment. In addition to improving patient comfort, it is important to reduce and immobilize fractures in a timely manner to minimize motion of the fracture fragments. This prevents further trauma to the surrounding muscles, soft tissues, and other underlying structures.

Reduction can be achieved in many ways depending on the type and severity of the fracture, the patient's underlying medical comorbidities, and any associated injuries. Noninvasive techniques of fracture manipulation are frequently used and include splinting, casting, or bracing. Other nonoperative and minimally invasive methods of reduction include skin and skeletal traction. More invasive reduction techniques involve both external and internal fixation. This chapter will focus on skeletal traction and external fixation, both of which are commonly utilized in the acute care setting.

38.2 Traction

When a bone is fractured or a joint is dislocated, the surrounding muscle spasm and contract, pulling the proximal and distal ends of the fracture. This causes further displacement of the fracture, limb shortening, and rotation. To counteract this, traction is one method used to maintain adequate limb length and gross fracture alignment. This technique is particularly useful in stabilizing long bone fractures, such as femoral shaft (Fig. 38.1), proximal femur and hip fractures, pelvic and acetabular fractures (Fig. 38.2).

Traction creates an opposing longitudinal or axial force that is applied to the affected extremity to counteract the muscle contraction that is causing the displacement of the fracture fragments. This technique counteracts these displacing forces and aligns the fracture and provides stabilization and immobilization until the fracture is amenable to definitive fixation.

J. Garofalo, MSN, FNP (✉) • M. Karunakar, MD
Carolinas HealthCare System, Charlotte, NC, USA

Department of Orthopaedics, Carolinas Medical Center, 1025 Morehead Medical Drive, Suite 300, Charlotte, NC 28204, USA
e-mail: Jenna.Garofalo@carolinashealthcare.org

D.A. Taylor et al. (eds.), *Interventional Critical Care*, DOI 10.1007/978-3-319-25286-5_38

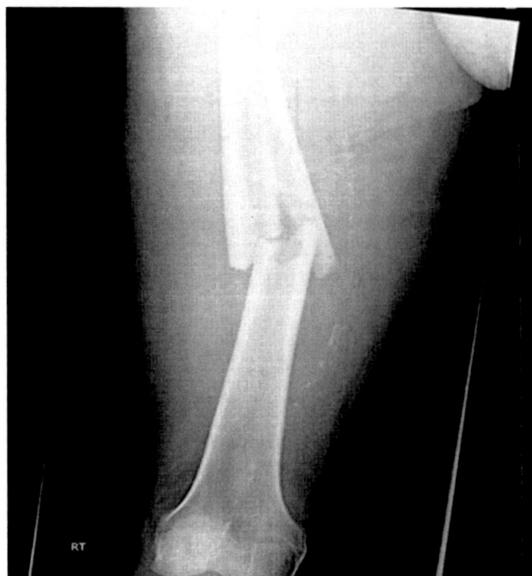

Fig. 38.1 Displaced femoral shaft fracture

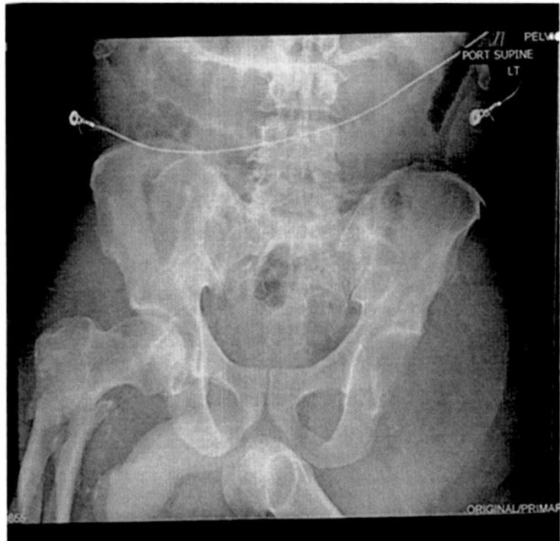

Fig. 38.2 Hip dislocation with contralateral comminuted proximal femur fracture

38.3 Skeletal Traction

Skeletal traction is a more invasive method of reduction that involves the insertion of a Kirschner wire (K-wire) or Steinmann pin through the bone. K-wires are smaller in diameter and require a tension bow with traction setup, while Steinmann pins are larger in diameter and a non-tension bow is used. There are several sites where this method of traction is used including the skull for unstable cervical spine injuries, distal femur, proximal tibia, distal tibia, calcaneus, and olecranon. For the purpose of this chapter, temporary skeletal traction of the distal femur and proximal tibia will be described in greater detail. One advantage of using skeletal traction over less invasive methods of traction is that it provides a more direct force to the fracture fragments allowing for a better reduction [1]. Skeletal traction can be performed at the bedside with local anesthetic with relative ease.

38.4 Materials and Supplies

1. K-wire (Fig. 38.3) or Steinman pin tray (Fig. 38.4)—contents are facility specific but should include pins or wires, drill, hammer, bow, and pliers
2. Sterile gloves
3. Betadine or ChloraPrep
4. Scalpel
5. Sterile towels
6. 4×4 gauze
7. 1 % Lidocaine
8. Syringe and needle
9. Tape

38.4.1 Skeletal Traction: Distal Femur

Distal femoral traction is most often indicated in acetabulum fracture dislocations, complex pelvic ring injuries including sacroiliac joint fracture dislocations, and proximal femur fractures. In patients with diaphyseal fractures of the femur and ipsilateral injury to the knee or proximal tibia, distal femoral traction is utilized as well since proximal tibial traction is contraindicated with these associated injuries [1].

38.5 General Considerations

- Obtain radiograph of the entire femur prior to placement to confirm traction pin is not inserted through a fracture or bony abnormality.
- Adequately identify landmarks, and always insert pin from medial to lateral to avoid injury to surrounding neurovascular structures [1]. If

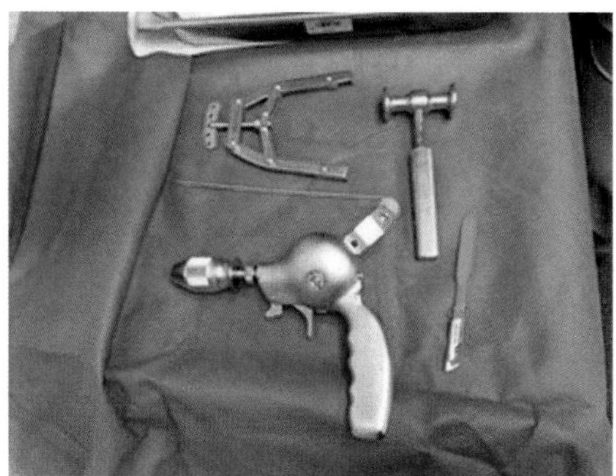

Fig. 38.3 Kirschner wire tray (clockwise from left: tension bow, hammer, scalpel, drill, K-wire)

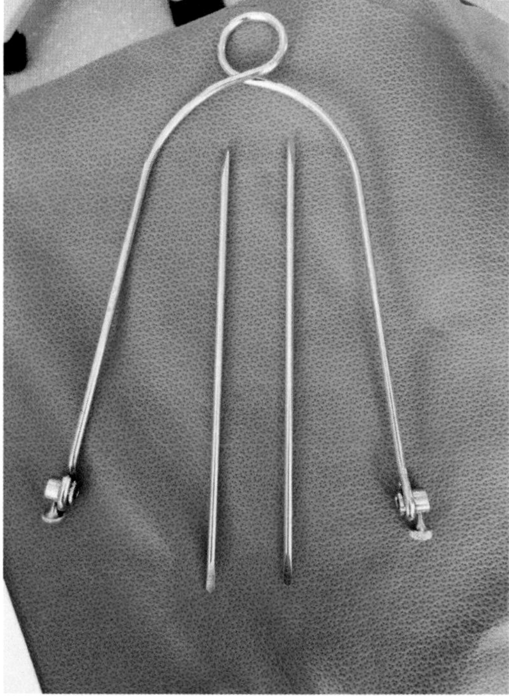

Fig. 38.4 Steinman pin with non-tension bow

inserted too distal, there is an increased risk of entering the knee joint at the intercondylar notch. Conversely, if inserted too proximal, there is a risk of damaging the neurovascular structures, such as the femoral artery [2].

- Traction pin should be inserted parallel to the knee joint [2].
- It is important to have someone help hold the patient's extremity in neutral alignment to ensure proper placement of traction pin.

38.6 Technique

1. With patient supine, position the affected extremity in neutral alignment, with knee flexed 30° over a bump and with the toes and patella pointing toward ceiling.
2. Identify the superior margin of the patella, and palpate along the medial aspect of the distal femoral condyle. The insertion point will be approximately 2 cm (2 fingerbreadths) proximal to the superior margin of the patella, and 2 cm medial, just proximal to the medial epicondyle or adductor tubercle (Fig. 38.5) [2]. Note that in an obese patient, these measurements will need to be adjusted to ensure that insertion point is in the middle of the bone.
3. Once the bony landmarks are identified, and marked if needed, begin preparing your sterile field and the extremity. Often, patients present with a temporary traction splint from the emergency department. Leave the extremity in traction during the procedure, but ensure that the sides are cut back or adjusted to allow adequate access.
4. Administer a local bolus of anesthetic to both the entrance (Fig. 38.6) and exit (Fig. 38.7)

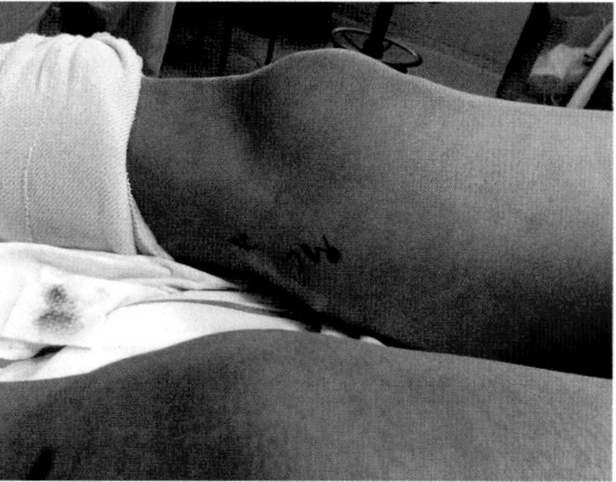

Fig. 38.5 Skin markings indicating insertion point of K-wire

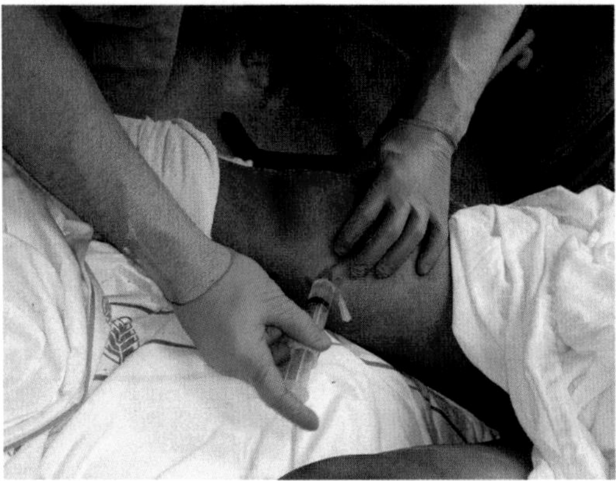

Fig. 38.6 Injection of Lidocaine into insertion point of K-wire, medial aspect of distal femur

points of the traction pin. The exit point will be on the lateral side of the distal femur, directly across from the insertion site. Use approximately 5 mL Lidocaine per side. Make sure to penetrate Lidocaine down to the bone. Cleanse area with Betadine or ChloraPrep solution, and drape surrounding portions of extremity with sterile towels, leaving only the immediate area exposed (Fig. 38.8) [3].

5. Select the appropriate K-wire pin size (usually 2 mm) or Steinmann pin (usually 4 mm) and place into drill [4].
6. Make a small stab incision using scalpel at insertion site along the medial aspect of the leg.
7. Insert K-wire into incision. Make sure wire is centered on bone. You may need to use the wire to identify the anterior and posterior cortices of the bone to locate center. Once appropriate position is confirmed, begin advancing using the drill (Fig. 38.9). Be sure that hand and drill are parallel to the bed to ensure pin is advancing in a straight line. Once the pin passes through the medial cortex, it will advance easily until it reaches the lateral cortex. When the tip of the pin exits the bone and tents the skin, make a small stab incision to expose the end of the pin.
8. Remove the drill. Using the hammer, lightly tap the medial end of the pin until there are equal parts of the pin exposed on both sides (Fig. 38.10). Do not hammer the pin through

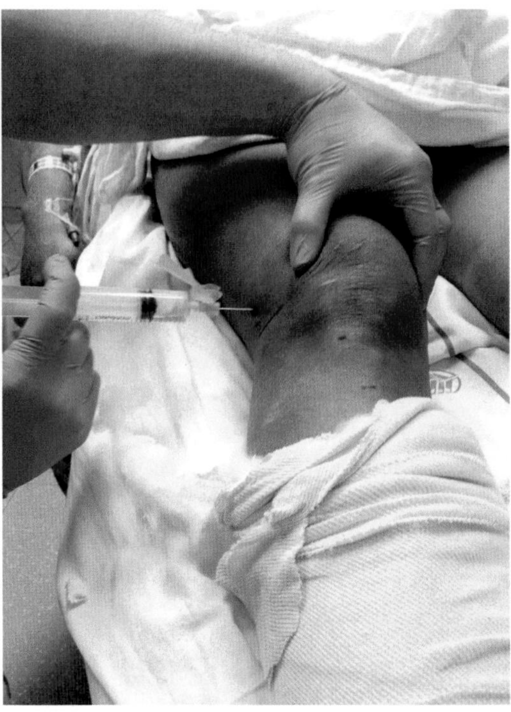

Fig. 38.7 Injection of Lidocaine into the projected exit point of the K-wire, lateral aspect of distal femur

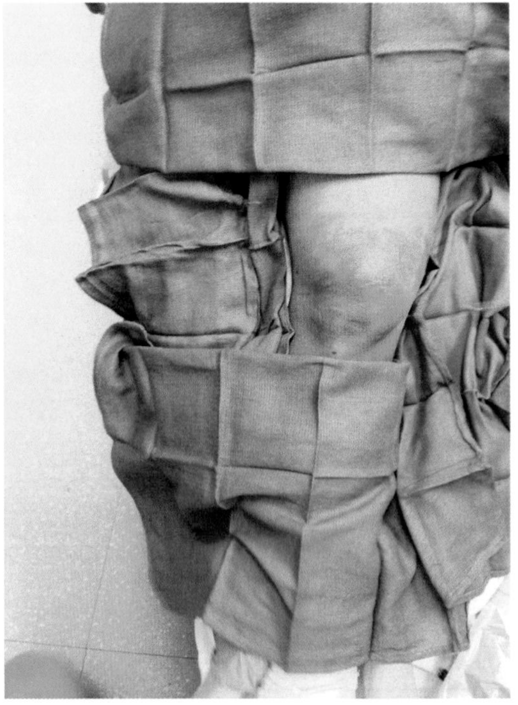

Fig. 38.8 Extremity prepped in sterile fashion

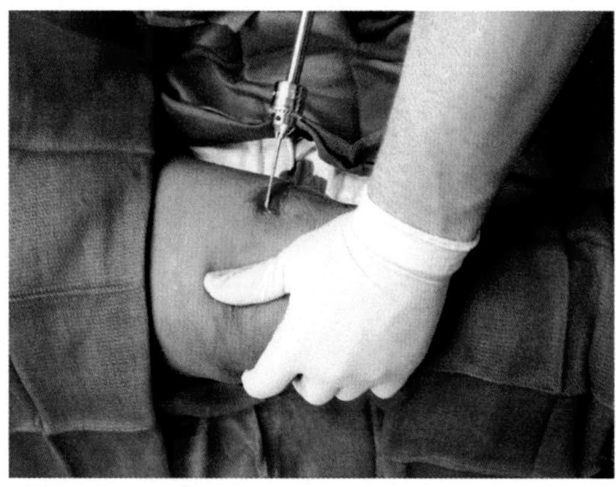

Fig. 38.9 K-wire advancing through medial cortex of the distal femur

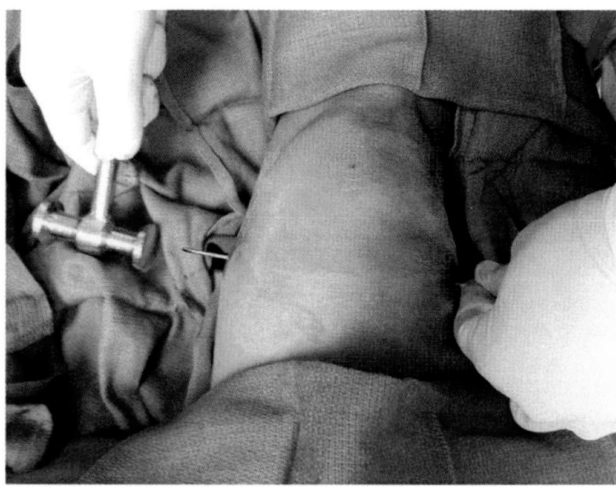

Fig. 38.10 Gently hammering K-wire

the bone; this could cause fracture around the pin site ([5], p. 122).

9. Attach bow to the traction pin and give it a gentle tug to make sure it is secure before the weights are attached.
10. Bend, cut, or cap the exposed portion of the traction pin to prevent injury from the sharp ends.
11. Wrap the towels around the bow to protect the soft tissues and bony prominences from pressure once weights are attached. Never leave bow lying directly on the leg, as this could cause skin breakdown and necrosis.
12. For an average-sized adult, the lower extremity can tolerate approximately 20 % of the individuals' body weight, which is usually 20–25 pounds of countertraction. This is applied using a trapeze and pulley apparatus attached to the patient's bed [1].

38.6.1 Skeletal Traction: Proximal Tibia

Proximal tibial traction is most often used in patients with diaphyseal fractures of the femur. This method is contraindicated in patients with associated fractures of the proximal tibia or ligamentous injuries to the knee. In addition, it should never be used in children as it could damage physeal bone, causing asymmetric closure of growth plates, resulting in deformity to the extremity [2].

38.7 General Considerations

- Obtain radiograph of the knee prior to procedure to confirm that traction pin is not inserted through a fracture or bony abnormality.
- Adequately identify landmarks for pin insertion. Always insert traction pin from lateral to medial to avoid injury to the common peroneal nerve [2].
- It is important to have someone help hold the patient's extremity in neutral alignment to ensure accurate placement of traction pin.

38.8 Technique

1. With patient supine, position the affected extremity in neutral alignment, with the toes and patella pointing toward ceiling (Fig. 38.11).

   Identify the patella, patellar tendon, tibial tuberosity (Fig. 38.12), and the fibular head, where the common peroneal nerve is located posteriorly; these will serve as the landmarks for proper pin insertion [6]. If needed, use a skin marker to identify the landmarks.
2. Measure 2.5 cm distal to the level of the tibial tuberosity (Fig. 38.13) and 2.5 cm posterior to the tibial tuberosity (Fig. 38.14) (aka 1–2 fingerbreadths) [2]. This will be the insertion site of the traction pin.
3. Once the bony landmarks are identified, and marked if needed, begin preparing your sterile field and the extremity. Often, patients present with a temporary traction splint from the emergency department. Leave the extremity in traction during the procedure,

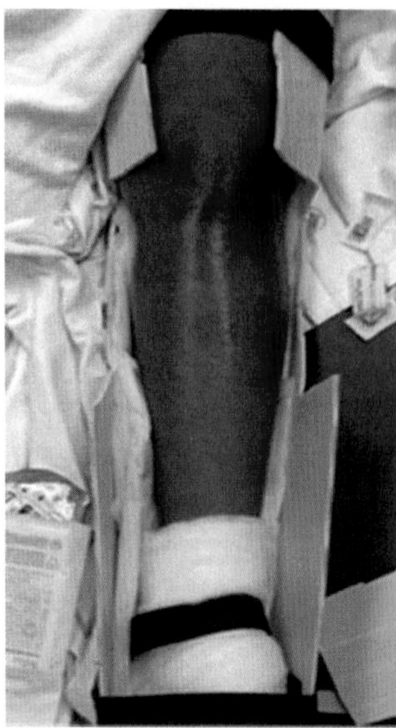

Fig. 38.11 Trauma patient with lower extremity in temporary traction splint

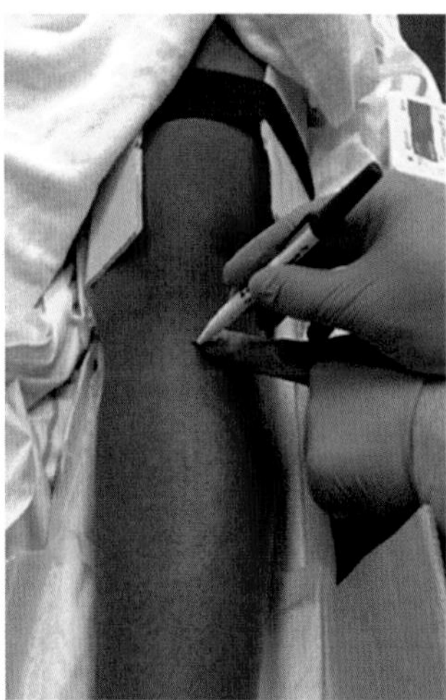

Fig. 38.12 Tibial tuberosity

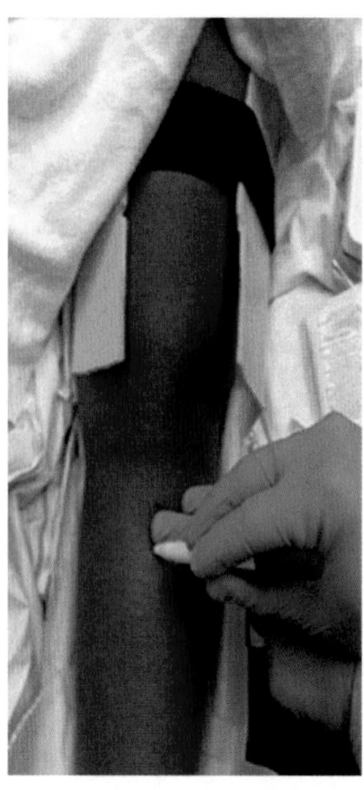

Fig. 38.13 2.5 cm distal to tibial tuberosity

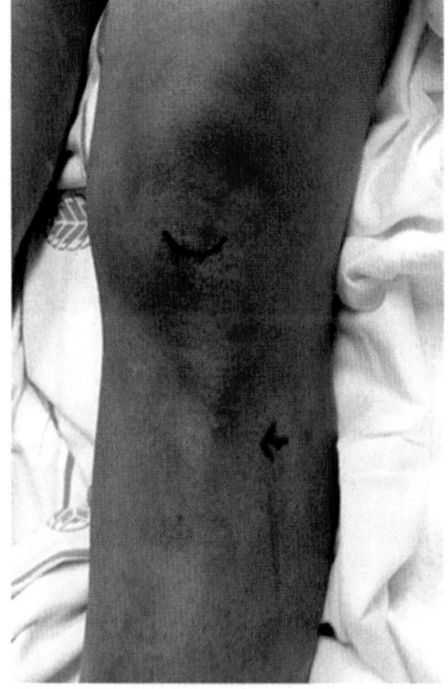

Fig. 38.14 2.5 cm posterior to tibial tuberosity

but ensure that the sides are cut back or adjusted to allow adequate access (Fig. 38.11).

4. Administer a local bolus of anesthetic to both the entrance and exit points of the traction pin. The exit point will be on the medial side of the proximal tibia, directly across from the insertion site. Use approximately 5 mL Lidocaine per side. Make sure to penetrate Lidocaine down to the bone. Cleanse area with Betadine or ChloraPrep solution, and drape surrounding portions of the extremity with sterile towels, leaving only the immediate area exposed [3].
5. Select the appropriate K-wire pin size (usually 2 mm) or Steinmann pin (usually 4 mm) and place into drill [4].

6. Make a small stab incision using scalpel at insertion site along the lateral aspect of the leg.
7. Insert K-wire into incision. Make sure wire is centered on bone. You may need to use the wire to identify the anterior and posterior cortices of the bone to locate center. Once appropriate position confirmed, begin advancing using the drill (Fig. 38.15). Be sure that hand and drill are parallel to the bed to ensure pin is advancing in a straight line. Once the pin passes through the lateral cortex, it will advance easily until it reaches the medial cortex. When the tip of the pin exits the bone and tents the skin, make a small stab incision to expose the end of the pin (Fig. 38.16).
8. Remove the drill. Using the hammer, lightly tap the lateral end of the pin until there are equal parts of the pin exposed on both sides (Fig. 38.17). Do not hammer pin through the bone as this could cause fracture at the pin site ([5], p. 122).
9. Attach the bow to the traction pin and give it a gentle tug (Fig. 38.18) to make sure it is tight before the weights are attached.
10. Bend, cut, or cap the exposed portion of the traction pin to prevent injury from the sharp ends (Fig. 38.19).
11. Wrap the towels around the bow to protect the soft tissues and bony prominences from pressure once weights are attached. Never leave bow lying directly on the leg, as this could cause skin necrosis.
12. For an average-sized adult, the lower extremity can tolerate approximately 20 % of the individuals' body weight, which is usually 20–25 pounds of counter traction. This is

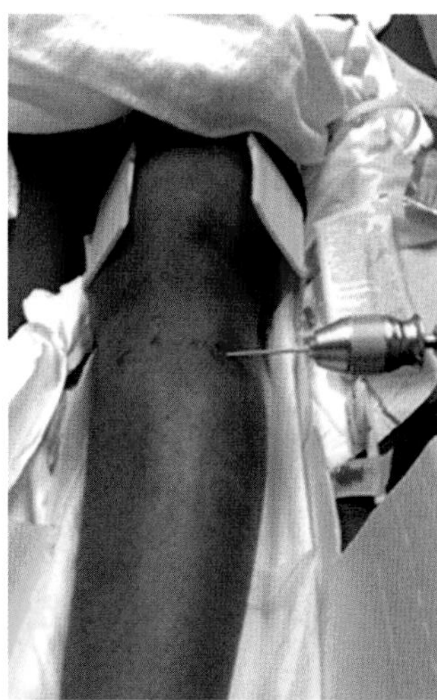

Fig. 38.15 Insertion of proximal tibia tissues traction pin—lateral to medial

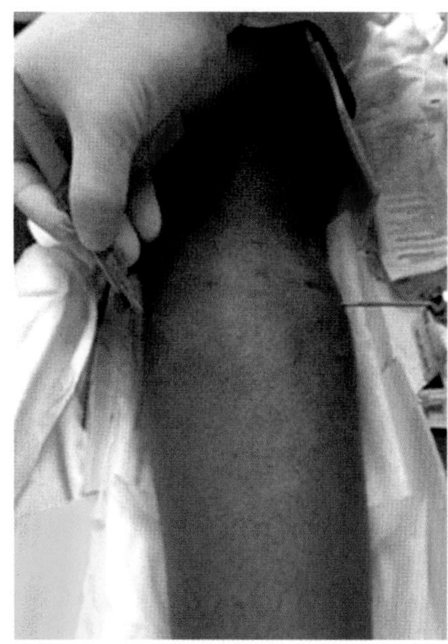

Fig. 38.16 Traction pin tenting medial soft tissues

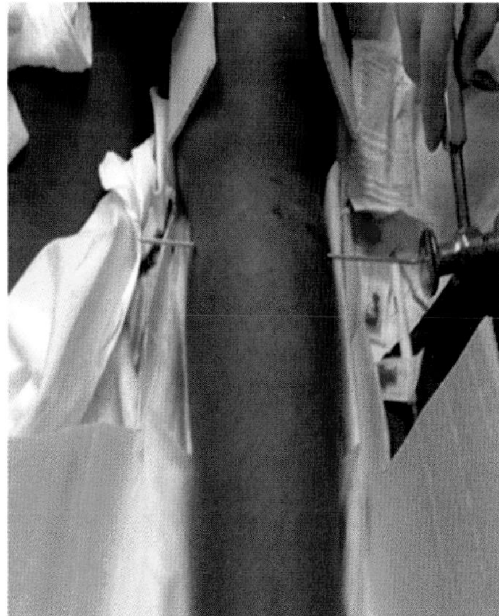

Fig. 38.17 Hammering of K-wire pin once lateral end exposed

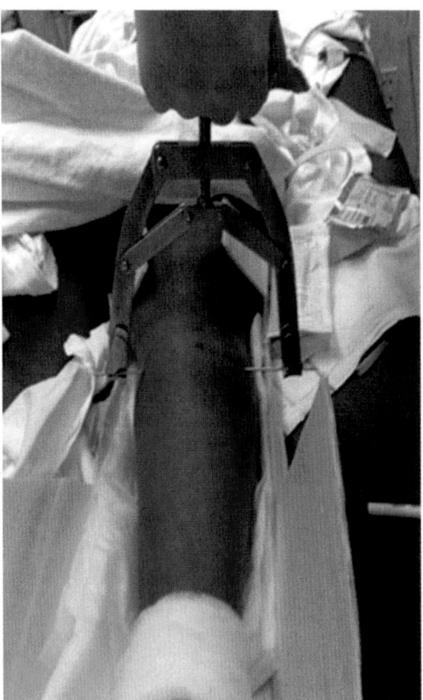

Fig. 38.18 Gentle tug of bow

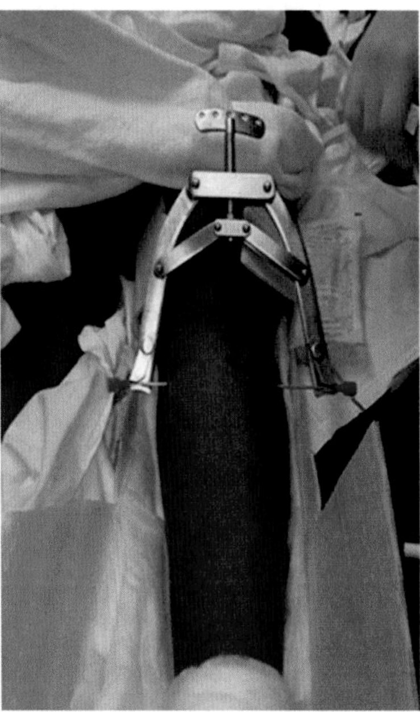

Fig. 38.19 Bow attached to K-wire

applied using a trapeze and pulley apparatus attached to the end of the patient's bed [1].

38.9 External Fixators: Principles

Frequently in the acute care setting, patients sustain fractures as a result of high-energy mechanisms. These fractures may be comminuted, displaced, and have associated soft tissue, nerve, or vascular injuries that require timely stabilization in the operating room (Fig. 38.20). In the event that the patient cannot undergo definitive internal fixation, whether it be due to soft tissue injury or concomitant comorbidities, an external fixator has proven to be an appropriate alternative.

An external fixator is essentially a scaffold that stabilizes and aligns fractures using external pins/wires, bars/rods, or rings and clamps. These devices are used to treat fractures in a variety of ways, with the primary goal being to restore anatomic length, alignment, and rotation Acutely, external fixators are used to temporarily or provisionally stabilize fractures until the patient's physiologic state or soft tissues surrounding the fracture are amenable to internal fixation. In individuals with multiple comorbidities from a medical or trauma standpoint, and who are unable to undergo operative fixation, and in fractures that are unable to achieve

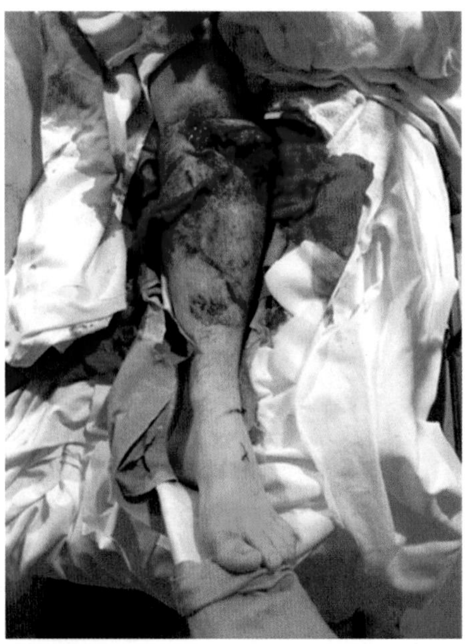

Fig. 38.20 Lower leg with fracture and overlying soft tissue injury

adequate reduction with casting or bracing, external fixators can function as definitive treatment (Figs. 38.21 and 38.22).

38.10 External Fixators: Indications

While internal fixation is the ultimate goal when discussing operative fixation for the majority of fractures, it is often not optimal as the initial treatment plan. As previously mentioned, in the unstable polytrauma patient, definitive fracture management is often delayed and requires staged fixation until adequate resuscitation has been achieved, especially in the setting of traumatic brain or chest injury. In these instances, the approach of damage control orthopedics (DCO) is put to use [7]. General trauma and orthopedic surgeons have adapted the basic concepts of damage control, which was a method initially utilized by the United States Navy, and applied it as a method used to manage patients in the acute care setting. DCO involves the initial stabilization of "major orthopedic injuries to stop the cycle of ongoing musculoskeletal injury and to control hemorrhage" primarily with the use of external fixation ([7], p. 543). External fixators are particularly appealing for use in polytrauma patients with orthopedic injuries requiring rapid stabilization as the application of this device is minimally invasive, can be applied rapidly (often in the intensive care unit in the severely injured patient), and results in minimal blood loss [8].

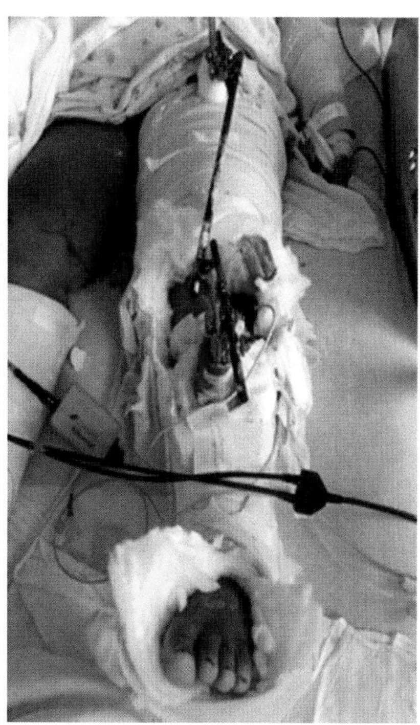

Fig. 38.22 Proximal tibia fracture treated definitively in an external fixator due to comminution and severe soft tissue injury

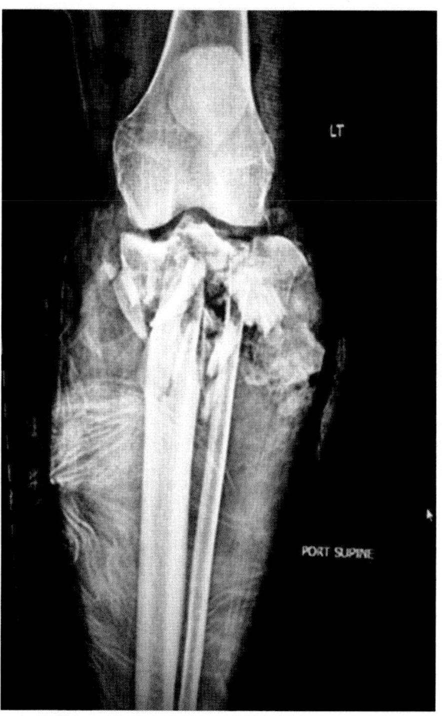

Fig. 38.21 Radiograph of severely comminuted proximal tibia and fibula fracture

When indicated, external fixators can be used to treat essentially every type of fracture. The most common fracture patterns this device is used on include intra-articular fractures of the distal and proximal tibia, severely comminuted long bone fractures, unstable knee dislocations, intra-articular distal femur fractures, unstable pelvic ring injuries, and complex intra-articular fractures involving the wrist and elbow.

External fixators are also used for fractures with associated soft tissue injuries, including open fractures with complex, contaminated wounds, and for closed fractures with significant soft tissue swelling or tissue compromise. The zone of injury not only pertains to the fracture itself but also to the surrounding tissues, which must also be considered when determining the appropriate course of treatment. Open fractures are at an increased risk of developing a deeper soft tissue and/or bony infection [1]. In open fractures with severe soft tissue injury or contamination (Figs. 38.23 and 38.24), initial treatment with internal fixation may not be the optimal choice for the patient. The advantage of using external fixators in fractures with associated open wounds is that the fracture can be manipulated and stabilized away from the actual site of injury, minimizing further contamination and trauma to the tissues (Fig. 38.25) [9, 10].

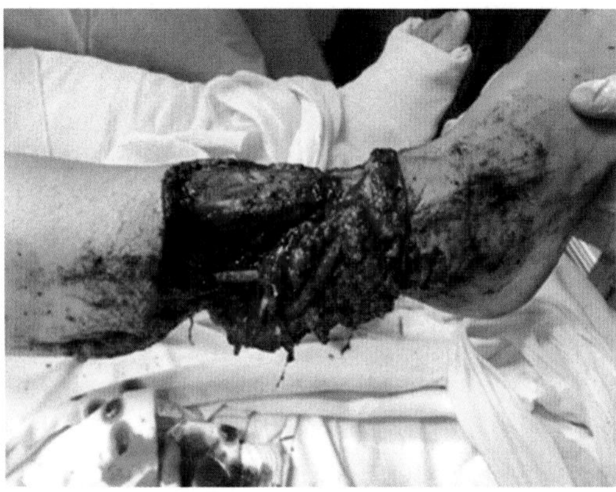

Fig 38.23 Patient with a severe soft tissue injury with gross contamination

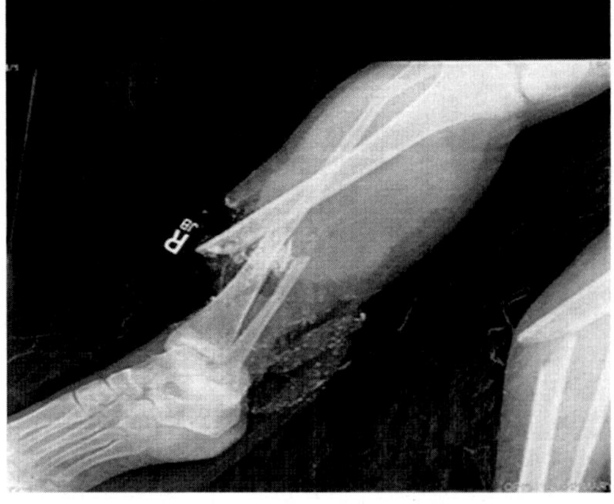

Fig. 38.24 Initial radiographs showing displaced diaphyseal tibia and fibula fractures

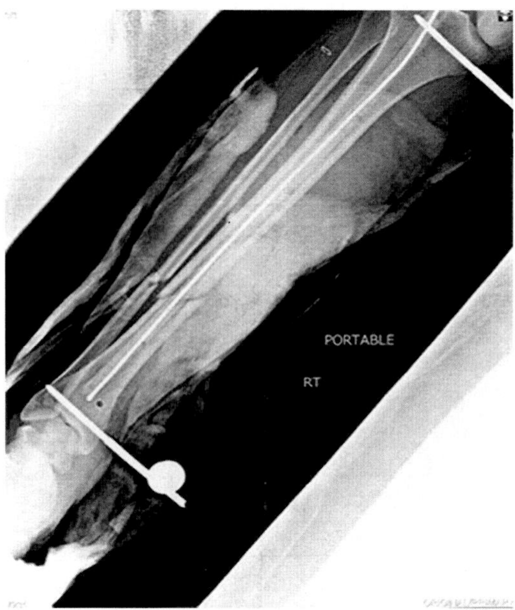

Fig. 38.25 Radiographs showing provisional fixation with external fixator and antibiotic nail

The device also allows the provider and nursing staff easier access to the wounds for assessment and dressing changes.

The orthopedic patient's journey does not end once they are discharged from the acute care setting. Often, in a patient who sustained injury to an extremity that required complex limb salvage, reconstruction is needed to correct the resultant deformity. External fixators can also be utilized to improve angular and rotational deformities associated with fracture malunion and substantial limb length discrepancies that result in cases with significant bone loss (Figs. 38.26 and 38.27; Table 38.1) [8].

38.11 External Fixators: Components and Mechanics

External fixators can be configured in a wide variety of ways to stabilize the fracture while accommodating the patient's associated soft

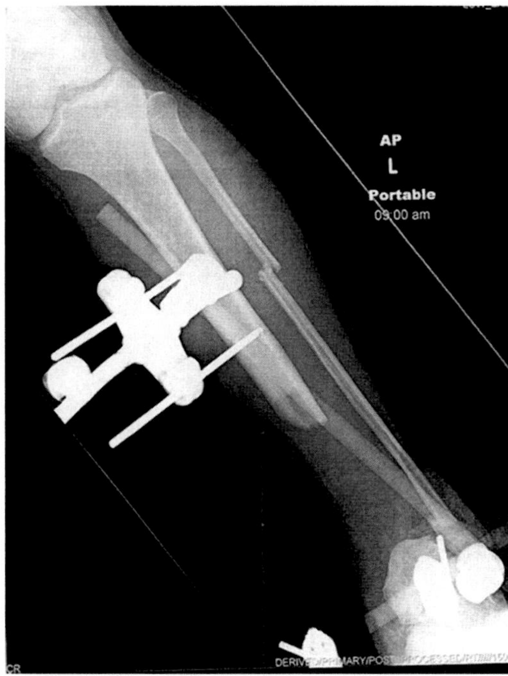

Fig. 38.26 Radiograph demonstrating substantial bone loss from the midshaft of the tibia extending distal to the ankle joint

Table 38.1 Indications for external fixators [8, 10]

• Severely comminuted long bone fractures (e.g., tibial shaft and femur fractures)
• Open fractures with soft tissue injury (Fig. 38.27)
• Complex, intra-articular fractures (e.g., Pilon, tibial plateau, distal femur, distal radius, and distal humerus fractures)
• Unstable pelvic ring injury (e.g., open book pelvis injury)
• Closed fractures with soft tissue injury
• Unstable ligamentous injuries (knee and elbow dislocations)
• Fractures with significant bone loss
• Critically ill patient unable to tolerate operative procedure
• High-risk patient for definitive treatment with internal fixation
• Reconstruction
– Malunion
– Nonunion
– Arthrodesis
– Osteomyelitis
• Deformity correction
– Limb lengthening
– Congenital deformities
– Acquired deformities

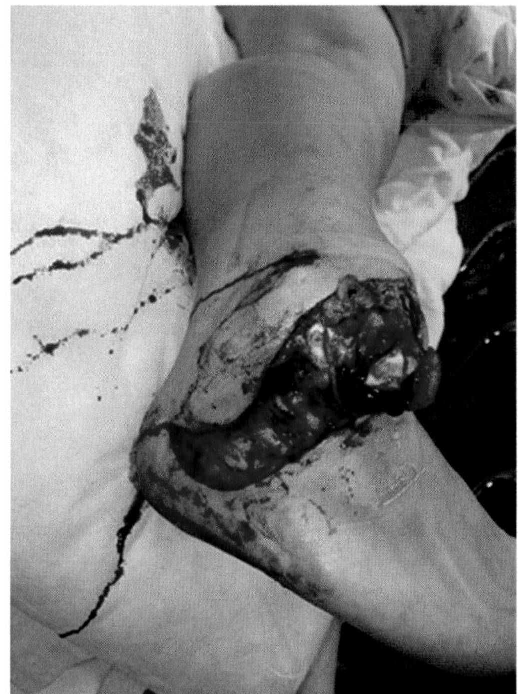

Fig. 38.27 Open fracture with associated soft tissue injury

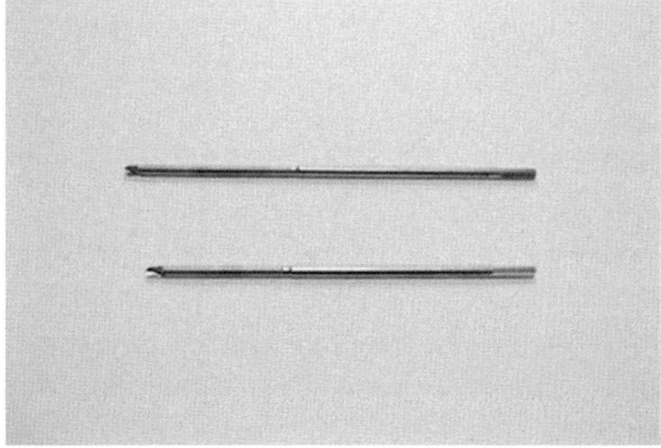

Fig. 38.28 Pins

tissue injuries and body habitus. As external fixators have continued to evolve, the same basic materials are used to build each frame. These devices are constructed using pins or wires (Fig. 38.28), clamps (Fig. 38.29), and bars or rings (Fig. 38.30).

Pins and wires serve to attach the fixator to the bone. There are several different pin types available, including different lengths and

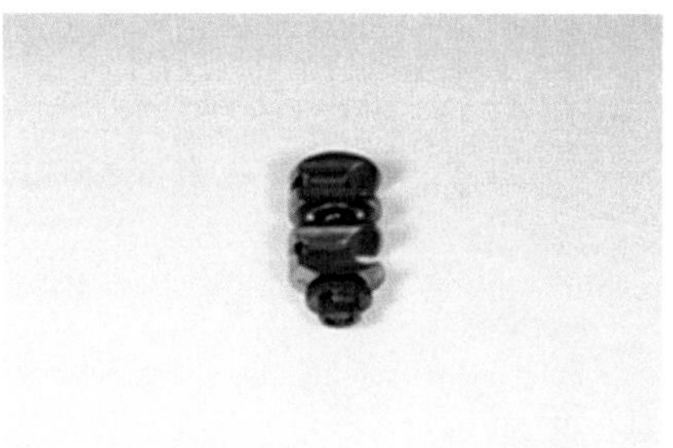
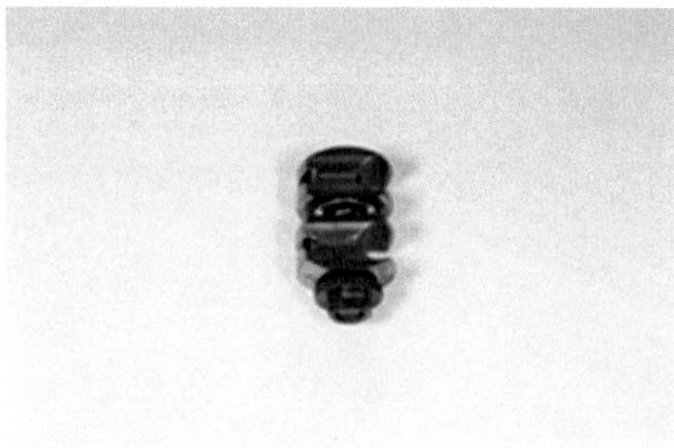

Fig. 38.29 Clamps

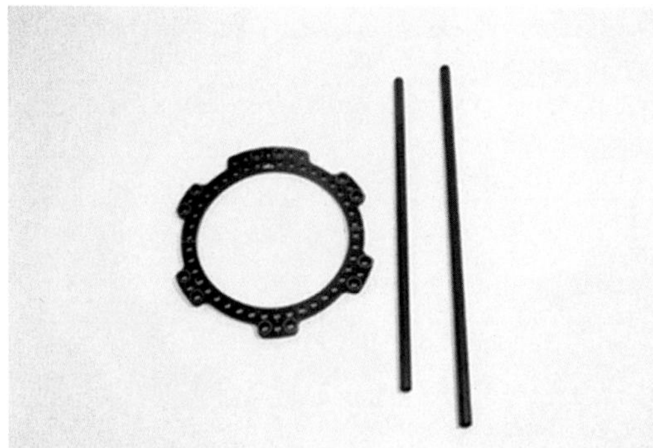

Fig. 38.30 Ring and bars

diameters, threaded or smooth pins, and many offer varying degrees of tapering. Most are made of stainless steel or titanium. The general rule is to select a pin whose diameter is less than 1/3 the diameter of the bone; selecting the appropriate pin diameter helps to decrease the risk of associated pin site fracture [9]. Clamps attach the pins or wires to the rods or rings of the frame. They also can attach two or more rods together, as seen with spanning external fixators. The bars or rings make up the frame itself. Bars span the fracture, stabilizing the proximal and distal fragments.

38.12 Frame Types

There are several different types of external fixation devices, each one able to be tailored to the location of injury, the fracture pattern, and to the patient. Fixators function to stabilize fractures by compression, distraction, or applying neutral forces [9]. The basic types of fixation devices include standard frames, joint spanning and articulated frames, and circular frames. Standard frames are primarily used to treat diaphyseal fractures, or fractures of the long bones, including the tibia, femur, humerus, and forearm, and allow for joint range of motion. Conversely, spanning external fixators are used for intra-articular fractures or in injuries with ligamentous instability, vascular injuries, or severe soft tissue compromise (Fig. 38.31).

With this type of fixation, the affected joints are immobilized to promote stability of the site of injury and surrounding tissues, to facilitate healing. Articulated frames are also utilized in ligamentous injuries, such as knee dislocations, and intra-articular fractures, although they do allow range of motion in the affected joint. These frames are more specialized with more specific indications than other devices. Circular or ring fixators, such as the Ilizarov frame, are used for limb salvage in severe acute injuries to the lower extremity and in cases of limb reconstruction or deformity correction. These frames are usually more complex and utilize rings, bars, struts, and telescoping rods (Figs. 38.32, 38.33, and 38.34) [9].

Struts are used to correct angular deformities, and telescoping rods are used for distraction to repair bone defects or limb length discrepancies. These techniques involve active participation by the patient, as they follow a program to adjust the struts and bone transporters on their own, mainly in the outpatient setting (Fig. 38.35).

As research and technology continues to evolve, the implications for further use of external fixators has become more commonplace in acute care hospitals worldwide.

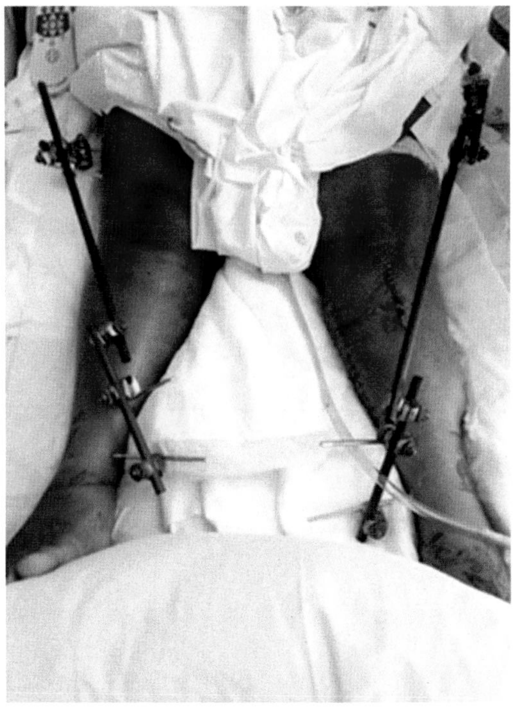

Fig. 38.31 Bilateral spanning external fixators in a polytrauma patient with associated soft tissue and vascular injury

38.13 Advantages

External fixators have become paramount in DCO due to their wide variety of indications, ease of application, and ability to stabilize fractures and soft tissues in the injured extremity. In the critically injured, polytrauma patient, these devices offer a minimally invasive solution to temporarily and effectively manage their orthopedic injuries until definitive treatment is amenable (Fig. 38.36). These devices provide stabilization away from the injury site, minimizing further damage to surrounding neurovascular supply [10].

38.14 Disadvantages

As with any type of fixation, external fixators have several associated risks. One common complication is pin site infections, which range in severity from superficial drainage from the pin tract, surrounding cellulitis, or deeper infections such as osteomyelitis [8]. Pin tracts provide a direct link from the outside environment to the bone and thereby can increase incidence of infections.

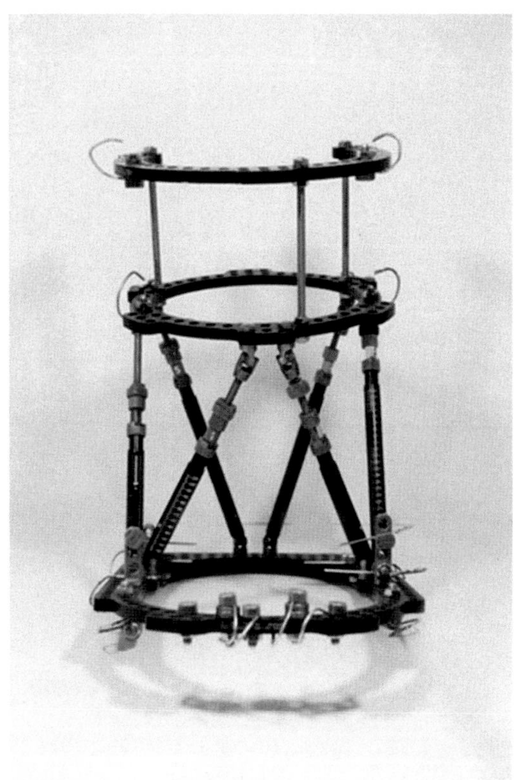

Fig. 38.32 Ring fixator utilizing struts

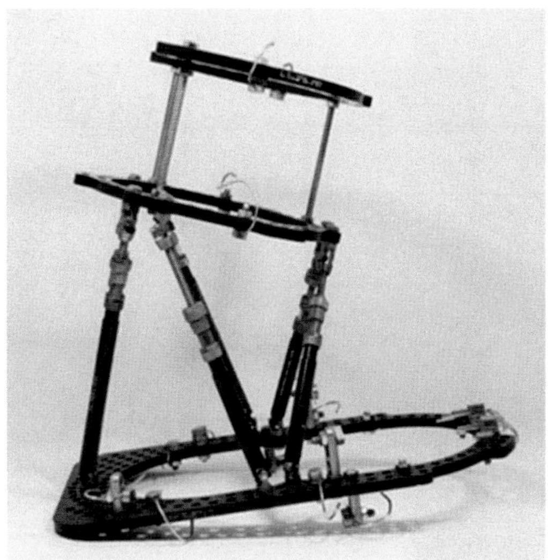

Fig. 38.33 Ring fixator utilizing struts—lateral view

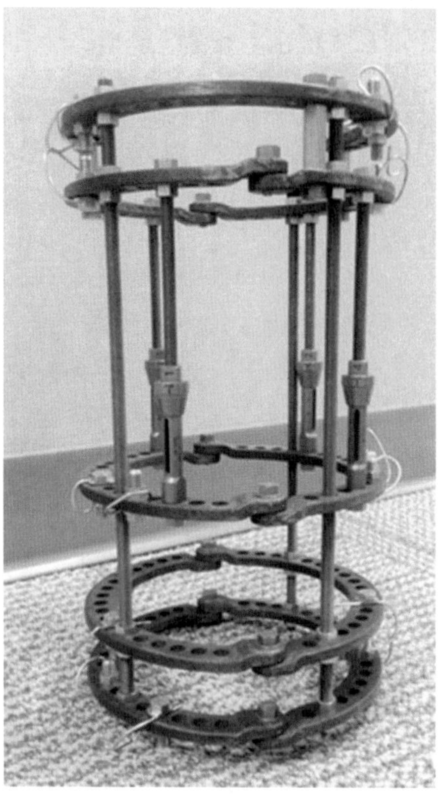

Fig. 38.34 Ring fixator utilizing telescoping rods for distraction

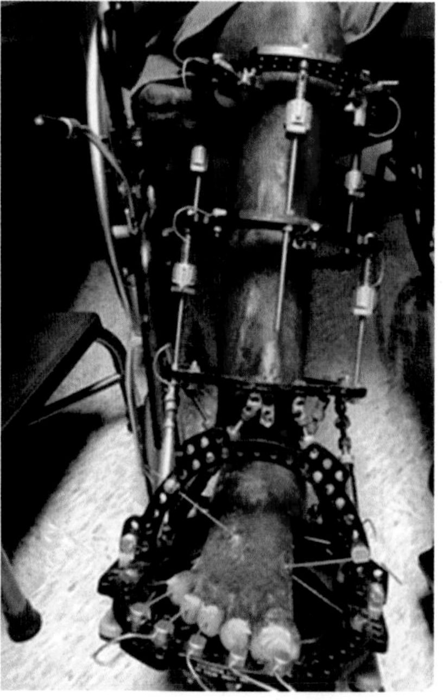

Fig. 38.35 Ring fixator used on a patient with limb length discrepancy as a result of bone loss from a prior trauma

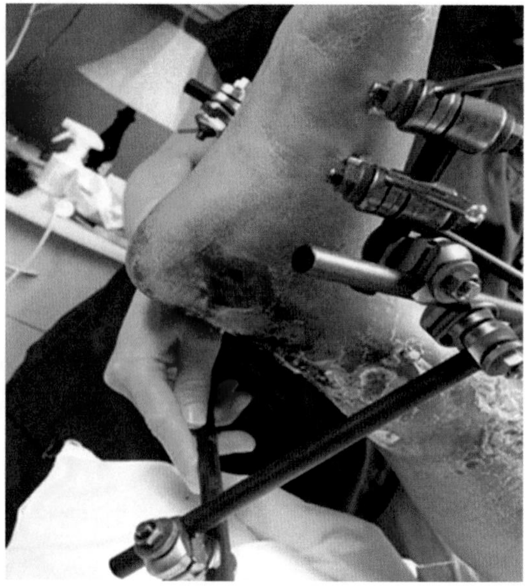

Fig. 38.36 Temporary external fixation due to associated soft tissue injury

Increased tissue mobility around the pin site also increases infection risk [8]. Usually pin site infections are superficial and localized, presenting with erythema around the pin site and purulent drainage. Once identified, early pin tract infections can be easily treated with proper hygiene, a short course of antibiotics, or removal of the pin or wire involved [8]. If the soft tissues are irritated due to increased mobility, wrapping a dressing around the pin site will help decrease tissue motion [8]. In cases where pin site infections track deeper into the bone, formal debridement or curettage of the pin site is often required coupled with antibiotic therapy [8]. If untreated, superficial pin site infections can progress to osteomyelitis. Early identification of pin tract infections is critical to minimizing further progression and long-term complications. Educating the patient, their families and caretakers, and clinical staff on the signs of potential pin site infection is important once discharged from the acute care setting. It is crucial to educate the patient and their families that keeping the pin sites clean and dry and minimizing tissue mobility, along with daily showers, are imperative to preventing pin site infections [8]. Institutions vary on specific methods of daily pin site care, but good basic hygiene is the underlying goal. Patients are encouraged to shower daily and

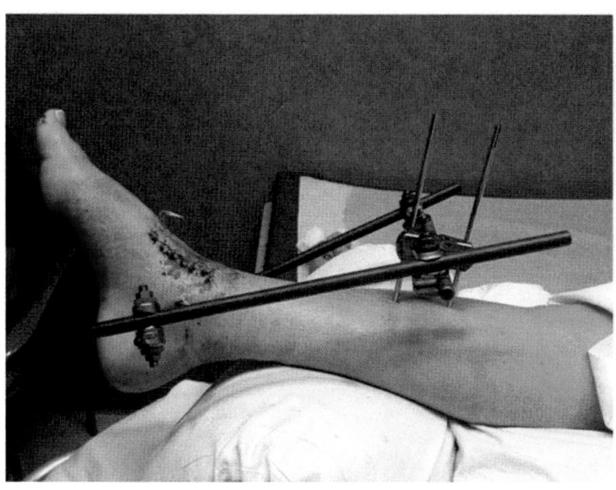

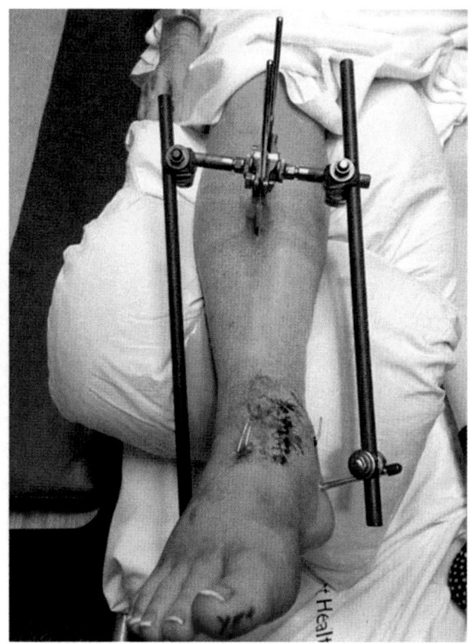

Fig. 38.37 Definitive treatment of a distal tibia intraarticular fracture using external fixation

Table 38.2 External fixation: advantages and disadvantages [5, 8]

Advantages	Disadvantages
• Wide variety of indications	• Pin tract infections
• Versatile	– Superficial → Osteomyelitis
• Minimally invasive	• Delayed union/ nonunion
• Rapid application	• Malunion
• Use in critically ill and polytrauma patients	• Injury to nerves/ vessels
• Can be temporary or definitive (Fig. 38.37)	• Failure of fixation
• Stable (depending on the construct)	• Joint stiffness, contractures
• Stabilize away from zone of injury	• Compartment syndrome
• Able to use with soft tissue defects or in the setting of infection	

cleanse both the affected extremity and the device with warm soapy water (Table 38.2).

While the relative stability of these devices is advantageous, if the construct is too rigid, the risk on fracture nonunion occurs. Bony callus is stimulated by micromotion at the fracture site. Without localized motion, callus formation is impaired and the fracture does not heal causing delayed or nonunion ([5], p. 130). Additional potential complications include fracture malunion, joint stiffness, injuries to surrounding nerves and vasculature, compartment syndrome, and hardware failure [8, 11].

References

1. Koval KJ, Zuckerman JD. Handbook of fractures. 3rd ed. Philadelphia: Lippincott Williams & Wilkins; 2006.
2. Wheeless, CR. Wheeless' textbook of orthopaedics: femoral and tibial traction pins. [Date of last update 18 Sept 2014]. http://www.wheelessonline.com/ortho/femoral_and_tibial_traction_pins.
3. Demmer P. AO handbook—nonoperative fracture treatment. Femoral shaft fractures—management with minimal resources. 2013. www.aosurgery.org.
4. Hessman M, Nork S, Sommer C, Twaddle B. AO surgery reference: traction (initial provisional stabilization). https://www2.aofoundation.org/wps/portal/surgery?showPage=redfix&bone=Tibia&segment=Distal&classification=43-C1&treatment=&method=Traction%20-%20(initial%20provisional%20stabilization)&implantstype

=&approach=&redfix_url=1285238987367&Language=en. Accessed 3 Dec 2008.
5. Dandy DJ, Edwards DJ. Methods of managing trauma. In: Essential orthopaedics and trauma. 4th ed. Philadelphia: Elsevier Science; 2003.
6. Florian G, Kregor P, Oliver C. AO surgery reference: temporary skeletal traction. https://www2.aofoundation.org/wps/portal/surgery?showPage=redfix&bone=Femur&segment=Distal&classification=33-C1&treatment=&method=Provisional%20treatment&implantstype=Temporary%20skeletal%20traction&approach=&redfix_url=1285238416489&Language=en. Accessed 3 Dec 2008.
7. Pape H-C, Tornetta P, Tarkin I, Tzioupis C, Sabeson V, Olson SA. Timing of fracture fixation in multitrauma patients: the role of early total care and damage control surgery. J Am Acad Orthop Surg. 2009;17(9):541–49.
8. Buccholz RW, Heckman JD, Court-Brown C, Koval KJ, Tornetta P, Wirth MA, editors. Rockwood and Green's fractures in adults. 6th ed. Philadelphia: Lippincott Williams & Wilkins; 2006. p. 257–95; 567–70.
9. Moss DP, Tejwani N. Biomechanics of external fixation: a review of literature. Bull NYU Hosp JT Dis. 2007;65(4):294–9.
10. Burgess AR, Poka A, Browner BD, First KR. Skeletal trauma: fractures, dislocations, ligamentous injuries. In: Principles of external fixation. Vol. 1. Philadelphia: W.B. Saunders Company; 1992.
11. Green SA. Browner: skeletal trauma. In: Principles and complications of external fixation. 4th ed. Philadelphia: W.B. Saunders Company; 2008.

39 Measurement of Compartment Syndrome

Dave Sander and Wayne Weil

39.1 Introduction

The procedure to check compartment pressures is relatively simple and is a quick way to ascertain if further workup may be needed. The reliability of the measurement can vary depending on the experience of the operator, so familiarity with your department's equipment is essential. In the lower leg, there are four compartments that may be at risk. Many texts advocate checking all four compartments for documentation purposes; however, a positive result in one or two compartments is a sufficient evidence to justify surgical intervention in the form of a fasciotomy.

The cause of compartment syndrome is often due to a posttraumatic event such as an acute crush injury or fracture or postoperative swelling, but it can be seen in other instances as well. These include chronic exertional compartment syndrome, chronic myeloid leukemia in children [1], abdominal compartment syndrome after a hip arthroscopy [2], burns and some bleeding disorders or medications, as well as bandages or casts that are too tight. Gunshot wounds have also been shown to be a relatively common cause of this condition in both the upper and lower extremities [3]. To be sure, many of these are quite rare, but in the critical care setting, it is important to recognize the signs and symptoms of the condition in order to treat a potentially rapidly developing problem.

Chronic exertional compartment syndrome is seen more often in athletes today and can be a long-term, recurring issue [4]. Upper extremity compartment syndrome, which is also quite rare, has been seen more often with the increase in popularity of Crossfit-type activities [5]. It can also be seen in motocross racers and in the intensive care setting from infiltrated intravenous lines or from radial arterial lines. Also, in the ICU setting, traction has been shown to cause lower extremity compartment syndrome after acute tibial fracture [3]. Traction causes the fascia to tighten, lowering the compartment volume. You can see how troublesome this would be in a patient that already has lower compartment volume due to traumatic swelling.

39.2 Indications for Measurement

Compartment syndrome is an expansion-type injury within a closed space that does not allow for that expansion. If untreated this will result in compromised tissue perfusion and could lead to permanent damage to the nerve and muscular structures underneath [6]. The lower leg is the

D. Sander, EMT-P, MPAS, PA-C (✉) • W. Weil, MD
Orthopedic Specialists of Seattle,
5350 Tallman Ave #500, Seattle, WA 98117, USA
e-mail: dsanderpac@gmail.com; d.sander@proliancesurgeons.com; w.weil@proliancesurgeons.com

D.A. Taylor et al. (eds.), *Interventional Critical Care*, DOI 10.1007/978-3-319-25286-5_39

most common and will be discussed here, but other sites include the hands, feet, forearm, thighs, buttocks, and abdominal cavity [7, 8]. The classic signs and symptoms of a patient who develops compartment syndrome include a fairly recent injury as described above, pain out of proportion to the findings on exam, increasing need for pain medicine, and pain on passive stretch on exam. Paresthesias may also be an early sign. The other classic symptoms are pulselessness, pallor, and poikilothermia; however, these are all late signs and irreversible damage may have already occurred. These symptoms are classically known as the "5 Ps" of compartment syndrome. In acute injury, the onset of symptoms can happen within 4–10 h but have been seen occurring as late as a week after the injury. In the obtunded patient, clinical suspicion should be high in extremities that demonstrate any of the "5 Ps" with an appropriate antecedent history. Chronic conditions causing compartment syndrome can cause symptoms for years before a patient seeks treatment [4].

39.3 Contraindications

There are no absolute contraindications in compartment syndrome measurement. It is recommended to avoid areas of open wounds and cellulitis on the overlying skin. As with all invasive procedures, there is a small risk of infection that can usually be negated by using proper technique. Due to the devastating sequelae of untreated compartment syndrome, practitioners should have a very low threshold to measure compartment pressures if there is suspicion of an emerging compartment syndrome.

39.4 Preparation

There are many measurement kits on the market. All work in largely the same way and use similar technique. Familiarize yourself with the specific kit used at your facility prior to attempting this procedure. The compression syndrome kit should be well located and within easy reach (Fig. 39.1).

The Stryker kit is the most common kit used to check for compartment syndrome. It includes the measuring device, the side-ported, noncoring needle, diaphragm compression chamber with one-way valve, and sterile saline come prepackaged together (Figs. 39.2, 39.3, and 39.4).

The monitor itself is not sterile, but the needle and fluid pathway are. The provider should always use sterile technique and keep the area of skin penetration as sterile as possible. The com-

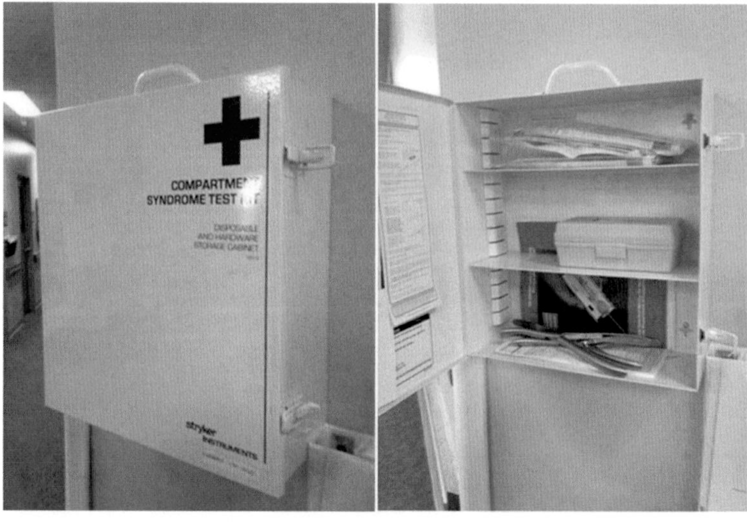

Fig. 39.1 An example of a compression syndrome kit station

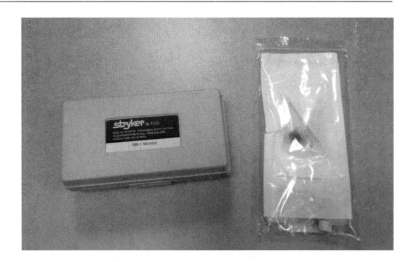

Fig. 39.2 The Stryker kit

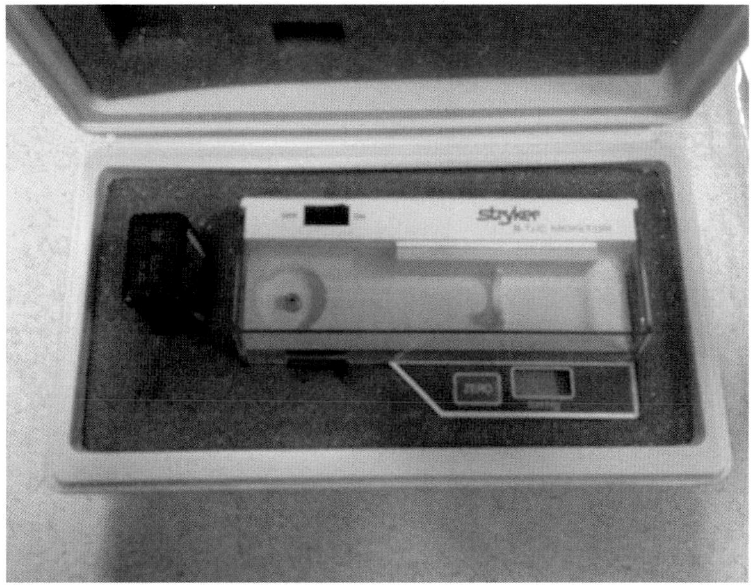

Fig. 39.3 The Stryker monitor and spare battery

pleted kit should be opened and assembled as per the instructions of the kit (Figs. 39.5 and 39.6). It is also important to always remember to zero out the monitor prior to use (Fig. 39.7).

39.4.1 Procedure: Patient Position and Comfort

Most patients are already quite uncomfortable when they present with the signs or symptoms of compartment syndrome. Pain levels can range from moderately uncomfortable to excruciating. Advancing a large needle into an area that is already very painful will only serve to increase their pain. Prior to the procedure, the site should be prepped with chlorhexidine or iodine (Fig. 39.8). Whenever possible, it is wise to anesthetize the area with a local anesthetic. 1–2 cc of 1 % lidocaine plain should be sufficient. Take care to stay in the superficial layers of the skin as deep infiltration may raise intracompartmental pressures, skewing the results. The patient's leg should be elevated off the table so that the pressure from

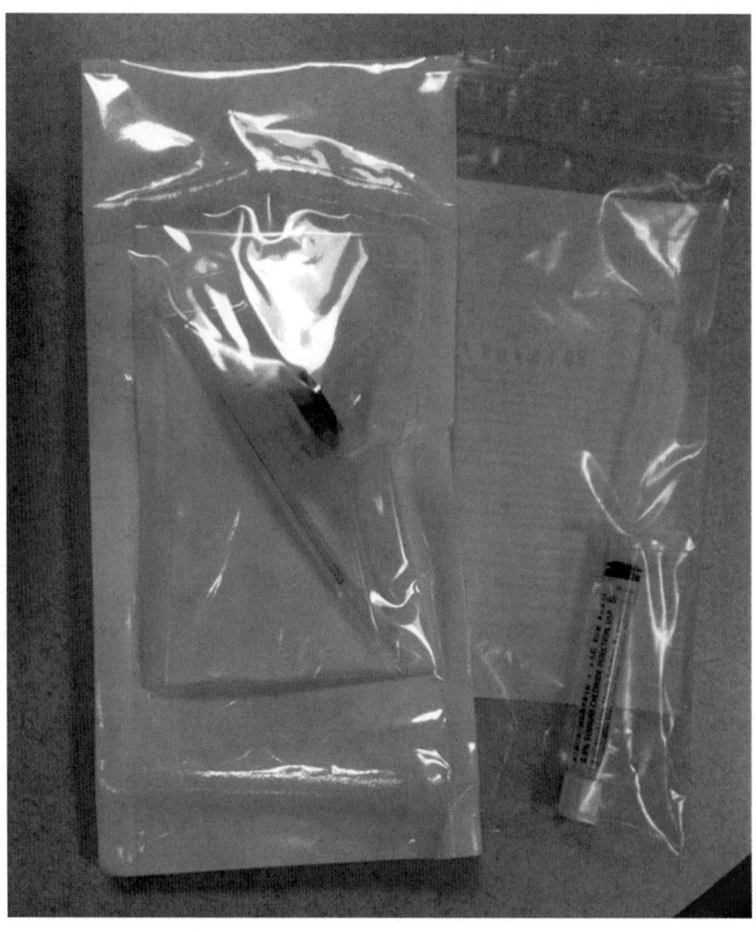

Fig. 39.4 Diaphragm chamber, needle, and prefilled syringe

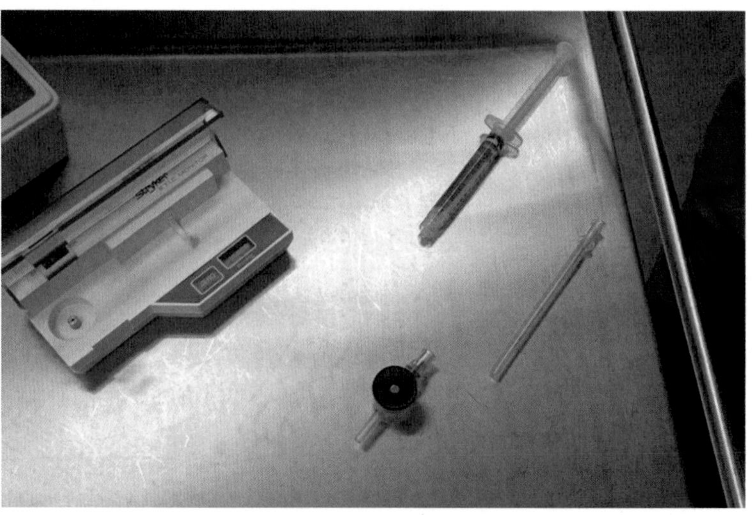

Fig. 39.5 Preassembly

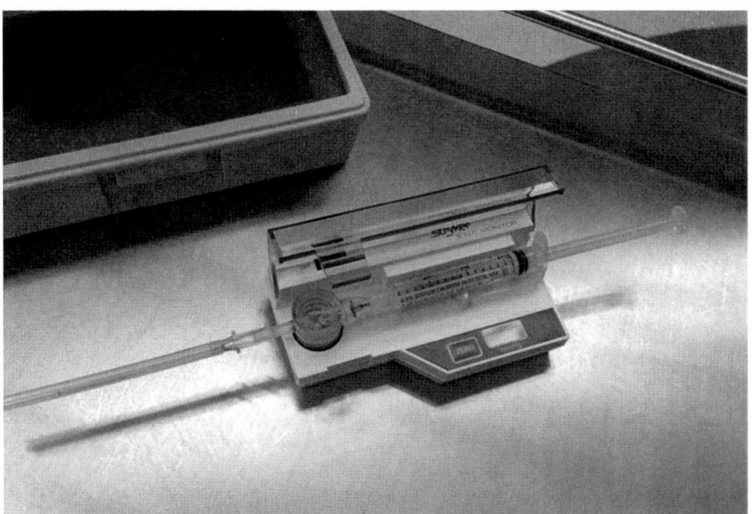

Fig. 39.6 The assembled Stryker monitor

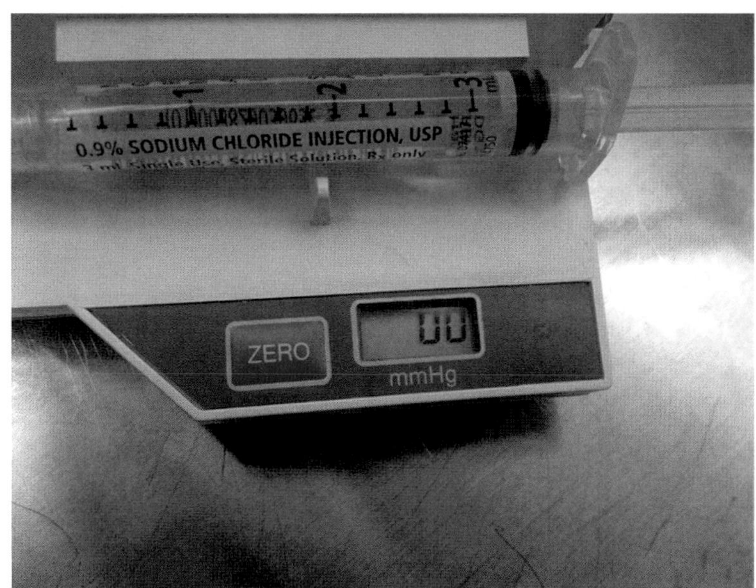

Fig. 39.7 Zeroing the monitor

the leg lying on the table does not contribute to a falsely elevated pressure measurement. This is especially important with the reading being borderline positive.

39.4.2 Site Selection and Prep

There are four main compartments in the lower leg that need to be considered when symptoms appear: the anterior compartment, lateral compartment, and deep and superficial posterior compartments (Fig. 39.9).

For entry into the anterior compartment (Fig. 39.10) or any compartment, the needle should enter the skin in a position that is nearly perpendicular to the compartment being tested. The extremity being tested should also be at the level of the heart whenever possible [8].

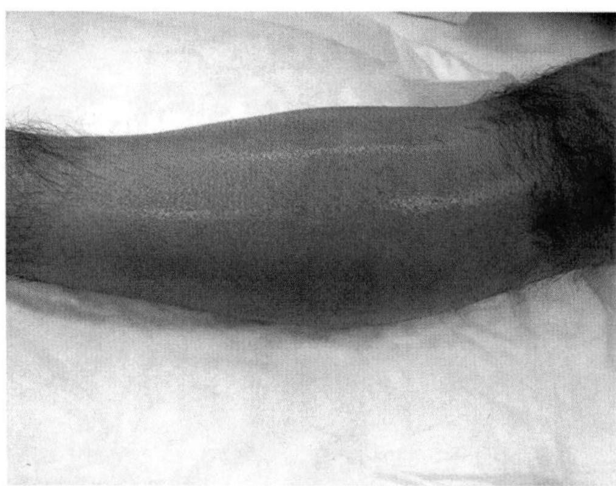

Fig. 39.8 Perping the insertion site. *Note*: This patient's leg had already been prepared for surgery. Shaving of hair is not necessary for a rapid measurement of compartment syndrome

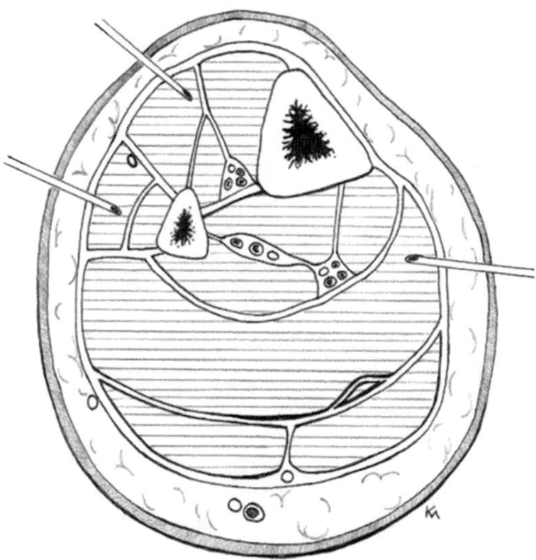

Fig. 39.9 The compartments. The upper left is the anterior compartment, and the lower left is the lateral compartment; the right shows access to the deep and the superficial posterior compartment

Pierce the skin until you feel the needle goes through the facial layer, usually 1–3 cm [8] (Fig. 39.11). Hold the monitor still and inject a small amount of saline. Usually 0.2–0.3 ml of saline is enough.

Entry to the lateral compartment is below the entry site of the anterior compartment. Note the position of the previous anterior compartment in Fig. 39.12.

From the approach in the previous figure, it is possible to reach the deep and superficial compartments (Fig. 39.13).

The criterion for a positive result in compartment syndrome measurement varies by source. In fact, animal models have shown sufficient perfusion with an absolute pressure of 59 mmHg [9]. The three most common criteria used are an absolute measurement of 30 or above, the perfusion pressure method, or an intracompartmental pressure within 20 mmHg below the diastolic pressure [8] (Fig. 39.14). The perfusion pressure method is the patient's current diastolic blood pressure minus the intramuscular pressure. For the perfusion pressure method, a value less than 30 mmHg is considered a positive result [7].

If one or all of the compartments come back with a positive result, the provider should arrange for an urgent fasciotomy. This is usually done in an Operating Room (OR) setting but can be done sterilely at bedside in remote or austere conditions with the proper equipment, medications, and training. While discussion of the technique of fasciotomy is not within the scope of this chapter, it is important to remember the importance of achieving at least 90 % release of the compartments if a fasciotomy is to be done [10].

39.5 Complications

Complications of this procedure are exceedingly rare. The most common reason for getting an inaccurate result is due to misuse or lack of familiarity with the equipment.

39.6 Pearls

Depressing the plunger too quickly and obstructing the needle with tissue after pulling the syringe back can cause falsely elevated

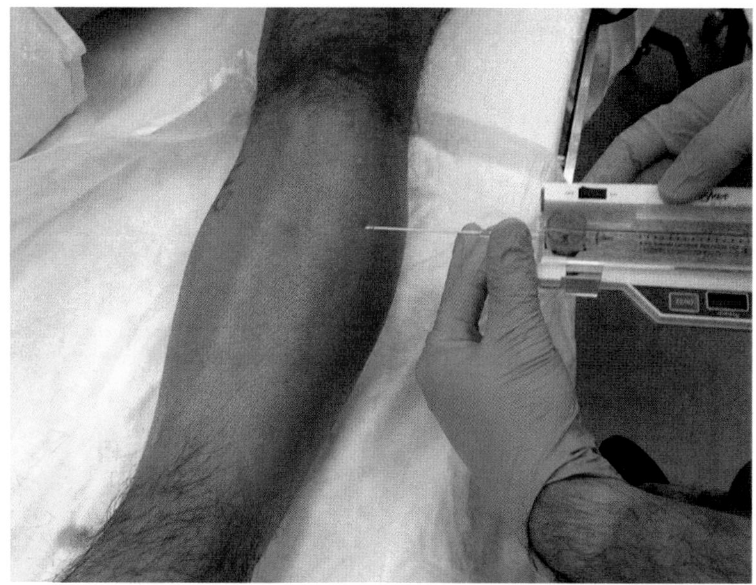

Fig. 39.10 Entry into the anterior compartment

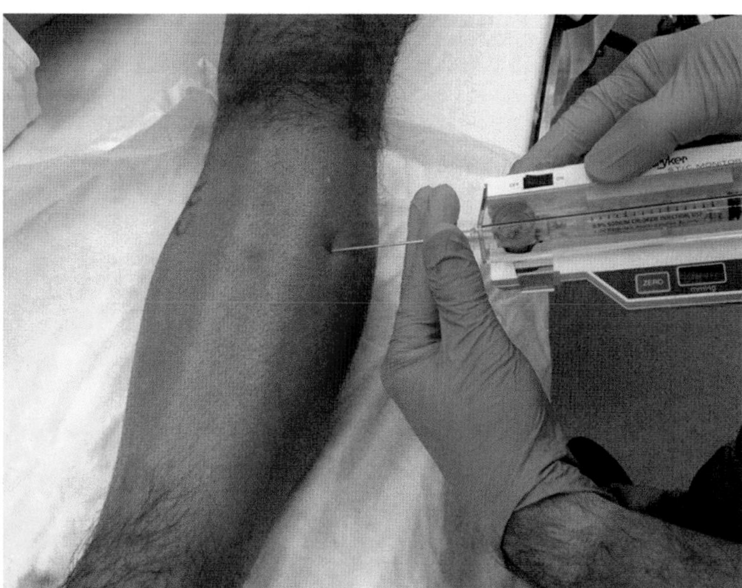

Fig. 39.11 Insertion into the skin

results [8]. In all cases, clinical exam must trump the measurement in cases where, even though the result was not positive, the patient's symptoms are consistent with compartment syndrome.

39.7 Conclusion

Compartment syndrome is a rare condition but must be evaluated quickly when symptoms present. This article has shown a reliable method in

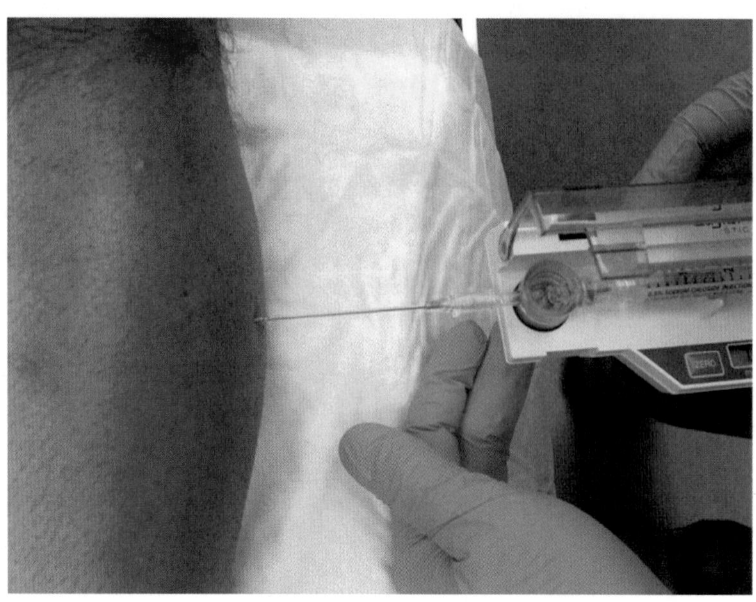

Fig. 39.12 Entry into the lateral compartment

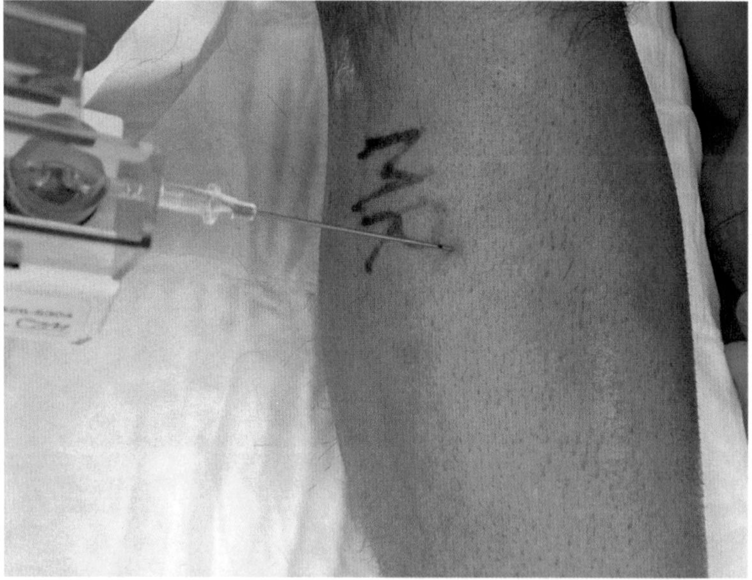

Fig. 39.13 Deep and superficial site entry

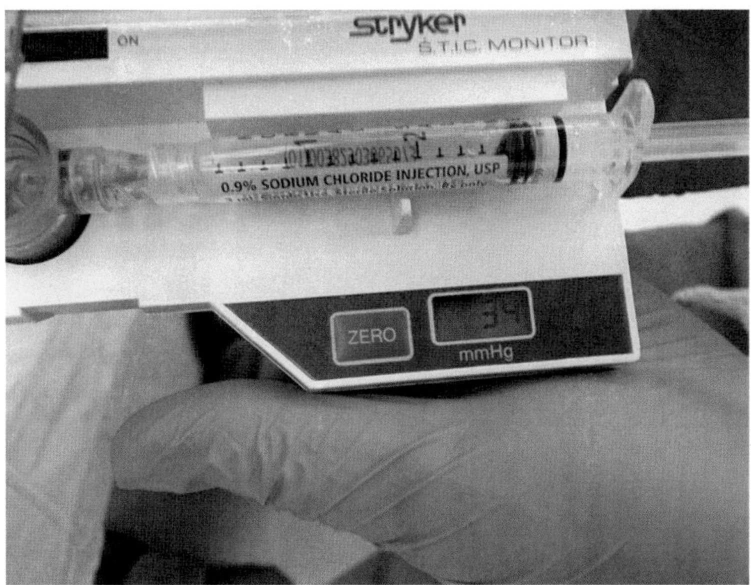

Fig. 39.14 Example of a positive test result using the absolute method

which to check compartment pressures using a common device. The procedure is quite safe and, with practice, very reliable.

References

1. Cohen E, Truntzer J, Klinge S, Schwartz K, Schiller J. Acute pediatric leg compartment syndrome in chronic myeloid leukemia. Orthopedics. 2014;37:e1036–9.
2. Ciemniewska-Gorzela K, Piontek T, Szulc A. Abdominal compartment syndrome—the prevention and treatment of possible lethal complications following hip arthroscopy: a case report. J Med Case Rep. 2014;8:368.
3. Olson S, Glasgow R. Acute compartment syndrome in lower extremity trauma. J Am Acad Orthop Surg. 2005;13:436–44.
4. Bhalla MC, Dick-Perez R. Exercise induced rhabdomyolysis with compartment syndrome and renal failure. Case Rep Emerg Med. 2014. http://www.hindawi.com/journals/criem/2014/735820
5. Robertson E. Crossfit's dirty little secret. Huffington Post. 28 May 2014.
6. Matsen FA. Compartmental syndromes. New York: Grune & Stratton; 1980.
7. Garner MR, Taylor SA, Gausden E, Lyden JP. Compartment syndrome: diagnosis, management and unique concerns in the twenty-first century. Hosp Spec Surg J. 2014;10:143–52.
8. Jagminas L. Compartment pressure measurement. Medscape Online. 13 May 2014.
9. Matava MJ, Whitesides Jr TE, Seiler 3rd JG, Hewan-Lowe K, Hutton WC. Determination of the compartment pressure threshold of muscle ischemia in a canine model. J Trauma. 1994;1:50–8.
10. Mathis JE, Schwartz BE, Lester JD, Kim WJ, Watson JN, Hutchinson MR. Effect of lower extremity fasciotomy length on intracompartmental pressure in an animal model of compartment syndrome: the importance of achieving a minimum of 90% fascial release. Am J Sports Med. 2015;43:75–8.

Fasciotomies

40

Daniel Geersen

40.1 Introduction

The use of fasciotomy for compartment syndrome has been described in countless articles and chapters as the only reliable method for treatment of acute compartment syndrome. In 1881, Volkmann described the relationship between ischemic events and late muscle contractures [1]. Dr. Paul Jepson demonstrated ischemic contracture in animals and that this may be prevented by prompt surgical decompression in 1924 [2].

Acute compartment syndrome is a surgical emergency and is defined as an elevation of the interstitial pressure in a closed osteofascial compartment that results in the decline in perfusion to the tissues of that compartment and eventual necrosis [3, 4]. This can result from blunt, crush, or penetrating trauma, exercise, reperfusion, prolonged immobilization, hematoma, intra-arterial injection, or massive fluid resuscitation.

The compartment's pressure can increase due to enlargement of the tissues within the compartment, such as reperfusion, or constriction of the compartments as in casting the limb. In reality it can take little pressure to make this happen. Hartsock et al. found a reduction in capillary inflow occurs at about 25 mmHg in rat models [5]. Most literature describes necessity to perform a release when the pressure exceeds 30 mmHg [6]. While normal pressures are about 10 mmHg, no definitive pressure measurement has been identified.

Irreversible damage has been described to be dependent upon perfusion pressure, more specifically when compartment pressures reach within 10–30 mmHg of the patient's diastolic pressure [7]. Two additional studies validated this pressure to be 30 mmHg with no missed cases including "unnecessary fasciotomies or significant complications" of acute compartment syndrome [3, 8, 9].

The diagnosis of acute compartment syndrome has been classically described as the five Ps: pain, pallor, pulselessness, paralysis, and paresthesia. The pain may be deep, burning, and constant. The patient often does not want to touch or move the limb.

Indications for fasciotomy have been described with clinical symptoms and signs of "pain out of proportion to palpation," passive stretch of the compartment's muscles, and increased narcotic demand with tense swelling and paresthesia. In all honesty, if the limb has loss of sensation or pulses, the critical point of recognition has already lapsed.

Flynn et al. looked at acute traumatic compartment syndrome in the pediatric population in two large tertiary care centers and noted that the average

D. Geersen, MPAP, PA-C (✉)
Division Vascular Surgery, Duke University Medical Center, Durham, NC, USA
e-mail: Daniel.geersen@duke.edu

D.A. Taylor et al. (eds.), *Interventional Critical Care*, DOI 10.1007/978-3-319-25286-5_40

time from injury to fasciotomy was 20.5 h. This raises the concern of proper diagnosis early and that speedy intervention occurs. Time delays can be seen across varying institutions [10].

If the clinical diagnosis can be made, then surgical intervention should be performed expeditiously. If there is still doubt, pressures can be taken. A transducer is connected to a catheter and inserted into the muscle bed via aseptic technique. There are several pressure measurement devices available. The more common devices are the Stryker Intracompartmental Pressure Monitor System, arterial line manometer, and Whitesides apparatus. These were all tested by Boody et al. with straight needle, side-port needles, and slit catheters. Their findings were that the arterial line manometer with a slit catheter showed the best correlation, while the Whitesides apparatus with the side-port needle showed the worse results. Overall the side port needles and slit catheters were more accurate than straight needles and that the arterial line manometer was the most accurate device with the Stryker being very accurate as well [11].

40.2 Treatment

Although definitive treatment is compartment release with fasciotomy, there are some conservative measures that can be performed. These include identifying and removing any constrictive dressings, devices, and other compressive items to expose the skin of the affected limb [3].

Further the limb should be level with the heart and not elevated. Elevation may decrease perfusion to the tissues although this is counterintuitive, with most cases of edema [12].

Further, the patient must be assessed for hypovolemia, metabolic acidosis, and myoglobinemia. This is most important to reduce the incidence of renal failure. Intravenous fluids should be given and regular labs drawn and monitored. The patient should maintain normotension, again for reducing the rate of hypoperfusion [3].

Medicinal management is uncommon. There was a case study for mannitol treatment in the setting of acute compartment syndrome, but this was in the setting of heat stroke and dehydration [13]. Trauma or prolonged ischemia requires surgical intervention.

The team must also be prepared for "crush syndrome" and its associated renal injury from myoglobinuria. Crush syndrome, also known as traumatic rhabdomyolysis, was first described by British doctor Eric Bywaters during the London Blitz [14]. When encountering thigh compartment syndrome, the mechanism of injury often leads to this condition.

When a fasciotomy is performed, it requires an adequate incision and facial release. Minimally invasive exposures should only be done by extremely knowledgeable staff as the full length of the fascia can be missed with the longitudinal incisions. All compartments must be released with preservation of vital structures, and a through debridement must be undertaken at the time of initial intervention and with subsequent debridements.

Remember to be liberal in obtaining consults from vascular, orthopedic, and plastic surgery when seeing these patients. Many times these are complex cases, and any fasciotomies undertaken must be performed with adequate supervision. Hand, foot, and buttock fasciotomies will not be discussed in detail due to their distinct specialization and need for expert intervention.

Fasciotomies are not performed when the extremity is nonviable from prolonged tissue ischemia, the patient is too unstable to tolerate intervention primarily from unstable hypoperfusion, and there is a large crush injury involving large portions of the tissue groups.

A clinically cold extremity with muscle rigor, complete neurological loss, and absent inflow by Doppler is known as grade 3 ischemia. This is irreversible and is generally contraindicated for reperfusion or other limb salvage.

40.3 Lower Extremity

If only one compartment is affected, it can be treated with a single incision and release. This is not recommended as most cases involve a greater cross section. In cases with arterial compromise and trauma, decompression of all major compartments must be pursued.

There was debate of a single- vs. double-incision fasciotomy in the 1970s. In World War II, two incision fasciotomies were standard of care [14]. In 1967 a fibulectomy through a single incision was advocated. The concern was that two incision fasciotomies neglected to fully decompress the deep posterior compartment [15]. This is no longer advocated due to risk of damage to the peroneal artery and nerve [16].

It was Murbarak and Owen who championed the double-incision fasciotomy and showed its effectiveness and advantages over fibulectomy [17]. It is recommended by the British Orthopaedic Association and British Association of Plastic, Reconstructive and Aesthetic Surgeons [3].
In the calf there are four anatomical compartments:

1. Anterior compartment: the tibialis anterior, extensor digitorum longus, extensor hallucis longus, and peroneus tertius with the anterior tibial artery and deep peroneal nerve.
2. Lateral compartment: the peroneus longus and brevis with peroneal nerve branches from the anterior compartment.
3. Posterior superficial compartment: the gastrosoleus complex with tibial nerve branches and arterial flow provided by the popliteal artery and posterior tibial and peroneal arteries.
4. Posterior deep compartment: the tibialis posterior, flexor hallucis longus, and flexor digitorum longus with the tibial nerve and posterior tibial and peroneal artery blood supply.

Two incisions are made, one medially and the other laterally. Each measures about 15 cm in length. A scalpel with electrocaudery can make the initial incision and dissection. The facial tissue should be cut with smooth-ended scissors like a Metzenbaum. The scissors should be angled slightly away from the muscle as not to bury the cutting edge into the tissue and inadvertently causing injury. Without moving the handles, the instrument can be pushed along the length of the incision from proximal to distal. This is similar to opening a cardboard box or cutting a wrapping paper. The medial incision is made about 2 cm medial to the tibial margin in a similar location to popliteal artery exposure. The length of the incision is dependent upon the extent of muscle protrusion/edema. However, this cannot be the sole judge as with revascularization procedures the edema may increase throughout the immediate postoperative period. The saphenous vein and nerve should be identified and injury be avoided. The superficial posterior compartment is opened by releasing the gastrocnemius fascia in a longitudinal fashion from proximal to distal. The deep posterior compartment is decompressed by dividing the attachments of the soleus muscle from the tibia.

The lateral incision is set between the shaft of the fibula and the crest of the tibia. The incision then is made over the intramuscular septum of the anterior and lateral compartments. The septum is palpable and feels like a dimpling of the tissue between the two muscle groups. The anterior compartment is decompressed and then the lateral fascia. The most common injury is to the common peroneal nerve and superficial peroneal nerve. Having the lateral incision too proximal to the tibial plateau or lateral condyle can injure the common peroneal nerve and, in many patients, the superficial nerve which rests in the septum of the anterior and the lateral intramuscular compartments.
In the thigh there are three compartments:

1. Anterior compartment: the quadriceps
2. Posterior compartment: the hamstrings
3. Medial compartment: the adductor muscles

A single lateral incision is commonly used as the lateral compartment is the one typically involved. Blunt trauma, crush injuries, and femur fracture are the most common causes [3]. A single lateral incision originating just distal from the intertrochanteric line and extending to the lateral epicondyle of the femur. The IT band and fascia of the vastus lateralis are incised the length of the skin incision to decompress the anterior compartment. The posterior compartment is decompressed by reflection of the vastus lateralis muscle medially, incising the intramuscular septum. The medial compartment is decompressed through a second incision overlying the adductor muscle group.

40.4 Upper Extremity

In the forearm there are three compartments:

1. Mobile wad: the brachioradialis, extensor carpi radialis longus, and brevis muscles, with the radial artery and nerve
2. Volar compartment: the superficial and deep flexors, with the ulnar artery and nerve and median nerve
3. Dorsal compartment: the extensor muscles

The radial or ulnar pulses are usually intact as their pressure of 120 mmHg is usually greater than the compartment pressures. This again is an unreliable marker for intervention. Most elevated pressures will be found in the volar compartment. Two separate incisions are often made to decompress the arm. Failure to do so may result in Volkmann's contracture, a permanent flexion of the hand at the wrist with the hand and fingers forming a claw.

Map out the medial aspect. From this position you can address the major nerve structures and expose the vascular beds to repair if necessary. If the clinical situation requires fasciotomy of the upper arm or hand and wrist, this can be taken in the same incision.

Start at the elbow and gently curve in an augmented S shape, the incision extending first out laterally and then coming medial with linear extension to the wrist. This can then join a lazy S of the hand if required and allow you to perform a carpal tunnel release if needed to preserve the median nerve.

From this location, the volar and mobile wad can be released. Using the same technique as described previously, a small incision can be made over the fascia with a snip of the scissors and then slide the cutting blades along the fascia to release. Separate muscle groups may require fasciotomies. Be careful not to injure the radial nerve and artery as you make a skin flap over the wrist. Skin flaps in this location can cover the median nerve and other vascular structures of the carpal tunnel for protection. Often a simple series of cuts can be made to free the tissue laterally and dorsally.

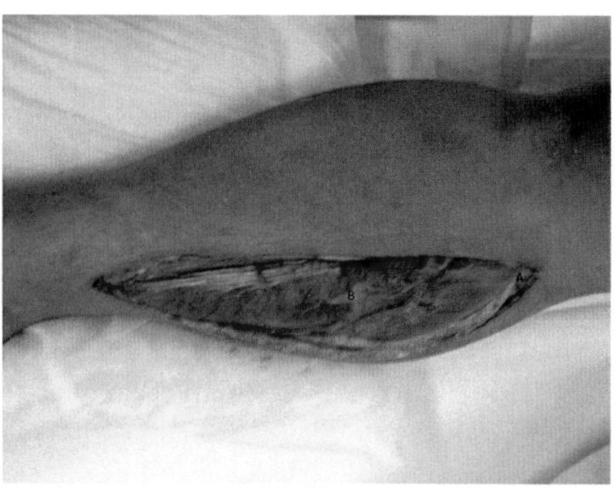

Fig. 40.1 (**a**) The fascial tissue seen cut and separated. (**b**) Muscle edema. Note how the muscle loses its structure once the fascia has been cut away

The dorsal incision is then made. Make sure after release is performed, a manual check confirms the origin and insertion points have been reached and the fascia is completely released (see Fig. 40.1).

40.5 Wound Care

All fasciotomy incisions are left open. Even though there is a movement that advocates fascial incision and then staple closure of the skin, complete tissue edema can take 24–48 h to occur and the muscle may require multiple debridements. It is therefore recommended to leave the wounds packed with sterile gauze or negative pressure dressing.

Bleeding may occur postoperatively and negative dressing pressures should be set with this in mind. 70–90 mmHg rather than 125 mmHg may be employed. Do not place the vac dressing directly on the muscle surface. Apply Vaseline gauze or Adaptic dressing to the tissue before sponge. After 48 h, intermittent suction is thought to promote healing quicker.

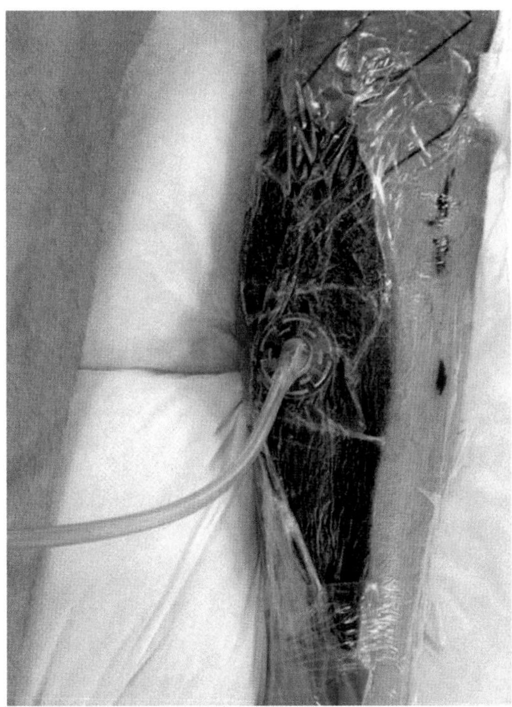

Fig. 40.2 Negative pressure dressing over fasciotomy site

If copious amount of drainage is experienced, the pressure may be increased to 150 mmHg or 200 mmHg and then reduced back to 125 mmHg (see Fig. 40.2).

40.6 Closure

After the tissues become soft and are more malleable, closure can be considered. A delayed secondary intention with wound vac or wet to dry dressings can be used. Split-thickness skin graft after an initial period of dressing changes is an alternative. The most ideal closure is primary.

Some recommend a shoe string technique that can be slowly tightened until closure. The initial sutures are run at the time of initial operation and then pulled closed as the edema resolves. This can be difficult given the need for tissue manipulation and pain management at the time of closure.

Others favor closure intraoperatively when tissues are able to be manipulated or local anesthetic with the vertical mattress-interrupted sutures. At times a skin flap needs to be demarcated. Granulation tissue can make this difficult to initially see. A finger can be run along the subdermal tissue and expose the planes between the fascia and subcutaneous tissue. Often freeing more generous amounts of subcutaneous tissue from the fascia below allows for an easier closure.

Large 1-0 vicryl sutures can be used. Braided is also available. Silk tends to pull into the skin more. Make generous bites of tissue to avoid skin necrosis with tightening and allow for proper elevation of the incision edges. Once the suture is in place, cut a proper length for tying and place a snap as this will allow for multiple sutures to be placed and then closed at once much like the laces of a football. Once the tissue is closed, staples can be used to better approximate the skin edges (see Figs. 40.3 and 40.4).

If more lymphatic drainage becomes an issue, a "strip vac" may be employed.

40.7 Chronic Issues After Fasciotomy

In a retrospective study of 60 patients who suffered upper or lower extremity fasciotomies, many complained of chronic issues associated with the procedure and/or injuries [18, 19] including:

Ongoing pain relating to the wound 10 %
Altered sensation 77 %
Dry skin 40 %
Pruritus 30 %
Discoloration 25 %
Edema 25 %
Tethered scars 26 %
Recurrent ulceration 13 %
Muscle herniation 13 %
Tethered tendons 7 %
Stigmatizing scars 23 %
Change in hobbies 28 %
Change in occupation 12 %

Chronic venous insufficiency due to lack of calf pump utilization is additionally noted in many patients, perhaps due to the lack of reapproximation of the fascia at time of closure. This occurs in patients equally despite vascular injury [20, 21].

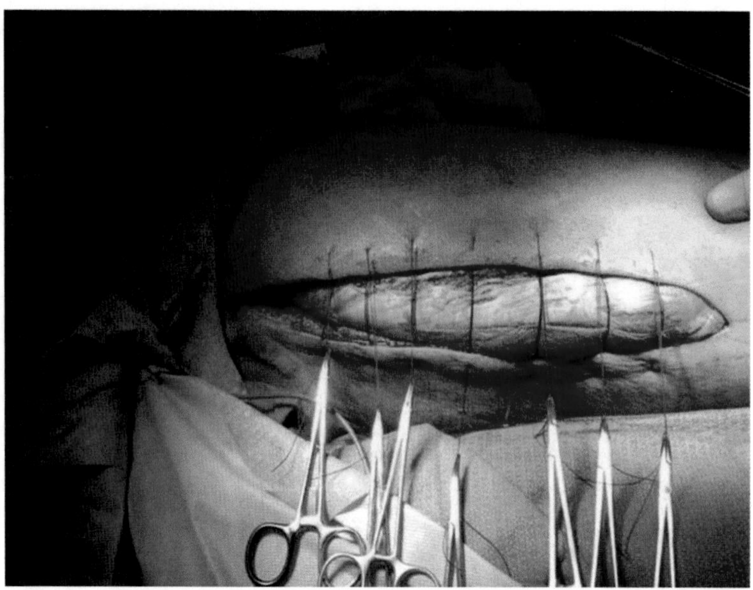

Fig. 40.3 Closure using braided nylon sutures in interrupted fashion

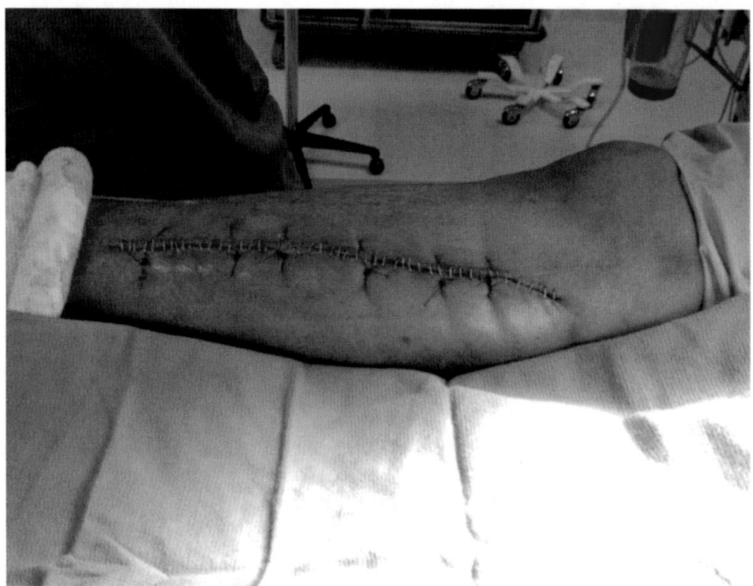

Fig. 40.4 Closure with the skin approximated with staples

40.8 Medicolegal Complications

Acute compartment syndrome is an extremely contested issue if not properly diagnosed and treated in a timely manner. Most often compartment pressures in these cases were not measured or measured incorrectly with malpositioning of the hardware. As stated previously, the diagnosis of compartment syndrome should be made clinically, if any doubt, the treating practitoner should trust their judgement rather than a number that may have been obtained incorrectly and perfrome the intervention.

40.9 Anticoagulation Therapy Contraindications

Many patients are on antiplatelets including aspirin, Plavix and Aggrenox, or Pletal. There is no contraindication with any of these agents.

Warfarin is also easily reversed if needed with vitamin K or fresh frozen plasma (FFP).

There is however a growing concern over Xa inhibitors including Xarelto, Eliquis, and Lixiana. There are no known reversal agents and FFP has no effect given the direct factor-inhibiting effect. However, the risk of limb loss, chronic limb dysfunction, or death with compartment syndrome is so high intervention should likely take place with meticulous hemostatic techniques being used. In these cases negative-pressure dressings should not be applied. Skin edge bleeding must be addressed and the use of thrombotic agents including Floseal, Tisseel, Surgicel, or StatSeal.

40.10 Conclusion

Acute compartment syndrome is a medical emergency requiring quick clinical decision making and clear understanding of the anatomy for successful compartment decompression. All patients with a clinical suspicion should be scrutinized, and delay can result in significant morbidity.

References

1. Volkmann R. Die ischaemischen Muskellahmungen und-Kontrakturen. Zentralbl Chin. 1881;8:801–5.
2. Jepson PN. Ischaemic contracture: experimental study. Ann Surg. 1926;84:785–95.
3. Donaldson J, Haddad B, Khan W. The pathophysiology, diagnosis and current management of acute compartment syndrome. Open Orthop J. 2014;8(Suppl 1:M8):185–93.
4. Ebraheim N, Abdelgawad A, Ebraheim M, Alla S. Bedside fasciotomy under local anesthesia for acute compartment syndrome: a feasible and reliable procedure in selected cases. J Orthop Traumatol. 2012;13:153–57.
5. Hartsock LA, O'Farrell D, Seaber AV, Urbaniak JR. Effect of increased compartment pressure on the microcirculation of skeletal muscle. Microsurgery. 1998;18:67–71.
6. Mubarak SJ, Owen CA. Double incision fasciotomy of the leg for decompression in compartment syndrome. J Bone Joint Surg Am. 1977;59-A:184–7.
7. Whitesides TE, Haney TC, Morimoto K, Harada H. Tissue pressure measurements as a determinant for the need for fasciotomy. Clin Orthop. 1975;113:43–51.
8. McQueen M, Court-Brown CM. Compartment monitoring in tibial fractures. J Bone Joint Surg Br. 1996;78-B:99–104.
9. White TO, Howell GE, Will EM, Court-Brown CM, McQueen MM. Elevated intramuscular compartment pressures do not influence outcome after tibial fracture. J Trauma. 2003;55:1133–8.
10. Flynn JM, Bashyal RK, Yeger-McKeever M, Garner MR, Launay F, Sponseller PD. Acute traumatic compartment syndrome of the leg in children: diagnosis and outcome. J Bone Joint Surg Am. 2011;93(10):937–41.
11. Boody A, Wongworawat M. Accuracy of the compartment pressures: a comparison of three commonly used devices. J Bone Joint Surg Am. 2005;87(11):2415–22.
12. Matsen FA, Wyss CR, Krugmire Jr RB, Simmons CW, King RV. The effects of limb elevation and dependency on local arteriovenous gradients in normal human limbs with particular reference to limbs with increased tissue pressure. Clin Orthop Relat Res. 1980;15:187–95.
13. Daniels M, Reichman J, Brezis M. Mannitol treatment for acute compartment syndrome. Nephron. 1998;79(4):492–3.
14. Bywaters EGI, Beall D. Crush injuries with impairment of renal function. Br Med J. 1941;1(4185):427–32.
15. DeBakey ME, Simeone FA. Battle injuries of the arteries in World War II. An analysis of 2,471 cases. Ann Surg. 1946;123:534–79.
16. Kelly RP, Whitesides RE. Transfibular route for fasciotomy of the leg. In proceedings of the American Academy of Orthopaedic Surgeons. J Bone Joint Surg. 1967;49-A:1022–3.
17. Patel RV, Haddad FS. Compartment syndrome in tibial fractures. J Orthop Trauma. 2009;23:514.
18. Fitzgerald AMI, Gaston P, Wilson Y, Quaba A, McQueen MM. Long-term sequelae of fasciotomy wounds. Br J Plast Surg. 2000;53(8):690–3.
19. Mubarak S, Owen C. Double-incision fasciotomy of the leg for decompression in compartment syndromes. J Bone Joint Surg. 1977;59-A:184–7.
20. Bermudez K, Knudson M, Morabito D, Kessel O. Fasciotomy, chronic venous insufficiency, and the calf muscle pump. Arch Surg. 1998;133:1356–61.
21. Morykwas MJ, Argenta LC. Non-surgical modalities to enhance healing and care of the soft tissue wounds. J South Orthop Assoc. 1997;6:279–88.

Amputations in the ICU Setting

41

Daniel Geersen

41.1 Amputations in the ICU Setting

Primary surgical amputation in the intensive care unit (ICU) is rare. However, in cases of severe sepsis or progressive limb ischemia where transportation to the operating room is of high risk, primary amputations can be seen. Causes are numerous, including diabetic foot infections, digitary ischemia, inotropic/vasopressor use, embolic events, arterial line placement, and trauma. While each of these has its own risk profile and treatment algorithms, the definitive intervention to eliminate the necrotic tissue in a hemodynamically unstable patient is the same.

Patients with diabetes are ten times more likely to have a lower extremity amputation [1]. With diabetes on the rise, the number of amputations attributed to diabetes is increasing as well. In 2003, it exceeded the number attributed to arterial inflow disease [2]. Although the number leveled off in 2005 to 71,000 [3], recent studies in Britain have demonstrated that the number of amputations attributed to diabetes mellitus (DM) type II is on the rise with a double in minor amputations and an increase of 40 % in major amputations. It is DM type I that has declined [4].

D. Geersen, MPAP, PA-C (✉)
Division of Vascular Surgery, Duke University Medical Center, Durham, NC, USA
e-mail: Daniel.geersen@duke.edu

In the *2012 Infectious Diseases Society of America Clinical Practice Guidelines for the Diagnosis and Treatment of Diabetic Foot Infections*, infection should be considered in any foot wound in a patient with diabetes. It will be warm and erythemic and have edema present locally or the entirety of the limb. Pain may or may not be present in a patient with severe neuropathy and should not be considered highly influential in decisions for treatment management.

Further note secretions, friability, and discolored granulation tissue. The odor may be important. Keep in mind that a deep musty, foul odor with a hint of sweet or fruity smell is classic for *Pseudomonas*. This will often fill an examination room and only get worse with the removal of bandages.

A probe-to-bone test in which you take the back end of a q-tip and slide it through the sinus tract to the firm bone is indicative of likely osteomyelitis [5]. With toe ischemia the great toe followed by the fourth toe is the most commonly affected in the diabetic population.

Wet gangrene is of particular concern in the diabetic patient. Unlike atherosclerotic arterial disease, most commonly associated with dry gangrene, the diabetic patient may still have patent tibial arteries. This results in preservation of inflow and can result in ischemia with surrounding tissue inflammation and a cytokine response, with bacterial infection.

D.A. Taylor et al. (eds.), *Interventional Critical Care*, DOI 10.1007/978-3-319-25286-5_41

Edema with blistering and a damp appearance are the common features of wet gangrene.

Gas gangrene is commonly associated with the bacterium *Clostridium perfringens*. It originates in the deeper necrotic or damaged tissue layers or compartments. The surface of the skin may initially appear normal, but as the condition deteriorates, it becomes pale and then a gray or purplish-red color with blistering of the skin. Subcutaneou s crepitation is not uncommon due to the subcutaneous emphysema, or gas within the tissue, when you press on it (see Figs. 41.1 and 41.2).

Digitary hand ischemia is less common. A 4-year study in 50 patients showed the pathophysiologic mechanism responsible for the ischemia to be emboli in 6 %, vasospasm in 10 %, thrombosis or "sludging" in 28 %, occlusive disease in 26 %, and occlusive disease associated with either vasospasm or external compression in 30 % [6] (see Figs. 41.3 and 41.4).

The treatment for digital ischemia associated with vasopressors is currently under investigation. Options include operative management if indicated and nonoperative strategies such as botulism toxin as seen in patient with Raynaud's disease [7].

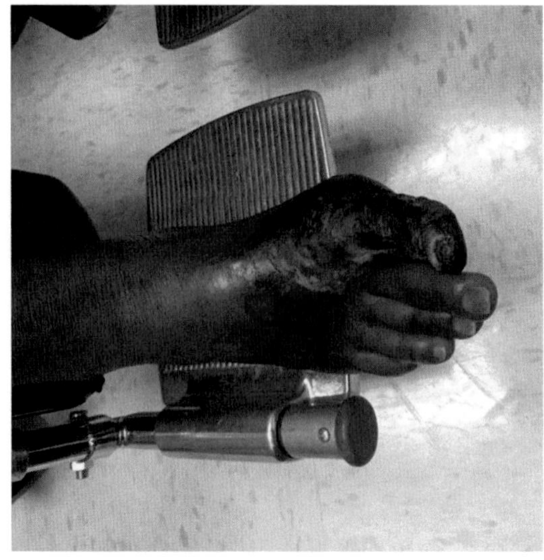

Fig. 41.2 Dry gangrene has no fluid air changes and appears flush with the skin with clear demarcation

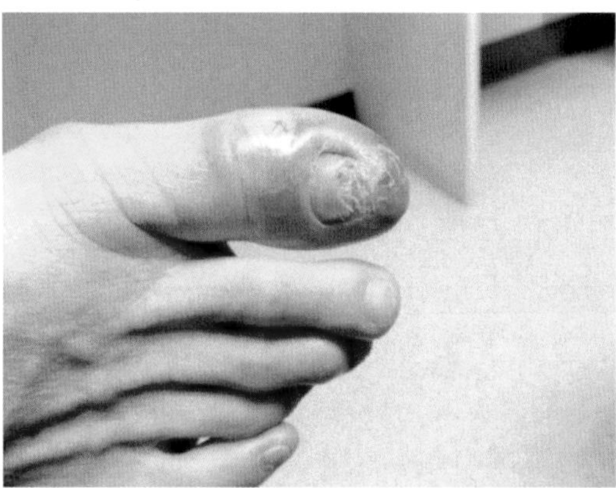

Fig. 41.3 Digital ischemia secondary to embolic event a.k.a. blue toe syndrome

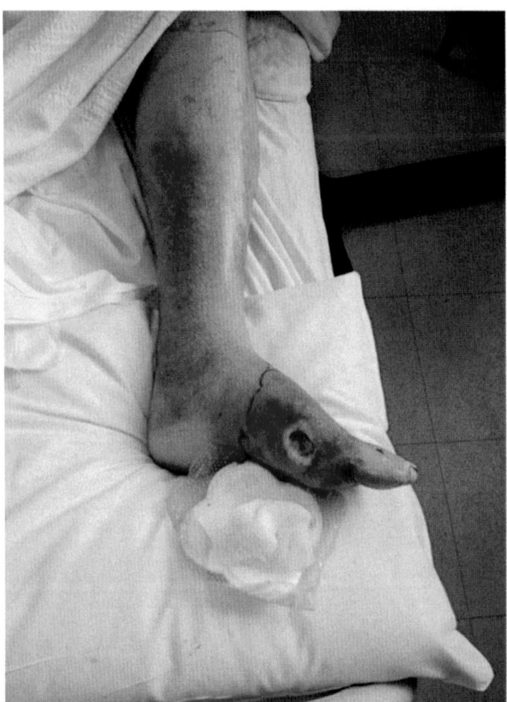

Fig. 41.1 Evidence of cellulitis extending proximally and progressing to wet gangrene

The complications associated with peripheral arterial catheters are rare, but when encountered are often in the ICU setting. These are used for hemodynamic monitoring and most commonly are placed in the radial, femoral, and axillary locations. The most common site is the radial location and the incidence of temporary occlusion is roughly 20 % [8]. Generally this has no significant sequelae.

Thrombotic complications are induced by changes to the integrity of the vessel wall caused by

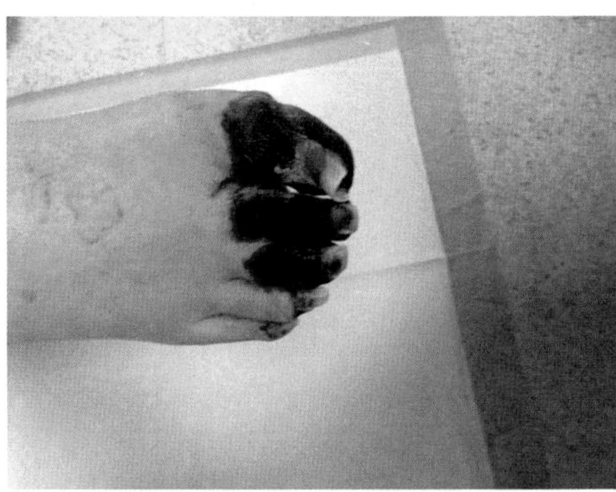

Fig. 41.4 Digital ischemia secondary to long-standing pressor use

the catheter [9]. Further the incidence of thrombus formation appears to correlate with the ratio of the catheter compared to the size of the artery [10]. The smaller the artery, the greater the risk. This is believed to increase the risk of thrombotic complication in females. There is also an increase in multiple punctures, hematoma formation, and catheter placement longer than 48–72 h [11]. There appears to be decreased risk of this with Teflon catheters as well as a decreased incidence of infection [11, 12].

If the tissue continues to be the source of infection and septicemia, a guillotine amputation can be considered in cases such as wet gas gangrene or fulminant osteomyelitis. If the wound flaps created at the stump can be approximated, no further intervention is required. In the above clinical scenarios, this is rare. These are conditions that prevent complete demarcation, yet this intervention provides the patient with a way to eliminate the source of infection.

We have seen in literature this to be a superior form of treatment. Panchbhavi and Schraga describe several studies to support this. They concluded that even with two interventions being required that with nonsalvageable foot amputations, guillotine interventions allow for better wound closure and reduce the risk of wound infection [13].

McIntyre et al. reviewed 75 below-the-knee amputations performed for nonsalvageable foot infections [14]. While these were not performed in ICUs, patients were placed in two distinct groups. The first underwent open-ankle guillotine amputations and then followed by definitive closures. The second underwent definitive amputations with primary closure. In group one, 97 % of the patients achieved primary healing after one revision, and none required a higher level of amputation. The second group only had 78 %, by contrast, primary healing. 11 % required revision to a higher level.

Fisher et al. randomized 47 patients to either one-stage amputation or a two-stage. 21 % in the first group had positive muscle cultures versus 43 % in the two-stage groups. 8 % in the first group had positive lymphatic cultures with 30 % in the two-stage group. Additionally, 21 % in the first group had wound complications attributed to the amputation technique, while none in the two-stage group [15].

Keep in mind the goal of therapy is to remove the necrotic tissue while minimizing risk of transport to the patient. Guillotine amputations provide an ability to perform this while keeping the patient in their current environment.

The counterargument is that a classical guillotine amputation below the knee may cause the infection or necrosis to spread to additional anatomical spaces between muscles and bones. Further, retraction of tissues after being transected will provide less real estate to create a flap in the future, and it is suggested that tibiotalar disarticulation with vertical crural incisions and secondary transtibial amputation as a first stage and then a transtibial amputation as a second [16].

Although it has been demonstrated that there is nearly a twofold increase in mortality of guillotine recipients [17], likely secondary to the patient's presentation, the guillotine amputation is a quick, safe, and reliable method for treating these high-risk patients that requires minimal resources.

41.2 Lower Extremity Guillotine Amputation

Performing an amputation in the ICU is not the optimal venue. They should be performed in extenuating circumstances, i.e., septic shock, and severe instability that precluded transportation out of the

ICU. This most commonly occurs in patients with high oxygen and ventilator demands and pressor requirements that would make even a short transport hazardous. Therefore the amputations performed in the ICU setting are typically limited to guillotine and digital amputations. Although a patient requiring a hip disarticulation may present with instability, this is a much larger surgery with both time and resources. It usually requires an operating room to be performed safely and effectively. Make sure to weigh the risks versus benefits.

Most ICU amputations will likely occur for sepsis as ischemic extremities can be packed in ice. Septic amputations will require reoperation as soon as feasible and hopefully within 24–48 h.

41.3 Preparation

These patients in the ICU may or may not be intubated. Although most are, proper participation by anesthesiology is key, especially in limb amputations rather than digital. In the ICU setting, there should be a specific individual team managing the anesthesia and resuscitation efforts which commonly include blood products.

Anesthetic options include general, spinal, epidural, or regional anesthetic. Regional is the preferred method to limit the stress on the cardiovascular system or in compromised situations such as shock, but is quite limited in the ICU setting.

In fact, it has been shown that peripheral nerve blocks are superior to general anesthesia (GA) in lower extremity amputations. Hypotension and the need for vasopressors was significantly more common in patients with GA as well as significant postoperative pain was increased in the GA group [18].

Make sure the room setup can accommodate respiratory and/or anesthesia at the head and if possible lower the bed rails and remove the footboard. A simple Mayo stand can be used for upper extremities to rest the limb on.

Assistance is required. Although the procedure can be performed by health-care providers with varying levels of experience, there remains a need to have an experienced practitioner available and mobilization of operating room (OR) staff including assistant and circulator to bring up the appropriate OR trays and remove the specimen.

41.4 Supplies

Prep kit: hospital specific (Hibiclens recommended), tourniquet, Gigli saw, electrocaudery if possible to have in place, 2-0 and 3-0 pop-off silk sutures, suture driver, pick-ups, hemostats, suction, and dressing (Xeroform or Vaseline gauze, abdominal gauze pads (ABDs), cotton cast padding, bias wrap, or negative pressure dressing, although this can result in increased risk of postoperative bleeding but may benefit in reducing edema).

41.5 Procedure

The patient should be lying in bed in supine position. If not already on scheduled antibiotics and therapeutic on a regimen, a single dose of prophylactic broad-spectrum antibiotics should be given. Open ulcers are prepped, and the foot is then covered with an impervious stocking and secured with a self-adherent wrap. The rest of the extremity should be prepped to a level well above the intended incision line. The limb is then prepped out with towels and if possible a limb isolation drape is brought up. If performing a below-the-knee amputation, have the knee exposed. If above the knee, drapes need to be placed at the inguinal ligament.

The surgeon should gown and then glove. Bring up the electrocaudery and suction devices. If you do not have these available, you can perform the procedure without them although skin edge bleeding will be more difficult to control. A portable battery-operated thermal cautery can be used. Large extremities will require electrocautery brought to the bedside. Then place the tourniquet pressurized above the systolic blood pressure, commonly 250 mmHg. This can reduce the initial bleeding and allows for better visualization of the vessels for ligation. Your decision to choose this may be influenced by your pulse examination or prior arterial inflow studies. For example, if the popliteal artery is occluded, you may decide to not use a tourniquet when performing a below-the-knee amputation. This should be removed prior to completing the procedure, so you can assess for any further bleeding before dressing the wound.

With severe infection of the limb, you do not want to use an Esmark for fear of spreading the bacteria proximally. It is, however, recommended routinely to compress and empty the venous system to reduce venous blood loss.

Mark the incision line and bring up the Gigli saw. You must be above the infected tissue and any tunneling gas in the deeper muscle compartments. This should be placed under the limb. Have an assistant hold a large DeBakey pickup or other large instrument like an Army/Navy over the superior aspect of the limb, so when cutting through the tissue the saw does not snap up. You can cut all the tissues initially with a Gigli saw. An amputation knife can also be used. Keep in mind that the secondary intervention will require fresh incisions above this line.

When operating the Gigli saw, hold the instrument more horizontally (see Figs. 41.5 and 41.6). You do not want to pull straight-up creating a U shape. Rather you want to use the instrument like a two-person lumberjack saw filing back and forth. A firm elevated approach will allow the saw to pass through the tissues. Do not stop at the bone. This can cause you to pinch the blade and makes starting more difficult. Complete the cut and remove the specimen.

Once removed you will have an opportunity to evaluate the tissue to make sure you are above the infected tissue. If a second more proximal amputation needs to be performed, then you should do it at this time. Then evaluate vessels for bleeding. Use the hemostat to stop the bleeding initially. You can then circumferentially ligate or use figure-of-eight stitches to achieve homeostasis. If the vessels are calcified, crunch the vessel with the hemostat first that will break the calcium surrounding the vessel wall and make them more pliable. Try not to encompass the nerves with these ligations if possible as this can cause pulsatile pain for the patient.

The peroneal artery, commonly, is the most difficult to ligate. It is located between the tibia and fibula and therefore a figure-of-eight stitch can be

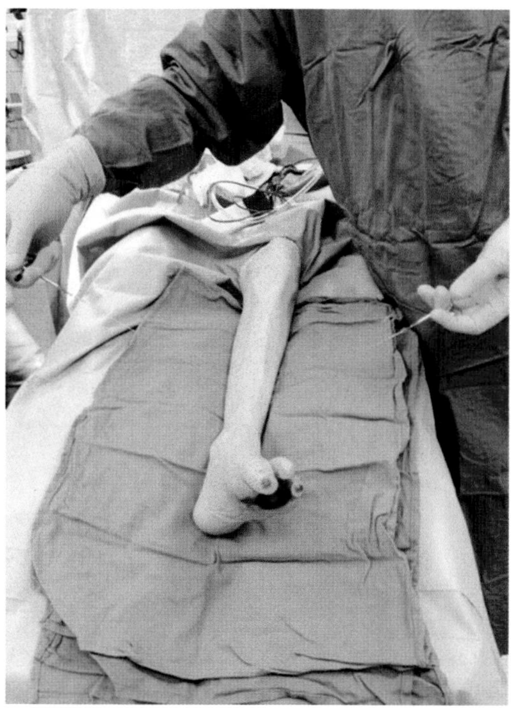

Fig. 41.5 A Gigli blade should be more horizontal with a gentle curve

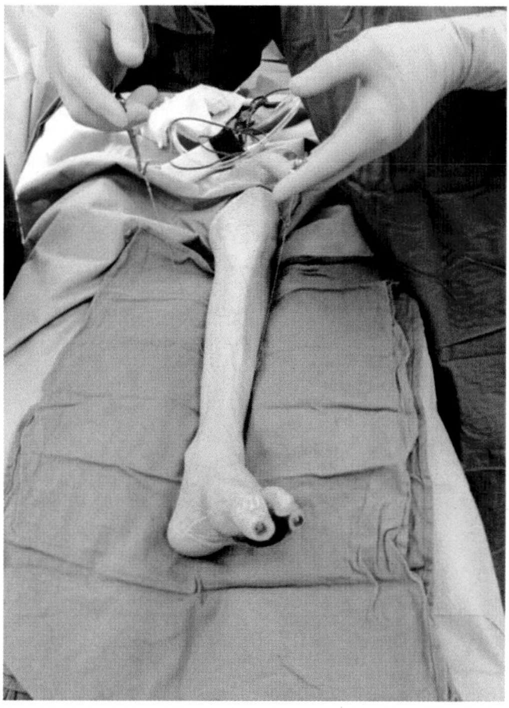

Fig. 41.6 The Gigli saw will pinch with use if arms are pulling up

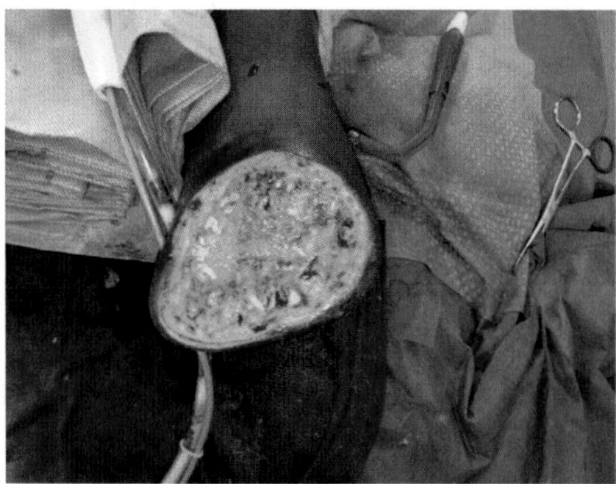

Fig. 41.7 Guillotine amputation; tissues are easily viewed for hemostasis evaluation

placed to close the vessel. The tibial nerve usually runs along the posterior tibial artery (see Figs. 41.7).

Once primary homeostasis is achieved, let down the tourniquet and observe for any additional bleeding. This is usually venous because arteries had already been identified. Skin edge bleeding should be cauterized and dressing can then be applied.

41.6 Dressing

If a negative pressure dressing is chosen, set the device to constant suction no greater than 75–90 mmHg of pressure. If intermittent or greater, this may cause postoperative bleeding. Make sure the staff is aware to monitor carefully for rapid filling of the chamber.

With conventional dressings, keep in mind that wound compression will help with reducing postoperative bleeding by tamponade. However, try not to make the circumferential compression too tight. This can cause skin edge bleeding. Plan on changing the dressing at least twice a day. Using a Xeroform or Vaseline gauze application on the tissues will reduce the rate of bleeding and pain with dressing changes. Elevate the limb to reduce the bleeding and edema. Many of these patients may be coagulopathic so use of Combat gauze or oxidized regenerated cellulose should be considered.

The risk of lower extremity contractures is rare, but can be seen with some regularity in the elderly and temporarily bedridden patients. A flexion contracture can occur with a 15° limitation in 3–5 % of major lower extremity amputations [19]. To prevent this a knee immobilizer can be incorporated to reduce this risk in transtibial amputations. Casting material can be used as well, but runs the risk of accidental patellar ulcerations or pressure ulcers and skin necrosis. If using a knee immobilizer, cut out the material for room around the patella and the corresponding Velcro strap. These can also be adjusted to accommodate the bulky dressings or negative pressure dressings used.

41.7 Digital Amputations

When performing an upper or lower extremity digital amputation, the mindset is to achieve primary closure at the same time if possible. This intervention is much less traumatic to the patient and family and can be performed in numerous settings including the emergency department. It does not require assistance and can be done in a matter of minutes if left open.

A digital nerve block or regional block can be employed to numb the area. Make sure to test the location of incision rather than the distal aspect of the digit for assured set up of the block.

41.8 Supplies

Prep kit: hospital specific(chlorhexidine recommended), tourniquet, knife 11 or 15 blade, electrocaudery if possible to have in place, 2-0 and 3-0 pop-off silk sutures, suture driver, pickups, hemostats, suction, rongeur, bone cutter, bone rasp, and dressing (petrolatum gauze, 4×4's, bias wrap).

41.9 Procedure

Depending upon the digit in question, a circumferential or modified racket incision can be employed (see Figs. 41.8). Make sure if your desire is to close the wound without having to bit

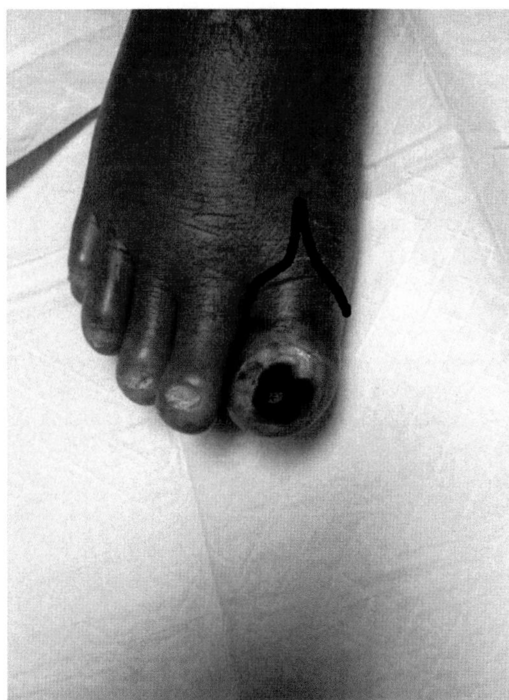

Fig. 41.8 Example of racket incision for digital amputation

back the metatarsal or metacarpal bones, you advance your incision more distal toward the gangrenous tissue. If you cannot do this safely without eliminating the entire tissue required, plan on leaving the wound open with packing versus using the rongeur to nibble the bone back.

Often the tissue will free itself enough to better mobilize the joint once the skin is incised. Retract the digit count to where you need to dissect and transect the ligament/tendon structures. Keep in mind you must retract these particular tissues and then transect them as they will interrupt wound healing if left in your closure. Be careful not to score the flap as you do so. Once the specimen is passed off you can use your Bovie or electric thermal cautery to stop any skin edge bleeding. Keep in mind much of this will tapenade with closure or dressings.

The flap can then be closed in layers using an absorbable suture to better approximate the subcutaneous tissues and the nylon sutures either with vertical matrice sutures or simple interrupted.

41.10 Dressing

The dressing should limit adherence to the sutures as this can be painful when removed for the patient. A silver product dressing can be used rather than Vaseline product if you desire a reduced risk of maceration to the tissues. Either silver sorb or silver alginates are common. Use a good amount of gauze to pad the tissues and avoid traumatic discomfort when the patient moves.

41.11 Postoperative Care

The management of these patients should be centered on supportive post-procedural care in conjunction with a multidisciplinary ICU team. Ventilator support, pain management, and fluid management should be administered by the primary unit team.

Antibiotics should be maintained postoperatively in two-staged procedures until completion is done. Often, as discussed above, perioperative management of diabetics with deep tissue infections are associated with other organisms than skin flora. Until identified what this is, broad-spectrum antibiotics should be administered with special attention given to anaerobic coverage for diabetics.

Thromboprophylaxis for venous thromboembolism (VTE) should be considered in all amputees. When examining a literature review, deep vein thrombosis (DVT) is reported in up to 50 % of all patients following a major lower extremity amputation when not on prophylactic anticoagulation [20]. The risk of major bleeding with VTE prophylaxis is less than 10 %. There appears to be no difference between heparin and low molecular weight heparin [21]. Keep in mind that even transmetatarsal amputations require limited weight-bearing activities, and although the surgery is more minor or less extensive, the risk for DVT is similar to below-knee amputations (BKAs) or above-knee amputations (AKAs).

The wound needs to be monitored for any signs of progressive infection. It is hoped that the edema will reduce over time. Compression wraps will assist in this. Any unexplained fever, increased pain in the amputated limb, erythema, warmth, purulent drainage, or superficial necrosis should be examined further to rule out infection progression. Keep in mind residual prosthetic material can be a nidus for infection.

The patients typically require a minimum of 2 days before consideration of closure can take place. This provides valuable time to allow the limb to drain foul material and gain the upper hand in clearing the patient's sepsis.

Pain management can often be difficult, and anesthesia is an essential player in controlling this. In the acute postoperative period, an epidural or regional block catheter may be the best option. When the patient is sedated and on the ventilator, placement of these is less critical. However, proper pain control preoperatively is critical in reducing the risk for phantom pain [22]. Care must be taken when placing these catheters as the patient is septic and also with causing hypotension. A consult with anesthesiologist should be obtained prior to moving forward with amputation to get the best option for the patient.

Perioperative mortality is directly attributed to the comorbidities involved. There is a higher risk in patients with cardiac complications, sepsis, pneumonia, end-stage renal disease, delirium, coagulopathy, and over 80 years old [17]. Mortality rates following major amputation range around 10 % with a higher level of amputation resulting in increased risk. The National Surgical Quality Improvement Program database demonstrated perioperative mortality as 12.8 % for AKAs and 6.5 % for BKAs. The foot is slightly less [23].

Amputations in the ICU setting are performed to remove infected, ischemic material. It is a lifesaving intervention that when performed can provide the patients with an avenue to recover and rejoin their life. It should not be taken lightly but do not avoid the need to remove the tissue. Patients and their families are looking for clear leadership and counsel when reaching this point in their lives.

References

1. Dillingham TR, Pezzin LE, Shore AD. Reamputation, mortality and health care costs among persons with dysvascular lower-limb amputations. Arch Phys Med Rehabil. 2005;86:480–6.
2. Centers for Disease Control and Prevention. Number (in thousands) of hospital discharges with ulcer/inflammation/infection (ULCER) as first-listed diagnosis and diabetes as any-listed diagnosis, 1980–2003. 2010. http://www.cdc.gov/diabetes/statisitics/hosplea/diabetes_complications/fig5.htm.
3. Centers for Disease Control and Prevention. Number (in thousands) of hospital discharges for nontraumatic lower extremity amputation with diabetes as a listed diagnosis, 1988–2006. 2010. http://www.cdc.gov/diabetes/statistics.lea/fig1.htm.
4. Vamos EP, Bottle A, Majeed A, Millett C. Trends in lower extremity amputations in people with and without diabetes in England, 1996–2005. Diabetes Res Clin Pract. 2010;87:275–82.
5. Lipsky BA, Berendt AR, Cornia PB, Pile JC, Peters EJ, Armstrong DG, et al. 2012 infectious diseases society of America clinical practice guideline for the diagnosis and treatment of diabetic foot infections. Clin Infect Dis. 2012;54(12):132–73.
6. Jones NF. Acute and chronic ischemia of the hand: pathophysiology, treatment, and prognosis. J Hand Surg Am. 1991;16(6):1074–83.
7. Neumeister MW, Chambers BB, Herron MS, Webb K, Wietfeldt J, Gillespie JN, et al. Botox therapy for ischemic digits. Plast Reconstr Surg. 2009;124(1):191–201.
8. Scheer BV, Perel A, Pfeiffer UJ. Clinical review: complications and risk factors of peripheral arterial catheters used for haemodynamic monitoring in anaesthesia and intensive care medicine. Crit Care. 2002;6:198–204.
9. Bedford RF, Wollman H. Complications of percutaneous radial artery cannulation: an objective study in man. Anesthesilogy. 1973;38:228–36.
10. Scheidegger D. Intravascular catheters. In: Benzer H, editor. Lehrbuch der Anasthesie und Intensivmedizin: Intensivmedizin. Berlin: Springer; 1993. p. 97–105.
11. Lopez-Lopez G, Pascual A, Perea J. Effect of plastic catheter material on bacterial adherence and viability. J Med Microbiol. 1991;34:349–53.
12. Davis FM. Radial artery cannulation: influence of catheter size and material on arterial occlusion. Anaesth Intensive Care. 1978;6:49–53.
13. Pranchbhavi VK, Schraga ED. Guillotine ankle amputation. Medscape Reference. http://emedicine.com/article/1894411.
14. McIntyre Jr KE, Bailey SA, Malone JM, Goldstone J. Guillotine amputation in the treatment of nonsalvageable lower-extremity infections. Arch Surg. 1984;119:450–3.
15. Fisher Jr DF, Clagett GP, Fry RE, Humble TH, Fry WJ. One-stage versus two-stage amputation for wet gangrene of the lower extremity: a randomized study. J Vasc Surg. 1988;8(4):428–33.
16. Altindas M, Kilic A, Cinar C. A reliable surgical approach for the two-staged amputation in unsalvageable limb and life threatening acute progressive diabetic foot infections: tibiotalar disarticulation with vertical crural incisions and secondary transtibial amputation. Foot Ankle Surg. 2011;17:13–8.
17. Aulivola B, Hile CN, Hamdan AD, Sheahan MG, Veraldi JR, Skillman JJ, et al. Major lower extremity amputation: outcome of a modern series. Arch Surg. 2004;139:395–9.

18. Gandhi K, Gadsden J, Xu D, Vandepidte C, Maliakal T. Peripheral nerve blocks are superior to GA in patients having lower extremity amputations. ASA: 2009. http://www.asaabstracts.com/strands/asaabstracts/abstract.htm;jsessionid=6BA44D4E0A9EA8C4953D05C5F55896CB?year=2009&index=17&absnum=1661
19. Wasiak K, Paczkowski PM, Garlicki JM. Surgical results of leg amputation according to Ghormley's technique in the treatment of chronic lower limb ischaemia. Acta Chir Belg. 2006;106:52–4.
20. Burke B, Kumar R, Vickers V, Grant E, Scremin E. Deep vein thrombosis after lower limb amputation. Am J Phys Med Rehabil. 2000;79:145–9.
21. Robertson L, Roche A. Primary prophylaxis for venous thromboembolism in people undergoing major amputation of the lower extremity. Chochrane Database Syst Rev. 2013;12, CD010525.
22. Karanikolas M, Aretha D, Tsolakis I, Monantera G, Kiekkas P, Papadoulas S. Optimized perioperative analgesia reduces chronic phantom limb pain intensity, prevalence, and frequency: a prospective, randomized, clinical trial. Anesthesiology. 2011;114:1144–54.
23. Nelson MT, Greenblatt DY, Soma G, Rajimanickam V, Greenberg CC, Kent KC. Preoperative factors predict mortality after major lower-extremity amputation. Surgery. 2012;152:685–94.

42 Wound Management in the ICU

Preston Miller, Ian M. Smith, and David M. White

42.1 Introduction

The management of wounds in the critical care setting is a complex task. Patient comorbidities, associated injuries, and systemic inflammation play critical roles in the healing process. The wound-healing process encompasses four basic phases. Initially, platelet function and the clotting cascade will begin the hemostasis phase. This begins immediately post injury as long as the patient is not coagulopathic. The inflammatory phase follows shortly thereafter as the capillaries become permeable, releasing plasma and neutrophils into the wound. The neutrophils, and subsequently macrophages, will begin to phagocytize bacteria and release enzymes that will degrade necrotic tissue. The macrophages will also begin to secrete growth factors and cytokines that lead into the proliferation phase. This phase will generally last for several weeks, although it may be substantially longer depending on the overall progress of the patient's critical illness. This phase is characterized by collagen deposition, granulation tissue formation, wound contraction, and epithelialization. Finally, the remodeling phase will occur as the collagen tissues are remodeled to produce greater tensile strength [1].

While primary closure is preferred to optimize the wound-healing process, this is often not feasible in the critically ill patient. Open wounds generally fall into two broad categories: the soft tissue defect and the open abdominal cavity. Large soft tissue defects occurring after injury may preclude primary closure, or closure may be deliberately avoided due to infection or significant contamination. Compartment syndrome and limb ischemia may make primary closure unsafe. The abdominal cavity may be deliberately left open for a number of reasons such as the use of damage control laparotomy or the management of abdominal compartment syndrome.

If primary closure is not an option, the two general options are wound packing and negative pressure dressings. In either case, the ideal dressing should absorb excessive fluid, while simultaneously keeping the wound moist. Both animal and human studies have shown accelerated healing, faster wound contraction, and faster granulation tissue in a moist environment [2]. The dressing should also eliminate dead space, as this can be a collection site for excessive fluid which may lead to infection and/or impaired healing. Additional considerations when choosing a dressing must include the amount of pain both during and between dressing changes, durability, and cost-effectiveness.

P. Miller, MD, FACS (✉) • I.M. Smith, MMS, PA-C
D.M. White, PA-C, MPAS
Surgery, Wake Forest Baptist Medical Center, Medical Center BLVD., Winston-Salem, NC 27157, USA
e-mail: pmiller@wakehealth.edu

D.A. Taylor et al. (eds.), *Interventional Critical Care*, DOI 10.1007/978-3-319-25286-5_42

42.2 Soft Tissue Wounds

42.2.1 Wound Packing

Traditionally, wound packing with wet-to-dry gauze dressings has been the modality of choice for large soft tissue defects [1]. Saline-soaked gauze is packed into the wound, eliminating dead space, allowing for wound drainage, and providing a moist environment for healing to occur. The gauze may be soaked in Dakin's solution, a mixture of diluted bleach, or other solutions when wound infection is a concern. All of these approaches may impede wound healing, and the practitioner must weigh the risks and benefits of the solution's anti-infective properties versus the potential for a longer healing process when deciding whether to use anything other than saline. The wet gauze is covered with dry gauze to prevent the wound from drying out. The wet gauze remains in place until dried. With each packing change, the removal of the dressing aids in debriding devitalized tissue. Dakin's solution is also thought to help further debride necrotic tissue. Wet-to-dry wound packing is especially useful in the case of dirty or infected wounds. The limited materials needed and expertise required also makes this wound therapy ideal for austere environments.

42.2.2 Negative Pressure Wound Therapy (NPWT)

Growing evidence indicates that NPWT promotes more rapid wound granulation when compared to wet-to-dry dressings. Recent studies have shown an even stronger indication for NPWT when wounds contain exposed tendon or bone [2]. NPWT has become commonplace in the critical care setting because of these improved results and the relative ease of patient care after application of NPWT [3].

The basic components of a NPWT system include a semipermeable conduit used to pack the wound, an occlusive dressing, a suction port, and a collection system. Commercially available kits are most commonly used (V.A.C.®, KCI, San Antonio, TX), and these utilize an open-pore polyurethane sponge as the fluid conduit, although other methods may be devised depending on the wound. The goal of the NPWT system is to eliminate the dead space, while the pressure gradient generated by the suction will promote excess fluid transport away from the wound, altering the inflammatory environment. The sponge will retain enough fluid to keep the wound moist, and the occlusive dressing will keep the wound warm and prevent leakage. The sponge will deform under the negative pressure, thus causing tissue deformation which will stimulate tissue remodeling.

42.2.3 Indications

In the critical care setting, NPWT is most commonly used for large soft tissue defects or when primary closure of a wound might contribute to development of compartment syndrome. Large soft tissue defects are commonly seen in the multi-trauma patient. The operational warfare of the recent conflicts in Iraq and Afghanistan has led to a marked increase in destructive blast injuries, and NPWT has been used quite successfully both in theater and in subsequent evacuation of these combat casualties [4]. In extremity trauma where compartment syndrome is a concern, NPWT may be employed as a safe dressing with a delayed primary closure once the initial risk of compartment syndrome has been alleviated [2]. Because NPWT is self-contained, and dressing changes are needed less frequently than when using wet-to-dry dressings, patients undergoing NPWT are generally considered easier to care for from a nursing standpoint.

42.2.4 Preparation and Setup

Negative pressure wound therapy dressing changes for soft tissue wounds are typically well tolerated by the patient. Appropriate analgesia should be provided; on occasion sedation may be required. If applicable, the previous dressing should be removed and discarded. If the previously placed sponge has adhered to underlying granulation tissue, it may be soaked in saline for several minutes to facilitate removal. The wound should be irrigated and any devitalized tissue debrided. The wound edges must be dry and hemostatic to ensure an optimal environment for the occlusive dressing to adhere properly and thus minimize the risk of the dressing leaking.

42.2.5 Application

Once the wound is prepared, the foam sponge is trimmed to fit the size of the wound, ensuring that the sponge edges do not extend past the wound edges. The sponge is packed into the wound, and an adhesive, occlusive covering is placed over the wound with at least a 3–5 cm margin covered around the wound edges. A small hole is created in the central portion of the occlusive dressing, and the suction port is placed over the defect. In the case of large wounds, more than one suction port may be placed strategically around the wound. The suction pump is then connected to the suction port, the pump initiated, and the dressing observed for any evidence that the dressing is not airtight. Most commercially available suction pumps will have an alarm that will alert the practitioner of a potential leak.

42.2.6 Wound Closure

As the patient's condition stabilizes, definitive wound closure is the goal. Depending on the circumstances surrounding the placement of the dressing, timing of the definitive closure can be quite variable. As the risk of compartment syndrome diminishes after an extremity fasciotomy, a delayed primary closure may be indicated. For a large soft tissue defect, serial dressing changes with either wound packing or NPWT may occur over weeks with a more complex definitive treatment required such as skin grafting or free flap reconstruction.

42.3 The Open Abdomen

Critical care providers are often charged with caring for patients with an open abdominal cavity. In the trauma setting, damage control laparotomy is a common procedure in the critically injured patient. In the hemodynamically unstable patient with abdominal trauma, a laparotomy is performed to control hemorrhage and intra-abdominal contamination. Often, these patients will become acidotic, hypothermic, and coagulopathic, exhibiting the aptly named "triad of death." In these instances, an abbreviated laparotomy is performed, where once the surgically correctable bleeding and contamination are controlled, the abdomen is left open with a negative pressure dressing in place, and the patient is moved to the critical care setting for aggressive resuscitation, limitation of further shock, and correction of the physiologic derangements. Leaving the abdomen open will hasten the trip to the intensive care unit (ICU) and prevent intra-abdominal pressure from increasing. After the physiologic shock is reversed, the patient will return to the operating suite for further definitive interventions. At that time, the surgical team will weigh several factors to decide whether to primarily close the abdomen or continue with serial negative pressure wound therapy dressings [5].

Emergency general surgery patients with intra-abdominal contamination or abscess formation may also be treated with an open abdomen requiring NPWT. The temporary abdominal dressing can aid in the removal of excessive fluid and pus and will facilitate easy access to reexplore and irrigate the abdomen at regular intervals [6].

Compartment syndrome is not limited to the extremities. The massive fluid resuscitation that the hemodynamically unstable patient often undergoes, combined with increased capillary permeability secondary to systemic inflammatory responses, increases the risk of abdominal compartment syndrome. Bowel wall edema will contribute to increased intra-abdominal pressures which may lead to cardiovascular, pulmonary, renal, hepatic, and gastrointestinal end organ damage through a variety of mechanisms. Several methods for measuring intra-abdominal pressure exist, but by far the most common is measuring intra-bladder pressures, with any value greater than 25 mm/Hg, commonly cited as an indication for surgical decompression [7].

In these cases, the use of a negative pressure wound therapy dressing meets the needs of an optimal dressing. The wound will remain warm and moist, enhancing healing. The negative pressure will help maintain fascial domain. In our published experience, this will facilitate definitive closure, avoiding the need for future intervention for a ventral hernia [8, 9]. It will maintain a sterile environment and will allow for excess fluid that may be detrimental to healing to be removed. Finally, it provides the critical care team the ability to reevaluate the intra-abdominal cavity regularly without having to reopen a closed wound.

42.3.1 Preparation and Setup

The placement of NPWT on an open abdomen may occur in the operating suite or bedside in the intensive care unit depending on the patient's current clinical status and availability of appropriate resources and staff. Placement may occur under general anesthesia, but may not be necessary if adequate analgesia and sedation can be achieved. Coordination with anesthesia, nursing, and respiratory therapy should thoroughly account for each particular patient situation regarding pain control and sedation if necessary. Once all necessary supplies and equipment have been gathered and the team is ready to begin, the previous NPWT should be removed, and the area should be prepped using Betadine or a similar agent and then draped using sterile technique. Good lighting is important as some defects are deep and hard to adequately visualize.

The wound should be carefully debrided of necrotic or devascularized tissue including the surrounding wound edge to ensure healthy tissue is available for the NPWT to effectively promote wound healing. Hemostasis should also be achieved to ensure a proper seal can be secured and continued blood loss does not occur in the critical care setting. Electrocautery and/or suture ligation may be used. Once hemostasis is achieved, the wound should be thoroughly washed out using warm saline and suction until clear fluid is returned and hemostasis is confirmed.

42.3.2 Technique

Application of the NPWT begins with a perforated polyethylene sheet, sometimes referred to as a "bowel bag" to overlie any viscera which is exposed in the wound. Scissors or a scalpel is used to perforate the sheet throughout with holes made approximately 3–5 cm apart, allowing for fluid to be drained through the bag (Fig. 42.1). If using the KCI ABThera system (ABThera™, KCI, San Antonio, TX), this corresponds to the visceral protective layer, which is pre-perforated. The bag or visceral protective layer is laid over any exposed viscera and tucked into the paracolic gutters along the wound edges to prevent direct suction being applied to vital structures and adhesion of the viscera to the abdominal wall (Fig. 42.2). Next, polyurethane sponge or sterile surgical towels are applied over the bowel bag (Figs. 42.3 and 42.4). The sponge should be measured and cut to fit the exact tissue deficit, or flat Jackson-Pratt drains should be placed overlying the towels to facilitate drainage and suction. Depending on the size of the wound, anywhere from 2 to 3 JP drains may be used, keeping in mind the extra requirements for wall suction or portable suction devices. If a sponge setup is chosen, the commercially available product from KCI (ABThera™, KCI, San Antonio, TX) contains all the necessary equipment for placement.

Once the overlying sponge or towel is in place, it must be covered with an adhesive drape. The surrounding wound edge and skin must then be cleaned and dried to ensure an effective seal is achieved. Drying and surgical adhesive agents such as Dermabond and/or Mastisol can be used to facilitate the adherence. The adhesive agent is applied to the dried skin of the surrounding area and allowed to set up. The adhesive drape should then be stretched tightly over the entire sponge or towel ensuring at least 3–5 cm of the surrounding tissue is covered. Most often, the adhesive drape used is Ioban® or dressings supplied by KCI (ABThera™, KCI, San Antonio, TX). For large areas, placement of the adhesive drape may be facilitated by overlapping several smaller drapes ensuring all of the seams are tight to avoid leaking.

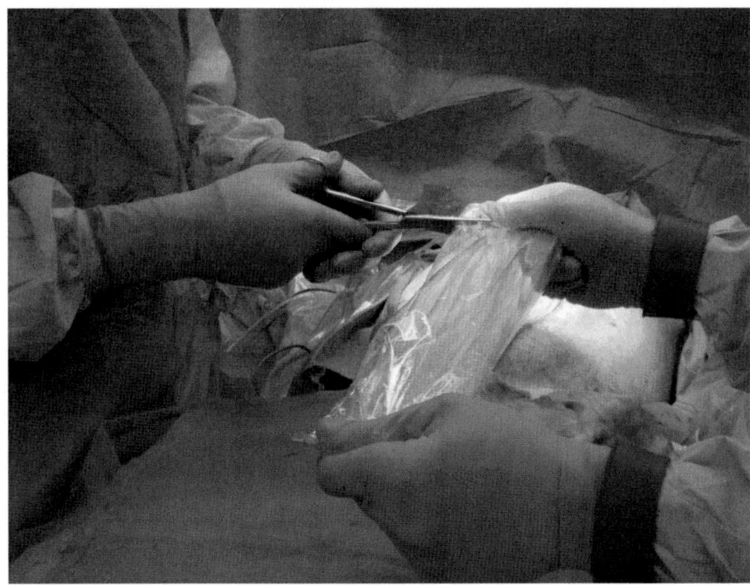

Fig. 42.1 Polyethylene sheet is perforated to allow egress of fluid

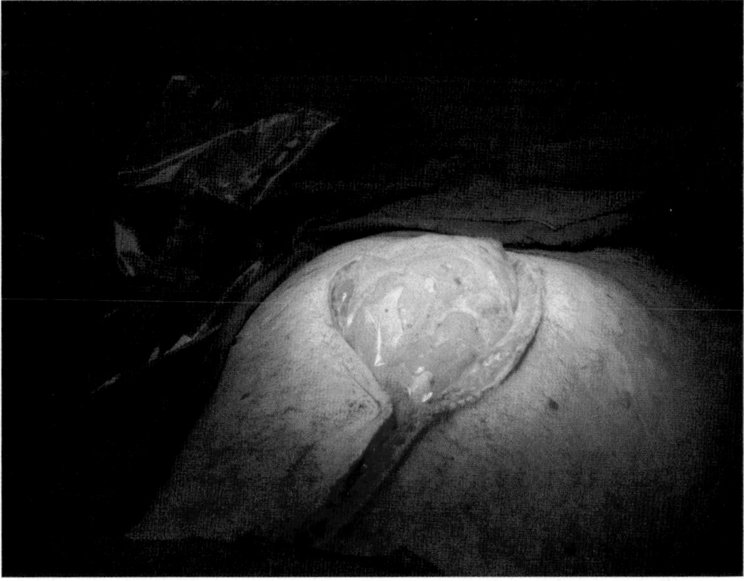

Fig. 42.2 Polyethylene sheet being placed over viscera and tucked into the paracolic gutters

Negative pressure should be quickly applied, either through the commercial adapter or the JP drains, to ensure seal is not lost as fluid begins to collect in the wound and sponge (Figs. 42.5 and 42.6). A KCI vacuum machine is often used to ensure proper constant negative pressure is applied and an adequate seal is maintained. Wall-mounted pressure regulators are used in the case of JP drain application. As pressure is applied, the sponge or towel should compress overlying the wound, more closely approximating the wound edges.

42.3.3 Contraindications

While no absolute contraindications exist for NPWT, caution must be exercised in several specific circumstances. If the negative pressure dressing is placed

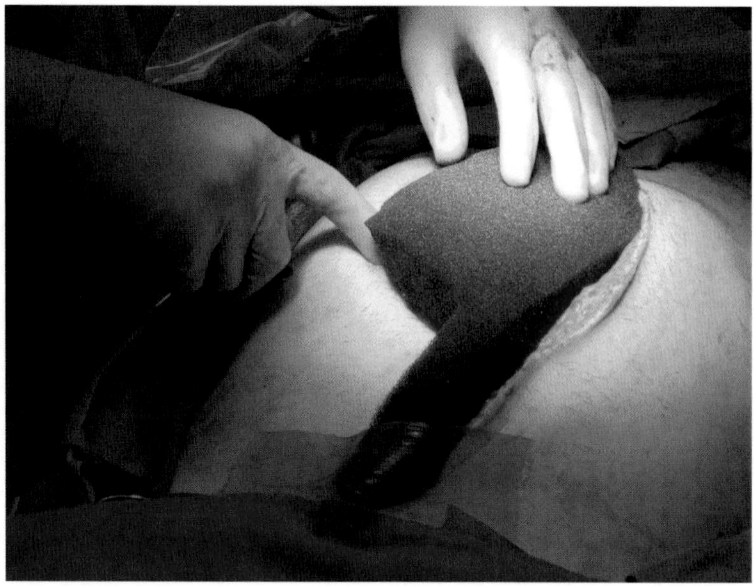

Fig. 42.3 Polyurethane sponge being laid over polyethylene sheet after being cut to size (note fascia has been partial closed with suture in this case)

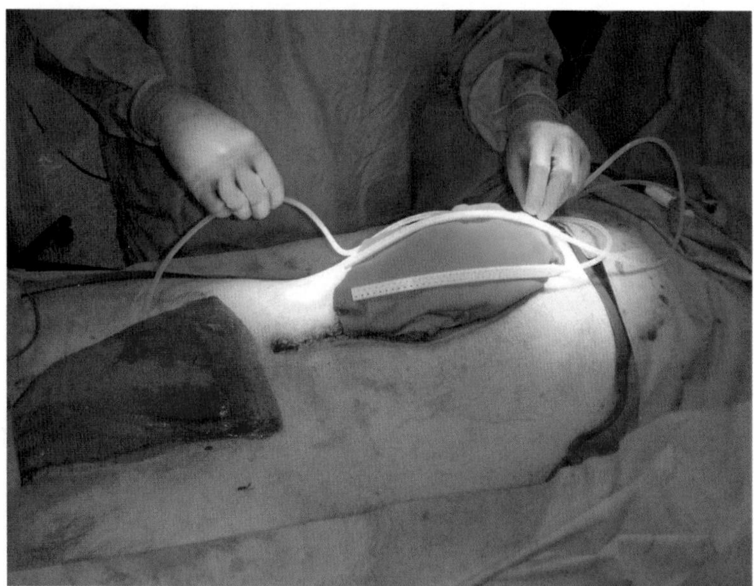

Fig. 42.4 Sterile surgical towel being laid over polyethylene sheet (note fascia has been partial closed with suture in this case)

directly on exposed organs, blood vessels, or vascular grafts, erosion may occur and catastrophic bleeding has been reported [1, 10]. Infection and devitalized tissue should be controlled prior to dressing application. Malignant tissue growth is promoted in the NPWT environment. Care should be taken in patients with fragile skin, as the occlusive dressing may cause skin tearing or necrosis.

42.3.4 Complications

Several complications may occur in the application of NPWT, including a poor seal or an air leak in the dressing, patient pain or discomfort, and fistula formation. Most often, inadequate coverage of the wound edges and application over wet skin will lead to a leak. If left unaddressed, air leaks and

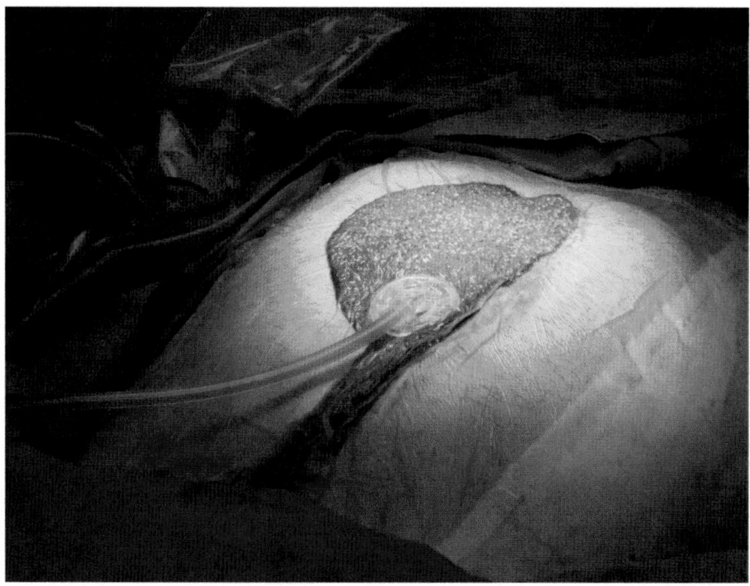

Fig. 42.5 Suction applied to final dressing with V.A.C. sponge (KCI, San Antonio TX)

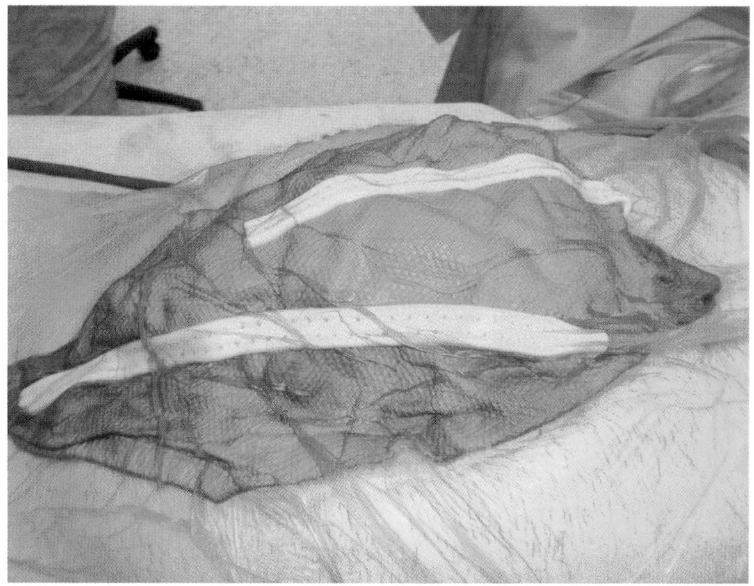

Fig. 42.6 Suction applied to final dressing with sterile surgical towel

poor seals will always worsen and so must be repaired quickly and effectively. Using surgical adhesive and more adhesive, drapes will often allow temporizing of the leak until the next change is scheduled. Occasionally a leak will be best addressed by changing the entire NPWT setup.

Rarely, patients will complain about pain or discomfort while undergoing NPWT. Usually this is associated with dressing changes rather than the NPWT itself. Adequate pain control prior to dressing changes is necessary. If pain occurs while undergoing NPWT, attention should be given to the device itself, ensuring negative pressure is not applied to vital structures or viscera underneath as this could lead to fistula formation or necrosis. Rarely, fistulas may occur if NPWT is applied directly to viscera [9, 11]. Always ensure adequate protection is applied via sponge or towel and bowel bag underneath.

42.3.5 Wound Closure

After temporary closure with NPWT or packing, the patient will be ready for delayed primary closure or permanent closure of the larger deficit using graft or flap. NPWT increases the chances of delayed primary closure in many cases, as NPWT continues to draw the wound edges closer with each vacuum change [11]. Some large soft tissue deficits cannot be closed primarily and must be covered using skin graft or free flap. Frequently, open abdominal wounds are too large to re-approximate and close primarily, and so Vicryl mesh and skin grafting or abdominal free flap must be used [11]. In some cases, abdominal hernia is accepted with correction understood to occur at a later point after the patient is stable [9].

42.4 Summary

The critical care practitioner can expect to be faced with the management of complex wounds on a regular basis. The team has access to a variety of modalities to care for these wounds, and the management plan should be customized for every patient and every wound individually. Factors to consider include patient comorbidities and current state of illness or injury, wound location and size, amount of contamination, presence or risk of compartment syndrome, and the stage of healing of the wound. The optimal dressing should promote an ideal healing environment and should keep the wound warm, moist, and sterile. The dressing should be durable, cost-effective, and well tolerated by the patient both between and during dressing changes.

Team members who care for patients with complex wounds must become familiar with the indications and contraindications in order to select the right dressing for the patient. They should be familiar with the removal and placement of the dressing and be able to troubleshoot and correct problems swiftly and efficiently. Whether dealing with an NPWT dressing on an extremity fasciotomy in a trauma patient, or a towel vac for intra-abdominal sepsis in an emergency general surgery patient, the provider needs to be comfortable and possess the skills to properly care for these complex wounds to optimize healing and improve the overall hospital course of the patient.

References

1. Orgill DP, Bayer LR. Negative pressure wound therapy: past, present and future. Int Wound J. 2013;10(s1):15–9. doi:10.1111/iwj.12170.
2. Putnis S, Khan WS, Wong JM. Negative pressure wound therapy—a review of its uses in orthopaedic trauma. Open Orthop J. 2014;8:142–7. doi:10.2174/1874325001408010142.
3. Robers DJ, Zygun DA, Grendar J, Ball CG, Robertson HL, Ouellet JF, Cheatham ML, Kirkpatrick AW. Negative-pressure wound therapy for critically ill adults with open abdominal wounds: a systematic review. J Trauma Acute Care Surg. 2012;73(3):629–39.
4. Fang R, Dorlac WC, Flaherty SF, Tuman C, Cain SM, Popey TL, Villard DR, Aydelotte JD, Dunne JR, Anderson AM, Powell ET. Feasibility of negative pressure wound therapy during intercontinental aeromedical evacuation of combat casualties. J Trauma. 2010;69 Suppl 1:S140–5. doi:10.1097/TA.0b013e3181e452a2.
5. Hatch QM, Osterhout LM, Ashraf A, Podbielski J, Kozar RA, Wade CE, Holcomb JB, Cotton BA. Current use of damage-control laparotomy, closure rates, and predictors of early fascial closure at the first take-back. J Trauma. 2011;70(6):1429–36. doi:10.1097/TA.0b013e31821b245a.
6. Perez D, Wildi S, Demartines N, Bramkamp M, Koehler C, Clavien PA. Prospective evaluation of vacuum-assisted closure in abdominal compartment syndrome and severe abdominal sepsis. J Am Coll Surg. 2007;205(4):586–92.
7. Anand RJ, Ivatury RR. Surgical management of intra-abdominal hypertension and abdominal compartment syndrome. Am Surg. 2011;77 Suppl 1:S42–5.
8. Miller PR, Meredith JW, Johnson JC, Chang MC. Prospective evaluation of vacuum-assisted fascial closure after open abdomen: planned ventral hernia rate is substantially reduced. Ann Surg. 2004;239(5):608.
9. Miller PR, Thompson JT, Faler BJ, Meredith JW, Chang MC. Late fascial closure in lieu of ventral

hernia: the next step in open abdomen management. J Trauma. 2002;53(5):843–9.
10. White RA, Miki RA, Kazmier P, Anglen JO. Vacuum-assisted closure complicated by erosion and hemorrhage of the anterior tibial artery. J Orthop Trauma. 2005;19(1):56.
11. Defranzo AJ, Pitzer K, Molnar JA, Marks MW, Chang MC, Miller PR, Letton RW, Argenta LC. Vacuum-assisted closure for defects of the abdominal wall. Plast Reconstr Surg. 2008;121(3):832–9. doi:10.1097/01.prs.0000299268.51008.47.

Part X

Special Procedures and Concepts

Inferior Vena Cava Filters Insertion in the Critically Ill

43

Judah Gold-Markel and Marcos Barnatan

43.1 Introduction

The use of inferior vena cava (IVC) filters is a common request in critically ill patients for the prevention of pulmonary embolism (PE). Caval interruption and advent of the IVC filter have progressed rapidly over the past 50 years in conjunction with the innovation of technology in the fields of vascular/endovascular surgery and radiology. The era of the modern optional IVC filter began in the United States in 1973; Lazar Greenfield first described the conical design that formed the basis for modern day design of percutaneous permanent and optional IVC filters. This conical filter was first implanted in humans in the 1980s. Since then there has been a rapid proliferation of multiple types of retrievable IVC filters (see Table 43.1) spurred by industry. As the ease of placement and retrieval has increased, many different specialists including vascular surgeons, interventional radiologists, cardiologists, trauma surgeons, and intensive care specialists have been documented to place these devices [1]. Facilitating this in 2003 and 2004, the United States Food and Drug Administration first approved changes to several permanent filters to permit percutaneous removal/retrievable IVC filters for caval interruption and protection from PE [2]. With this came the increased use of these filters [3] with little clinical data to support or refute the efficacy and safety of retrievable IVC filters. To date there have been no large prospective randomly controlled trials supporting the use of IVC filters [4]. We do know from smaller non-randomized trials and clinical series that the ability to successfully place and retrieve these devices has been shown to be safe and seems to have led to the increased use of them [5]; however, the number of filters actually being retrieved has remained quite low [3,6]. This paper will focus on permanent and optional filters that are defined as IVC filters designed to remain permanently or IVC filters designed to be partially or completely removed, respectively (see Fig. 43.1). The purpose of this paper is to discuss IVC filter technology, its evolution, and the different means of bedside placement of IVC filters in the critically ill.

43.2 Indications

The sole indication for the placement of an IVC filter is to prevent PE and migration of deep venous thrombus by filtration of return blood from the IVC. This is achieved by the trapping of embolic venous clots at the IVC filter prior to their reaching the cardiopulmonary system and causing systemic

J. Gold-Markel, PA-C, MMSc (✉)
• M. Barnatan, MD
Department of Vascular and Endovascular Surgery, Legacy Health System, 501 North Graham Street, Suite 415, Portland, OR 97227, USA
e-mail: jgold@lhs.org; mbarnata@lhs.org

D.A. Taylor et al. (eds.), *Interventional Critical Care*, DOI 10.1007/978-3-319-25286-5_43

Table 43.1 Types of IVC filters

	Types of IVC filters			
Filter	Type	Sheath	Access	Maximum caval diameter
TrapEase (Cordis)	Permanent	6 Fr	Femoral, jugular, antecubital	30 mm
Stainless steel and titanium Greenfield filters (Boston Scientific)	Permanent	12 Fr	Femoral, jugular	28 mm
Bird's Nest (Cook)	Permanent	12 Fr	Femoral, jugular	40 mm
Vena Tech LP and LGM filters (B. Braun)	Permanent	9 Fr	Femoral, jugular	28 mm
Celect (Cook Medical)	Optional	7 Fr	Femoral, jugular	30 mm
OpTease (Cordis)	Optional	6 Fr	Femoral, jugular, antecubital	30 mm
Gunther Tulip (Cook Medical)	Optional	7 Fr	Femoral, jugular	30 mm
Crux (Volcano)	Optional	9 Fr	Femoral, jugular	28 mm
Option (Argon)	Optional	5 Fr	Femoral, jugular	30 mm
Denali (Bard)	Optional	8.4 Fr	Femoral, jugular	28 mm

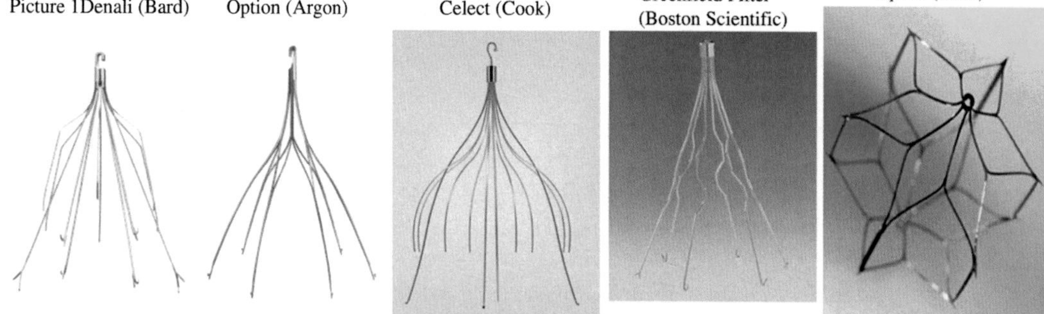

Fig. 43.1 Types of IVC filters

cardiovascular collapse. IVC filters should not be considered a primary treatment for venous thromboembolism (VTE) as it is well documented throughout the literature that pharmacological VTE and the use of external compression devices are the first-line therapy [7]. However, the risk factors of VTE and PE are many and can increase, decrease, or remain at a steady state depending on the patient's condition. Such risk factors include but are not limited to major surgery, trauma, malignancy, morbid obesity, thrombophilia, and acute major illnesses with prolonged inactivity. The placement, duration of IVC filter therapy, and removal of the filter are mitigated by the patient's condition and the ability to treat primarily with systemic anticoagulants.

For many institutions there is no clear consensus on indication and patient selection leading to wide area of standards of practice. This is further influenced by the ever-changing technology around IVC filters that has evolved and the role that industry plays in the market. What is known is that there is a lack of high-quality prospective randomly controlled trials. General consensus breaks the indication for IVC filters down into three categories: absolute, relative, and prophylactic [2]. Absolute indications have a documented VTE/PE and have a contraindication or failure of primary therapy. Relative indications for IVC filters are patients with a documented VTE/PE who are considered at high risk despite primary therapy (VTE/PE with limited pulmonary reserve, large iliocaval thrombus), inability to maintain on primary therapy (poor compliance), or at high risk for anticoagulation (elderly, falls). Prophylactic IVC filters are placed in patients who are felt to be at high risk for VTE and/or PE, but have not yet had a documented incident of either. They are often most likely unable to be started on primary therapy for VTE due to some other significant clinic risk, e.g., need for major surgery, trauma, intracranial hemorrhage, critically ill patients with history of VTE, and inability to anticoagulate.

There has been a noted increase in the use of IVC filters particularly in the realm of prophylactic IVC filters. From 1998 to 2005 the use of IVC filters doubled with the number of prophylactic filters exceeding 21 % [3,5]. Due to the lack of guidelines and rigorous data surrounding IVC filters, several large organizational bodies have come out with their recommendations. Both the Society of Interventional Radiology (SIR) and the Eastern Association for the Surgery of Trauma (EAST) have put out guidelines regarding the indications and the use of IVC filters. The SIR indications are listed below in Table 43.2, while the EAST recommendations simply state that there is no Class I evidence for prophylactic IVC filters; however there is Class II and III evidence, and they note that they recommend placement of an IVC filter in high-risk patients who cannot be anticoagulated [8]. It should be noted in contraindication to this, the American College of Chest Physicians do not recommend prophylactic filters.

Patients in the intensive care unit (ICU) represent an important and select population that may benefit from IVC filter placement. While the indications for IVC filter placement remain the same, these patients tend to be at higher risk for VTE/PE due to many different comorbidities including age, obesity, recent surgeries, trauma, immobility, central venous catheterization, and proinflammatory/prothrombotic states. The ability to achieve full primary pharmacological VTE anticoagulation is difficult due to their multiple comorbidities, impending or recent surgeries, obesity, and metabolism [9].

Table 43.2 SIR indications and contraindications for all vena cava filters (reprinted with permission from Elsevier)

Indications and contraindications for all vena cava filters
Absolute indications (proven VTE)
Recurrent VTE (acute or chronic) despite adequate anticoagulation
Contraindication to anticoagulation
Complication of anticoagulation
Inability to achieve/maintain therapeutic anticoagulation
Relative indications (proven VTE)
Iliocaval DVT
Large, free-floating proximal DVT
Difficulty establishing therapeutic anticoagulation
Massive PE treated with thrombolysis/thrombectomy
Chronic PE treated with thromboendarterectomy
Thrombolysis for iliocaval DVT VTE with limited cardiopulmonary reserve
Recurrent PE with filter in place
Poor compliance with anticoagulant medications
High risk of complication of anticoagulation (e.g., ataxia, frequent falls)
Prophylactic indications (no VTE, primary prophylaxis not feasible[a])
Trauma patient with high risk of VTE
Surgical procedure in patient at high risk of VTE
Medical condition with high risk of VTE
Contraindications to filter placement
No access route to the vena cava
No location available in vena cava for placement of filter

[a]Primary prophylaxis not feasible as a result of high bleeding risk, inability to monitor the patient for VTE, etc.

43.3 Anatomical Considerations

Understanding of the venous system is necessary for safe and efficacious placement of IVC filters. The IVC is the final pathway for blood return to the heart and lungs from the lower extremities, pelvis, and abdomen. The IVC originates at the confluence of the iliac veins around L5 (lumbar) level. It typically runs to the right of the aorta and the right of the vertebral bodies. It has multiple branches from the lumbar veins, and between L1 and L2, the left and right renal veins join the IVC. This divides the IVC into suprarenal and infrarenal segments. In the suprarenal segment, there are typically hepatic branches and then the IVC will go into the right atrial-caval junction. Preprocedural imaging such as CT scans, ultrasounds, or cavagrams should be thoroughly reviewed to assess the anatomical landmarks of the IVC and to note any variations or anomalies.

Knowledge of the most common anatomical variants of the IVC is important when planning for placement of the IVC filter. The most common variants include transposition or a left-sided IVC, duplication of the IVC, and a circumaortic left renal vein. Typically these common anomalies are due to differences in embryological development of the cardinal veins into the mature venous system. The infrahepatic IVC develops between the sixth and eighth weeks in utero. It is a composite structure formed from three paired embryonic veins: the posterior cardinal, the subcardinal, and the supracardinal veins. With the maturation and regression of these veins, the IVC is formed. Persistence of any of these structures can lead to the abovementioned anomalies [10].

Transposition of the IVC is due to the persistence of the left supracardinal vein. It is also recognized as a "left-sided" IVC. Typically it will run to the left of the aorta and then cross over at the junction with the left and right renal veins. It will then join into the atrial-caval junction on the usual right side. Prevalence is felt to be 0.2–0.5 %. Duplication of the IVC is felt to be slightly more common with a prevalence of 0.2–3 % in the general population. This results from a persistence of both supracardinal veins. The duplicated left IVC will typically run into the left renal vein, which will proceed in its normal anatomical tract to join the "normal" right-sided IVC anterior to the aorta. The left-sided or duplicate IVC will typically originate from the left iliac vein. Many times two caval filters will be required to ensure adequate protection from DVT. Finally, the most common variant is the circumaortic left renal vein. This results from the embryological persistence of the dorsal limb of the embryonic left renal vein and of the dorsal arch of the renal collar. It is found in up to 9 % of the population. The superior renal vein receives the left adrenal vein and crosses the aorta anteriorly. The inferior renal vein receives the left gonadal vein and crosses posterior to the aorta approximately 1–2 cm inferior to the normal anterior vein. Care must be taken to place the IVC filter either below the anomalous take off the left renal vein or in a suprarenal position in order to provide adequate protection from DVT embolization [1]. With regard to anatomy within the normal IVC and the iliac veins, there are several other factors that should be noted prior to the placement of an IVC filter. These include length, diameter, and the presence of thrombus within the IVC or iliac veins. Manipulation of the venous system with prior thrombus burden must be undertaken with appropriate precaution.

43.4 Bedside Insertion of Vena Cava Filters

Insertion of the IVC filter has traditionally taken place in the angiography suites, but in critically ill or morbidly obese patients, the option to travel to the angiography suites may not exist. Furthermore, technical consideration of the weight limits on the angiography table must be taken into account for the morbidly obese. The ability to place IVC filters with a portable c-arm using ionizing radiation or the utilization of ultrasound has allowed not only vascular surgeons or interventional radiologists to place these devices but also trauma surgeons, critical care intensivists, and other specialists [3]. More recently the use of both intravascular ultrasound (IVUS) and transabdominal ultrasound has allowed IVC filters to be inserted safely and effectively at the bedside in various settings including the ICU [11]. There is an abundance of literature concerning the practice of bedside IVC filter insertion using portable fluoroscopy, IVUS, or transabdominal ultrasound [12,13]. While there are no established criteria for insertion of IVC filters, there have been some suggestions that the use of bedside insertion of IVC filters has less cost associated with it and reduced risk associated with transportation of critically ill patients [11]. What is established is that the procedure should be done in the setting for which the operator has the most experience and their staff is most experienced to minimize risk of iatrogenic injury, filter misdeployment, or other incidents.

Prior to the insertion of an IVC filter, several aspects need to be considered. First, lab values need to be surveyed. These labs include coagulation markers including prothrombin time, partial thromboplastin time, and international normalized ratio. Abnormal coagulation status does not preclude insertion of the IVC filter and maybe preferred in some circumstances. Renal status should also be assessed as the use of potentially nephrotoxic contrast could be utilized. The patient's creatinine can be used as a marker of their renal status. Different steps can be done to mitigate abnormal lab values from correcting coagulation pathways to extra hydration or limiting the use of contrast for patients with poor renal function. Other techniques such as the use of carbon dioxide instead of nephrotoxic contrast or the use of ultrasound to guide in the placement of the IVC filter can eliminate the need for contrast and has been shown to safe and efficacious [14]. Finally, for critically ill patients, any current medications or drips should be noted as these may affect cardiovascular status, sedation status, and coagulation.

The next step is to review prior imaging. Most patients by the time they have arrived in the ICU will have CT scans. Often a CT scan of the abdomen can be reviewed to locate the renal veins and the infrarenal portion of the IVC in relation to the lumbar vertebral bodies. Also any congenital anomalies of the IVC can be noted at this time. While dependent on many factors such as hydration status and respiratory cycle, the diameter of the IVC can also be measured to determine the presence of a "megacava" greater than 30 mm as there are very few IVC filters indicated for greater than 28 mm. The length of the IVC can be measured to assure the filter will not intrude into the common iliac vein. The presence of thrombus should be noted, as manipulation of the thrombus by instrumentation should be avoided. These steps can also be done at the time of the cavagram.

Selection of access site can now be determined. The most commonly utilized sites include the right femoral vein and the right internal jugular vein. The right femoral vein and right jugular veins are used preferentially as it offers easier access to the IVC and minimizes chances of angulation/tilt of the filter during deployment. Furthermore, the selection of the access site can be dictated by body habitus, the presence of thrombus in the vein, and mechanism of deployment of the device. The use of ultrasonography has improved central venous and vascular access to allow more definitive puncture of the appropriate vessel. Ultrasonography is especially helpful in a challenging situation due to body habitus, anticoagulated patients, or patients with prior surgeries to the access areas.

For bedside fluoroscopic insertion, the use of a portable fluoroscopy machine or "c-arm" with technician is required. A fluoroscopically compatible bed is required to allow ease of movement of the machine and prevent radiopaque regions. Safety concerns within the ICU for radiation exposure must be addressed with proper protective gear and personnel that have been trained in radiation safety. Typical safety items include the use of thyroid and torso protection from radiation. Lead shields or aprons are used to protect the body, and thyroid shields protect the neck region. The use of lead-lined glasses is also recommended to protect the eyes. Healthcare providers should follow their institutions' radiation safety policies. Recent studies suggest that radiation exposure/scatter for healthcare professionals can be kept at levels that are safe and acceptable within the ICU even when routine and invasive procedures are done utilizing ionizing radiation [15]. While beyond the scope of this chapter, the key concepts with regard to radiation safety include fluoroscopic time, distance of personnel and patient from imaging equipment, and suitable garments for radiation protection.

The next step after insertion of the IVC filter deemed necessary at bedside is the "pause" or "time-out" in line with institutional practices. All team members involved in the procedure will review the pertinent aspects of the procedure including identification of the procedure, identification of the patient, relevant laboratory, or diagnostic findings and insuring that the proper materials needed for the procedure are available. Once this is complete the patient is prepped and draped in a sterile manner that allows the access site to be fully visualized. Seldinger technique utilizes standard angiographic needles that allow a wire to be threaded through the needle into the vessel and ultimately the IVC. Typically a 4 or 5 French (Fr) micropuncture needle with guidewire will be utilized for gaining vascular access. This can be further confirmed with ultrasound or under fluoroscopic imaging. A small stab wound incision is made with a #11-blade scalpel to ease insertion of the catheter/sheath. The micropuncture sheath is then placed over the wire. The initial guidewire is then exchanged for a 0.035 in. × 180 cm floppy-tipped or J-tipped wire, and under fluoroscopic imaging the guidewire is placed into the suprarenal portion of the IVC. Next, the micropuncture sheath is removed, and the sheath and dilator for the IVC filter is placed in the distal vena cava around L3 or L4 lumbar bodies. Many IVC filter sheaths and dilators allow for a standard cavagram to be performed and have radiopaque markers allowing for accurate measurement of the IVC. A standard cavagram under digital subtraction fluoroscopy is then preformed using as minimal contrast as needed. Due to volume and diameter of the IVC, this can require 15–30 ml of contrast injected over several seconds. The renal veins are located, and any anatomical anomalies, the presence of thrombus, and dimensions are then taken into account. As mentioned prior the IVC should be measured to determine both the diameter of the cava and its length. Most IVC filters cannot be placed in a cava greater than 28 mm. Any presence of thrombus should be noted, as manipulation of the thrombus by instrumentation should be avoided. The device is selected depending on whether it will be a permanent or optional filter and then placed over a guidewire just caudally from the renal veins and superior to the iliac vein confluence. The guidewire is then removed, and the device is deployed. The venous catheter/sheath is removed, and pressure is maintained until hemostasis is achieved (see Fig. 43.2).

The use of transabdominal ultrasound or IVUS at the bedside has been shown to be safe and efficacious [16]. For both transabdominal ultrasound and IVUS, the limitations to the utilization of this technology lie with experience and expertise of the practitioner and their ability to interpret the imaging. When placing an IVC filter under ultrasound, it is highly recommended to review any preexisting imaging in order to get help gauge relevant landmarks, congenital anomalies, and boney anatomy vis-à-vis the renal caval junction. Placement of IVC filters utilizing transabdominal ultrasonography is very difficult and relatively contraindicated in the morbidly obese due to the difficulty of obtaining reliable imaging of the IVC and renal veins. For placement of the IVC filter using transabdominal ultrasound, standard venous access with Seldinger technique is preformed, and a venous sheath is placed in the femoral vein. The use of the right jugular vein is more difficult due to the inability to track the wire through the right atrium into the IVC in real time. A 0.035 in. guidewire is passed into the IVC under visualization with the ultrasound probe in both longitudinal and transverse axis. The renal veins are found in the transverse axis, and the venous sheath is then advanced just caudal/inferior to the renal veins. The device is then deployed and visualized in both transverse and longitudinal manners with the ultrasound probe. An abdominal x-ray is then obtained to confirm positioning, degree of angulation, and assurance of proper insertion of the device.

For deployment of IVC filters using IVUS, once again it is very dependent on the practitioner being familiar with vascular ultrasound imaging and the IVUS machine. One advantage IVUS has over traditional ultrasonography is that it can be used in the morbidly obese. Both a single stick and double stick method has been described in the literature; however the single stick method seems to be the more prevalent means at this date in time. For the single stick method, access is ideally obtained using Seldinger technique from the right common femoral vein. A radiopaque 8 Fr delivery sheath is then placed over the wire into the femoral vein, and the IVUS catheter is then placed into the suprarenal portion of the IVC. A slow retraction or pullback of the IVUS catheter is then done to assess vascular landmarks. Typically the practitioner will be able to identify both renal veins, the right renal artery running behind the IVC and caudally/inferiorly to the veins (Fig. 43.3). Also identified is the confluence of the IVC and the iliac veins. The renal veins are typically 35–40 cm from the femoral vein access. The iliac confluence is usually 15–20 cm to femoral access. Once the IVUS catheter is positioned

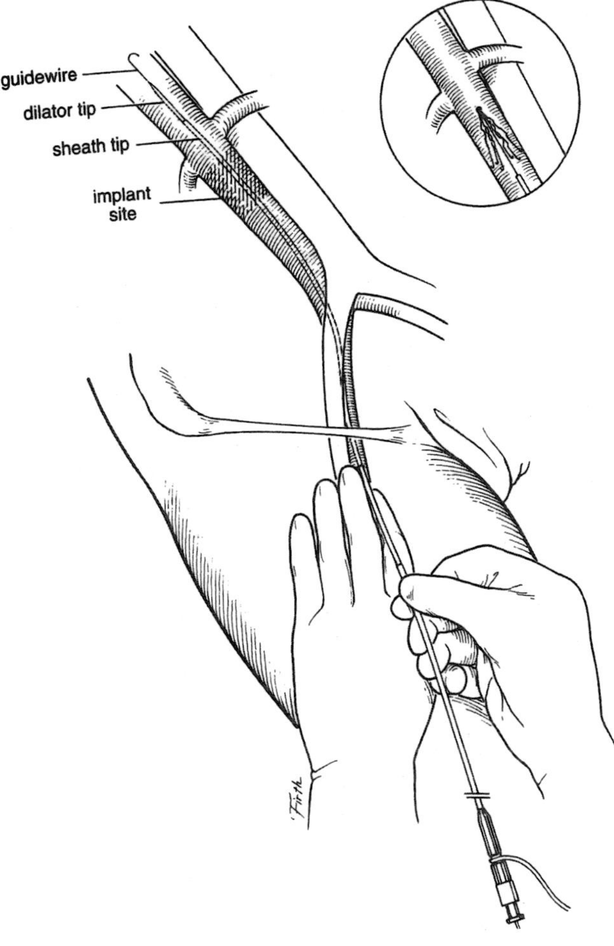

Fig. 43.2 Insertion of an inferior vena cava filter via the right femoral vein (reprinted with permission from Dr. Demetrios Demetriades)

just below the lowest renal vein, the 8 Fr radiopaque sheath is then advanced over the IVUS catheter until the radiopaque tip shadows the ultrasound image of the IVUS catheter. The sheath is then held in that position while the IVUS catheter and wire are removed in a standard pin and pull maneuver. The IVC filter is then passed into position. The IVC filter is placed into the 8 Fr sheath and advanced with a blunt-tipped dilator until the filter is positioned with the top of the filter at the tip of the sheath. The sheath which has not been moved should be just below the renal veins, and the filter is then in the correct position for deployment. The dilator is then held secure with slight forward pressure while the sheath is withdrawn once again utilizing the pin and pull method to deploy the IVC filter in an infrarenal position. Filter position can then be confirmed with a plain abdominal radiograph or through reintroduction of the IVUS over a wire and through a catheter into the IVC (see Fig. 43.4) [17].

43.5 Conclusion

The judicious use of IVC filters and the increased ease of insertion have allowed specialists in different fields of medicine to place IVC filters. The evolution of IVC filter technology has played an integral role in not only the prevention of PEs but also the ability to place them in multiple settings including at the bedside in the critically ill. IVC filters have been shown to be safely and effectively inserted in the critically ill patient at the bedside

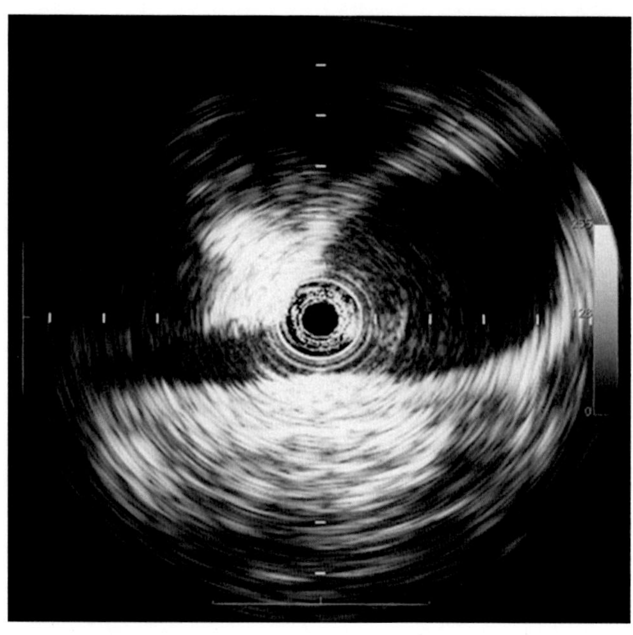

Fig. 43.3 IVUS identification of the right and left renal veins

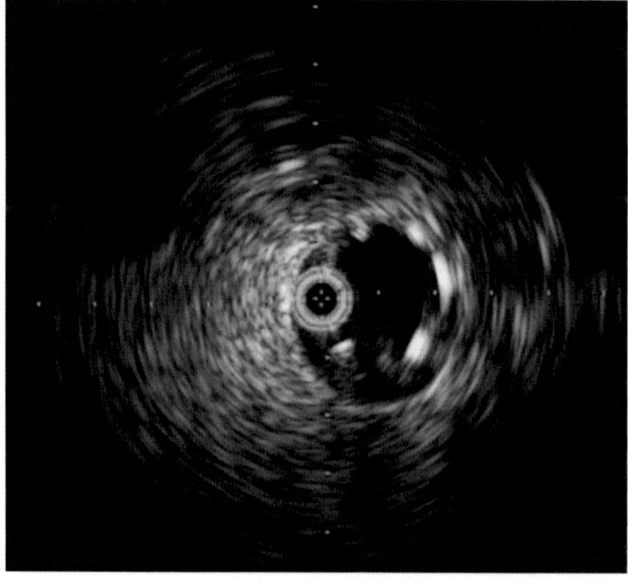

Fig. 43.4 IVUS placement of an inferior vena cava filter (Reprinted with permission from Volcano Corporation)

with either the use of portable fluoroscopy or ultrasound guidance [4]. Indications for placement at bedside include decreasing risks associated with transportation to angiography suites (decreased risk of both venous and arterial line dislodgement, unplanned endotracheal extubations, dislodgement of drains, and the potential risk of hemodynamic instability during transportation) and the theoretical cost savings associated to the patient of doing the procedure at the bedside [4].

References

1. Martin M, Blair K, Curry T, Singh N. Vena cava filters: current concepts and controversies for the surgeon. Curr Probl Surg. 2010;47(7):524–618.
2. Kaufman J, Kinney T, Streiff M, Sing R, Procter M, Becker D, et al. Guidelines for the use of retrievable and convertible vena cava filters: report from the Society of Interventional Radiology Multidisciplinary Consensus Conference. J Vasc Interv Radiol. 2006;17:449–59.
3. Duszak R, Parker L, Levin DC, Rao VM. Placement and removal of inferior vena cava filters: national trends in the medicare population. J Am Coll Radiol. 2011;8(7):483–89.
4. Paton BL, Jacobs DG, Heniford BT, Kercher KW, Zerey M, Sing RF. Nine-year experience with insertion of vena cava filters in the intensive care unit. Am J Surg. 2006;192(6):795–800.
5. Moore P, Andrews JS, Craven TE, Davis RP, Corriere MA, Godshall CJ, et al. Trends in vena caval interruption. J Vasc Surg. 2010;52(1):118–25.
6. Karmy-Jones R, Jurkovich GJ, Velmahos GC, Burdick T, Spaniolas K, Todd SR. Practice patterns and outcome of retrievable vena cava filters in trauma patients: an AAST multicenter study. J Trauma. 2007;62(1):17–25.
7. February 2012; 141(2_suppl) Antithrombotic therapy and prevention of thrombosis, 9th ed: American College of Chest Physicians Evidence-Based Clinical Practice Guidelines. https://www.chestnet.org/Guidelines-and-Resources/Guidelines-and-Consensus-Statements/Antithrombotic-Guidelines-9th-Ed
8. Rogers FB, Cipolle MD, Velmahos G, Rozycki G, Luchette F. Venous thromboembolism: role of vena cava filter in the prophylactic treatment of PE. J Trauma. 2002;53(1):142–64.
9. Pastores SM. Management of venous thromboembolism in the intensive care unit. J Crit Care. 2009;24:185–91.
10. Giordano JM. Embryology of the vascular system. In: Rutherford RB, editor. Rutherford vascular surgery. 6th ed. Philadelphia: Elsevier Saunders; 2005.
11. Haley M, Christmas B, Sing RF. Insertion of inferior vena cava filters by a medical intensivist: preliminary results. J Intensive Care Med. 2009;24(2):144–47.
12. Sing RF, Jacobs D, Heniford BT. Bedside insertion of inferior vena cava filters in the intensive care unit. J Am Coll Surg. 2001;192:570–6.
13. Wellons ED, Rosenthal D, Shuler FW, Levitt AB, Matsuura J, Henderson VJ. Real-time intravascular ultrasound-guided placement of a removable inferior vena cava filter. J Trauma. 2004;57(1):20–3. discussion 23–5.
14. Sing RF, Stackhouse DJ, Jacobs DG, Heniford BT. Safety and accuracy of bedside carbon dioxide cavography for insertion of inferior vena cava filters in the intensive care unit. J Am Coll Surg. 2001;192(2):168–71.
15. Mostafa G, Sing RF, McKeown R, Huyn TT, Heniford BT. The hazard of scattered radiation a trauma intensive care unit. Crit Care Med. 2002;30:574–76.
16. Nunn CR, Neuzil D, Naslund T, Bass JG, Jenkins JM, Pierce R, et al. Cost-effective method for bedside insertion of vena caval filters in trauma patients. J Trauma. 1997;43(5):752–58.
17. Jacobs D, Motaganahalli RL, Peterson BG. Bedside vena cava filter placement with intravascular ultrasound: a simple, accurate, single venous access method. J Vasc Surg. 2007;46(6):1284–6.

Left Ventricular Assist Devices 44

Robert Molyneaux, Nimesh Shah, and Anson C. Brown

Abbreviations

Afib	Atrial fibrillation
Aflutter	Atrial flutter
AI	Aortic insufficiency
AoV	Aortic valve
AVM	Arteriovenous malformation
AVNRT	AV nodal reentry tachycardia
AVRT	AV reciprocating tachycardia
BSA	Body surface area
BTT	Bridge to transplant
CHF	Congestive heart failure
CO	Cardiac output
CPR	Cardiopulmonary resuscitation
CT	Computed tomography
CVP	Central venous pressure
DBP	Diastolic blood pressure
DDAVP	desmopressin
DT	Destination therapy
ECMO	Extracorporeal membrane oxygenation
EKG	Electrocardiogram
EP	Electrophysiology
FDA	US Food and Drug Administration
FRC	Functional residual capacity
IABP	Intra-aortic balloon pump
ICD	Implantable cardiac defibrillator
IVC	Inferior vena cava
IV	Intravenous
LA	Left atrium
LPM	Liters per minute
LV	Left ventricle
LVAD	Left ventricular assist device
LVEDV	LV end-diastolic volume
LVEF	Left ventricular ejection fraction
MAP	Mean arterial pressure
MCS	Mechanical circulatory support
MV	Mitral valve
NYHA	New York Heart Association
PA	Pulmonary artery
PAM	PA mean
PAC	Premature atrial contraction
PAP	PA pressure
PCWP	Pulmonary capillary wedge pressure
PDE	Phosphodiesterase
PVC	Premature ventricular contraction
RA	Right atrium
RPM	Revolutions per minute
RV	Right ventricle
RVAD	Right ventricular assist device
RVEDV	RV end-diastolic volume
RVEF	RV ejection fraction

R. Molyneaux, PA-C (✉)
Procedure Service, Surgical Critical Care Services/MedStar Washington Hospital Center, Washington, DC, USA
e-mail: robert.e.molyneaux@medstar.net

N. Shah, MD
Medical Director Cardiovascular Recovery Room, Surgical Critical Care Services/MedStar Washington Hospital Center, Washington, DC, USA

A.C. Brown, PA-C, MS
Surgical Critical Care Services/MedStar Washington Hospital Center, Washington, DC, USA

D.A. Taylor et al. (eds.), *Interventional Critical Care*, DOI 10.1007/978-3-319-25286-5_44

RVFAC	RV fractional area of change
RVSWI	RV stroke work index
SBP	Systolic blood pressure
SV	Stroke volume
SVT	Supraventricular tachycardia
TAPSE	Tricuspid annular plane systolic excursion
TEE	Transesophageal echocardiogram
TV	Tricuspid valve
TR	Tricuspid regurgitationVAD Ventricular assist device
MRI	Magnetic resonance imaging
WHO	World Health Organization
PH	Pulmonary hypertension
UTI	Urinary tract infection
MRSA	Methicillin resistant *Staphylococcus aureus*
vWF	Von Willebrand factor
LDH	Lactate dehydrogenase
tPA	Tissue plasminogen activator

44.1 Introduction

Patients with one or both failing ventricles are increasingly offered mechanical circulatory support (MCS) with a ventricular assist device (VAD). These may be temporary devices to bridge the acutely ill patient to decisions on continued care, recovery, transplant, or a durable VAD implantation. Patients on a slower decline may be similarly offered a durable left VAD as a bridge to transplant (BTT) or as destination therapy (DT) for those ineligible for transplant. More accurately all of these may be referred to as bridge to decision, as 5 % of durable VAD patients have resolution of the underlying heart failure (myocarditis, peripartum cardiomyopathy) resulting in explants of the device; 17 % of DT patients underwent heart transplant after a mean of 10 months on a left ventricular assist device (LVAD), as secondary renal and hepatic insufficiency resolved. Further, BTT patients may develop stroke or sepsis negating their eligibility for heart transplant [1–4].

Current devices use various methods of providing a continuous flow MCS to assist the failed ventricle. This is in distinction to early devices that relied on pulsatile flow.

This chapter will provide an awareness of types of temporary and durable VADs currently available with the indications for each device. In addition, continuous flow physiology will be presented to help with the management of these patients whether acutely ill, in a postoperative implant period, or presenting with a separate illness.

A significant focus will be placed on the durable devices and their management, as these will be the most likely for the clinician to encounter. Once the physiology is understood, many of the principles of management can be transferred to the temporary device management.

Common complications and their avoidance plus pitfalls in management of these patients will also be addressed.

Finally, we will provide resources available to assist the clinician who is unfamiliar with the devices and physiology or is facing complex challenges that may involve the devices.

44.2 Background

a. The prevalence of congestive heart failure (CHF) is high and likely to go up. Stages 3 and 4 CHF are deadly with a 5-year survival rate of 29 % [5], worse than many types of cancers [6]. MCS devices can lower mortality [7] and improve functional status and quality of life [8–10].
b. Indications
    i. Advanced systolic heart failure from:
        1. Nonischemic cardiomyopathies (NICM)—viral cardiomyopathy, postpartum, amyloid, etc.
        2. Ischemic cardiomyopathy (ICM)
c. Pulsatile MCS is rarely used aside from the intra-aortic balloon pump (IABP). Two exceptions (CorWave disk membrane and tubular membrane pump and C-pulse periaortic cuff) [11, 12] are still in clinical trials: US Food and Drug Administration (US FDA)-approved

devices in commercial use, and almost all others in the US and European trials at this writing now use *continuous* flow LVADs in two pump styles and two intended durations:

i. Temporary: all commercial devices are US FDA approved for up to 6 h for acute decompensating heart failure; however, there are many reports of off-label use of up to 2–3 weeks.
   1. Centri-Mag:
      a. Centrifugal pump flow via a magnetic-levitation (mag-lev) motor with normal speed ranging from 1500 to 5500 revolutions per minute (RPM) and max flows of 9.9 liters per minute (LPM) [4].
      b. Cardiac output (CO) is measured with an in-line probe.
      c. LVAD use requires anticoagulation to avoid arterial embolic phenomena.
      d. Right ventricular assist device (RVAD) use does not require anticoagulation and approved for cardiogenic shock from RV failure up to 30 days [4].
      e. Approved for use to support circulation in short term, while longer-term options are considered. Use as *bridge* to recovery or decision (i.e., durable device, transplant, weaning from cardiopulmonary bypass or withdrawal of care) is in evaluation period [4] (Fig. 44.1).
   2. Impella
      a. Axial pump flow (high velocity Archimedes' screw) ranging from 2000 to 40,000 RPM in 9 gradations of speed.
      b. Three sizes available: 2.5, 2.5 plus, and 5.0 with flows of 2.5, 3.3, and 5 LPM, respectively [8, 9].
      c. Placed in retrograde fashion into the left ventricle (LV) from the aorta via femoral access in a standard arterial catheterization procedure. May be placed in open procedure into the ascending aorta near the innominate bifurcation.
         i. The blood inlet is near the tip of the pump in the left ventricle.
         ii. The blood outlet is in the ascending aorta, with the body crossing the aortic valve (AoV).
      d. May be used for RV failure
         i. Pump flow is reversed compared to LV with inflow at the base in the right atrium and the outflow at the tip in the pulmonary artery.
         ii. FDA approved for up to 14 days based on RECOVER-RIGHT trial [14].
   3. TandemHeart
      a. Centrifugal pump on a hydrodynamic bearing suspended by 10 ml/h saline infusion that lubricates and cools pump.
      b. Pump is external to the patient.
      c. It is placed in venous side [3].
      d. Designed to eject blood within 1.5 revolutions to minimize hemolysis at <5500 RPM.
      e. Transonic flow sensor.
      f. Two insertion options:
         i. Percutaneous: 5 LPM max. Femoral venous access is obtained, and then a cannula is inserted via transseptal procedure across the fossa ovalis to place the tip in the left atrium (LA). Blood is returned to the patient in the femoral artery providing preload reduction and systemic perfusion.
         ii. Surgical: 8 LPM flow max. LV apex or direct LA intake, then outflow returned directly via the aorta. Must be performed in the operating room (Fig. 44.2).

ii. Durable: FDA-approved devices: HeartMate II (BTT and DT) and HeartWare (BTT; DT trials ongoing)
   1. BTT: approved for patients who are listed as candidates for heart transplantation
   2. DT: approved nontransplant candidates with chronic end-stage heart failure (New York Heart Association (NYHA) Class IV LV failure) with LV ejection fraction (LVEF) <25 % and failed pharmacologic management for at least 45 of last 60 days

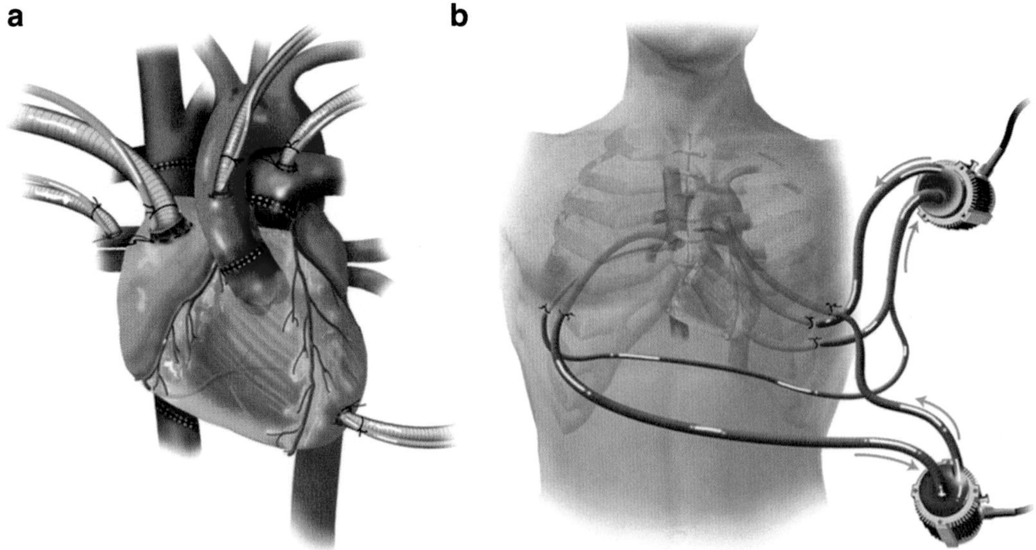

Fig. 44.1 (**a**) Biventricular VAD cannulation; (**b**) CentriMag circuits for both LVAD and RVAD; images A and B reproduced with permission from Kaczorowski et al. [13].

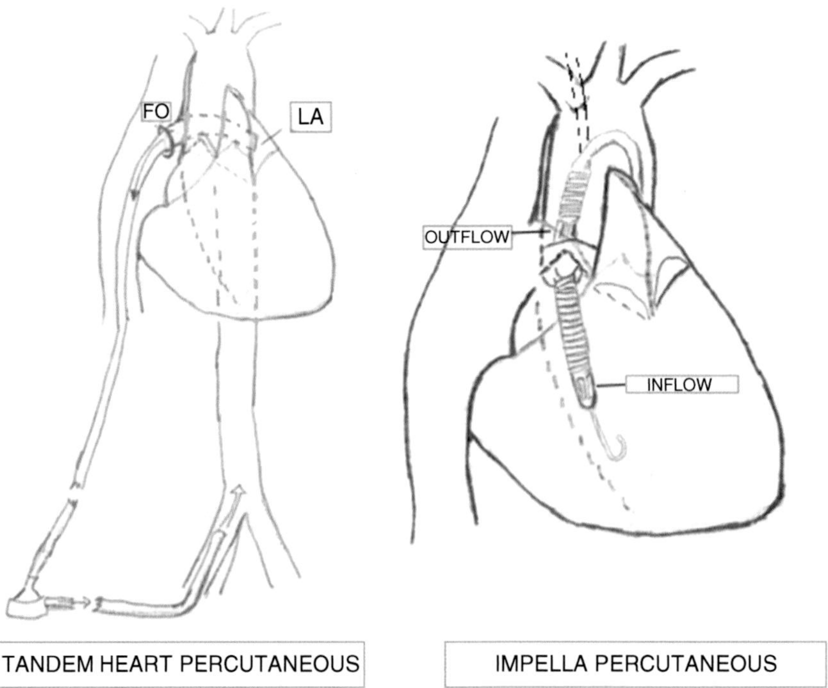

Fig. 44.2 Temporary percutaneous VAD examples. *FO* foramen ovalis, *LA* left atrium. *TandemHeart* percutaneous schematic of inflow through left atrium via atrial septal perforation/foramen ovalis from venous side; *Impella* percutaneous and optional open through ascending aorta approaches

or IABP dependent for 7 days or inotrope dependent for 14 days [15]
3. CO is *calculated* based on a complex algorithm incorporating speed (RPM), power (watts), and hematocrit (accounting for blood viscosity)
4. Can last for >5 years [10]
5. Requires full systemic anticoagulation within days after implant, but can run safely without for the first few postoperative days
6. HeartMate II
   a. Uses axial flow like an Archimedes' screw at 6000–15,000 RPM [16].
   b. Sits on two bearings that can erode.
   c. The implanted pump sits outside of the chest, in a preperitoneal pocket with the driveline tunneled.
7. HeartWare
   a. Uses centrifugal pump flow within a normal range of 2000–3000 RPM [17].
   b. It is a frictionless system in which the impeller floats by magnetic levitation and hydrodynamic thrust. The *hematocrit must be >20 %*, as *higher viscosity is required* to keep the impeller floating [in a conversation with Stephen Boyce, MD. Investigator ADVANCE bridge to transplant trial. 7/24/2014].
   c. The small pump and inflow cannula size allow for pericardial placement and avoid the need for intra-abdominal access.

d. Anatomy of LVAD (or RVAD)
   i. Illustrations (Fig. 44.3). The inflow cannula is placed in the left (or right) ventricular apex, and the outflow cannula is placed in the ascending aorta (or pulmonary artery (PA)). LVAD: apical inflow cannula is directed perpendicular to the plane of the mitral valve (MV) annulus.
   ii. Cannulation bypasses the AoV, that is why some patients have no pulse.

44.3 Physiology (Same for Temporary and Durable)

a. Pulse—the patient with a continuous flow left ventricular device may not have a palpable pulse. As long as the patient has physical signs of adequate blood flow (mentation, appropriate renal function, and warm skin, etc.), it is not a problem and indicates full support by the LVAD. The lack of pulse implies that the AoV does not open during ventricular systole [18–21].
   i. How to check blood pressure without a palpable pulse:
      1. Sphygmomanometer—Korotkoff sounds cannot be heard. Auscultate constant, nonpulsatile blood flow with a Doppler probe over the brachial artery before the cuff is inflated. Starting at a pressure of 130 mmHg, the cuff is manually deflated with the Doppler carefully positioned over the brachial artery.
         a. When the continuous sound is heard, the cuff pressure approximates the mean arterial blood pressure.
         b. This method cannot assess systolic or diastolic blood pressure.
         c. Automated blood pressure cuffs should not be used and are unreliable without a pulse.
      2. Arterial catheter—gold-standard method to measure blood pressure. This invasive method is useful in the immediate postoperative period or when reliable measurements are necessary [22].
         a. Cannulation of the artery must be guided by ultrasound imaging.
         b. Measures mean arterial pressure (MAP).
         c. Systolic blood pressure (SBP).
         d. Diastolic blood pressure (DBP).
         e. A pulsatile waveform on the arterial line tracing should be visualized.
      3. Pulse pressure (SBP—DBP): Even the weakest heart (unless fibrillating) will have some arterial pulsatility due to

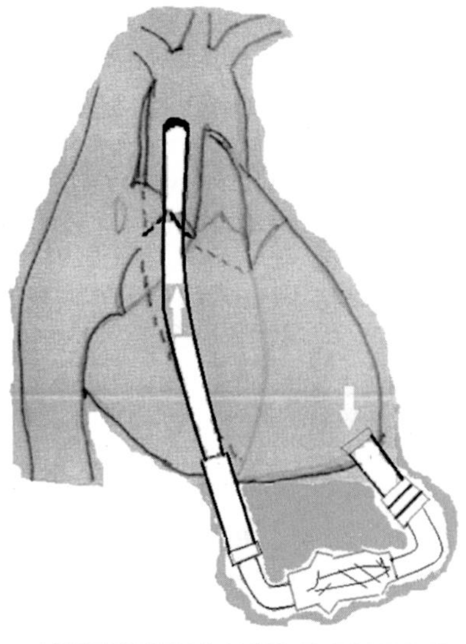

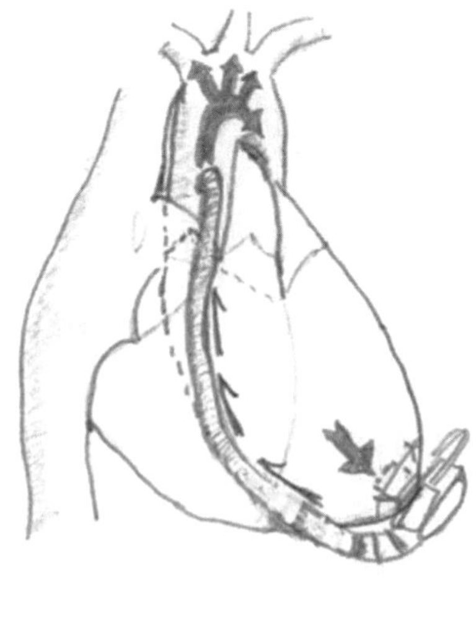

Fig. 44.3 Durable continuous flow LVADs commercially available

systolic contraction. If pulse pressure is larger than 25 mmHg, the AoV is likely opening, but requires confirmation by echocardiography. A small pulse pressure indicates a severely weak left ventricle or excessive RPM.

ii. Pulse oximetry is unreliable without a pulse. Arterial blood gas must be used to confidently determine hemoglobin oxygen saturation.

iii. How to check blood pressure if palpable pulse—this is no different than measuring blood pressure in a patient without an LVAD.

1. Auscultation—listen for Korotkoff sounds with a stethoscope or Doppler to obtain SBP and DBP.
2. Automated noninvasive blood pressure monitor can be used.
3. A palpable pulse implies that the AoV is opening.

b. Blood flow—depends on cardiac loading conditions and underlying myocardial function [17, 19, 23, 24].

i. Pressure vs blood flow (HQ curve) has an inverse relationship as depicted in Fig. 44.4.

1. Head pressure (H) on the ordinate is the difference in aortic pressure (afterload) and LV chamber pressure (preload). Head pressure is the pressure the rotor must generate to pump blood out of the left ventricle.
2. Blood flow (Q) on the abscissa is inversely proportional to the head pressure for a fixed RPM.
3. Preload (i.e., left ventricular pressure) is the greatest determinant of head pressure; higher LV pressure will improve flow through the LVAD.

a. Even severely myopathic left ventricle still follows Frank-Starling curve

i. Increase in LV volume will increase LV systolic contraction (up to a limit of distention).

b. Increased myocardial contraction will increase left ventricular pressure.

4. Afterload (i.e., MAP) also impacts flow; higher MAP will reduce flow through the LVAD.
5. Increase RPM will increase blood flow if there is enough left ventricular preload.

ii. Blood flow through the LVAD is greater during myocardial contraction, and thus it is pulsatile.

a. During systole, left ventricular pressure is higher (i.e., head pressure is lower) and blood flow increases.

i. Blood flow increases during systole with inotropic agents.

b. Pulsatile flow is present even if the AoV is closed.

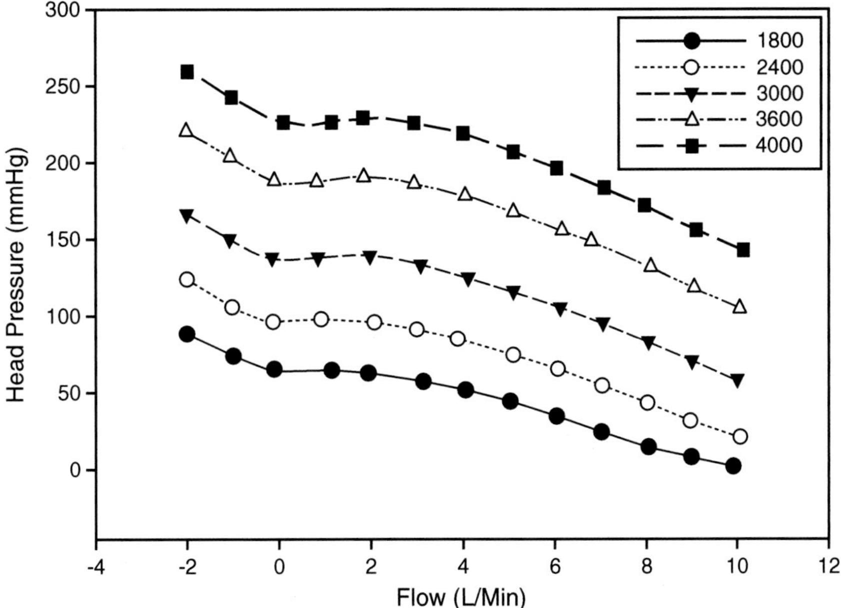

Fig. 44.4 Flow-pressure (HQ) curve for the HeartWare pump at a constant blood viscosity during the entire range of operating speeds in RPM. This HQ curve is used to estimate blood flow. Reproduced with permission from Larose et al. [25]. Adaptations are themselves work protected by copyright. So in order to publish this adaptation, authorization must be obtained both from the owners of the copyright in the original work and from the owner of copyright in the translation or adaptation

c. Power consumption is proportional to blood flow. Energy consumption (i.e., Watts) by the LVAD is higher during systole.

44.4 LVAD Device Parameters

There is only one variable to manipulate for both durable and temporary continuous flow devices—rotor speed (RPM). All other variables displayed by the machine (blood flow, power, and pulsatility index (PI)) are either calculated or measured based on the physiology of the patient [17, 19, 23].

a. Blood flow in LPM—The displayed value may not reflect true total CO related to the patient's physiology and device limitations.
   i. Physiologic conditions related to AoV. Knowledge of the AoV function is compulsory to determine degree of LVAD support. This is best determined by visualization of AoV with echocardiography [26].
      1. AoV opens during systole—the displayed value will underestimate true blood flow.
         a. If AoV is opening then blood travels from the LV into the aorta by a parallel circuit. Blood flows through the LVAD continuously in the cardiac cycle and also ejected through the AoV during systole.
            1. Total CO is sum of the blood flow through the LVAD and AoV. However, it is not easy to assess the actual flow across the AoV.
            2. In steady state, the total CO will equal the venous return to the right heart. Thus, the best approximation of the total CO in the

presence of an opening AoV is by calculation of CO (Fick or thermodilution) with a pulmonary artery catheter.

b. If AoV is closed, then blood flows only through the LVAD and the displayed blood flow is more likely to approximate true CO.

2. AoV insufficiency [27, 28].
   a. Blood flow displayed by the LVAD overestimates the true CO delivered to the body.
      1. AoV insufficiency creates recirculation phenomenon. A portion of the output from the aortic outflow graft will reenter the LV. This leads to heart failure despite adequate function of the LVAD.
      2. Often develops in long-term LVAD implant.
   b. True CO is measured by pulmonary artery catheterization. See Table 44.1 for management.

ii. Inaccuracy of the devices. The durable devices (HeartWare and HeartMate II), the CO is calculated [30, 31].
   i. Each device uses a unique algorithm that integrates Watts and RPM.
      1. HeartMate II algorithm is not accurate.
      2. HeartWare function also depends on blood viscosity and hematocrit also another variable in flow.
      3. Clot in the motor will overestimate blood flow.

b. Power—the value displayed is the actual amount of energy consumed (in Watts) to spin the motor [17, 19, 32].
   i. Power consumption is directly proportional to the amount of blood flow through the LVAD (with one exception). The following device conditions relate to the power consumption:
      1. The more blood flows through the LVAD, the more power is necessary to pump it.
      2. Power usage is higher during systole because more blood flows across the LVAD.
      3. If there is an obstruction of the in inflow or outflow cannula or graft, then less flow will go through the pump and less power will be consumed.
   ii. Exception to the power—blood flow relationship. If a clot is present in the motor itself, power usage will increase for same amount of flow across the LVAD.
      1. High power consumption (>10 Watts) can be a sign of pump thrombus. This is usually accompanied with signs of hemolysis.

c. Pulsatility index (PI)—It represents the contractility of the left ventricle in relation to its loading conditions (preload and afterload) [16, 17, 19, 33].
   i. Calculation.
      1. PI = (peak flow − through flow)/mean flow
   ii. Device differences.
      1. HeartMate II—displayed PI continuously; normal range 3.5–5.5.
      2. PI is not available on temporary devices (i.e., CentriMag).
      3. HeartWare device—the pulsatility is visually represented as flow vs time graph. The PI is not calculated or displayed. Normal flow amplitude is > 4 LPM.
   iii. High pulsatility is seen in the following physiologic conditions.
      a. Increase left ventricular preload.
      b. Myocardial recovery or inotropic medications—this is often accompanied by opening of the AoV (i.e., LV pressure > aortic pressure).
      c. Reduced afterload.
      d. Hyperdynamic states—exercise or sepsis.
   iv. Low pulsatility is seen in the following physiologic conditions:
      1. Reduced LVAD preload from:
         a. Hypovolemia
            i. Bleeding
            ii. Dehydration
         b. RV failure
            i. In setting of existing cardiomyopathy

Table 44.1 Treatment recommendation for early postoperative hemodynamic management

Cardiac index (liters/min/m^2)	MAP (mm Hg)	LV ejection	Primary recommendation	Alternative
<2.2	<65	No	Epinephrine	Dopamine
			Vasopressin	
			Norepinephrine	
		Yes	Increase pump speed	Volume for low CVP
	>65	No	Dobutamine	Milrinone
		Yes	Increase pump speed	
	>90	No	Milrinone	Sodium nitroprusside
		Yes	Nitroglycerin	Nicardipine
			Hydralazine	
>2.2	<65	No	Norepinephrine	Vasopressin
		Yes	Norepinephrine	Vasopressin
	>65 and <90	No	No intervention	
		Yes	No intervention	
	>90	No	Sodium nitroprusside	Milrinone
			Nitroglycerin	Nicardipine
			Hydralazine	
		Yes	Sodium nitroprusside	Nicardipine

CVP central venous pressure, *LV* left ventricular, *MAP* mean arterial pressure

Treatment recommendations in the early post-op period. Feldman et al. [29] Open source document

ii. Existing pulmonary hypertension from chronic LV systolic failure
iii. RV geometry change
    1. Due to ventricular interdependence, the septum shift can change geometry of the tricuspid valve (TV) annulus
        a. Increase TR
    2. Increased venous return—LVAD improves LV ouput and thus increases preload on struggling RV
2. Excessive pump speed
    a. Can contract LV chamber size outpacing preload
3. Inflow cannula malposition
    a. If cannula shifts orientation may get partial occlusion effectively reducing LVAD preload.
    b. Inflow or outflow cannula obstruction (Fig. 44.5).

44.5 Troubleshooting and Complications (Fig. 44.6: Algorithm)

44.6 Complications

a. Early postimplantation LVAD complications
    i. RV dysfunction leading to failure is associated with significant morbidity and mortality after LVAD implantation [34]. Some degree of RV dysfunction should be expected, and therefore, management should be both proactive and preventative [15]. If the patient is decompensating postoperatively, rapid measures to diagnose and treat RV dysfunction should be instituted (note: when RV dysfunction requires prolonged inotropic support and/or inhaled nitric oxide >1 week or RVAD implantation, then it is considered RV "failure") [35].

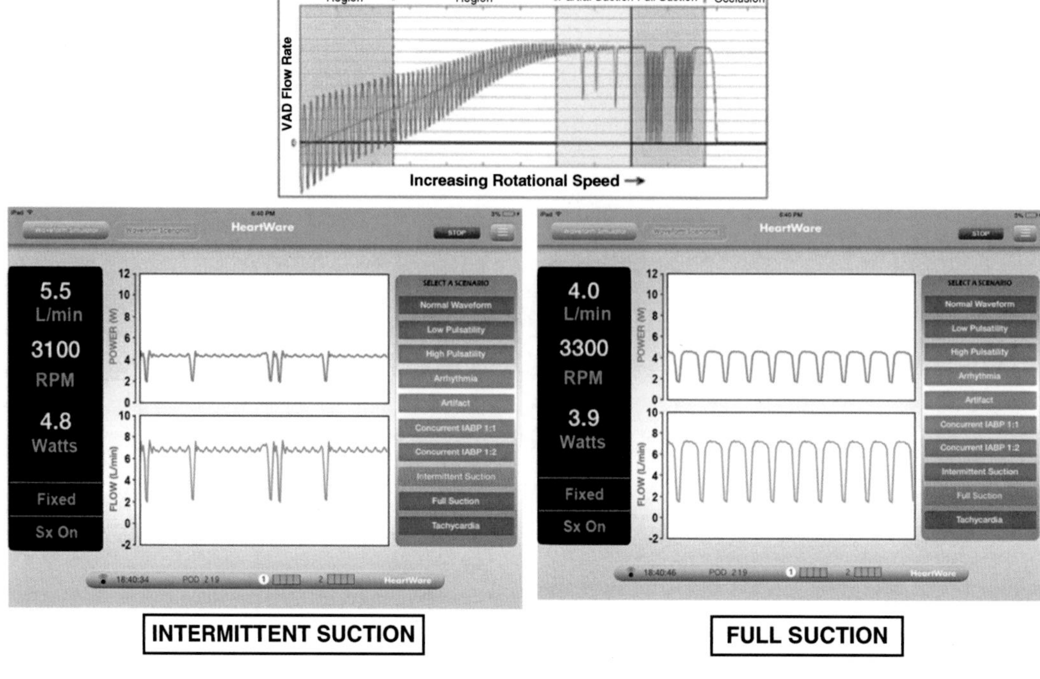

Fig. 44.5 Suction event negative deflection examples. Image permissions from HeartWare

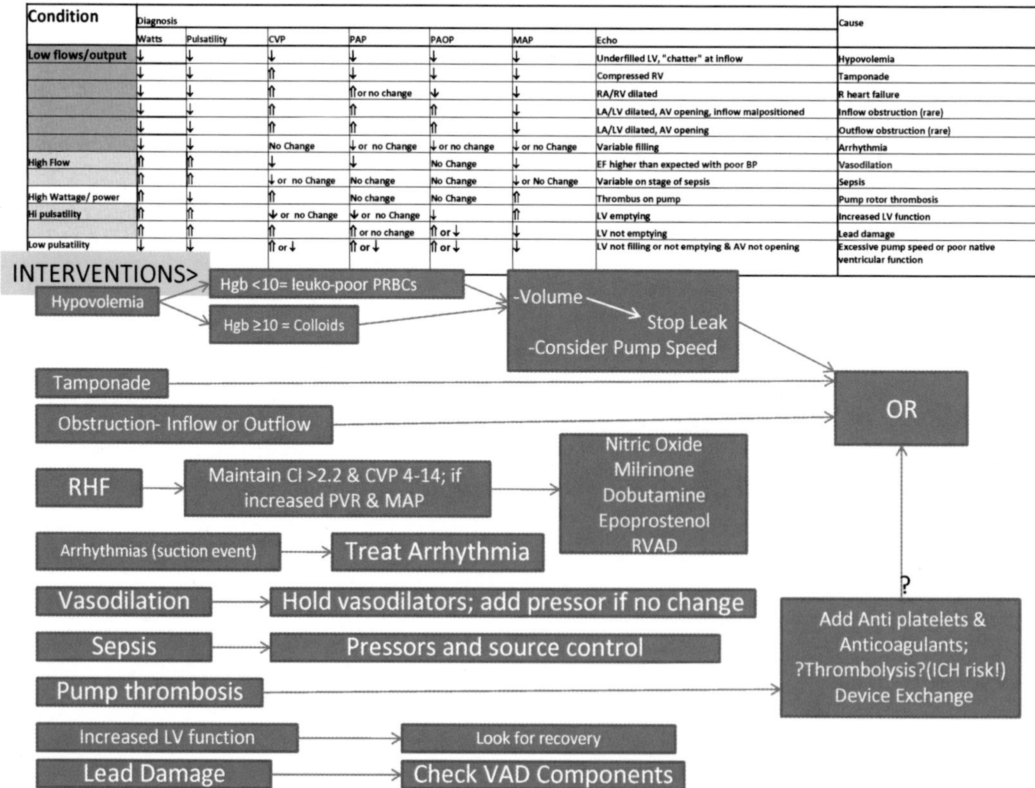

Condition	Diagnosis							Cause
	Watts	Pulsatility	CVP	PAP	PAOP	MAP	Echo	
Low flows/output	↓	↓	↓	↓	↓	↓	Underfilled LV, "chatter" at inflow	Hypovolemia
	↓	↓	⇑	↓	↓	↓	Compressed RV	Tamponade
	↓	↓	⇑	⇑ or no change	↓	↓	RA/RV dilated	R heart failure
	↓	↓	⇑	⇑	⇑	↓	LA/LV dilated, AV opening, inflow malpositioned	Inflow obstruction (rare)
	↓	↓	⇑	⇑	⇑	↓	LA/LV dilated, AV opening	Outflow obstruction (rare)
	↓	↓	No Change	↓ or no Change	↓ or no change	↓ or no Change	Variable filling	Arrhythmia
High Flow	⇑	⇑	↓	↓	No Change	↓	EF higher than expected with poor BP	Vasodilation
	⇑	⇑	↓ or no Change	No change	No Change	↓ or No Change	Variable on stage of sepsis	Sepsis
High Wattage/ power	⇑	↓	⇑	No change	No Change	⇑	Thrombus on pump	Pump rotor thrombosis
Hi pulsatility	⇑	⇑	↓ or no Change	↓ or no Change	↓	⇑	LV emptying	Increased LV function
	⇑	⇑	⇑	⇑ or no change	⇑ or ↓	↓	LV not emptying	Lead damage
Low pulsatility	↓	↓	⇑ or ↓	⇑ or ↓	⇑ or ↓	↓	LV not filling or not emptying & AV not opening	Excessive pump speed or poor native ventricular function

Fig. 44.6 Troubleshooting algorithm. Once cause is determined in matrix, move to flowchart for interventions. Chart adapted from Feldman et al. [29]. Open source document

1. RV function depends largely on septal positioning and LV contraction. As the LVAD decompresses the LV, the septum shifts to the left, thereby increasing RV compliance but decreasing RV contractility [36].
2. Increased CO provided by the LVAD increases right heart venous return, which can overwhelm a chronically dysfunctional RV.
3. Additionally, chronic pulmonary hypertension from left heart failure increases RV afterload.
4. As with any operation requiring cardiopulmonary bypass (CPB), ventricular stunning can occur from inadequate myocardial protection during cardiac diastolic arrest, further contributing to RV dysfunction in the postoperative period.
5. Care should be guided by PA catheter monitoring, as changes in central venous pressure (CVP), CO, and PA pressures can be useful in assessment of RV preload, contractility, and afterload, respectively.
6. Echocardiographic evaluation should be performed intraoperatively and as needed postoperatively to evaluate RV function, chamber size, and ventricular septum position.
7. Focus should be on preventing RV failure, rather than treatment alone.
8. Judicious use of volume infusion immediately postoperatively is prudent as the RV receives increased preload from LV unloading and the RV may become over distended.

ii. Shock (see Table 44.1 and Fig. 44.6)—evidence of malperfusion (oliguria, lactic acidosis, low mixed venous saturation, mottling) in the setting of low CO and/or MAP; patients may have multiple etiologies of shock concomitantly.
   1. Cardiogenic: RV dysfunction.
      a. Diagnostic features
         i. Hemodynamics
            1. High CVP
            2. Evidence of severe TR: On CVP waveform may see large c-v waves with loss of y-decent as the incompetent TV elevates toward the right atrium and atrial filling pressures are increased during ventricular systole
            3. Low pulmonary arterial mean pressure (PAM) (unless chronic pulmonary hypertension)
            4. Low pulmonary capillary wedge pressure (PCWP)
            5. Low CO (thermodilution or Fick method)
            6. Low RV stroke work index (RVSWI). RVSWI = [(mean PAP − mean CVP) × SV]/BSA
         ii. Echocardiogram (transesophageal echocardiogram (TEE) best)
            1. Dilated RV estimated by RV end-diastolic volume (RVEDV)
            2. Reduced RV systolic function evaluated by:
               i. Tricuspid annular plane systolic excursion (TAPSE)
               ii. RV ejection fraction (RVEF)
               iii. RV fractional area change (RVFAC) = (end-diastolic area − end-systolic area)
            3. Moderate to severe tricuspid regurgitation (TR)
            4. Septal bowing toward small LV cavity in systole and diastole
            5. Large inferior vena cava (IVC) (caution as positive pressure from mechanical ventilation alone can cause IVC distention due to increased intrathoracic pressure)
         iii. LVAD
            1. Low PI, power, and flow amplitude (due to the RV's inability to provide LV preload).
            2. "Suction" events (See Fig. 44.5): same as above with additional temporary drop in RPMs due to severely

low LV end-diastolic volume (LVEDV) causing the endocardial tissue to obstruct LVAD inflow. The RPMs will gradually increase back to the set speed.

b. Treatment/intervention
   i. Preload optimization—In the setting of significant preoperative diuresis for acute decompensated heart failure, some volume may be needed postoperatively if low CO/flows associated with low filling pressures; however, for reasons aforementioned, it is common for the RV to become dilated and volume overloaded.
      1. Volume removal—In severe RV dysfunction, hypotension may improve with volume removal as the Frank-Starling curve shifts up and to the left causing increased CO with decreased RV preload.
         i. Diuretics—bolus or continuous dosing
         ii. Ultrafiltration
      2. Avoid excessive infusion of volume by concentrating drips.
      3. Reduce RPM—Decrease the amount of preload returned to RV by decreasing RPM (may reduce CO).
   ii. Afterload reduction.
      1. Pulmonary vasodilators
         a. Inhaled nitric oxide. Significantly reduces pulmonary vascular resistance and may improve LVAD flow [37, 38]
         b. Inhaled prostacyclin: epoprostenol. Can reduce PA pressures but may exacerbate blood loss given its platelet inhibition properties [39]
         c. Intravenous (IV) PDE type 3 inhibitor: milrinone. Can reduce PA pressures but may cause systemic hypotension
         d. IV peripheral arterial and venous dilator: sodium nitroprusside. Caution as causes hypotension and risk of cyanide toxicity
         e. Oral PDE type 5a inhibitor: sildenafil [40]. Can cause systemic hypotension
      2. Techniques of mechanical ventilation
         a. Judicious use of positive pressure ventilation
         b. Attempt to keep lungs at functional residual capacity (FRC) as atelectasis and alveolar overdistention increase pulmonary vasoconstriction
         c. Avoid hypoxemia and hypercarbia, which cause pulmonary vasoconstriction [41]
   iii. Increase contractility.
      1. IV PDE type 3 inhibitor: milrinone
      2. IV Beta agonist
         a. Dobutamine—provides both inotropy and chronotropy to improve CO
         b. Epinephrine—excellent inotrope but may cause lactic acidosis
         c. Isoproterenol—may be better choice if patient has only fixed amount of RV stroke volume, by increasing HR
      3. Improve RV geometry
         a. Reduce LVAD speed if septum shifted leftward and RV is volume overloaded
      4. Coronary perfusion pressure
         a. RV systolic function may improve with increased coronary blood supply.
            i. RV myocardial oxygen delivery dependent on pressure differential of RV chamber pressure and MAP
            ii. RV coronary artery perfusion pressure = MAP − mean RV pressure
            iii. Keep MAP higher particularly if CVP is also high

iv. RVAD or extracorporeal membrane oxygenation (ECMO)—use if severe RV failure not amenable to medical therapy above (i–iii) [42]

2. Hypovolemia or bleeding.
   a. Diagnostic features
      i. Hemodynamics
         1. Low CVP
         2. Low PAP (unless baseline pulmonary HTN)
         3. Low PCWP
         4. Low CI
      ii. Bleeding
         1. In immediate postoperative period, the most likely source is at surgical sites.
            a. Check mediastinal/pleural chest drains for output
            b. New or worsening anemia
      iii. Echocardiography
         1. Small RV and LV chamber sizes
         2. IVC small
      iv. LVAD
         1. Low PI, power, and flow that will improve with volume infusion.
         2. "Suction events" may occur.
   b. Treatment/intervention
      i. IVF in small bolus increments if concern of hypovolemia
      ii. Bleeding
         1. Treat anemia with autologous blood or packed red blood cell transfusions (leukocyte reduced if bridge-to-transplant (BTT) patient). If HeartWare LVAD, adjust hematocrit level on monitor accordingly to ensure accurate flow estimation.
         2. Treat coagulopathy.
         3. Permissive mild hypotension to prevent bleeding exacerbation.
         4. Avoid/treat hypothermia with warming blanket, heated IV fluids, and heated ventilator circuit.
         5. Treat acidosis if pH < 7.25.
         6. Mediastinal exploration is imperative if ongoing bleeding refractory to medical therapy.
3. Cardiac tamponade—blood clot can accumulate anywhere in the pericardium and has compartmentalized compression of any chamber; therefore, the typical "equalization of pressures" is not observed. Ultimately, high suspicion based on the clinical exam and scenario should alert the bedside practitioner of this critical diagnosis.
   a. Diagnosis
      i. Hemodynamics
         1. High CVP
         2. High or normal PCWP
         3. Low CO
         4. Hypotension, gradual or precipitous, and frequently requires high dose vasopressors
      ii. Echocardiography
         1. May see pericardial effusion or clot compressing any chamber
         2. RV/right atrial (RA) collapse during diastole
      iii. LVAD
         1. Low PI, power, and flow that transiently improve or not at all
         2. May have "suction event" if left atrial (LA) compression
4. Vasodilatation—likely cause immediately postoperatively is postcardiac surgery systemic inflammatory response. Sepsis is a consideration but less likely.
   a. Postcardiac surgery systemic inflammatory response syndrome
      i. Diagnosis of exclusion (i.e., ruled out tamponade, RV dysfunction, hypovolemia, sepsis)
      ii. Mediated by complement activation, endotoxin, and cytokine release [43]
   b. Side effects of inotropic medication
      i. PDE3 inhibition of milrinone and beta-2 agonistic effects of

        dobutamine causing vascular smooth muscle relaxation

      ii. Hemodynamics
         1. Low CVP
         2. Low PCWP
         3. Normal to high CO
      iii. Echocardiographic—nonspecific
   c. Sepsis
      i. Consider infection in recent hospitalized patient
         1. Pneumonia if in hospital >48 h [44]
         2. Old central lines

5. Arrhythmia—rhythm optimization is important if perfusion is inadequate.
   a. Atrial (i.e., narrow QRS complex tachycardia, premature atrial contractions (PAC), rarely: supraventricular tachycardia (SVT) with aberrancy causing wide QRS complex)
      i. Etiologies
         1. Atrial fibrillation (Afib) and atrial flutter (Aflutter)—often preexisting; particularly with chronic structural heart abnormalities (dilated atria, valvular disease)
         2. SVT: AV node reentry tachycardia (AVNRT), AV reciprocating tachycardia (AVRT), atrial tachycardia—may be new onset or known history of SVT exacerbated by critical illness and inotropic/chronotropic medications
      ii. Diagnosis
         1. Atrial electrogram: touch epicardial atrial wire to ECG surface lead and discern any organized atrial activity; if there is no discernable atrial rhythm, then likely Afib
         2. ECG or telemetry
      iii. Treatment
         1. Pharmacologic cardioversion—if adequate perfusion but new onset Afib, can use amiodarone IV bolus and/or continuous infusion to achieve sinus rhythm.
         2. Synchronized cardioversion—if SVT or new onset Afib or Aflutter with inadequate perfusion (decrease MAP, CO, LVAD PI, power, and flow).
         3. Rate control—can use amiodarone to slow the rapid ventricular response [45].
         4. Avoid calcium channel blockers and beta-blockers in acute period as they are negative inotropes.
         5. Correct electrolyte derangements.
         6. Maze procedure (long-term possibility).
   b. Ventricular (i.e., wide QRS complex tachycardia, premature ventricular contractions (PVC))
      i. Etiologies
         1. Underlying cardiomyopathy (often have implantable cardioverter defibrillator (ICD) preoperatively)
         2. Arrhythmogenic inotropic medications
         3. Suction events if RV failure, hypovolemia, excess RPM, LVAD malposition
         4. Aberrant myocardial depolarization from LVAD insertion site
         5. Electrolyte derangements
      ii. Diagnosis
         1. EKG and telemetry
         2. LVAD waveform and history screen—look for suction events and low flow alarms
         3. May need electrophysiology (EP) consultation for mapping and potential ablation (rarely done in the acute setting after LVAD)
         4. If suspicion for LVAD cannula malposition can get chest

computed tomography (CT), cardiac magnetic resonance imaging (MRI), or TEE

iii. Treatment

1. Antiarrhythmics (usually amiodarone and lidocaine are safest in setting of low EF).
   a. Any other antiarrhythmic should have EP consultation (dofetilide, mexiletine).
2. Wean or change inotropes if possible.
3. If related to suction events, treat underlying cause (i.e., RV failure, hypovolemia, etc.) and consider decreasing RPMs.
4. Correct electrolyte derangements.

b. Late postimplantation LVAD complications

i. After months, the RV becomes a passive conduit for blood into the LV. RV systolic function generally does not improve much, but the pulmonary vascular resistance improves (assuming it was World Health Organization (WHO) group 2 pulmonary hypertension (PH)); i.e., Fontan physiology; thus RV failure tends not to be an issue for late problems post-LVAD implantation [46, 47].

ii. Shock.

1. Aortic insufficiency (AI)—over time as MAP (i.e., aortic pressure) is greater than LV chamber pressure, it places the AoV in an unnatural pressure gradient and contributes to AI.
   a. Mitigate this by gradually decreasing RPMs so that the AoV opens regularly during the post-perioperative period.
      i. Diagnosis
         1. Echocardiogram-regurgitant flow across AoV
      ii. Treatment
         1. When AoV develops AI, it is difficult to manage.
            a. Creates recirculation phenomenon
               i. Recirculation may get worse if flow/RPM increased.
               ii. Lowering RPM may contribute to worsening CHF.
         2. Transplant.

2. Sepsis
   a. Etiologies
      i. Driveline infection—characterized by erythema, warmth along the subcutaneous driveline tract, may have fluctuance or draining fluid around the site
         1. Use CT scan and u/s to see fluid pockets.
      ii. Pump pocket infection—deeper-seated infection
      iii. Bloodstream infections
         1. Can be from central lines or other organ systems
         2. Thorough exam for source
      iv. Pneumonia
      v. Any reason to get infected (e.g., urinary tract infection (UTI), skin/soft tissue structure, joint implant)
   b. Diagnosis
      i. Culture data
   c. Treatment
      i. Assume that the LVAD patient is colonized with nosocomial pathogens and should get initial empiric abx coverage for methicillin-resistant Staphylococcus aureus (MRSA), Pseudomonas, and common local nosocomial organisms.
      ii. Tailor antibiotics to sensitivities and pathogen as soon as possible.
      iii. Must have source control: Any concern should be treated quickly and aggressively so not to contaminate LVAD.
         1. Pump pocket and driveline—debridement.
         2. Bloodstream infections—pull out infected catheter or

treat through if not able to remove.
3. Surgical excision of infected area or incision and drainage of any collection of suspect fluid in body.
iv. May need to increase anticoagulation (increased thrombosis in setting of infection).
3. Bleeding
   a. Usually arteriovenous malformations (AVMs)—LVAD develop AVM likely related to continuous flow physiology.
      i. GI bleed—can be common and requires endoscopy and may require surgical intervention
      ii. Nose bleeds—rarely requires packing or embolization
   b. Acquired von Willebrand factor (vWF) deficiency—shear stress contributes to breakdown of vWF multimers.
      i. Stop antiplatelet agents
      ii. Desmopressin (DDAVP)
      iii. Cryoprecipitate (contains vWF)
   c. Blood products.
      i. Be mindful of status (BTT vs DT). BTT does not want to acquire sensitization to blood products.
      ii. When in doubt, use leukoreduced blood products.
4. Clotting
   a. Pump thrombosis
      i. Diagnosis
         1. Evidence of hemolysis (high lactate dehydrogenase (LDH) and plasma free hemoglobin)
         2. High power surges
         3. Multislice CT scan with contrast
         4. Evidence of embolic phenomena
      ii. Treatment
         1. Antiplatelet tagents (Eptifibatide[Integrilin])
         2. Antifibrinolytics (low-dose tissue plasminogen activator (tPA))
         3. Increased anticoagulation (particularly in setting of infection)
         4. Device exchange

iii. Stroke.
   1. Hemorrhagic—predisposed because on anticoagulation ± aspirin
      a. Also associated with MAP >90; to avoid hemorrhagic strokes, LVAD patients should have good BP control.
      b. Aggressive reversal of anticoagulants.
      c. Neurosurgical evaluation if appropriate.
   2. Ischemic—occurs about 10 % of patients
      a. Etiologies
         i. Embolic—atrial fibrillation, pump thrombus, or clot at AoV
         ii. Atherosclerotic disease
            1. Carotid
            2. Intracranial
         iii. Hypoperfusion

iv. Cardiac arrest—generally traditional chest compression cardiopulmonary resuscitation (CPR) is not performed for patients who have LVADs. The algorithm does not apply here as many LVAD patients do not have palpable pulse.
   1. Chest compressions are not advised if arrest is not related to device malfunction.
      a. If there is some power output from the LVAD, flow must be going across the pump and other reversible etiologies should be sought [17, 19].
      b. Chemical medications, cardioversion, and treatment of underlying process should be instituted without chest compressions. Case reports of abdomen show only CPR is successful [48].
   2. If device malfunction is suspected, CPR is appropriate
      a. Fractured driveline.
      b. Pump thrombosed.
      c. CPR does risk dislodgment of cannulation sites.

v. Fractured driveline

1. Etiologies include, but not limited to:
   a. Motor vehicle collisions and accidental movement
   b. Rough housing/wrestling/falls
   c. Malfeasance/suicide attempt
2. Complex problem. Refer to tertiary care center that has active VAD program. May require:
   a. Explant with implant of new device
   b. Heart transplant—may move patient up on list.
   c. Termination of LVAD support or withdrawal of intervention

44.7 Resources: Where to Get Help

Patients and families are trained and experienced in the function and features of their VAD and should be considered a first-line resource when able. The patient's clinical center where the device was placed typically has a team member on-call at all times. They may facilitate support at the closest qualified center as well. Below is North American contact information for device manufacturers. Outside of North America, company websites typically guide you to your region for local contact information:

Berlin Heart, Inc. Telephone: 281-863-9700 http://www.berlinheart.de/index.php/kontakt/content/kontakt_berlin_heart_us

HeartWare, HVAD, MVAD. 24 Hour Clinical/Technical Support US: (888) HW-INFO-5 or (888) 494-6365. http://www.heartware.com/contact-us

Jarvik Heart, Jarvik 2000. Phone (212) 397-3911 **http://www.jarvikheart.com/home.asp?id=Contact**

MicroMed, DeBakey VAD: assumed by ReliantHeart (see below)

MiTiHeart Corporation, MTIHeartLVAD. Phone: 301-869-9720 http://mitiheart.com/#/contact-us/4556245704

ReliantHeart—formerly MicroMeds HeartAssist 5(US investigational use only) Phone: (713) 592-0913. http://reliantheart.com/about/contact-us/

Sunshine Heart, C-pulse. Phone +1 952 345 4200 http://www.sunshineheart.com/contact-us/

Terumo, DuraHeart. Phone: 800-803-8385 http://www.terumoheart.com/us/index.php/contact

Thoratec—HeartMate series XVE, II, and III;PVAD, IVAD, VentrAssist (formerly made by Ventracor). Customer Service & Technical Support: HeartLine™ (800) 456-1477 http://www.thoratec.com/about-us/contact-us.aspx

Acknowledgement The authors would like to acknowledge Steven Boyce, MD of MedStar Heart and Vascular Institute and Alexandra Pratt, MD of MedStar Washington Hospital Center Surgical Critical Care Services for their review and input on this chapter.

References

1. Wilson SR, Mudge Jr GH, Stewart GC, Givertz MM. Evaluation for a ventricular assist device: selecting the appropriate candidate. Circulation. 2009;119(16):2225–32. Epub 2009/04/29.
2. Miller LW, Guglin M. Patient selection for ventricular assist devices: a moving target. J Am Coll Cardiol. 2013;61(12):1209–21. Epub 2013/01/08.
3. TandemHeart escort controller 510(k) summary. August 2006. http://www.accessdata.fda.gov/cdrh_docs/pdf6/K061369.pdf. Accessed 14 July 2014.
4. Thoratec Centrimag and PediMag Blood Pump Fact Sheet. http://www.thoratec.com/downloads/CentriMag_Product_Fact_Sheet-B100-0812.pdf. Accessed 11 June 2014.
5. Cleland JG, Gemmell I, Khand A, Boddy A. Is the prognosis of heart failure improving? Eur J Heart Fail. 1999;1(3):229–41. Epub 2000/08/10.
6. Heart failure patients living longer, but long-term survival still low. 2013. http://newsroom.heart.org/news/heart-failure-patients-living-longer-but-long-term-survival-still-low. Accessed 15 May 2013.
7. Starling RC, Naka Y, Boyle AJ, Gonzalez-Stawinski G, John R, Jorde U, et al. Results of the post-U.S. Food and Drug Administration-approval study with a continuous flow left ventricular assist device as a bridge to heart transplantation: a prospective study using the INTERMACS (Interagency Registry for Mechanically Assisted Circulatory Support). J Am Coll Cardiol. 2011;57(19):1890–8. Epub 2011/05/07.
8. 510(k) Summary Imepella 2.5 Plus. 2012. http://www.accessdata.fda.gov/cdrh_docs/pdf11/k112892.pdf. Accessed 14 July 2014.
9. 510(k) Summary Impella 5.0. 2009. http://www.accessdata.fda.gov/cdrh_docs/pdf8/K083111.pdf. Accessed 14 July 2014.

10. Starling RC. Advanced heart failure: transplantation, LVADs, and beyond. Cleve Clin J Med. 2013;80(1):33–40. Epub 2013/01/05.
11. CorWave. www.corwave.com. Accessed 14 July 2014.
12. C-Pulse Heart Assist System. www.sunshineheart.com/c-pulse/. Accessed 14 July 2014.
13. Kaczorowski DJ, Datta J, Kamoun M, Dries DL, Woo YJ. Profound hyperacute cardiac allograft rejection rescue with biventricular mechanical circulatory support and plasmapheresis, intravenous immunoglobulin, and rituximab therapy. J Cardiothorac Surg. 2013;8:48. doi:10.1186/1749-8090-8.
14. ABIOMED press release. http://investors.abiomed.com/releasedetail.cfm?sh_print=yes&releaseID=893135. Accessed 29 January 2015.
15. Slaughter MS, Pagani FD, Rogers JG, Miller LW, Sun B, Russell SD, et al. Clinical management of continuous-flow left ventricular assist devices in advanced heart failure. J Heart Lung Transplant. 2010;29(4 Suppl):S1–39. Epub 2010/02/26.
16. Griffith BP, Kormos RL, Borovetz HS, Litwak K, Antaki JF, Poirier VL, et al. HeartMate II left ventricular assist system: from concept to first clinical use. Ann Thorac Surg. 2001;71(3 Suppl):S116–20. Discussion S4–6. Epub 2001/03/27.
17. Larose JA, Tamez D, Ashenuga M, Reyes C. Design concepts and principle of operation of the HeartWare ventricular assist system. ASAIO J. 2010;56(4):285–9. Epub 2010/06/19.
18. Potapov EV, Loebe M, Nasseri BA, Sinawski H, Koster A, Kuppe H, et al. Pulsatile flow in patients with a novel nonpulsatile implantable ventricular assist device. Circulation. 2000;102(19 Suppl 3):III183–7. Epub 2000/11/18.
19. HeartMate II LVAS Left Ventricular Assist System [Operating Manual]. Thoratec Corporation. 2013. http://www.thoratec.com/_assets/download-tracker/103884F-HMII-LVS-Operating-Manual.pdf. Accessed 22 July 2014.
20. Christensen DM. Physiology of continuous-flow pumps. AACN Adv Crit Care. 2012;23(1):46–54. Epub 2012/02/01.
21. Myers TJ, Bolmers M, Gregoric ID, Kar B, Frazier OH. Assessment of arterial blood pressure during support with an axial flow left ventricular assist device. J Heart Lung Transplant. 2009;28(5):423–7. Epub 2009/05/07.
22. Bennett MK, Roberts CA, Dordunoo D, Shah A, Russell SD. Ideal methodology to assess systemic blood pressure in patients with continuous-flow left ventricular assist devices. J Heart Lung Transplant. 2010;29(5):593–4. Epub 2010/01/12.
23. Butler KC, Dow JJ, Litwak P, Kormos RL, Borovetz HS. Development of the Nimbus/University of Pittsburgh innovative ventricular assist system. Ann Thorac Surg. 1999;68(2):790–4. Epub 1999/09/04.
24. Hayward CS, Salamonsen R, Keogh AM, Woodard J, Ayre P, Prichard R, et al. Effect of alteration in pump speed on pump output and left ventricular filling with continuous-flow left ventricular assist device. ASAIO J. 2011;57(6):495–500. Epub 2011/10/13.
25. LaRose JA, Tamez D, Ashenuga M, Reyes C. Design concepts and principle of operation of the HeartWare ventricular assist system. ASAIO J. 2010;56:285–9. doi:10.1097/MAT.0b013e3181dfbab5.
26. Rasalingam R, Johnson SN, Bilhorn KR, Huang PH, Makan M, Moazami N, et al. Transthoracic echocardiographic assessment of continuous-flow left ventricular assist devices. J Am Soc Echocardiogr. 2011;24(2):135–48. Epub 2011/01/18.
27. May-Newman K, Enriquez-Almaguer L, Posuwattanakul P, Dembitsky W. Biomechanics of the aortic valve in the continuous flow VAD-assisted heart. ASAIO J. 2010;56(4):301–8. Epub 2010/06/19.
28. Tuzun E, Rutten M, Dat M, van de Vosse F, Kadipasaoglu C, de Mol B. Continuous-flow cardiac assistance: effects on aortic valve function in a mock loop. J Surg Res. 2011;171(2):443–7. Epub 2010/09/11.
29. Feldman D, Pamboukian SV, Teuteberg JJ, Birks E, Lietz K, Moore SA, et al. The 2013 International Society for Heart and Lung Transplantation Guidelines for mechanical circulatory support: executive summary. J Heart Lung Transplant. 2013;32(2):157–87. Epub 2013/01/29.
30. Lund LH, Gabrielsen A, Tiren L, Hallberg A, El Karlsson K, Eriksson MJ. Derived and displayed power consumption, flow, and pulsatility over a range of HeartMate II left ventricular assist device settings. ASAIO J. 2012;58(3):183–90. Epub 2012/03/08.
31. Ozbaran M, Yagdi T, Engin C, Nalbantgil S, Ayik F, Oguz E, et al. New circulatory support system: heartware. Transplant Proc. 2012;44(6):1726–8. Epub 2012/07/31.
32. Kikugawa D. Motor current waveforms as an index for evaluation of native cardiac function during left ventricular support with a centrifugal blood pump. Artif Organs. 2001;25(9):703–8. Epub 2001/11/28.
33. Jacquet L, Vancaenegem O, Pasquet A, Matte P, Poncelet A, Price J, et al. Exercise capacity in patients supported with rotary blood pumps is improved by a spontaneous increase of pump flow at constant pump speed and by a rise in native cardiac output. Artif Organs. 2011;35(7):682–90. Epub 2011/05/28.
34. Kormos RL, Teuteberg JJ, Pagani FD, Russell SD, John R, Miller LW, et al. Right ventricular failure in patients with the HeartMate II continuous-flow left ventricular assist device: incidence, risk factors, and effect on outcomes. J Thorac Cardiovasc Surg. 2010;139(5):1316–24. Epub 2010/02/06.
35. Holman WL. Interagency Registry for Mechanically Assisted Circulatory Support (INTERMACS): what have we learned and what will we learn? Circulation. 2012;126(11):1401–6. Epub 2012/09/12.
36. Pratt AK, Shah NS, Boyce SW. Left ventricular assist device management in the ICU. Crit Care Med. 2014;42(1):158–68. Epub 2013/11/19.
37. Kukucka M, Potapov E, Stepanenko A, Weller K, Mladenow A, Kuppe H, et al. Acute impact of left ventricular unloading by left ventricular assist device on the right ventricle geometry and function: effect of

nitric oxide inhalation. J Thorac Cardiovasc Surg. 2011;141(4):1009–14. Epub 2010/10/05.
38. Argenziano M, Choudhri AF, Moazami N, Rose EA, Smith CR, Levin HR, et al. Randomized, double-blind trial of inhaled nitric oxide in LVAD recipients with pulmonary hypertension. Ann Thorac Surg. 1998;65(2):340–5. Epub 1998/03/04.
39. Groves DS, Blum FE, Huffmyer JL, Kennedy JL, Ahmad HB, Durieux ME, et al. Effects of early inhaled epoprostenol therapy on pulmonary artery pressure and blood loss during LVAD placement. J Cardiothorac Vasc Anesth. 2014;28(3):652–60. Epub 2013/10/10.
40. Tedford RJ, Hemnes AR, Russell SD, Wittstein IS, Mahmud M, Zaiman AL, et al. PDE5A inhibitor treatment of persistent pulmonary hypertension after mechanical circulatory support. Circ Heart Fail. 2008;1(4):213–9. Epub 2009/10/08.
41. Balanos GM, Talbot NP, Dorrington KL, Robbins PA. Human pulmonary vascular response to 4 h of hypercapnia and hypocapnia measured using Doppler echocardiography. J Appl Physiol. 2003;94(4):1543–51. Epub 2002/12/17.
42. Scherer M, Sirat AS, Moritz A, Martens S. Extracorporeal membrane oxygenation as perioperative right ventricular support in patients with biventricular failure undergoing left ventricular assist device implantation. Eur J Cardiothorac Surg. 2011;39(6):939–44. Discussion 44. Epub 2010/11/13.
43. Wan S, LeClerc JL, Vincent JL. Inflammatory response to cardiopulmonary bypass: mechanisms involved and possible therapeutic strategies. Chest. 1997;112(3):676–92. Epub 1997/10/07.
44. American Thoracic Society, Centers for Disease Control and Prevention, Infectious Diseases Society of America. American Thoracic Society/Centers for Disease Control and Prevention/Infectious Diseases Society of America: controlling tuberculosis in the United States. Am J Respir Crit Care Med. 2005;172(9):1169–227. Epub 2005/10/27.
45. Clemo HF, Wood MA, Gilligan DM, Ellenbogen KA. Intravenous amiodarone for acute heart rate control in the critically ill patient with atrial tachyarrhythmias. Am J Cardiol. 1998;81(5):594–8. Epub 1998/03/26.
46. Salzberg SP, Lachat ML, von Harbou K, Zund G, Turina MI. Normalization of high pulmonary vascular resistance with LVAD support in heart transplantation candidates. Eur J Cardiothorac Surg. 2005;27(2):222–5. Epub 2005/02/05.
47. Zimpfer D, Zrunek P, Roethy W, Czerny M, Schima H, Huber L, et al. Left ventricular assist devices decrease fixed pulmonary hypertension in cardiac transplant candidates. J Thorac Cardiovasc Surg. 2007;133(3):689–95. Epub 2007/02/27.
48. Rottenberg EM, Heard J, Hamlin R, Sun BC, Awad H. Abdominal only CPR during cardiac arrest for a patient with an LVAD during resternotomy: a case report. J Cardiothorac Surg. 2011;6:91. Epub 2011/07/19.

45 Extra Corporal Membrane Oxygenation and Extracorporeal Life Support

Jon Van Horn

45.1 Introduction

Extracorporeal membrane oxygenation (ECMO) is the cornerstone therapy of extracorporeal life support (ECLS) which encompasses all of the care of the critically ill or injured patient in need of oxygenation when conventional therapies are failing. ECMO itself involves the cannulation of the central circulation, siphoning of the blood into a closed circuit, external oxygenation and removal of CO_2, and return of the blood to the patient (Fig. 45.1). ECMO has been utilized in neonates for many years, but is being increasingly utilized in the adult population, and this will be the primary focus of this chapter. Early decisions can be lifesaving in those with cardiogenic shock, massive pulmonary insult due to trauma or infection, or refractory acute respiratory distress syndrome. In the adult population, ECMO has been historically viewed as a bridge to transplant, but more recently, it is being used as a bridge to recovery after the initial insult has resolved.

The main goals of ECMO are:

- Oxygenation and removal of CO_2 from the circulating blood and subsequent delivery to coronary vessels and tissues.
- Myocardial rest
- Continued efforts during ECMO to ventilate, clearance of secretions, and oxygen supplementation using conventional techniques [1]

Relative contraindications include:

High-pressure ventilation (plateau airway pressures over 30 cm of water) for more than 7 days

High Fraction of Inspired Oxygen (FIO_2) requirements (over 80 % for more than 7 days)

Limited vascular access

Inability to accept blood products

Any condition or organ dysfunction that would limit the likelihood of overall benefit from ECMO, such as severe, irreversible brain injury or untreatable metastatic cancer

Patients who cannot be anticoagulated

Absolute contraindications include:

Patients with irreversible organ damage and multiorgan failure or those who are not candidates for transplantation will usually not benefit from ECMO support.

Severe aortic regurgitation or aortic dissections are contraindications for venoarterial (VA) ECMO.

45.2 Initiation of Therapy

The mode of ECMO is determined largely by the underlying organ system affected and the degree of hemodynamic stability. Primary respiratory

J. Van Horn, MPAS, PA-C, FAASPA (✉)
Trauma Services, Legacy Emanuel and Randall Children's Hospital, Portland, OR, USA
e-mail: jvanhorn@lhs.org

D.A. Taylor et al. (eds.), *Interventional Critical Care*, DOI 10.1007/978-3-319-25286-5_45

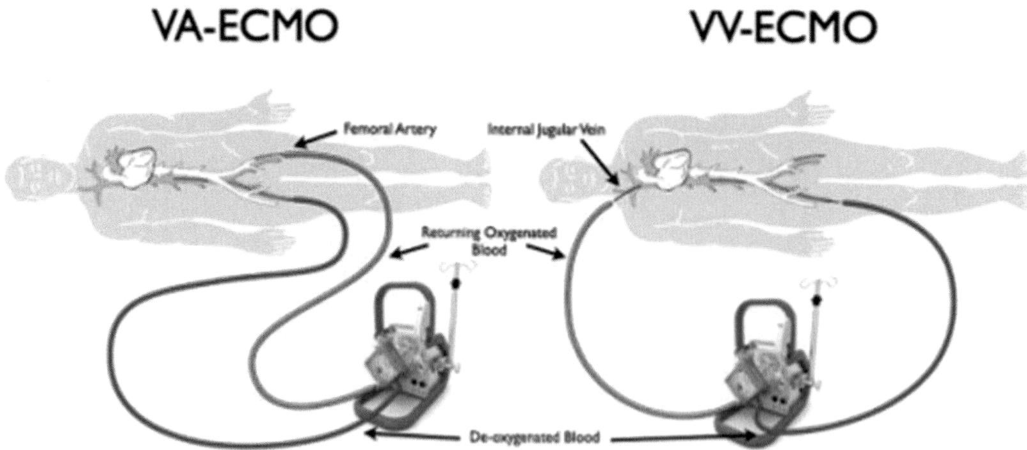

Fig. 45.1 ECMO techniques

failure with hemodynamic stability can be managed with venovenous (VV ECMO). Cardiac failure and hemodynamic instability should be managed with VA ECMO support. This will determine the cannulation sites chosen and subsequent direction of flow.

Blood draining from central venous circulation determines pump preload, and this limits pump flow, regardless of the type of perfusion used. The amount of gas exchange across the oxygenation membrane is known as the "sweep rate."

Cannula sizes are chosen that will allow:
120 ml/kg/min for neonates
90 ml/kg/min for pediatrics
50–60 ml/kg/min for adults (see Percutaneous Cannulation for sizes)

The shortest length and largest diameter cannula should be chosen to reduce resistance to flow. This is best determined by the rated flow capacity of the ECMO lung compared to the flow rates intended for the patient. Arterial cannula should be large enough to allow for calculated flow and to avoid high circuit pressures and blood shearing due to excessive flow through narrow cannula.

45.3 Modes

45.3.1 Venovenous

VV ECMO is "in series" with native circulation (blood is siphoned, oxygenated/CO_2 removed, and returned before leaving the right side of the heart) (Fig. 45.1).

45.3.2 Venoarterial

VA ECMO is "in parallel" to native circulation and is true cardiopulmonary bypass as blood is siphoned, oxygenated/CO_2 removed, and returned to the arterial side of the circulatory system (Fig. 45.1).

45.4 Neonates/Pediatrics

A single-site double-lumen cannula is placed in the right internal jugular and advanced to the level of the right atrium (Fig. 45.2). A newer cannula technique (Avalon, Inc.) utilizes two drainage lumens (1 IVC, 1 SVC) and a single return lumen directed at the tricuspid valve. Although this technique provides excellent flow with minimal recirculation, it requires echocardiography or fluoroscopy for optimal placement and may

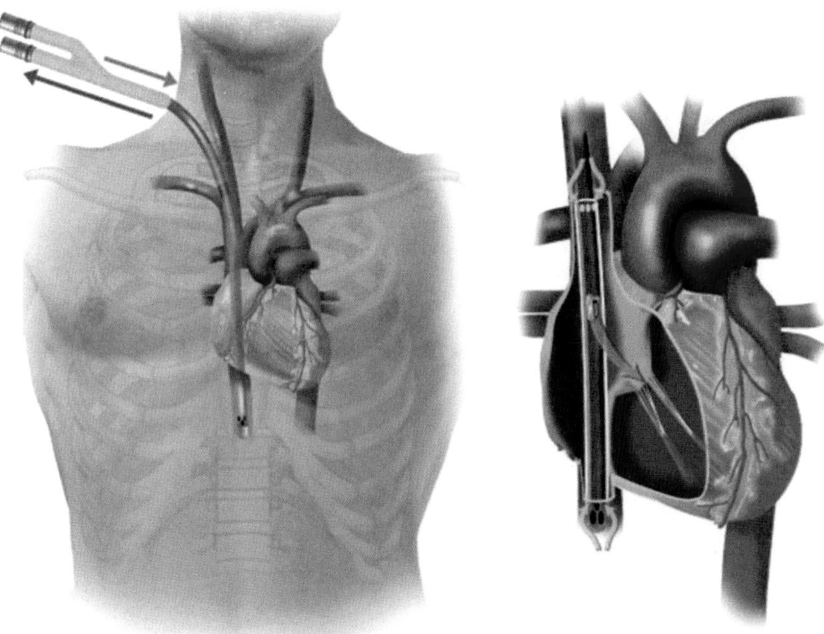

Fig. 45.2 Single-site, double-lumen cannulation

limit its use if these modalities are not available. This technique has seen increased use in adults with the development of adult-sized cannulae.

45.5 Adult Patients

These patients usually require two-site cannulation unless as described above for single-site cannulation. Cannulae are usually placed in the right internal jugular and either right or left femoral vein for VV and femoral artery for VA. Alternate sites are discussed later. The direction of flow is determined by the ECMO physician and is based on anatomical factors (obesity, vessel size, etc.) that would impact the ability to siphon sufficient blood to meet the patient's oxygenation demands.

45.6 Open Chest Cannulation

For those patients who undergo open heart surgery and are unable to be weaned off of the bypass circuit, there is indication for central cannulation (Fig. 45.3). In this technique, the aortic and right atrial cannula is directly connected to the ECMO circuit in VA flow. The chest is then covered and the cannulae are secured to the patient.

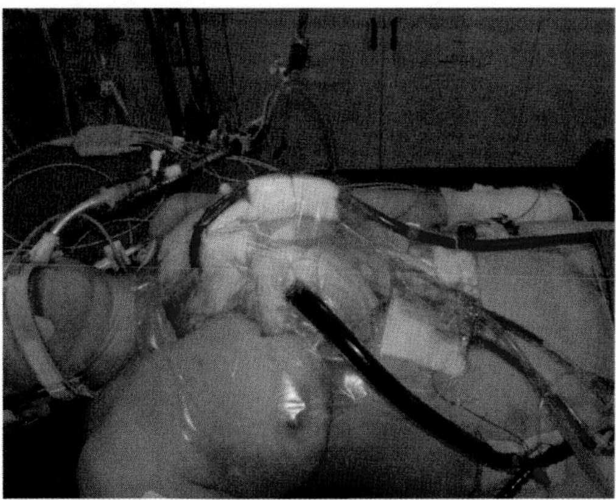

Fig. 45.3 Open chest cannulation

45.7 Open Cannulation/Direct Visualization

If time allows, CT angiography of vessels should be reviewed prior to cannulation (Fig. 45.4). For those patients that are noted to have severe

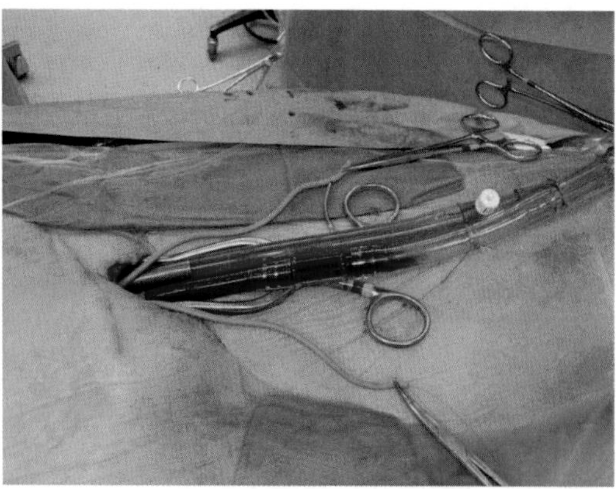

Fig. 45.4 Open femoral cannulation

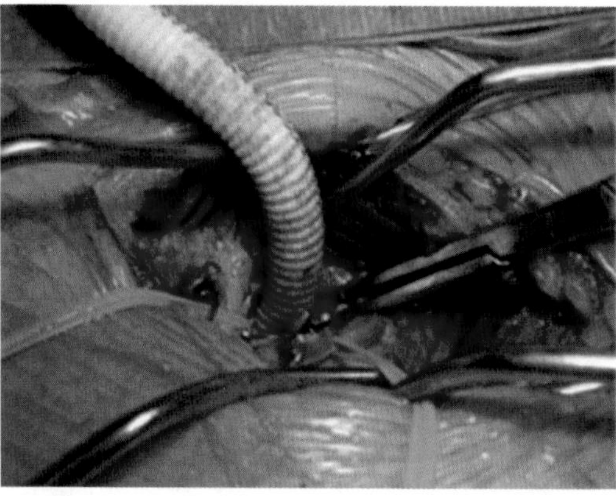

Fig. 45.5 "Stovepipe" cannulation

peripheral artery disease or other contraindication for femoral cannulation, axillary cannulation using a side graft of Dacron sewn to the artery allows cannulation by "stovepipe" and reduces risk of limb ischemia (Fig. 45.5). After removal of the cannula, a "diamond" patch of Dacron is used to repair the artery to reduce risk of future stenosis.

45.8 Percutaneous Cannulation Procedure

Step 1: Get your gear—initial setup and preparation

- Quiet down the room.
- Prep the patient with full-barrier, sterile scrub and drapes.

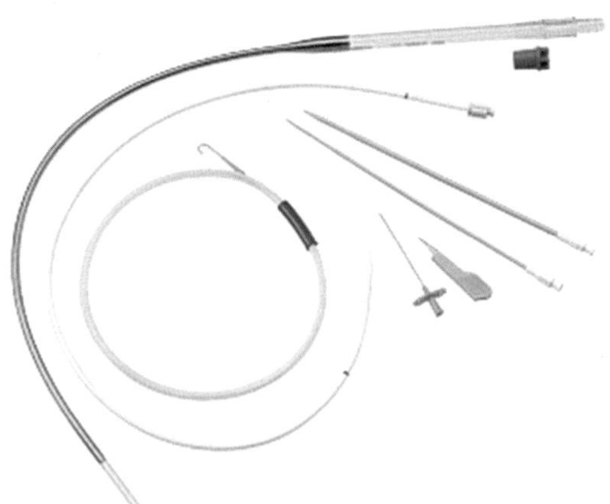

Fig. 45.6 Cannulation kit

- Heparinize the patient: 3000–5000 units (100 units/kg).
- Fill a large, sterile bowl with NS and have a 60 cc bulb syringe ready for cannula irrigation and flushing.
- Initial vascular access.
  - Be efficient: While setting up the circuit and the team is gathering supplies, start by obtaining vascular access (Fig. 45.6).
  - Initial access: Place a right femoral CVC, a left femoral a-line, and a right IJ CVC under ultrasound guidance. If you already have an a-line, you can suture a femoral arterial wire in place for future use.
  - At this time, also determine any other lines that need placement and determine site of access (arterial, CVC, or PA catheter) (Fig. 45.7).
  - Pitfall: Not placing these lines under ultrasound guidance, as we all know, in the critically ill or critically hypoxic patient, arterial blood can look the same color as venous blood. Don't count on appearance alone. Even using a pressure column can be misleading.
  - Double check: Confirm wire placement in the lumen of the vessel.
- Cannulation Equipment
  - Cannulae

    Venous cannulae: sizes range from 23–29 French steel wire reinforced

    Arterial cannulae: sizes range from 19–21 French steel wire reinforced

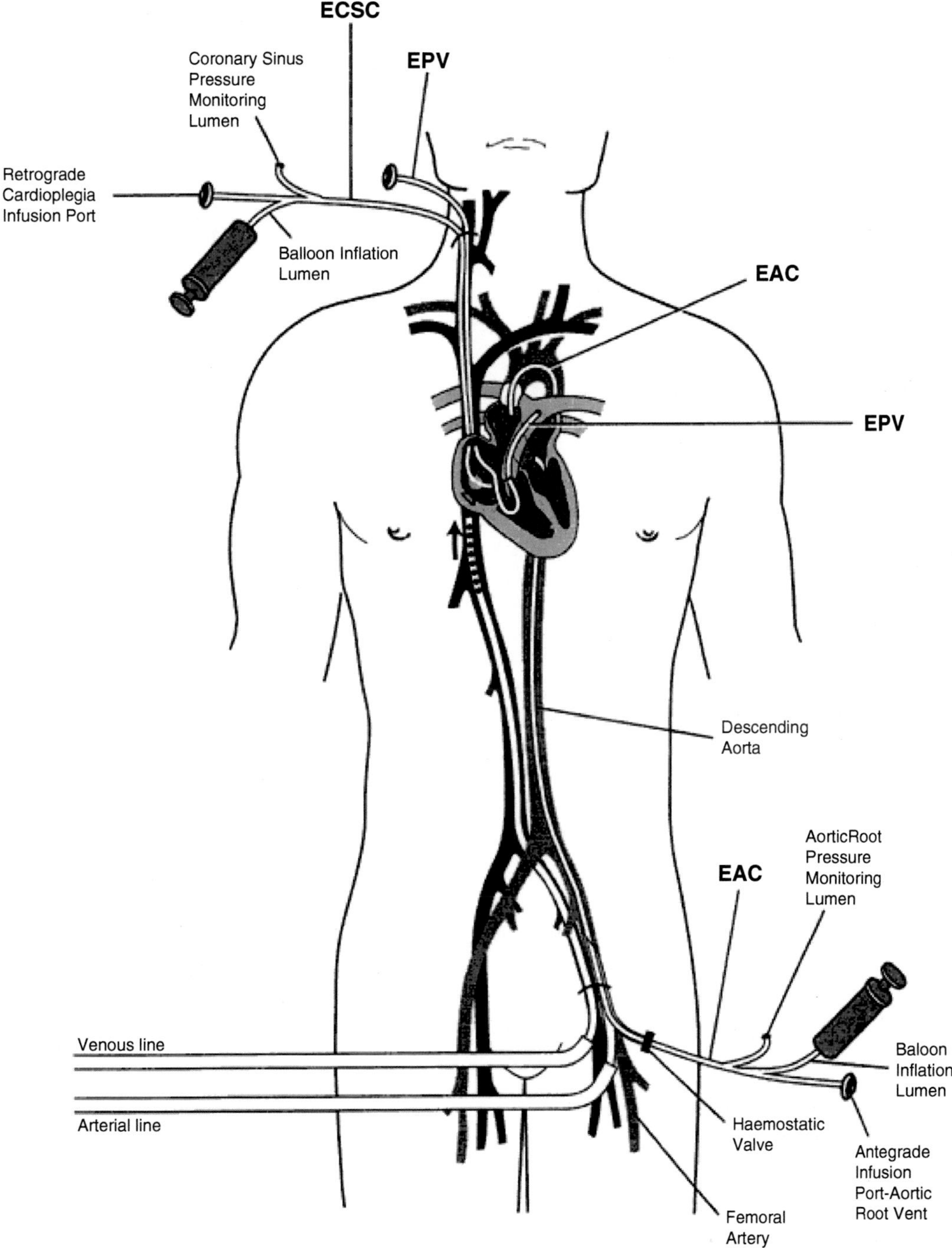

Fig. 45.7 Venous and arterial access needs

Different insertion lengths: range from 15–55 cm (depending on manufacturer) (Fig. 45.8)

Lock introducer

The size of the venous cannula directly determines blood flow. The largest possible venous cannula should be used to maximize flow and easily achieve target output:

- Some will choose cannula size on flow goals alone.

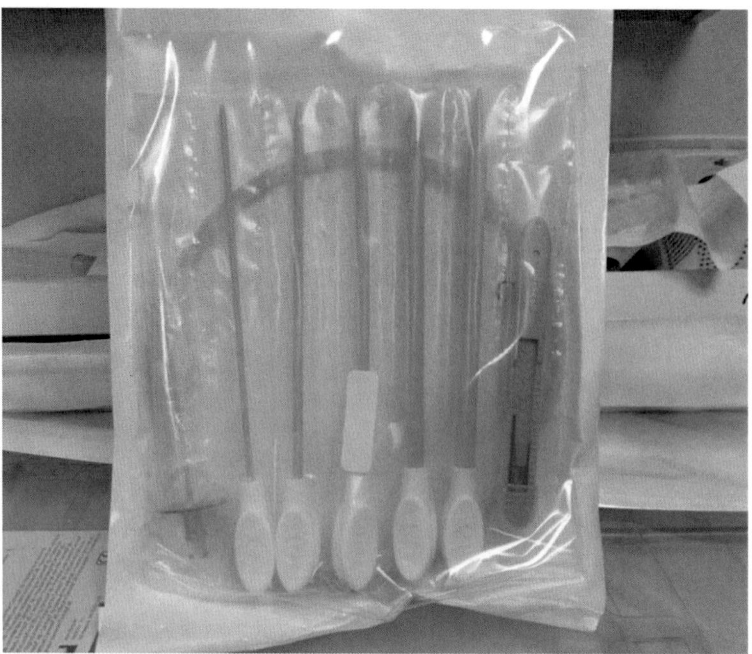

Fig. 45.8 Cannulation dilators

- Some data to suggest the use of US may be helpful to determine vessel lumen size and appropriate cannula size [2].

Venous cannula length targets:

- Femoral: Distal tip rests in the IVC, generally at the level of T10–T11. You do not want to advance the cannula past the hepatic vein, as this can cause an obstruction and hepatic congestion.
- Internal jugular: Distal tip to rest in the SVC.
- Try to measure the lengths with the cannulae beforehand, so when advancing, you know when to stop!

Note: For VV ECMO, circuit of a femoral drainage (deoxygenated blood) and internal jugular return cannulae (oxygenated blood) is believed to provide less recirculation than the reverse (see Recirculation).

Dilators: Series of 8, 12, 16, 20, and 24 French dilators

Step 2: Dilate up the initial insertion sites

- Insert the 150-cm guide wire through the distal port of the femoral CVC.
- Remove the CVC and hold pressure over the insertion site to prevent excessive bleeding.
- Load the 8 French dilator onto the introducer wire and advance it just to the skin.
  - Prior to advancing the dilator, you will have to extend your initial incision.
  - Extend the incision by about 1 cm just smaller than the size of your dilator.
  - This will provide adequate hemostasis each time you dilate the soft tissue.
- Introduce the dilator in a corkscrew-wise fashion, advancing the dilator at the level closest to the skin.
- As you advance the dilator, periodically check to make sure your guide wire freely moves within the dilator itself. If you develop a kink or difficulty passing the dilator, you run the risk of lacerating the vessel.
- Repeat this step for each dilator up until you reach the appropriate size for your chosen cannula.

Step 3: Inserting the ECMO cannula

- After your final dilation, load your introducer onto the 150-cm guide wire.
- Advance the introducer through the soft tissue, far enough that you actually dilate the wall of the femoral vein.

- Remove the introducer and hold lots of pressure.
- Load your venous cannula onto the introducer, then onto the 150-cm guide wire.
- Finally, advance your cannula to the prede-cided distance.
- Remove the dilator and wire and double clamp the open end of the cannula.
- Flush your cannula with a copious amount of sterile saline.
- Pearl: There is a slight step-off between the cannula and the introducer due to the actual thickness of the wire-reinforced cannula itself. If your dilation is inadequate, this step-off can get hung up on the soft tissue while attempting to insert it into the vessel.
- Pearl: You can use your ultrasound to visualize cannula placement in the IVC! Use it.

Step 4: Connect to the cannula to the circuit

- Check the circuit tubing: Remove all twists and coils. Make sure that there is plenty of length between the circuit and the cannulae themselves.
- Irrigate the ends of the tubes: As you attach the cannulae to the circuit tubing, use the bulb syringe to irrigate the ends to prevent air from getting trapped in the tubing (Fig. 45.9).

Step 5: The same steps above for the return cannula

Step 6: Turn on the circuit

- Goal flow for VV ECMO (in adults) about 50–60 cc/kg/min. You can start at around 2 l and titrate up, usually to a goal of 4–5 lpm.
- Start the sweep at about 2 lpm (for CO_2 clearance) and titrate (Fig. 45.10).

Step 7: Cleanup and confirmation

- Order a chest and abdominal XR to confirm cannula location.
- While you are waiting, you can also perform a bedside ultrasound to visualize the cannula tip in the IVC.
- Make sure your cannulae are secure. Usually, place at least two stabilizing sutures (for IJs) and three to four for the femoral cannulae with a 0 silk suture. Cover the sites with a sterile dressing [2].

45.9 Weaning and Discontinuation of ECMO

For patients with isolated respiratory failure, indications that the patient may be ready for weaning from ECMO would be improvements in pulmonary compliance, arterial oxygen saturation using standard ventilation modalities, and improved radiographic appearance.

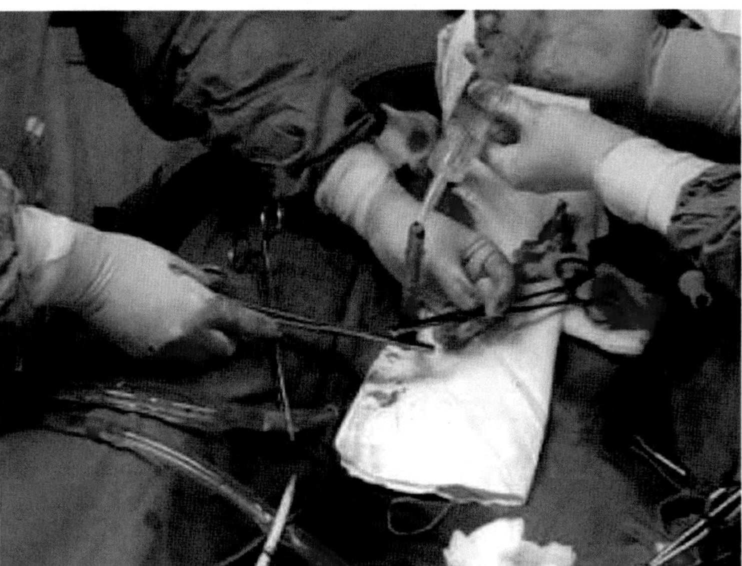

Fig. 45.9 Cannula filling

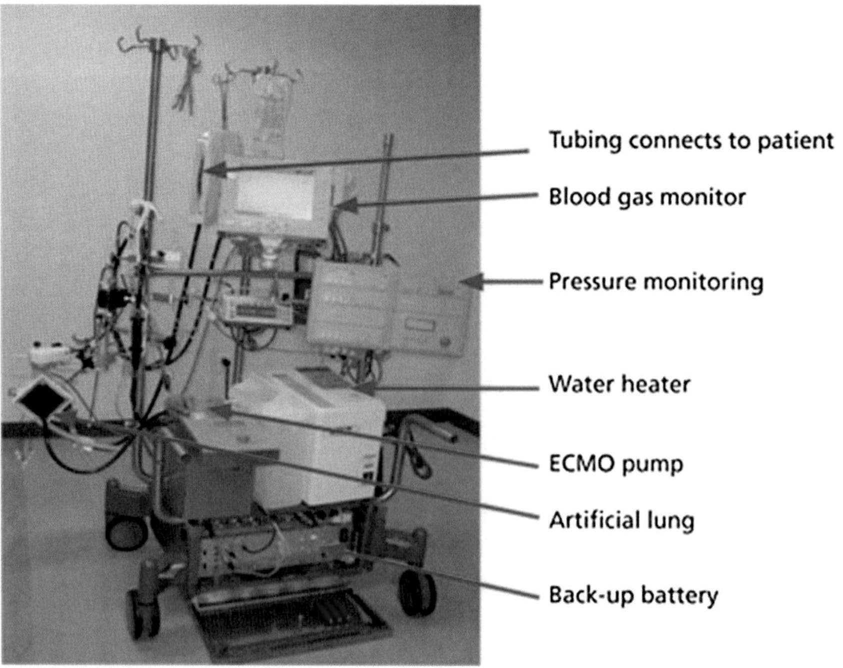

Fig. 45.10 ECMO module

This is accomplished by slowly reducing gas exchange through the oxygenator in the circuit and then eventually stopping all gas exchange. Although ECMO circulation continues, no gasses are exchanged. If the patient tolerates this, they may be decannulated.

Similarly, for patients on ECMO for cardiac failure, indications that the patient is ready to come off of ECMO would be enhanced aortic pulsatile wave form and improved left ventricular function. However, the technique for weaning is different than in VV ECMO. VA ECMO trials require temporary clamping of both the drainage and infusion lines while allowing the ECMO circuit to circulate through a bridge between the arterial and venous limbs. This bridge prevents thrombosis of stagnant blood within the ECMO circuit. Because of the increased risk of thrombus formation in the VA circuit, VA ECMO weaning trials are usually shorter than in VV ECMO and require constant heparinization of the circuit during weaning. If the patient continues to fail, they may be candidates for a ventricular assist device (VAD) [3].

45.10 Decannulation

For open cannulation techniques, arterial vessels are repaired with patch, and veins are repaired or ligated. For percutaneous cannulation, direct pressure is usually sufficient with close observation for development of pseudoaneurysm or arteriovenous (AV) fistula.

45.11 Complications

The complications due to ECMO are mainly attributed to vascular injury due to cannulation and anticoagulation side effects.

Cannulation injuries include limb ischemia and potential amputation, vessel laceration or dissection, pseudoaneurysm, and AV fistula formation.

Anticoagulation side effects range from spontaneous intracranial hemorrhages and ischemic watershed infarcts to spontaneous solid organ hemorrhage and subsequent life-threatening hemorrhage [4].

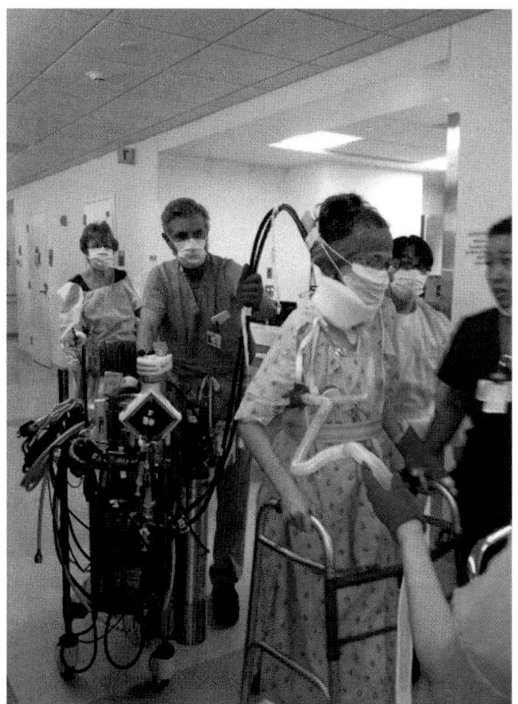

Fig. 45.11 Aggressive mobilization with patient on ECMO and ventilator

45.12 Recirculation

Recirculation is the inadvertent siphoning of oxygenated blood from the circuit that is pulled into the venous cannula. This is common during ECLS when using VV circulation only and can occur in both single and double cannula circuits. Due to mixing of the blood, circuit SVO_2 is invalidated. Additionally, when recirculation occurs, the effectiveness of the VV circuit is reduced as that portion of the blood never reaches the native circulation. To counteract this effect, higher flow rates are required; however, flows >400–500 ml/min will result in further recirculation and may actually reduce oxygenation. Clinically, recirculation is evidenced by falling arterial oxygen saturation (SPO_2) and concurrent rise in circuit mixed venous oxygenation (SVO_2). Troubleshooting may simply involve repositioning the patient's head when a double-lumen cannula is used. Recirculation in two-cannula systems is likely due to the cannulae being in close proximity and may be solved by cannula repositioning. Another option would be to change the direction of flow with a decrease in the incidence of recirculation using drainage from a femoral vein and return to the IJ cannula [3].

45.13 Conclusion

ECMO remains an option for those patients who fail conventional ventilation modalities and those in cardiogenic shock. Most recently, ECMO has been shown to improve survival of some patients diagnosed with the H1N1 influenza virus [5]. Early involvement of an ECMO center and team is essential for improved outcomes in these patients (Fig. 45.11). Entire ECMO courses are available to assist the practitioner in managing these complex patients.

Bibliography

1. Annich, G. ECMO: extracorporeal cardiopulmonary support in critical care. 4th edn. 2012.
2. Anatomy of an percutaneous ECMO cannulation (femoral vein cannulation): Part I. 2014. http://marylandccproject.org/education/anatomy-percutaneous-ecmo-cannulation-femoral-vein-cannulation/.
3. Short, BL. ECMO specialist training manual.
4. Martinez G, Vuylsteke A. Extracorporeal membrane oxygenation in adults. Contin Educ Anaesth Crit Care Pain. 2012;12:57–61.
5. Zangrillo A, Biondi-Zoccai G, Landoni G, Frati G, Patroniti N, Pesenti A, Pappalardo F. Extracorporeal membrane oxygenation (ECMO) in patients with H1N1 influenza infection: a systematic review and meta-analysis including 8 studies and 266 patients receiving ECMO. Crit Care. 2013;17:R30.
6. Russo MJ, Merlo A, Eton D, Patel PJ, Fedson S, Anderson A, Shah A, Jeevanandam V. Successful use of ECMO in a Jehovah's witness after complicated re-heart transplant. ASAIO J. 2013;59(5):528–9.

Index

D.A. Taylor et al. (eds.), *Interventional Critical Care*, DOI 10.1007/978-3-319-25286-5

R

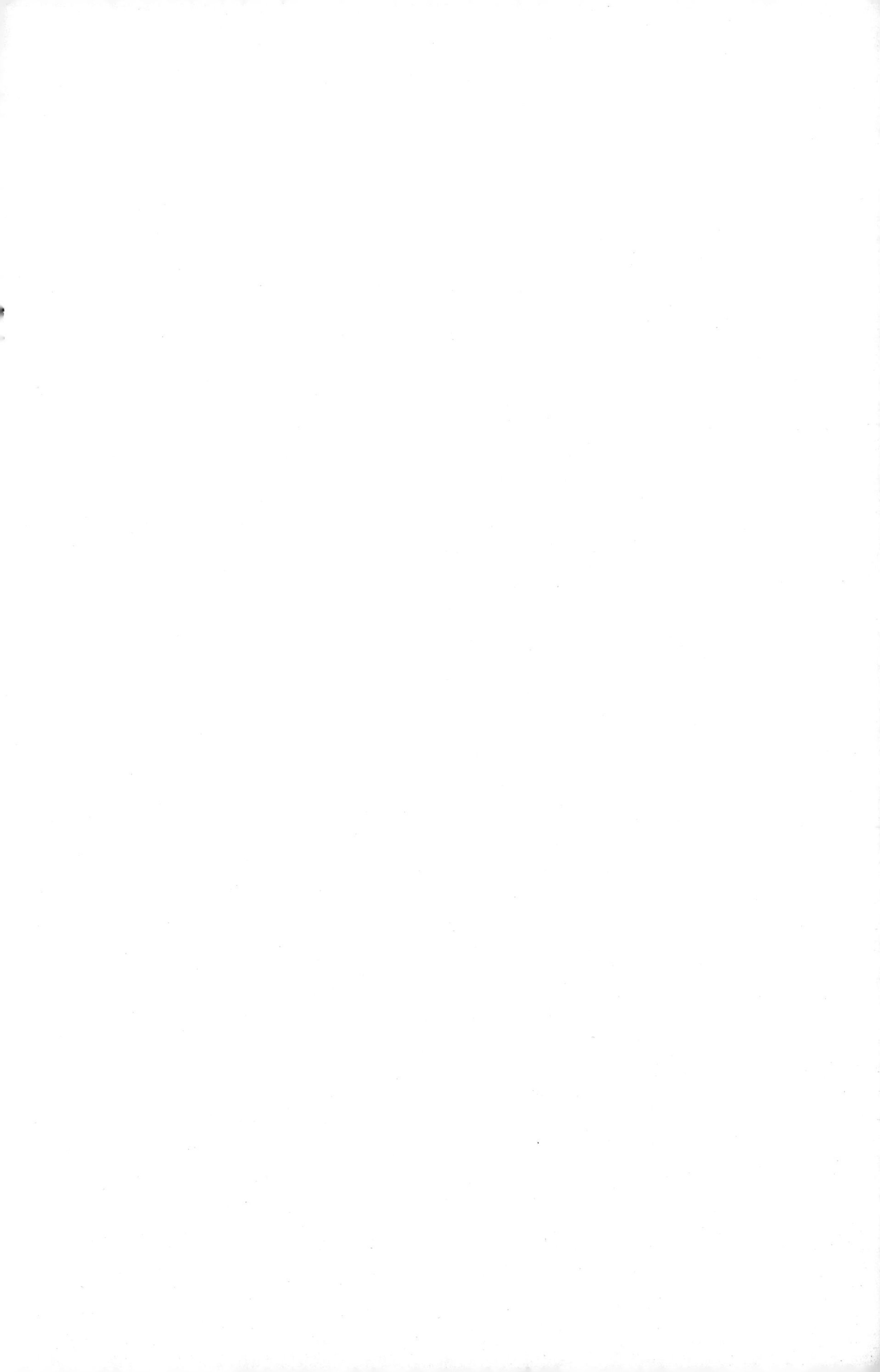

Made in the USA
Columbia, SC
21 April 2021